AMBULATORY GYNECOLOGY

AMBULATORY GYNECOLOGY

SECOND EDITION

Edited by

David H. Nichols, MD
Visiting Professor of Obstetrics, Gynecology, and
    Reproductive Biology
Harvard Medical School
Chief of Pelvic Surgery
Vincent Memorial Gynecologic Service
Massachusetts General Hospital
Boston, Massachusetts

Patrick J. Sweeney, MD, PhD
Professor of Obstetrics and Gynecology
Brown University School of Medicine
Director of Ambulatory Care
Women and Infants Hospital of Rhode Island
Providence, Rhode Island

41 Contributors

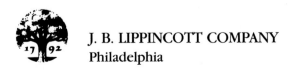

J. B. LIPPINCOTT COMPANY
Philadelphia

Acquisitions Editor: **Lisa McAllister**
Sponsoring Editor: **Emily M. Linkins**
Project Editor: **Bridget C. Hannon**
Indexer: **Maria Coughlin**
Design Coordinator: **Kathy Kelley-Luedtke**
Cover Designer: **Larry Pezzato**
Production Manager: **Caren Erlichman**
Production Coordinator: **David Yurkovich**
Compositor: **Compset Inc.**
Printer/Binder: **Quebecor/Kingsport**
Color Insert Printer: **Walsworth Publishing Company**
Color Pre-Press: **Mandarin Offset**
Pre-Press: **Jay's Publishers Services, Inc.**

2nd Edition

6 5 4 3 2 1

Library of Congress Cataloging in Publication Data

Ambulatory gynecology / edited by David H. Nichols, Patrick J.
    Sweeney; 41 contributors.—2nd ed.
        p.   cm.
    Includes bibliographical references and index.
    ISBN 0-397-51325-9 (alk. paper)
    1. Gynecology.   2. Generative organs, Female—Diseases.
3. Ambulatory medical care.   I. Nichols, David H., 1925–
II. Sweeney, Patrick J., 1945–
    [DNLM: 1. Genital Diseases, Female—diagnosis.   2. Genital
Diseases, Female—surgery.   3. Ambulatory Care—methods.   WP 140
A4971 1995]
RG103.A644   1995
618.1—dc20
DNLM/DLC
for Library of Congress   94-34437
                                                                    CIP

This paper meets the requirements of ANSI/NISO 239.48-1992 (Permanence of Paper).

The authors and publisher have exerted every effort to ensure that drug selection and dosage set forth in this text are in accord with current recommendations and practice at the time of publication. However, in view of ongoing research, changes in government regulations, and the constant flow of information relating to drug therapy and drug reactions, the reader is urged to check the package insert for each drug for any change in indications and dosage and for added warnings and precautions. This is particularly important when the recommended agent is a new or infrequently employed drug.

To
Lorraine and Eve

Contributors

Gloria A. Bachmann, MD
Professor of Obstetrics and Gynecology
Chief, Division of General Obstetrics and
    Gynecology
University of Medicine and Dentistry of
    New Jersey
Robert Wood Johnson Medical School
New Brunswick, New Jersey

Kevin E. Bachus, MD
Assistant Professor
Division of Reproductive Endocrinology and
    Infertility
Department of Obstetrics and Gynecology
Duke University Medical Center
Durham, North Carolina

Robert L. Barbieri, MD
Kate Macy Ladd Professor of Obstetrics,
    Gynecology and Reproductive Biology
Harvard Medical School
Chairman, Department of Obstetrics and
    Gynecology
Brigham and Women's Hospital
Boston, Massachusetts

Louis Burke, MD
Associate Professor of Obstetrics, Gynecology
    and Reproductive Biology
Harvard Medical School
Associate Director Emeritus
Department of Obstetrics and Gynecology

Director, Laser/LEEP Colposcopy Clinic
Boston Beth Israel Hospital
Boston, Massachusetts

Stephen Mark Cohen, MD
Associate Professor
Department of Obstetrics and Gynecology
University of Massachusetts Medical School
Associate Chairman, Department of Obstetrics
    and Gynecology
University of Massachusetts Medical Center
Worcester, Massachusetts

M. Yusoff Dawood, MD
The Berel Held Professor and Director
Division of Reproductive Endocrinology
Department of Obstetrics, Gynecology and
    Reproductive Sciences
University of Texas Medical School at Houston
Attending Obstetrician and Gynecologist
Herman Hospital
Houston, Texas

Alan H. DeCherney, MD
Professor and Chairman
Department of Obstetrics and Gynecology
Tufts University School of Medicine
Chairman, Department of Obstetrics and
    Gynecology
New England Medical Center
Boston, Massachusetts

Jeffrey S. Dungan, MD
Assistant Professor
Division of Human Genetics
Department of Obstetrics and Gynecology
University of Maryland Medical Center
Baltimore, Maryland

Sherman Elias, MD
Professor
Department of Obstetrics and Gynecology
Division of Reproductive Genetics
University of Tennessee College of Medicine
Memphis, Tennessee

Sebastian Faro, MD, PhD
Professor and Chairman
Department of Obstetrics and Gynecology
University of Kansas Medical Center
Kansas City, Kansas

David C. Foster, MD
Assistant Professor
Department of Obstetrics and Gynecology
Director, Division of General Gynecology
The Johns Hopkins School of Medicine
Baltimore, Maryland

James A. Grifo, MD, PhD
Assistant Professor, Obstetrics and Gynecology
Cornell University Medical College
The Center for Reproductive Medicine and
    Infertility
The New York Hospital-Cornell Medical Center
New York, New York

Charles B. Hammond, MD
E.C. Hamblen Professor and Chairman
Department of Obstetrics and Gynecology
Duke University Medical Center
Durham, North Carolina

Dorothy J. Hicks, MD
Professor, Department of Obstetrics and
    Gynecology
University of Miami School of Medicine
Director, Pedi-Gyn Clinic
Department of Obstetrics and Gynecology
Jackson Memorial Hospital
Miami Beach, Florida

Peter J. Julian, MD
Associate Clinical Professor
University of Texas Southwestern Medical School
Presbyterian Hospital of Dallas
Dallas, Texas

Frank W. Ling, MD
Associate Professor and Acting Chairman
Department of Obstetrics and Gynecology
University of Tennessee, Memphis
Memphis, Tennessee

Jacquelyn S. Loughlin, MD
Assistant Professor
Department of Obstetrics and Gynecology
University of Medicine and Dentistry of
    New Jersey
The New Jersey Medical School
Newark, New Jersey

Veronica T. Mallett, MD
Assistant Professor
Department of Obstetrics and Gynecology
Division of Gynecologic Specialties
Wayne State University Medical School
Hutzel Hospital
Department of Obstetrics and Gynecology
Detroit, Michigan

Charles M. March, MD
Professor
Department of Obstetrics and Gynecology
University of Southern California School of
    Medicine
Los Angeles, California

Karen L. McGoldrick, MD
Clinical Instructor in Obstetrics and Gynecology
Brown University School of Medicine
Women and Infants Hospital of Rhode Island
Providence, Rhode Island

George W. Mitchell, Jr., MD
Chief of Gynecology and Clinical Professor
Department of Obstetrics and Gynecology
University of Texas Health Science Center
San Antonio, Texas

Ana Monteagudo, MD
Assistant Professor
Clinical Obstetrics and Gynecology
Columbia University
Columbia-Presbyterian Medical Center
New York, New York

David Muram, MD
Associate Professor and Chief
Section of Pediatric and Adolescent Gynecology
Director, Division of Gynecology
Department of Obstetrics and Gynecology
University of Tennessee
Memphis, Tennessee

David H. Nichols, MD
Visiting Professor of Obstetrics, Gynecology, and
    Reproductive Biology
Harvard Medical School
Chief of Pelvic Surgery
Vincent Memorial Gynecologic Service
Massachusetts General Hospital
Boston, Massachusetts

Donald R. Ostergard, MD
Professor of Obstetrics and Gynecology
Director, Division of Urogynecology
University of California, Irvine
Associate Medical Director of Gynecology
Women's Hospital
Long Beach Memorial Medical Center
Long Beach, California

Joseph G. Pastorek, II, MD
Professor of Obstetrics and Gynecology
Chief, Section of Infectious Disease
Member Section of Maternal-Fetal Medicine
Louisiana State University Medical Center
Clinical Director of Perinatal Medicine
Medical Center of Louisiana/Charity Hospital
New Orleans, Louisiana

Jeffrey F. Peipert, MD, MPH
Assistant Professor of Obstetrics and Gynecology
Brown University School of Medicine
Physician-in-Charge
Obstetrics and Gynecology Emergency Services
Women and Infants Hospital
Providence, Rhode Island

Beth E. Quill, RN, CPNP, MPH
Director of Health
Northeast District Department of Health
Brooklyn, Connecticut.

Harry Reich, MD
Wyoming Valley GYN Associates
Nesbitt Memorial Hospital
Kingston, Pennsylvania

David A. Richardson, MD
Assistant Professor
Department of Obstetrics and Gynecology
Division of Gynecologic Specialties
Wayne State University Medical School
Hutzel Hospital
Department of Obstetrics and Gynecology
Detroit, Michigan

Zev Rosenwaks, MD
The Revlon Distinguished Professor of
    Reproductive Medicine in Obstetrics and
    Gynecology
Professor of Obstetrics and Gynecology
Cornell University Medical College
Director, Program of In Vitro Fertilization
Division of Reproductive Endocrinology
The New York Hospital-Cornell Medical Center
New York, New York

Isaac Schiff, MD
Joe Vincent Meigs Professor of Gynecology
Department of Obstetrics, Gynecology and
    Reproductive Biology
Harvard Medical School
Chief of the Vincent Memorial Obstetrics and
    Gynecology Service
Massachusetts General Hospital
Boston, Massachusetts

Kristen L. Stoops, MS
Department of Obstretrics and Gynecology
New England Medical Center
Boston, Massachusetts

Thomas G. Stovall, MD
Associate Professor and Head
Section on Gynecology
Department of Obstetrics and Gynecology
Bowman Gray School of Medicine
Wake Forest University
Winston-Salem, North Carolina

Anne A. Stulik, MSN
Clinical Teaching Associate
Department of Obstetrics and Gynecology
Brown University School of Medicine
Adjunct Faculty, College of Nursing
University of Rhode Island
Nurse Practitioner
Department of Obstetrics and Gynecology
Women and Infants Hospital of Rhode Island
Providence, Rhode Island

Khalid M. Sultan, MD
Clinical Instructor of Obstetrics and Gynecology
Cornell University Medical College
Assistant Attending, Obstetrics and Gynecology
The New York Hospital-Cornell Medical Center
New York, New York

Patrick J. Sweeney, MD, PhD
Professor of Obstetrics and Gynecology
Brown University School of Medicine
Director of Ambulatory Care
Women and Infants Hospital of Rhode Island
Providence, Rhode Island

Steven E. Swift, MD
Assistant Professor
Department of Obstetrics and Gynecology
Medical University of South Carolina
Charleston, South Carolina

Ilan E. Timor-Tritsch, MD
Professor of Clinical Obstetrics and Gynecology
Columbia University College of Physicians and
　　Surgeons
Director of Obstetric and Gynecologic Ultrasound
Co-director of Obstetrical Service
Columbia-Presbyterian Medical Center
New York, New York

May M. Wakamatsu, MD
Instructor in Obstetrics, Gynecology and
　　Reproductive Biology
Harvard Medical School
Assistant in Gynecology
Massachusetts General Hospital
Boston, Massachusetts

Brian W. Walsh, MD
Assistant Professor of Obstetrics, Gynecology,
　　and Reproductive Biology
Harvard Medical School
Director, Menopause Center
Brigham and Women's Hospital
Boston, Massachusetts

Susan A. Wolf, MD
Assistant Professor
Department of Obstetrics and Gynecology
University of Medicine and Dentistry of
　　New Jersey
The New Jersey Medical School
Newark, New Jersey

J. Donald Woodruff, MD
Professor Emeritus
Department of Gynecology and Obstetrics
Johns Hopkins University School of Medicine
Baltimore, Maryland

Preface

Many changes in the discipline of ambulatory gynecology have occurred since the publication of the first edition of this text. The most significant of these are the widespread acceptance and applicability of computerized axial tomography (CAT scan), transvaginal ultrasound, and the greater use of magnetic resonance imaging (MRI) as it becomes affordable as alternatives to diagnostic radiation, and the vast refinements in laparoscopic surgical techniques.

The gynecologist recognizes that an ever-increasing proportion of his or her professional activities is devoted to ambulatory gynecology. The advent of new technology has made ambulatory procedures safer and more practical, has altered individual practice patterns, and has elevated the practice of office gynecology to even higher levels of sophistication.

New techniques and technologies represent challenges to those practitioners who completed their formal postgraduate educations as recently as five to ten years ago. There have been refinements in the indications for methods of urodynamic testing.

The epidemics of HIV and HPV have captured the attention of both patients and providers, and have generated new research into the treatment of sexually transmitted diseases. New formulations of oral contraceptives continue to be introduced, while recently approved injectable and implantable hormonal preparations offer attractive alternatives for patients seeking long-term protection.

We are also responsible for the care of a greater number of older women. For these women, the quality of life is the essence of enjoyment of their longevity. As primary care physicians to women, we must assume responsibility for the problems our patients face throughout their lives.

With much sorrow we note that Dr. John Evrard, former colleague, friend, and co-editor of the First Edition of Ambulatory Gynecology, has passed away. It is with pleasure that Patrick J. Sweeney is welcomed as co-editor of this Second Edition.

David H. Nichols, MD
Patrick J. Sweeney, MD, PhD

Preface to the First Edition

Efficient and cost-effective ambulatory and office care now occupies a place of increasing importance in the health care of women. Increased public awareness, enthusiasm, and acceptance of this alternate to traditional, longer stay care, has further stimulated its attractiveness.

The technical details of providing this care are different from those generally learned in residency programs in the past—indeed, many modalities such as colposcopy, lasers, and endoscopy were then for all practical purposes unknown or unavailable. Evaluation of the total woman, not just her birth canal, has become a conceptual responsibility. *Ambulatory Gynecology* is intended to bridge the gap between yesterday's knowledge in this field and the wealth of new techniques and information currently available and essential to practice. Contributing authors have been especially selected for their authoritative expertise in particular topics and have responded generously to our invitation to share their experience and recommendations.

For ease of reference the book has been arranged more or less chronologically, both by the patient's age and by development of the concept of thorough and adequate diagnosis and individualized appropriate treatment.

It should therefore be of value to the seasoned practitioner who wishes to update his ability to respond effectively to the new challenge and mandate of ambulatory care. To the medical student, house officer, other health practitioner, and health care administrator, it details a blueprint for the future of gynecological care and embraces effective use of both the physician's office and the short stay unit or ambulatory center as the setting for both diagnosis and therapy. The reader will find here in a single book the latest practical information to fill this vast need. Topics have been cross-indexed for ready reference.

We wish to thank the J. B. Lippincott Company for all of its assistance in first recognizing the need for this publication and for its encouragement and skills in the book's manufacture. Particularly, we would like to express our gratitude to editors Lisa Biello and Richard Winters and former editor Rebecca Rinehart, who was so valuable during the early formative stages.

David H. Nichols, MD
John R. Evrard, MD

Acknowledgements

Thanks and special appreciation are extended to Lisa McAllister, Emilie Linkins, and Bridget Hannon of J. B. Lippincott for their patience, tolerance, forbearance, assistance, understanding, and enthusiasm during the planning and preparation of this text.

Contents

AMBULATORY GYNECOLOGY

Ambulatory Gynecology, Second Edition,
edited by David H. Nichols and Patrick J. Sweeney.
J. B. Lippincott Company, Philadelphia, © 1995.

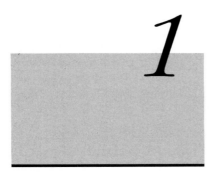

Patient Education and Informed Consent

Jeffrey F. Peipert

PATIENT EDUCATION

Obstetrics and gynecology residency programs devote a great deal of time to surgical techniques, procedures, and medical management, with considerably less time devoted to patient education. In fact, patient education is not a formal component of medical school curricula, although it is well established in colleges of nursing and other health-profession disciplines. Much of medical student teaching and resident education occurs in the inpatient setting, and issues of patient education and compliance have traditionally been linked to ambulatory care. As the emphasis shifts from in-hospital care to ambulatory care, issues and techniques of patient education will begin to receive the attention they rightfully deserve.

In this brief chapter, the necessary components and theory of patient education and informed consent are outlined and illustrated with examples in ambulatory obstetrics and gynecology. The importance of patient education is emphasized as a necessary ingredient in the practitioner–patient relationship and in the care of individual patients.

A Historical Perspective

The concept of patient education as a necessary component of health care is relatively new. Although there are early references to patient education in the medical literature dating back to the 1950s, the objective of patient education was not outlined until the American Medical Association held a conference on health education goals in 1964. At this conference, one objective specified for health education was to educate individuals to assume responsibility for maintaining personal health. It is this objective that we refer to as patient education.

In 1973, the Patient's Bill of Rights was published by the American Hospital Association. This document outlines the patient's right to information regarding his or her diagnosis, treatment, and prognosis of a given medical condition. The document also stresses that the information be presented in terms understandable to the patient and be complete enough to enable informed decisions about treatment options and procedures. This document by the American Hospital Association resulted in the widespread acceptance of education as a patient's right and led to the concept of informed consent. Informed consent is addressed separately later in this chapter.

In the 1970s, the importance of patient education in effecting behavioral change and improving health outcomes was recognized by many organizations, including the Joint Commission on American Hospitals, the American Medical Association, the American Nurses Association, the American Society for Hospital Pharmacists, and the American Dietetic Association.[1] Over the past two decades, the subject of patient education has been studied and taught in nursing schools but has been slow to enter medical school curricula. As medical schools begin to look to the new curriculum of the 21st century, increased emphasis is being placed on the physician as an effective communicator and educator.[2]

The Clinician's Responsibility

Patient education refers to the ability to educate individuals to assume responsibility for maintaining personal health. As clinical preventive services assume greater importance, the need for obstetrics–gynecology practitioners to teach patients how to improve health habits is greater than ever.[3] All members of the health care team can participate and contribute to the education of the patient but it is ultimately the responsibility of the primary provider to be sure the patient understands her condition and can follow the prescribed plan of management. From a legal standpoint, it is primarily the responsibility of the physician to be sure the patient is appropriately informed.

Numerous barriers exist that deter physicians from involvement in health promotion. These barriers include lack of confidence in the outcome of educational efforts, time pressures, disease orientation of physicians, and lack of reimbursement for educational efforts. Despite these barriers, patient education is clearly a physician's responsibility.

Although the word "doctor" means teacher, few physicians spend time actually teaching. When physicians do give instruction or counseling, there

is evidence that they do it poorly.[4,5] When trained in communication or when equipped with structured programs and material, physicians can have a significant impact on a patient's health habits and learning.[6,7] There is convincing evidence linking patient satisfaction with physician communication skills. As a result, satisfied patients are more likely to comply with treatment plans and follow-up.[8] Therefore, from both a clinical and a business perspective, involvement of the physician as a health educator is essential.

Patient Education in Ambulatory Gynecology

Patient education is an extremely important component of ambulatory care. Studies of patient compliance with medications and treatment plans repeatedly demonstrate its importance. Treatment regimens in the ambulatory setting depend on patient adherence to recommended therapy. Compliance is positively correlated with patients' self-reported understanding of their condition and with their satisfaction with the amount of information received.[9] For example, in a randomized controlled trial, women receiving mailings of written educational materials were more likely to adhere to follow-up after an abnormal Pap smear.[10]

Several studies demonstrate that knowledge is necessary but not sufficient to assure behavior change.[8,11–13] If the patient is expected to make a lifestyle change such as a daily medication routine or a change of diet or smoking habits, more than information is necessary.[14] Motivation, direction and cues to action are also important components of patient counseling for behavioral change.

A patient's understanding of the information received is affected by the level of language used, by the use of supportive materials, and by the readability of the educational materials provided to the patient. About 20% of Americans are "functionally illiterate" and lack the literacy skills necessary to function in today's society.[15] An additional 33% have only marginal reading competence.[15] Because typical educational handouts require at least an 8th-grade education, many patients have difficulty understanding these patient education materials.[16] Adolescents, the elderly, and non–English speaking patients have special needs in terms of literacy.[17,18]

Studies evaluating recall of information demonstrate high recall failures, ranging from 40% to 70% of the information presented within a short time after visits.[5,19] One of the main problems is that providers assume the patient can understand common medical terminology. Commonly used terms such as Pap smear, virus, tumor, and hypertension were misunderstood by 24% to 72% of patients in one study.[20] Age, educational level, and cultural background must all be considered when providing information to patients. It is extremely important to deliver the message at an appropriate level to the individual patient.

Guidelines for Providing Information to Patients

There are some basic rules to follow to facilitate patient education. First, be sure the patient's agenda is addressed in the physician–patient encounter. This is the initial step in establishing a favorable relationship and rapport. Second, have the patient play an active role in the learning process, either by having the patient demonstrate her understanding or through role playing. Third, limit the number of take-home messages. A typical patient is able to absorb a maximum of three major points in a given encounter with her provider. Finally, keep in mind that different educational styles may be necessary for different individuals. One patient may learn through computer-assisted instruction, whereas another may require personal interaction with a health care provider to address specific concerns.

Recommendations for patient education and counseling have been outlined by the United States Preventive Services Task Force.[3] In their report on clinical preventive services, the task force listed the key components necessary for effective counseling, targeting specific behavioral changes. These recommendations are summarized in Table 1-1.

The ability to educate patients is not an inherent skill. Physicians and health care providers can improve their teaching effectiveness by learning and adopting a few fundamental instructional techniques. Even small changes in a clinician's teaching behavior can translate into large gains for patients. One problem relating to both compliance and patient recall of information concerns the number of recommendations that run together when information is presented to the patient.[9] An important principle is to *present each category of information separately*. Categorizing information can increase patient recall by nearly 50%.[7] Organizing and clustering information is consistent with instructional design principles and is an effective way of achieving positive behavior changes.

An example of categorizing information is illustrated, using an example of an abnormal Pap smear.

Table 1–1
United States Preventive Services Task Force: Key Components for Effective Counseling for Behavioral Change

1. Develop a therapeutic alliance
2. Counsel all patients
3. Ensure that patients understand the relationship between behavior and health
4. Work with patients to assess barriers to behavior change
5. Gain commitment from patients to change
6. Involve patients in selecting which risk factors to change
7. Use a combination of strategies
8. Design a behavior modification plan
9. Monitor progress through follow-up contact
10. Involve office staff

Data from Stenchever MA: Too much informed consent? Obstet Gynecol 77:631, 1991

One example dialogue could be, "Your Pap smear is abnormal and I would recommend we proceed with a colposcopic examination of the cervix."

Alternatively, the provider can use explicit categorization of information: "I am going to explain the problem and what further tests will be necessary. First, the problem is that your Pap smear was read as abnormal. Second, the next appropriate step in the evaluation would include a colposcopic examination of the cervix."

This technique of communicating information illustrates several other important principles. One is to *preview the message*. Tell the patient what you are going to tell her. An example preview could be, "I am going to explain the problem that was detected. Next, I will describe further tests that will be necessary; then I will explain the plan of action."

Patients are better able to absorb information if they know the scope and sequence of the information to be provided.[7]

Another important principle is to *summarize major points*. Repetition is at the core of instructional methodology. In essence, you tell the patient what you just told her. The patient is more likely to remember those points that the physician mentions more than once in the dialogue.

In addition to the above principles of instructional design, the clinician should be sure to *establish rapport* with the patient before initiating the discussion. Be sure the patient is able to devote full attention to the advice and is not occupied with getting dressed or another activity. *Use lay terms and avoid professional jargon.* Often, the educational level of the patient is overestimated, and the explanation is not simple enough or understandable. For a variety of reasons, many patients are reluctant to ask for clarification.

Providing *supplemental patient education materials* is also helpful, especially if illustrations are provided to demonstrate the important points. Because patients only retain about half of the essential information communicated at an office visit, some written information should be provided after most visits.[21] This information must be at an appropriate reading level for the patient and also must be in a language the patient can understand.

It is also helpful to *put instructions and information in writing.* Either the patient can "take notes" or the provider can draw simple diagrams or spell out diagnoses or instructions for the patient to refer to at a later time. Individual patient instructions, such as when to arrange subsequent visits and how to call for results, should be provided. Consider having the patient sign the instructions to indicate comprehension and agreement with the plan. It is a good practice to personalize preprinted instructions by highlighting or underlining important points and adding additional information when appropriate. These techniques are also likely to increase a patient's understanding of her condition and any plans for follow-up.

At the end of the provider–patient encounter, it is helpful to *check for patient comprehension* of the most important points that have been conveyed. Patients tend to recall the diagnosis better than the proposed treatment, so it is important to determine retention of the plan at management.[21] In an effort to avoid offending the patient, it may be helpful to use a phrase indicating your interest such as, "It would help me if you would tell me what you understand to be the plan," rather than, "Now repeat the plan back to me."

The above guidelines for providing information to patients in an ambulatory gynecologic setting are by no means exhaustive but a brief list that can assist the busy practitioner. A summary of the guidelines outlined above is provided in Table 1-2.

Role of Support Staff and Group Programs

Hospitals and large clinics often have health education departments or staff members who can assist in providing physicians and practitioners with tools

Table 1–2
Guidelines for Providing Information to Patients

1. Establish rapport with the patient
2. Use lay terms and avoid professional jargon
3. Preview the message
4. Present each category of information separately
5. Summarize the major points
6. Provide supplemental materials
7. Put information in writing
8. Check for patient comprehension

to improve their ability as teachers. Providers with an interest in patient education have a continuous need for materials that are current, readable, and understandable.

Integrating patient education into an office practice can be facilitated by support staff and by addressing some practical management issues. Nurses, for example, frequently have considerable interest in patient education and can be an invaluable asset to the office setting. Involving nurses in patient education can save physician time and enhance the effectiveness of care. Educating patients regarding preventive measures such as breast self-examination, family planning, and cancer screening are just a few examples. In other settings, nurses may work with specific chronic problems or conditions such as diabetes or preterm labor–prevention programs. It is important to outline in advance which information will be covered by the nurse and which will be covered by the physician to avoid omissions. In addition, care teams should decide who will give information and what information is to be given. This minimizes conflicting information and resulting confusion and unnecessary anxiety to the patient.[22]

Nurses, office staff, and patient educators can help to convert the waiting room into an important source of patient information with the addition of a pamphlet rack that contains some of the most common conditions encountered in a clinic or practice. Some examples in ambulatory gynecology practice would include smoking cessation, weight reduction, exercise, sexually transmitted diseases, endometriosis, fibroids, estrogen replacement therapy, cancer screening, and family planning. The American College of Obstetricians and Gynecologists is an excellent source for patient education handouts covering the gamut of gynecologic and obstetric conditions. Some practices also find it helpful to use a bulletin board for health-related news clippings. Removal of ashtrays and a no-smoking policy in the waiting room are also important ways of communicating important health messages to patients.

Structured systems for physician-directed patient education also have an impact on health-related behavior. Reminder systems such as problem lists in the medical record or color codes are used to indicate smokers and quitting attempts. Computerized cancer-screening trigger mechanisms both improve physicians' educational efforts and subsequent patient behaviors.[21] Physicians are reluctant to use precious clinical time to educate patients about an intractable behavior such as smoking. They must realize, however, that these efforts may be highly cost-effective, even when compliance rates with advice are low.[23]

Group programs and support groups may be useful for providers who see many patients with similar conditions. In a survey of 340 members of a health-maintenance organization, group programs are the most broadly accepted component of health promotion in a clinical setting.[24] Considering, however, the relatively small percentage of patients interested in attending classes and the absence of data indicating that classes are more effective than other interventions, group programs should be one choice among many educational options.[25] Physician-directed intervention, materials-based intervention, media campaigns, and computer-assisted instruction all warrant consideration.

Computer-Assisted Patient Education

Medical computer reference systems have grown to include extensive patient handouts that can be customized by clinics and individualized for patients. Individualized handouts can serve as both a patient education aid and as a supplement to informed consent forms. Acceptance of theses systems has been slow but as computerized systems for accessing laboratory and radiology data become more broadly available, the use of computer-based patient education resources will increase.

Computers can also serve as reminder systems to automatically flag and alert practitioners that a patient is due for a clinical preventive service such as a Pap smear, mammogram, or immunization. Personalized exercise, diet, or other health habit prescriptions can be developed, and the automated system could provide feedback and progress reports as an individual works toward a health-directed goal.

Interactive computer programs have been developed to teach patients about health risks and to generate a health-risk profile. The programs may make suggestions regarding recommended therapy. These interactive systems can be used by patients and by health educators. An interactive computer program developed by Brown University students Atul Butte and Anne Andrade, called *Personal Choice*, was created to assist students interested in learning about reproductive physiology and contraceptive choices (Fig. 1-1). The interactive system allows students to learn at their own pace and obtain details of various family planning methods.

In addition to computer-assisted educational devices, an increasing number of videotapes have been developed that are devoted to patient education. These videotapes address numerous indications, ranging from a description of family planning methods to detailed information about a surgical procedure.

In summary, patient education in ambulatory gynecology is not only an essential component of patient care but also a legal obligation. The legal obligations of patient education are obvious in the discussion that follows concerning informed consent.

INFORMED CONSENT

Every human being of adult years and sound mind has the right to determine what shall be done with his own body.[26]

The right of individual self-determination so forcefully summarized by Justice Cardozo in the Schloendorff case 80 years ago underpins the doctrine of informed consent.[26] The doctrine requires the physician to disclose information to the patient so that decisions about therapy and care can ultimately be resolved by the person most directly affected—the patient.

Informed consent has been defined as "the willing and uncoerced acceptance of a medical intervention by a patient after adequate disclosure by the physician of the nature of the intervention, its risks and benefits, as well as alternatives with their risks and benefits."[27] The protection of patient autonomy is the primary purpose of the consent process. By communicating with the patient and informing her of the potential risks and benefits of the proposed treatment and alternatives, the physician

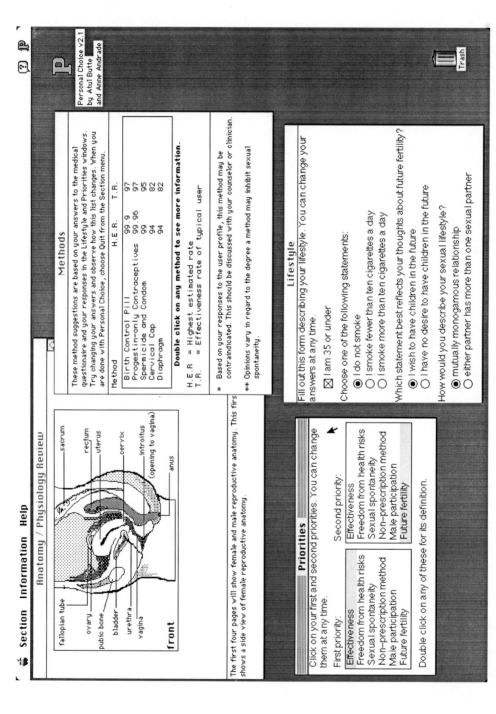

Figure 1-1. Selected screens from *Personal Choice*, version 2.1, an interactive computer program used to educate students about reproductive physiology and contraceptive choices. (Figure courtesy of Atul Butte and Anne Andrade. *Personal Choice*, version 2.1, is copyrighted by Brown University Health Services.)

enables the patient to exercise personal choice in the decision-making process. This communication is central to the physician–patient relationship.[28]

The doctrine of informed consent was developed in the early years of this century to deal with situations in which the patient consented to surgical procedures and was aware of what was going to be done but was not fully informed of the inherent risks or possible adverse side effects. The failure to disclose known risks to the patient was deemed to vitiate the consent given and in effect, to make the procedure one that was performed without the patient's consent.

In the 1960s, many judicial innovations in the doctrine of informed consent began to assess not only the quantity of information but also the quality of information provided by physicians to patients. The physician must not only give technically accurate information to the patient but must also relay the information *effectively*. These judicial innovations in informed consent developed as medicine entered a new era of rapid advances and technical innovation. Informed consent assumes great importance, especially in teaching hospitals and other medical research institutions. Thus, as is often the case, judicial reform mirrored changes occurring in the society at large—in this case, the medical community.

The premise underlying the doctrine of informed consent is the basic inequality inherent in the patient–physician relationship. This inequality stems from both the physician's extensive and usually superior knowledge of medicine and from the patient's need for care without any real ability to bargain for it. Each patient needs the physician's services more than the physician needs the particular patient. This inequality creates a fiduciary relationship between the physician and the patient. The physician, as trustee of the patient's welfare and of society's general well-being, must satisfy a relatively stringent obligation to provide information to the patient to allow her to make an informed, intelligent, and voluntary choice of treatment.

The doctrine of informed consent imposes a duty on the physician that is completely separate and distinct from his or her responsibility to skillfully diagnose and treat the patient's illness. Liability for failure to obtain the patient's informed consent does not require any negligence on the part of the physician in the choice of treatment or in the manner in which it was administered. Liability is based on the patient not being informed of certain inherent risks of the procedure, one of those risks actually coming to pass, and that the patient would not have consented to the procedure had she been informed of the risks.

From a legal standpoint, the standards of informed consent were traditionally based on the amount of information that a physician would typically divulge to a patient in customary practice. Since the 1972 court decision of Nathanson versus Kline, courts have gradually changed their perspective of what a patient needs to know to make an informed choice regarding treatment.[29] This shift from a paternalistic to a partnership model was driven by societal forces and the patients' rights movement.

Necessary Components of Informed Consent

Certain components of informed consent have been deemed essential in the dialogue between the physician and patient. These components are summarized in the mnemonic *BRAIDED* and listed in Table 1-3.[30] Every discussion should include (1) a description of the procedure and why it is recommended; (2) risks and benefits of the procedure; (3) alternative treatments, including taking no action; (4) projected outcome and relative chances of success with the treatment and its alternatives; and (5) information about costs and necessary follow-up care. Patients should have adequate time and op-

---

Table 1–3
Necessary Components of Informed Consent: BRAIDED

B—The **benefits** of the treatment

R—The potential **risks**

A—The **alternatives**

I—**Inquiries** are the patient's right and responsibility

D—The patient's **decision** may be altered or consent withdrawn

E—An **explanation** is owed to the patient

D—**Documentation** in the medical record of each of the above

---

Hatcher RA, Trussel J, Stewart F, et al: Contraceptive technology 16th ed. New York, Irvington Publishers, 1994

portunity to ask questions, and they also have the right to change their mind and withdraw consent.

Most informed consent litigation cases arise because a risk or complication occurs that the physician has not discussed with the patient. All known material risks must be disclosed. The frequency and gravity of the risk determine materiality. If a risk is not grave but occurs frequently, it is material. If a risk is grave yet seldom occurs, it may still be considered material by the court. A balance must be struck between the gravity of harm, the frequency of the occurrence, the patient's need to know the risks to make an intelligent choice, and the desire to not cause the patient undue anxiety. Courts have held that any risk of death, however slight, is material. Even a 1% chance of paralysis has been considered to be material.[31]

Problems may also arise if the physician places too much emphasis on unrealistically positive projections in an effort to develop an optimistic outlook in the patient. A realistic assessment of potential outcomes is crucial to informed consent. Examples would include the probability of failure for various contraceptive methods, the possibility that stress urinary incontinence may not be alleviated with a surgical procedure, and the failure rate of treatment modalities for cervical neoplasia. It is important to know that a patient can sue and win, even though the treatment produced no harm, if the plaintiff reasonably relied on the physician's representations and the promised result did not occur. Physicians have an obligation to disclose to the patient both their own personal professional experience and that of the medical community in general, if known.

In addition to providing information regarding alternative procedures, patients should have an understanding of the outcome of the disease should nothing be done. An example in ambulatory gynecology would include the treatment of low-grade squamous intraepithelial lesions of the cervix. Before consenting to an ablative procedure, a patient should be informed that most of these lesions may regress on their own without therapy.[32]

Documenting Informed Consent

Rather than simply having a signature on a consent form, it is preferable to have documentation that a process has occurred in which information was provided and the patient had adequate opportunity to ask questions and to gain an understanding of the recommended treatment or procedure. The most effective means of reducing exposure to professional liability is to maximize the quality of the communication between the patient and physician. This not only prevents misunderstandings and inaccurate expectations but also prevents lawsuits. Attending to details and carefully documenting discussions in the patient's medical record requires an additional expenditure of time but may ultimately save time, energy, and significant psychological burden from litigation. Allow adequate time for uninterrupted discussions with the patient, encourage the patient to ask questions or to write them down for subsequent discussions, see that the patient follows instructions and is a participant in her care, and finally, document all conversations (including telephone conversations) in the patient's record.

When Disclosure Is Not Required

There are exceptions to the informed consent disclosure requirements. When faced with an emergency in which disclosure is not practical and the need for immediate treatment overrides the concern for consent, it is reasonable to proceed without consent. There are also circumstances wherein disclosure would prove a threat to the patient's well-being. These situations are rare and reserved for when there is strong reason to believe that full disclosure would make the patient so emotionally upset and distraught as to foreclose rational decision-making, impede treatment, or actually cause psychological harm. When faced with this potential conflict, the clinician should obtain a psychological consultation, if possible. Lastly, if a patient prefers not to be told of the risks of a procedure, disclosure can be waived. A prudent physician should obtain a waver of disclosure signed by the patient, however.

There may be times when a patient's capacity to comprehend and process the medical information presented to her may be in doubt. In addition, most states have statutes specifying when a minor is permitted to give consent for medical care without parental permission. In either case, the physician should obtain consultation when necessary and attempt to clarify the patient's capacity to provide consent. If a patient is unable to provide consent, a guardian or substitute decision-maker should be sought.

Simple Guidelines for Informed Consent

As with patient education, there are some simple suggestions that can improve the physician's technique of obtaining informed consent. To begin with, *effective communication* is essential. Communication that reaches the patient in simple, understandable, and nonthreatening language, manner, and circumstances is not only good but required practice. Not just *what* is said but *how* it is said is important.

The discussion between the physician and patient should be a dialogue, not a monologue. Encourage the patient to ask questions and to play an active role in the discussion rather than just listening to what is said. Develop the conversation so that it is easy for the patient to ask questions and make judgments; the resulting rapport will further ensure her understanding of the situation. As the patient's comfort increases, so does her comprehension. Avoid a paternalistic or judgmental demeanor that may make the patient feel uneasy about asking questions. Be available to the patient, in person or by telephone, to discuss questions that may arise regarding the diagnosis or proposed treatment.

A physician can help to eliminate the patient's fear, anxiety, or defensiveness by being receptive to the patient as a person. It is important to understand the patient's feelings as well as the factual content of her words. It is equally important to communicate understanding of and empathy for the patient's point of view.

If forms are used for informed consent in the office setting, they should be drafted in simple nontechnical language, describing only the medical issues in question. Using language that attempts to limit legal liability only instills fear and distrust in the patient.

Perhaps most important is to recognize the emotional response of the patient who is confronted with a new diagnosis and potential procedures and treatment. Strong emotional stimuli always cloud perception. The validity of informed consent is directly related to the circumstances in which it is given. It is important to pay attention to the psychological and emotional state of the patient, both generally and when information is given. Try to determine the patient's level of understanding about her condition and plans for therapy. If a patient is fearful or embarrassed or if she feels vulnerable, she is less likely to comprehend. Patients also tend to react to certain words with anxiety. Careful wording when discussing problems such as cervical neoplasia, cancer, birth defects, and sterility is essential for patient understanding of informed consent information.

SUMMARY

In summary, patient education and the doctrine of informed consent are essential components of ambulatory gynecology. Education is a critical component of prenatal care, prevention of preterm birth, family planning, sexually transmitted diseases, and compliance with medications and cancer screening. Physicians and all health care providers should strive to improve their skills as patient educators and work together with patients to enhance well-being and promote preventive health maintenance.

REFERENCES

1. Falvo DR: Effective patient education: a guide to increased compliance. Rockville, MD, Aspen Publications, 1985
2. Brown University School of Medicine: An educational blueprint for the Brown Univerisity School of Medicine. Competency-based curriculum, 1993
3. United States Preventive Services Task Force: "Guide to Preventive Services." Baltimore, Williams & Wilkins, 1989
4. McClellan W: Current perspectives: patient education in medical practice. Patient Educ Couns 8:151, 1986
5. Ley P: Satisfaction, compliance and communication. Br J Clin Psychol 21:241, 1982
6. Kottke T: Attributes of successful smoking cessation interventions in medical practice. JAMA 261:75, 1988
7. Ley P, Bradshaw, et al: A method for increasing patients' recall of information presented by doctors. Psychol Med 3:217, 1973
8. Haynes RB: Strategies in improving compliance with referrals, appointments, and prescribed medical regimens. In Haynes RB, Taylor DW, Sackett DL (eds): Compliance in health care, p 123. Baltimore, Johns Hopkins University Press, 1979
9. Terry PE: Health education. In Barnett AE, Gilbert Mayer G (eds): Ambulatory care management and practice. Gaithersburg, MD, Aspen Publications, 1992
10. Paskett ED, White E, Carter WB, Chu J: Improving follow-up after an abnormal Pap smear: a randomized controlled trial. Prev Med 19:630, 1990
11. Baile WF, Engel BT: A behavioral strategy for the treatment of noncompliance following myocardial infarction. Psychosom Med 40:413, 1978

12. Closson R, Kikuwago C: Noncompliance with drug class. Hospitals 49:89, 1975

13. Hackett TP, Cassem NH: White-collar and blue-collar responses to heart attack. J Psychosom Res 20:85, 1976

14. Golden A, Grayson M, Bartlett E, Barker LR: The doctor-patient relationship: communication and patient education. In Barker LR, Burton JR, Zieve PD (eds): Principles of ambulatory medicine, 2nd ed, p 36. Baltimore, Williams & Wilkins, 1986

15. Doak CC, Doak LG, Root JH: Teaching patients with low literacy skills. Philadelphia, JB Lippincott, 1985

16. Davis TC, Crouch MA, Wills, et al: The gap between patient reading comprehension and the readability of patient education materials. J Fam Pract 31:533, 1990

17. Zion AB, Aiman J: Level of reading difficulty in te American College of Obstetricians and Gynecologists patient education pamphlets. Obstet Gynecol 74:955, 1989

18. Hussey LC: Overcoming the clinical barriers of low literacy and medication noncompliance among the elderly. J Gerontol Nurs 17:27, 1991

19. Brody D: An analysis of patients' recall of their therapeutic regimens. J Chron Dis 33:75, 1980

20. Spiro D, Heidrich F: Lay understanding of medical terminology. J Fam Pract 17:277, 1983

21. Ley P: Psychological studies of doctor-patient communication. In Rachman S (ed): Contributions to medical psychology, I. Oxford, UK, Pergamon Press, 1977

22. Stenchever MA: Too much informed consent? Obstet Gynecol 77:631, 1991

23. Cummings SR, Nowakowski TA, Schwandt JR: The cost-effectiveness of counseling smokers to quit. JAMA 261:75, 1989

24. Bernton CT: What is the future of health promotion in HMOs? Am J Health Promotion 1:24, 1987

25. Terry PE, Pheley A: Health risks and educational interests of members of a state-wide HMO. HMO Practice 5:3, 1991

26. Schloendorff v Society of New York Hospital, 211, NY 125 (1914)

27. Jonsen AR, Siegler M, Winslade WJ: Clinical ethics: a practical approach to ethical decisions in clinical medicine, 2nd ed. New York, Oxford University Press, 1989

28. American College of Obstetricians and Gynecologists: Ethical decision-making in obstetrics and gynecology. ACOG Technical Bulletin. Number 136, November 1989

29. Roberts DK, Raines E: Informed consent and medicolegal problems. In Sciarra J (ed): Gynecology and obstetrics, vol 1. Philadelphia, JB Lippincott, 1992

30. Hatcher RA, Trussel J, Stewart F, et al: Contraceptive technology, 16th ed. New York, Irvington Publishers, 1994

31. Cantebury v Spence, 464 F2d 772 (DC Cir 1972)

32. Nasiell K, Roger V, Nasiell M: Behavior of mild cervical dysplasia during long-term follow-up. Obstet Gynecol 67:665, 1986

The author would like to thank Atul Butte for providing Figure 1.

Ambulatory Gynecology, Second Edition,
edited by David H. Nichols and Patrick J. Sweeney.
J. B. Lippincott Company, Philadelphia, © 1995.

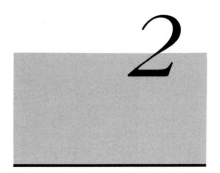

Pediatric and Adolescent Gynecology

David Muram

Most physicians are aware of the various gynecologic disorders that may affect female infants, children, and adolescents. Therefore, many perform a routine inspection of the external genitalia during a well-child examination, allowing early detection of infections, labial adhesions, congenital anomalies, and even genital tumors. The reproductive tract in children differs in structure and in function from the genital organs of the adult female. Thus, the physician caring for young patients should be familiar with these differences. Moreover, the anatomic differences require the use of specially designed equipment (eg, vaginoscope or virginal vaginal specula) if the examination is to be completed without causing undue discomfort and subsequent anxiety about future examinations.

ANATOMIC AND PHYSIOLOGIC CONSIDERATIONS

Newborns

Immediately after birth and during the first few weeks of life, the female newborn responds to maternal estrogens. The effects of such stimulation may be seen for perhaps 6 weeks and sometimes even longer. The most obvious sign, breast budding, occurs in nearly all children born at term. Sometimes the breast enlargement is marked and may be accompanied by a discharge from the nipples. This breast enlargement requires no treatment, and repeated examinations may lead to bruising of the breast tissue or infection.

The external genitalia are also affected by maternal estrogens. The labia major are bulbous and the labia minor are thick and protruding (Fig. 2-1). The clitoris is relatively large but with a normal index of 0.6 cm^2 or less. The effects of maternal estrogens are particularly evident in the hymen, which initially is thick and turgid and projects from the slightly gaping vulva. The vaginal mucosa is thick and appears pink and moist. Vaginal discharge is common because the cervical glands secrete considerable amounts of mucous, which mixes with exfoliated vaginal cells.

Maternal estrogens also affect the internal genital organs. The vagina is 4 cm in length and the vaginal secretions are acidic. The uterus is enlarged, has no axial flexion, and the ratio between cervix and corpus is 3:1. The columnar epithelium protrudes through the external cervical os to produce a reddened zone of "physiologic eversion." The ovaries, which are derived from T_{10} level, are abdominal organs in early childhood and not palpable on rectoabdominal examination. Occasionally, after birth and subsequently declining estrogen levels, the stimulated endometrial lining sheds and vaginal bleeding occurs. Such bleeding stops within a week to 10 days of life, however.

Early Childhood

During early childhood (age, birth to 7 years), the genital organs receive little estrogen stimulation and the external genitalia assume a different appearance from that of the newborn. The labia major are flat and labia minor are thin (Fig. 2-2). There is minimal separation between the labia majora and minora. The clitoris, no longer turgid, is hidden in the small cleft of the vulva. The mucous membranes of the introitus and vagina are thin, pink, and atrophic. On cross-section, they may be only two to three cell layers thick. The mucosal surfaces appear redder than the vaginal epithelium of a woman in the reproductive years because the blood vessels underneath the thin mucosa are closer to the surface. The thin vaginal lining has relatively few rugae and therefore, the distensibility is limited. These atrophic tissues have little resistance to trauma and infection. The secretions are neutral or slightly alkaline and contain mixed bacterial flora. The cervix is no longer distinct but flush with the vaginal vault. Occasionally, it is difficult to visualize the cervix.

Late Childhood and Adolescence

During late childhood (age 7 to 10 years), the external genitalia begin to show early signs of estrogen stimulation; the mons thickens, the labia majora fill out, the labia minora become rounded, and the hymen becomes thicker. The hymenal orifice increases in size. The vaginal mucosa becomes thicker, and the vagina elongates and measures 8 cm in length. Exfoliative cytology may show (in addition to the basal cells) some parabasal cells and occasionally, superficial cells. The corpus uteri grows also and is as large as the cervix, with the ratio of cervix to corpus being 1:1.

During early puberty (ages 10 to 13), the external genitalia finally assume an adult appearance. The major vestibular glands (Bartholin's) begin to produce mucous just before menarche. The vagina reaches its adult length (10 to 12 cm), the mucosa becomes thick and moist, the vaginal secretions become acidic, and lactobacilli reappear. With the development of vaginal fornices, the cervix separates from the vault. Uterine growth is pronounced but affects mainly the corpus, which is twice as large as the cervix. The ovaries descend into the true pelvic cavity. Secondary sex characteristics often develop rapidly during the late childhood period. The body habitus becomes rounded, especially in the shoulders and hips. Accelerated somatic growth (adolescent growth spurt) occurs, followed by breast development and sexual hair growth.

GYNECOLOGIC EXAMINATION OF INFANTS, CHILDREN, AND YOUNG ADOLESCENTS

An infant girl should have her first gynecologic examination in the delivery suite or nursery as part of the routine newborn evaluation. Most gynecologic abnormalities (clinically important to be recognized in the prepubertal period) are limited to the external genitalia; therefore, they should be recognized at birth or soon afterward. In most cases, it is unnecessary to perform an internal examination. Some isolated abnormalities require immediate correction, whereas other malformations may alert the physician to the possibility that the baby suffers from other disorders (eg, ambiguous genitalia caused by congenital adrenal hyperplasia) that require immediate medical therapy to prevent potentially lethal complications. Even if the management of the

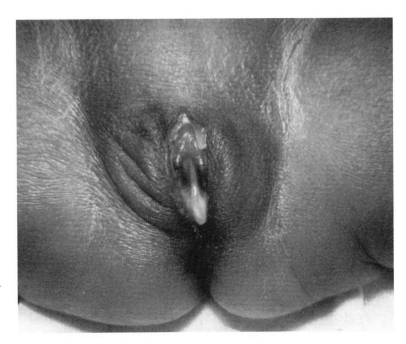

Figure 2–1. The external genitalia of a newborn female. Note the hypertrophy and turgor of the vulvar tissue. Note also the large amount of vaginal secretions.

anomaly can be safely delayed until early adulthood, early diagnosis allows better planning and therapy for conditions amenable to treatment and emotional support for patients for whom treatment is unavailable.

Gynecologic examination is indicated at any age when the child presents with genitourinary symptoms. In the absence of such symptoms, inspection of the external genitalia should be incorporated into every well-child examination.

A comprehensive gynecologic examination, even in asymptomatic girls, is warranted when sexual activity is contemplated or initiated. In addition, girls who are at increased risk (eg, in utero diethylstilbestrol [DES] exposure) should be examined immediately after menarche or at age 13 (whichever comes first), even if completely asymptomatic.

Newborns

A careful general examination may reveal somatic abnormalities that suggest a genital anomaly (eg, webbed neck, abdominal mass, edema of the hands and legs, coarctation of the aorta). The genital examination that follows consists primarily of inspection and palpation of the external genitalia. The clitoris deserves particular attention because enlargement in the newborn is frequently associated with other anomalies; most often, the infant has congenital adrenal hyperplasia but other causes must be considered (eg, true hermaphroditism). The vaginal orifice should be evident when the labia are separated. If not, it can be found by gently inserting a small well-lubricated pediatric feeding tube. When an opening cannot be found, the infant most likely has an imperforate hymen or vaginal

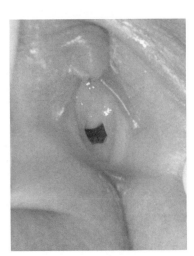

Figure 2–2. The external genitalia of a child 3 years of age.

agenesis. Infrequently, associated inguinal hernias, particularly when there is a mass in the hernial sac, suggest the possibility that the child is a genetic male. A rectoabdominal examination is performed to complete the primary evaluation. Usually, the uterus and adnexa cannot be palpated on rectal examination. Occasionally, because of stimulation by maternal estrogens, a small central mass can be felt. The ovaries are located at the pelvic brim; when an ovary is palpable, it denotes marked enlargement, which warrants further investigation. Finally, the rectal examination confirms patency of the anorectal canal.

Young Children

Young children are sensitive to the physician's attitude. They withdraw from a doctor or a nurse who is hurried, brusque, or indifferent. They react positively to someone who is kind, warm, interested, and patient. These young patients must be assured that the examination, although perhaps uncomfortable or embarrassing, will not be painful. The mother, who often accompanies the girl to the examination room, may be helpful during the examination because she provides comfort and a sense of security. Young children (younger than 5 years of age) may become apprehensive when placed on the examination table. Thus, placing the patient on the mother's lap reduces the anxiety. The mother may further assist by supporting the child's legs, permitting an unimpaired view of the genital area (Fig. 2-3). Older children are asked to lie on the examination table but the use of stirrups is generally not necessary. The patient is asked to flex her knees and abduct her legs. The patient should be asked to support her legs by placing her hands on the dorsal aspects of the lower thighs. Asking for a child's help is of definite value, with her involvement lessening the apprehension and providing a sense of control over the examination.

The examination begins with an evaluation of the child's general appearance, nutritional status, body habitus, and gross congenital anomalies. General uncleanliness suggests an associated poor perineal hygiene, which may contribute to vulvovaginitis. The child's breasts should be inspected and palpated. The breasts usually do not begin budding until age 8 to 9 years. It is common and normal for a small, firm, flat "button" to form beneath the nipple at the onset of breast growth. Prominence of the nipple and breast development at an earlier age may be the first sign of sexual precocity.

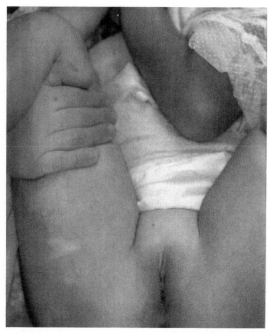

Figure 2–3. The examination of a young girl while seated on mother's lap. The mother supports the child's legs, thereby providing an excellent view of the genital area.

Inspection and palpation of the abdomen should precede examination of the genitalia. Light palpation and slow movement from one area to the another elicits most needed information. The ovary of a premenarcheal child is situated high in the pelvis. In addition, the small size of the pelvic cavity tends to force ovarian tumors toward the mid-abdomen. Thus, large ovarian neoplasms are often mistaken for other abdominal masses (eg, polycystic kidney). The vulva and vestibule may be exposed by light lateral and downward pressure of each side of the perineum. Particular attention should be paid to presence of vaginal discharge and general perineal hygiene. The examiner should also look for skin lesions, perineal excoriations, ulcers, and tumors. Signs of hormonal stimulation in early childhood or their absence when they should be evident are significant because many endocrine disorders are associated with abnormal pubertal development. Enlargement of the clitoris is also of diagnostic significance. In addition, the patency of the hymenal orifice must be assured.

It is impossible to perform a digital vaginal examination in a child if the size of the hymenal opening is normal for age. Gentle rectal digital examination can be easily accomplished, however, and should not cause pain. Nonetheless, accurate intra-pelvic evaluation is often difficult because of the relatively small size of the uterus and ovaries and the firmness of the abdominal wall. The examiner may assume that if uterus and ovaries are not palpable, the child does not have a genital tumor. If the presence of a pelvic tumor is suspected but cannot be palpated on rectal examination, other diagnostic procedures such as sonography should be performed.

Vaginoscopy

Vaginal instrumentation is not a routine part of the pelvic examination of young patients. It is required when the upper third of the vagina requires evaluation (eg, vaginal bleeding, DES screening). It may also be required in some patients to confirm patency of the genital tract, to observe and remove foreign bodies, and to assess vaginal trauma after penetrating injuries. In most children, the examination is done under general anesthesia. Numerous instruments have been used to perform vaginoscopy; I prefer the use of a water cystoscope, which distends the vagina and at the same time irrigates secretions, blood, and debris. Additional instruments, such as biopsy forceps, may be inserted through the operative channel.

Adolescents

The adolescent's first trip to the gynecologist is often fraught with fear and apprehension. Girl-friends may have told her harrowing stories they have heard about vaginal examinations. Therefore, time spent in putting the patient at ease and winning her confidence saves time and frustration in the examining room. One must impress on the adolescent that she, not her mother, is the patient. The girl, not her mother, is asked for routine information required for the medical record. Questions about sexual behavior and venereal diseases require a delicate approach and obviously, such questions should not be asked with the mother present. After the history-taking, the girl is given a brief description of what the examination entails. She and her mother may need to be assured that her hymen will not be injured and that the examination, although perhaps uncomfortable or embarrassing to her, will not be painful.

The examination is performed in the presence of a female assistant, who must constantly reassure the young patient. Examination of the breasts is an integral part of the physical examination of every female patient. In addition, instructions for self-examination and pamphlets for patient-education should be given at this time. Explanations of what is being done are given throughout the genital examination, and the physician may wish to use a mirror to show the girl her own genitalia.

After an inspection of the external genitalia, a speculum is inserted into the vagina. The introitus of most adolescents is about 1.0 cm in diameter and admits a narrow speculum without difficulty. In an adolescent, the Huffman-Graves long-bladed instrument is preferable to the short-bladed Graves speculum. The adolescent vagina is 10 to 12 cm long, and this particular speculum is so designed to allow an easy inspection of the cervix. In a patient with a large hymenal opening, bimanual examination is performed by inserting a finger into the vagina. Those who have a hymenal orifice too small for digital examination are examined rectally.

After the examination, the girl is given an opportunity to talk privately with the examiner. This is a prime opportunity to form a secure patient–physician relationship. The adolescent should be assured that she may discuss intimate issues and that her confidence will be respected. The examination and findings are discussed with the parent or parents only after the physician and the patient have completed their discussion and agreed on what should be held in confidence. Under no circumstances should the physician violate the patient's request for privacy. If the physician believes the parents should be aware of certain details, the patient must be so advised and persuaded that for her own benefit this information should be discussed with her parents.

COMMON DISORDERS IN THE PREMENARCHAL CHILD

Vulvovaginitis

Vulvovaginitis is the most common gynecologic disorder in children.[1] The young child is susceptible to infections for the following reasons:

Lack of estrogen
Contamination by stool and other debris
Possible impaired immune mechanisms of the vagina.

In young children, perineal hygiene is often less than adequate and contamination by stool and other debris is common. The vaginal mucosa is thin and atrophic because of the lack of estrogen and is therefore less resistant to infectious organisms.[2]

Vulvovaginitis can be divided into three major etiologic groups:

1. Nonspecific vulvovaginitis; a polymicrobial infection associated with disturbed local homeostasis (eg, poor perineal hygiene, foreign body)
2. Secondary inoculation; vaginal infection resulting from inoculation of the vagina with pathogens affecting other areas of the body by transfer through contact or blood (eg, urinary tract infections)
3. Specific infections; specific primary vaginal infection, most commonly sexually transmitted (eg, gonorrhea)

The symptoms of vulvovaginitis vary from minor discomfort to relatively intense perineal pruritus, a sensation of burning accompanied by a foul smelling discharge. Vaginal discharge may vary from minimal to copious. The irritating discharge inflames the vulva and often causes the child to scratch the area to the point of bleeding. Acute vulvovaginitis may denude the thin vulvar or vaginal mucosa but bleeding is usually minimal and as a rule, the discharge is little more than bloodstained. Inspection of the vagina usually reveals an area of redness and soreness, which may be minimal or may extend laterally to the thighs and posteriorly to the anus.

Evaluation of secretions should include:

1. Smears for Gram stain
2. Bacterial cultures
3. Cultures for mycotic organisms
4. Wet preparation for:
   A. Mycotic organisms
   B. White and red blood cells
   C. Vaginal epithelium (estrogen effect)
   D. Trichomonas
   E. Parasitic ova

The treatment of vulvovaginitis requires determination of the exact etiology. If a specific organism is found, sensitivity tests determine which antibiotics will be most effective. Generally, broad-spectrum antibiotics such as ampicillin are extremely useful. In all instances, appropriate instructions are given to both mother and child concerning vulvar hygiene. When the infection is severe and extensive mucosal damage is observed, a short course of topical estrogen cream may pro-

mote healing of vulvar and vaginal tissues. When irritation is intense, hydrocortisone cream may be necessary to alleviate the itching. Vaginoscopy is useful to exclude a foreign body or tumor. In girls with (1) recurrent vaginal infections, (2) infection refractory to treatment, or (3) a foul-smelling bloody discharge, vaginoscopy should be performed to investigate the source of infection and to exclude other pathologic conditions (eg, neoplasm). In children in whom an infection is documented for the first time, however, vaginoscopy may be delayed.

Foreign Bodies

Foreign bodies in the vagina induce an intense inflammatory reaction and result in a blood-stained foul-smelling discharge. Usually, the child does not recall inserting the foreign object or will not admit to it. The most commonly found foreign bodies are rolled pieces of toilet paper, which appear as amorphous conglomerates of grayish material. They are usually found on the posterior vaginal wall (Fig. 2-4). Because many foreign bodies are not radiopaque, radiographs are of little value. Vaginoscopy is essential, not only to discover and remove objects situated in the vagina, but also to exclude other causes for the bleeding. Although a foreign body that is situated in the lower third of the vagina can be washed out with warm saline, vaginoscopy is still indicated to confirm that no other foreign bodies are present in the upper vagina.

Lichen Sclerosus

Vulvar pruritus may be caused by any of several vulvar or perineal dermatologic disorders. These conditions are often not limited to the vulva but affect other body areas as well. Lichen sclerosus of the vulva is a hypertrophic dystrophy. Although it affects women mainly in the postmenopausal age group, it is occasionally seen in young children.[3] The symptoms consist of vulvar irritation, dysuria, and pruritus. Examination of the vulva shows flat ivory-colored papules, which may coalesce into plaques and may have pronounced vascular markings. In extreme cases, the lesion may involve the entire vulvar surface (Fig. 2-5). The lesion does not extend laterally beyond the middle of the labia majora nor does it encroach into the vagina. Nonetheless, the clitoris, posterior fourchette, and the anorectal area are frequently affected. The lesions tend to bruise easily, forming bloody blisters sus-

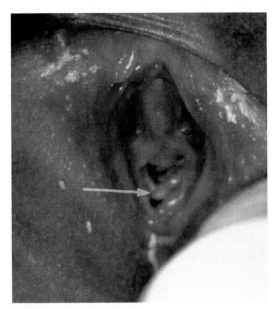

Figure 2–4. A foreign body (*arrow*) in the lower vagina.

ceptible to secondary infections.[3] Histologically, the skin shows flattening of the rete pegs, hyalinization of the subdermal tissues, and keratinization. In children, hyperplastic lichen sclerosus has no known malignant potential. Treatment consists of improved local hygiene, reduction of trauma, and the short-term use of hydrocortisone creams to al-

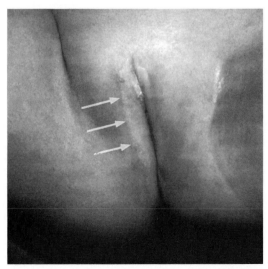

Figure 2–5. Lichen sclerosus of the vulva of 6-year-old child. The margins of the lesion are clearly defined (*arrows*).

leviate the intense pruritus. Treatment may be repeated when exacerbations occur.

Marked improvement in symptoms and appearance of the skin lesions after puberty is described. Review of the literature suggests that up to 50% of the children improve significantly or recover during puberty, 30% to 45% have no change, and in 5% to 10% of affected girls, the disease worsens.[3,4]

Labial Adhesions

Labial adhesions in prepubertal children are believed to be a relatively common finding. Among 1500 girls followed-up for routine care for 3 years by Ben-Ami and colleagues, labial adhesions developed in nine girls younger than age 3 years.[5] Huffman considers girls age 2 to 6 years most likely to be affected; however, others find the highest frequency to be in children younger than 2 years of age.[5,6,8] Labial adhesions are usually asymptomatic and thus are unreported in many youngsters.

The etiology is not known but is probably related to the low levels of estrogen in the prepubertal child. It is suggested that the thin skin covering the labia may be denuded as a result of local irritation and scratching. The labia then adhere in the midline, stick to each other, and as reepithelialization occurs on both sides, the labia remain fused in the midline (Fig. 2-6). Studies show that labial adhesions are more prevalent in prepubertal girls who are sexually abused.[7,8]

Most children with small degrees of labial adhesion are asymptomatic. When symptoms do occur, they usually relate to interference with urination or to the accumulation of urine behind the adhesed labia. Dysuria and recurrent vulvar or vaginal infections are the presenting symptoms. On rare occasions, when complete occlusion is present, urinary retention may occur.[9]

If asymptomatic, a minimal to moderate degree of labial fusion does not require treatment. When the degree of fusion is significant or the child is symptomatic, a short course of treatment with Premarin cream, applied twice daily for 7 to 10 days, may separate the labia. When such medical treatment fails or if severe urinary symptoms exist, surgical division of the fused labia is indicated.[10] Recurrence of labial adhesions is common because the estrogen deficiency exists until puberty. After puberty, the condition usually resolves spontaneously. Improved perineal hygiene and removal of irritants from the vulva may prevent recurrences, however.

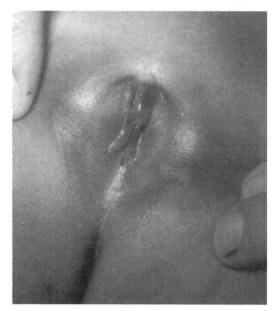

Figure 2–6. Labial adhesions in a young girl. Note the translucent vertical line in the center where the labia are fused together.

Urethral Prolapse

The urethral mucosa protrudes through the meatus and forms a hemorrhagic, tender vulvar mass that bleeds easily (Fig. 2-7). The urethral orifice can be identified in the center of the mass, which is separated from the vagina. When the lesion is small and

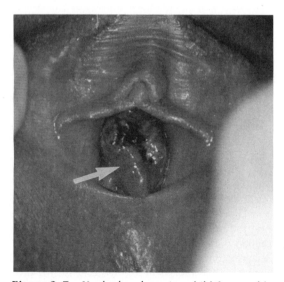

Figure 2–7. Urethral prolapse in a child 6 years old.

urination is unimpaired, a short course of topical estrogens is beneficial.[11] Resection of the prolapsed tissue should be considered if urinary retention occurs, the lesion is large and necrotic, or if the child is examined under anesthesia.[12,13]

Genital Tumors

Although uncommon, genital tumors must be considered whenever a girl is found to have a chronic genital ulcer, a nontraumatic swelling of the external genitalia, tissue protruding from the vagina, foul smelling bloody discharge, abdominal pain, genital enlargement, virilization, or premature sexual maturation. Despite their rarity, virtually every type of genital neoplasm reported in adults has also been found in girls younger than 14 years, and about half of these are malignant.

Vulvar and Vaginal Tumors

Most benign tumors of the vagina in children are unilocular cystic remnants of the mesonephric duct. Other benign neoplasms include teratomas, hemangiomas, simple cysts of the hymen, retention cysts of the paraurethral ducts, benign granulomas of the perineum, and condylomata acuminata.

Small cysts of the mesonephric (Gartner's) duct do not require surgery when asymptomatic. Large cysts may interfere with urination or vaginal drainage, however, thereby requiring surgical treatment. The cyst is opened, most of the accessible cyst wall is removed, and the edges are marsupialized to prevent future accumulation of fluid. Obstruction of a paraurethral duct may form a relatively large cyst, distorting the urethral orifice. Simple excision or marsupialization is again the recommended treatment. Teratomas usually present as cystic masses arising from the midline of the perineum. Although a teratoma in this area may be benign, local recurrence may be a problem. Therefore, a generous margin of healthy tissue should be excised around its periphery. Capillary hemangiomas usually disappear as the child grows older and require no therapy. In contrast, cavernous hemangiomas are composed of vessels of considerable size, and injury to them may cause serious hemorrhage. For this reason, cavernous hemangiomas are best treated surgically.

Embryonal carcinoma of the vagina (botryoid sarcoma) is seen most commonly in the very young age group (younger than 3 years old). In these young children, the tumor is often situated in the lower vagina, whereas in an older child (over age 10) the tumor more often affects the upper vagina or the cervix. The tumors arise in the submucosal tissues and spread rapidly beneath an intact vaginal epithelium. The vaginal mucosa then bulges into a series of polypoid growths, which may protrude through the vaginal orifice (Fig. 2-8). The diagnosis is confirmed by histologic examination of a biopsy specimen.[14]

Initial treatment of embryonal carcinoma consists of combination chemotherapy (usually vincristine, actinomycin D, and cyclophosphomide), which has been employed with success. After the course of chemotherapy, the tumor is reexamined and rebiopsied. If it is then amenable to surgical removal, radical hysterectomy and vaginectomy with preservation of the ovaries is performed. Exenteration is not recommended, although it may be required in some patients who do not respond to other treatment modalities.[14] If the tumor is still unresectable after chemotherapy, radiotherapy is employed to further assist in shrinking and controlling tumor growth.[14]

Ambiguous Genitalia

Anomalies of the genitalia may be divided into two major categories: those that suggest sexual ambiguity (intersex problems) and those that do not.

When significant ambiguity of the external genitalia is present, the true gender cannot be immediately determined (Fig. 2-9).

Ambiguous genitalia denotes partial or incomplete virilization of the external genitalia. Ambiguous genitalia may be seen, therefore, in genetic females who were virilized in utero, in undervirilized males, or in true hermaphrodites. Generally, exposure to androgens after 12 weeks of gestation leads only to clitoral hypertrophy. Examination of the genitalia reveals an enlarged clitoris, with a normal vestibule, urethra, and vagina. The labia majora are altered by redundancy, wrinkling, and skin pigmentation. Exposure at progressively earlier stages of embryologic development also leads to clitoral hypertrophy but additionally to retention of the urogenital sinus and to fusion of the labioscrotal folds. In these severely virilized individuals, the labia are fused in the midline to form a median raphe. The area of fusion may be partial or extend the entire distance from the perineum to the phallus. When extensive, the fused labia form a wrinkled pouchlike structure, which resembles the scrotum in a cryptorchid male. The vaginal opening is absent. Instead, a single opening is present, which extends to a common passage connecting the urethra and

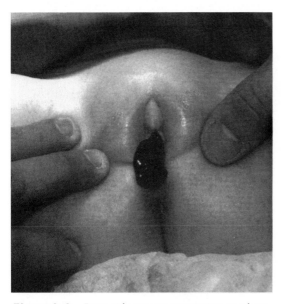

Figure 2–8. Botryoid sarcoma presenting as a hemorrhagic growth extruding from the vagina.

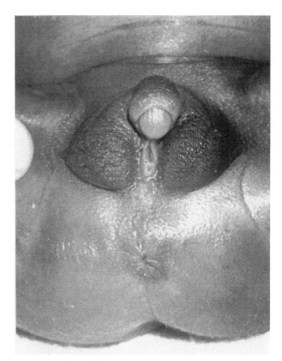

Figure 2–9. Ambiguous genitalia of a female child, caused by congenital adrenal hyperplasia.

vagina. Müllerian duct and gonad development remain unaffected because neither is androgen-dependent.

The surgical correction of genital ambiguity should be performed only after the completion of the medical evaluation. Reconstruction of the female external genitalia is best accomplished in two stages. The first, performed before the infant's discharge from the hospital, consists of clitoral reduction. The purpose of the surgical reduction is to attain female appearance to the external genitalia. When a reduction clitoroplasty is performed, the surgeon should attempt to preserve the neurovascular connections to the glans. In this manner, a functional clitoris of normal size can be created. Removal of the entire clitoris is rarely indicated. Vaginal reconstruction should be delayed until after pubertal development. Generally, division of the labia is all that is required if only labial fusion is present. Minor degrees of narrowing of the vaginal introitus can be easily corrected. When a significant narrowing is present, enlargement of the introitus may require the use of rotated skin flaps or a split-thickness skin graft.

Genital Trauma

Most injuries to the genitalia during childhood are accidental but some are the result of child abuse. The physician must determine how the child sustained the injury because abused children must be removed from an unsafe environment. Many genital injuries are of minor significance but a few are life-threatening and require major surgical procedures. With severe trauma or in very young children, it may be necessary to perform the examination under general anesthesia.[15]

Vulvar and Vaginal Injuries

Because the perineum and vulva are extremely vascular and the subcutaneous tissues are loosely arranged, an injury may cause blood vessels underneath the perineal skin to rupture. Blood accumulates under the skin and forms a hematoma, producing a rounded, tense, and tender swelling, the size of which depends on the amount of bleeding. A contusion of the vulva does not usually require treatment. A small vulvar hematoma can usually be controlled by pressure with an ice pack. A large hematoma or one that continues to increase in size should be incised, the clotted blood removed, and bleeding points ligated. If the source of the bleeding cannot be found, the cavity should be packed with gauze and a pressure dressing applied. The pack is removed in 24 hours. Prophylactic broad-spectrum antibiotics are advisable. The vulva should be kept clean and dry. When the urethra is obstructed by the hematoma, it is necessary to insert a suprapubic catheter. Pelvic x-ray may be necessary in some patients to rule out a fracture of the pelvis.

Most vaginal injuries occur when an object penetrates the vagina through the hymenal opening. Such penetration results in a laceration or a tear of the hymenal ring (Fig. 2-10). Usually, there is little bleeding from a hymenal injury but it indicates va-

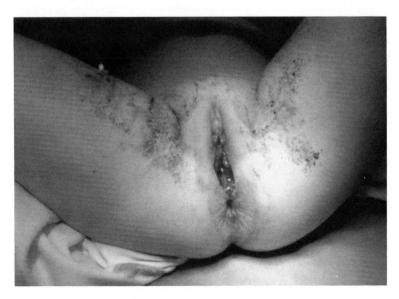

Figure 2–10. Vaginal laceration following sexual assault in a 2-year-old infant.

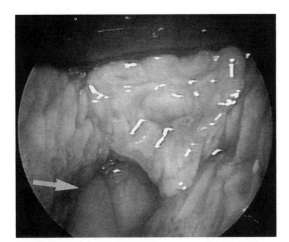

Figure 2–11. Vaginoscopy in a child, showing loops of small bowel in the vagina following sexual assault.

Table 2–1
Early Sexual Maturation

Incomplete Forms

Premature thelarche

Premature adrenarche

Premature menarche

Premature pubarche

Complete Forms

Immature hypothalamic–pituitary–ovarian axis
    Exposure to estrogens
        In the food chain
        Medications
    Endogenous estrogen production
        Functional ovarian cysts
        Ovarian neoplasms
        Other hormone-producing neoplasms

Mature hypothalamic–pituitary–ovarian axis
    Constitutional precocious puberty
    Central nervous system lesions
    McCune–Albright syndrome

ginal penetration and thus the possibility of additional vaginal injuries. Therefore, a detailed examination is necessary to exclude injuries to the upper vagina (Fig. 2-11). When a vaginal laceration extends to the vaginal vault, a laparotomy is indicated to exclude extension of the tear into the broad ligament or the peritoneal cavity. Bladder and bowel integrity must also be confirmed.

Most vaginal wounds involve the lateral walls. Generally, there is relatively little blood loss, and the child does not have much pain if the damage is only mucosal. The child complains of intense pain when a lacerated blood vessel retracts underneath the vaginal mucosa and forms a hematoma. If the torn vessel is small, bleeding may stop spontaneously. Larger vessels may form large, tense hematomas, which may distend the vagina and require evacuation and ligation of the bleeding vessel.

Early Pubertal Development

Puberty is the process by which the sexually immature organs become capable of reproduction. These changes occur largely as a result of the maturation of the hypothalamic–pituitary–gonadal axis. Puberty may be truly precocious if the stimuli for such change is due to early hypothalamic–pituitary activity. Conversely, similar-appearing physiologic alterations may be the result of stimulation by estrogens of exogenous or endogenous origin without hypothalamic–pituitary maturation (Table 2-1). As a rule, breast development, cornification of

the vaginal mucosa, and the growth of genital hair precede uterine bleeding by about 2 years.

The normal sequence of events in sexual development has been well described. Usually, growth acceleration occurs first. The breast bud develops between ages 9 and 11 and is followed by pubarche and the adolescent growth spurt. The first menstrual period occurs at an average of 12.8 years in American girls. Regular ovulation, 20 months later, marks the end of the pubertal cycle.

Sexual precocity is the onset of sexual maturation at any age that is 2.5 standard deviations earlier than normal. The appearance of any of the secondary sexual characteristics before 8 years of age or onset of menarche before age 10 is considered precocious.

Early Sexual Development— Incomplete Forms

Occasionally, for reasons that remain unclear, only one sign of pubertal development is present (breast development, pubic hair, or menstruation). It is possibly the result of transient elevations in the levels of circulating steroid hormones or alternatively, may be caused by extreme sensitivity of the end organ to the low prepubertal levels of sex hormones. Such isolated development may be the first sign of precocious puberty; reevaluation at regular intervals is thus indicated.

PREMATURE THELARCHE.   Premature the-larche is the isolated development of breast tissue before age 8 years. It may occur at an earlier age but is most common between 1 to 3 years. It may affect one or both breasts. Although the exact eti-ology is unknown, such breast development may reflect increased end-organ sensitivity or alterna-tively, a response to transient elevation of plasma estrogens. On examination, somatic growth pattern is not accelerated, bone age is not advanced, and vaginal smear fails to show estrogenic effect. The diagnosis is made by exclusion of other disorders such as hypothyroidism. Surgical biopsy of the breast is contraindicated because a relatively large portion of breast tissue may be unwittingly excised and cause permanent damage of the breast. Follow-up is necessary to identify those patients in whom such breast development heralds the onset of true precocious puberty.

PREMATURE PUBARCHE.   Premature pubarche is the isolated development of pubic or axillary hair before age 8 years, without other signs of preco-cious puberty. Such hair growth may be idiopathic and of no clinical significance. These individuals, in some series, tend to be slightly taller, have margin-ally advanced bone age, and have slightly elevated blood levels of dehydroepiandrosterone sulfate.[16]

Early pubarche may be a sign of excess andro-gen production, however, due to an enzyme defi-ciency (eg, congenital adrenal hyperplasia) or tu-mor (eg, Leydig cell tumor). Thorough evaluation of adrenal and gonadal function in addition to as-sessment of androgen production is necessary to exclude such abnormalities. Thus, the diagnosis of idiopathic premature pubarche is made only after such an evaluation fails to detect a developmental abnormality.

PREMATURE MENARCHE.   Premature men-arche denotes the appearance of cyclic vaginal bleeding in girls younger than age 10 years in the absence of other signs of secondary sexual devel-opment. The etiology is unknown but may be in-creased end-organ sensitivity (in this case, the en-dometrium) to the low estrogen levels, which are in the prepubertal range. Alternatively, the endome-trial shedding may reflect cyclic, transient eleva-tions of serum estrogens produced by gonadotro-pin-independent ovarian follicles.

Examination of these children is usually normal, and the genital appearance and cytologic vaginal smears show lack of constant estrogenic stimula-tion. Growth and development are appropriate for age, and the bone age is not advanced. When these girls are given gonadotropin-releasing hormone (GnRH), the response of the pituitary gland is sim-ilar to that seen in prepubertal children.

The diagnosis is formulated by exclusion after a complete evaluation of other causes of vaginal bleeding. With time, the diagnosis is confirmed when the cyclic nature of the bleeding becomes ap-parent. Prognosis for these girls is excellent; adult height is uncompromised, future menstrual pattern is normal, and fertility potential remains unim-paired.[17]

Early Sexual Development— Complete Forms

EXOGENOUS ESTROGENS.   Accidental inges-tion of estrogens or the prolonged use of creams containing estrogens is a possible (yet uncommon) cause of early feminization. If such exposure is doc-umented, prompt discontinuation is proper treat-ment.

ENDOGENOUS ESTROGEN PRODUCTION. The ovary of a newborn contains 1 to 2 million primordial follicles, most of which undergo atre-sia during childhood without producing significant quantities of estrogen. Occasionally, however, large follicular cysts capable of estrogen production oc-cur and may lead to early feminization. In addition, other benign tumors of the ovary (eg, teratoma, cystadenoma) are capable of either producing es-trogens or inducing surrounding ovarian tissue to produce sex steroids. Finally, granulosa cell tumors capable of estrogen production are a rare cause of feminization of a prepubertal child. Other tumors of extragonadal origin may produce estrogens, includ-ing adrenal adenomas and hepatomas, but they are extremely rare.

CONSTITUTIONAL PRECOCIOUS PUBERTY. Constitutional precocious puberty is most com-monly seen in individuals who are nearing the age of menarche, usually at age 6 or 7 years. These pa-tients have no abnormality except for the early de-velopment of pubertal changes, which progress in an orderly sequence (Fig. 2-12). Precocious puberty may occur in a younger child, 2 or 3 years of age; in these girls, computed tomography (CT) scanning of the brain occasionally demonstrates the presence of small hamartomas in the hypothalamus. Whether a patient with small hamartoma should be consid-ered to have idiopathic precocious puberty or alter-natively, a central nervous system (CNS) lesion, is unclear.

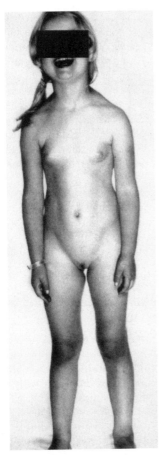

Figure 2–12. Precocious puberty in a child 4 years of age.

Girls with idiopathic precocious puberty have some loss of adult height due to an accelerated bone maturation. In other respects, however, prognosis is favorable and future menstrual pattern and fertility in this group of patients is expected to be normal.[18]

CENTRAL NERVOUS SYSTEM LESIONS. Patients with CNS lesions such as tumors, severe head injuries, meningitis, or encephalitis occasionally have early sexual development, possibly due to an irritative phenomenon on the hypothalamus, resulting in an earlier than normal activation of the hypothalamic–pituitary–ovarian axis. Usually, pubertal development is slower than normal and progresses gradually over many years. The clinical findings (apart from the early pubertal development) are related to the nature of the primary CNS lesion. When such lesions are large, concurrent

neurologic deficit may be present. Treatment is directed toward the primary disorder and precocious puberty treated symptomatically. Prognosis is determined by the nature of the primary CNS lesion.

McCUNE–ALBRIGHT SYNDROME. An association of polyosthotic fibrous dysplasia, irregular cutaneous pigmentation, and precocious puberty are the cardinal signs of McCune–Albright syndrome. These children usually present at a younger age than those with idiopathic precocious puberty. Vaginal bleeding occurs early and in most is the first sign of puberty. The diagnosis is made by skin pigmentation and the demonstration of bone lesions or pathologic fractures. The exact etiology of McCune–Albright syndrome is unknown but it has been suggested that it may be the result of a primary ovarian abnormality, with premature estrogen production.

The prognosis is unfavorable. Adult height is significantly reduced, not only because of the early epiphyseal closure but also because of pathologic bone fractures. In addition, most adults have menstrual abnormalities and infertility.[18]

Evaluation of the Patient With Accelerated Sexual Development

The evaluation of a child presenting with early sexual maturation requires a detailed history—in particular, onset and progression of growth and secondary sexual features, use of medications, history of head injury or CNS lesions, and family history of early sexual maturation. A complete physical examination should include height, weight, and Tanner staging of breast and pubic hair development. Growth should be plotted on standard growth charts as well as on growth-velocity charts. Careful inspection of the skin should be performed in search of pigmented nevi or neurofibromata. Inspection of the genitalia is required to determine degree of estrogenic stimulation. A rectoabdominal palpation is required to delineate large ovarian lesions. Initial laboratory evaluation in patients with isolated breast development consists of plasma estrogen levels, prolactin levels, and when clinically indicated, thyroid function tests. A left hand and wrist x-ray is obtained to determine bone age. If all these tests are normal, the diagnosis of premature thelarche is highly likely. These patients require follow-up to determine whether progression occurs. Absence of further development confirms the diagnosis.

Initial laboratory evaluation in patients with isolated pubic hair development consists of plasma androgen levels, 17-α-hydroxyprogesterone, and when clinically indicated, adrenocorticotropic hormone stimulation and suppression tests. A left hand and wrist x-ray is obtained to determine bone age. If all these tests are normal, the diagnosis of premature adrenarche is highly likely. These patients require follow-up to determine whether progression occurs. Absence of further development confirms the diagnosis.

Initial laboratory evaluation in patients with suspected precocious puberty consists of plasma estrogen levels (or an evaluation of vaginal smear for estrogen effects), a left hand and wrist x-ray to determine bone age, a pelvic sonogram, and a CT or magnetic resonance imaging scan of the skull. Diagnosis is confirmed by a pubertal response to a GnRH challenge test.

Treatment of the Patient With Accelerated Sexual Development

Treatment of early sexual development depends on the exact etiology. Patients with premature thelarche and premature adrenarche require no therapy. In patients with gonadal or adrenal neoplasms, the treatment consists of surgical excision of the neoplasm. Patients with congenital adrenal hyperplasia require steroid replacement therapy. Patients with CNS lesions may require surgery or irradiation, depending on the histologic features and the location of the lesion.

Treatment of patients with idiopathic precocious puberty is aimed at suppression of gonadotropin secretion. The most common treatment today is the administration of GnRH agonists. These lower production and secretion of gonadotropins by the pituitary gland. If GnRH agonists are not available, 50 to 100 mg every 2 to 4 weeks of medroxyprogesterone acetate may be given intramuscularly weekly or twice monthly.

Delayed Sexual Maturation

Delayed sexual development is defined as the absence of normal pubertal events at an age 2.5 standard deviations from the mean. The absence of thelarche by age 13 or of menarche by age 15 both qualify as delayed sexual maturation by that definition and therefore require investigation. The physician need not always delay evaluation until such strict criteria are met, however. The concern of the

patient, her family, or the referring physician are reasons enough for initiating an evaluation. Because some degree of sexual maturation occurs in more than 30% of patients with gonadal dysgenesis, an investigation is necessary when a girl presents after thelarche with delay in progression of pubertal development.[19]

Patients presenting with abnormal puberty may be classified according to gonadal function. Thus, patients are divided into three major clinical groups according to secondary sexual development.

1. Delayed menarche, with adequate secondary sexual development
2. Delayed puberty, with inadequate or absent secondary sexual development
3. Delayed puberty and heterosexual secondary sexual development.

Patients With Adequate Secondary Sexual Development

Patients with functioning ovaries and delayed sexual maturation usually consult a physician in their mid-teens for amenorrhea. Most have a well-formed female configuration, with developing breasts. In addition, most patients with apparent normal sexual development suffer from inappropriate luteinizing hormone feedback and subsequent anovulatory cycles, unopposed estrogens, and in some patients, an excess of androgens. The resulting endocrine disturbance (namely, distortion of the estrogen:androgen ratio) is also encountered in adolescents with postnatal adrenogenital syndrome and patients with polycystic ovary disease. The signs and symptoms are similar in these conditions; when hyperandrogenism is present, evaluation of adrenal function should be performed. Primary amenorrhea may also persist until the patient is challenged with a progestin. Additionally, patients should be monitored for continued menstrual shedding. Persistent amenorrhea is treated with progestins administered every other month to assure endometrial shedding and to prevent potentially heavy menstrual bleeding (10 mg p.o. daily for 5 days). Obviously, if the patient is sexually active, birth control pills are preferred to cyclic progestins.

Congenital anomalies of the paramesonephric (müllerian) structures are often seen in patients with amenorrhea.[20] The most frequent defect is congenital absence of the uterus and vagina. Other anatomic causes of amenorrhea include imperforate hymen, transverse vaginal septa, agenesis of the cervix, and partial or complete agenesis of the vagina. Gynecologic examination supplemented by sonography establishes the diagnosis of these congenital anomalies.

IMPERFORATE HYMEN. Sometimes the hymen forms a solid membrane without an aperture—what is known as imperforate hymen. It is believed that an imperforate hymen represents a persistent portion of the urogenital membrane and occurs when the mesoderm of the primitive streak abnormally invades the urogenital portion of the cloacal membrane.[20]

Because the vagina is obstructed by this solid membrane, accumulation of vaginal secretions or menstrual blood may distend the vagina and uterus, forming, respectively, a mucocolpos or hematocolpos (Fig. 2-13). Unless the correct diagnosis is established, the distended vagina forms a large mass, which may fill the pelvis. Careful gynecologic examination is required to determine the true nature of such masses and to prevent enlargements of this type from being mistaken for abdominal tumors.

An imperforate hymen without accumulation of fluid (as may be seen in prepubertal children) forms a fibrous, smooth surface between the labia minora, which may be difficult to differentiate from an absent vagina. Sonographic evaluation of the pelvis

may identify the uterus, cervix, and vagina and thus distinguish between these two conditions.

Imperforate hymen often is not diagnosed until an adolescent girl reports primary amenorrhea and recurrent pelvic pain. Occasionally, the first symptom may be urinary retention, caused by pressure of a large hematocolpos on the bladder and urethra. Inspection of the vulva generally reveals a dome-shaped purplish-red hymenal membrane bulging outward in response to the collection of blood above it. On rectal examination, the vagina is palpable as a large cystic mass.

The blood fills the vagina (hematocolpos) and then the uterus (hematometra) and may spill through the tubes into the peritoneal cavity. Endometriosis and vaginal adenosis are potential but not inevitable complications in such patients.

An imperforate hymen must be corrected. In infants, the central portion of the membrane is lifted up and snipped away. Sutures usually are not necessary. In postmenarcheal girls with an imperforate hymen, a portion of the membrane should be removed because when the hymen is only incised, the edges tend to coalesce after draining the hematocolpos. Follow-up evaluation of the vagina and pelvis should be deferred for 4 to 6 weeks to reduce the risk of introducing infection.

TRANSVERSE VAGINAL SEPTUM. Transverse vaginal septa are the result of faulty canalization of the embryonic vagina and therefore are present at birth. They are usually found in the mid-vagina but may occur at any level. When the septum is located in the upper vagina, it is likely to be patent, whereas those located in the lower part of the vagina are more often complete.

An asymptomatic complete vaginal septum in a child should be at least incised before menarche, converting it to an incomplete septum to allow egress of vaginal secretions and later of menstrual blood. An undiscovered imperforate transverse septum may lead to the formation of a large mucocolpos in infancy or to an obstruction of menstrual flow in the adolescent.

After the initial incision, these septa and incomplete vaginal septa discovered during childhood should not be treated further until after puberty because of the technical difficulties in performing intravaginal surgery on the immature structures of a young child. Once drainage is secured, I prefer to wait until after menarche to complete septal extirpation, at which time the membrane may be excised and vaginal narrowing, which may be present at the level of partition, corrected.

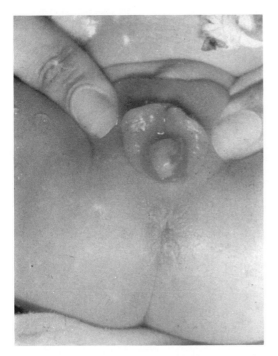

Figure 2–13. Mucocolpos secondary to an imperforate hymen.

VAGINAL AGENESIS. The external genitalia of patients with vaginal agenesis (Rokitansky syndrome) appear normal. A ruffled ridge of tissue represents the hymen, inside of which an indentation marks the spot where the vagina should be found. Instead, only a dimple or a short blind vagina is found. In most patients, the uterus and tubes are absent or rudimentary. In addition, other developmental defects may be present, affecting the urinary tract (45% to 50%), the spine (10%), or less frequently, the middle ear. Therefore, at some time during childhood, there should be an evaluation of the urinary tract, the spine, and audiometric evaluation.[21]

Individuals with the Rokitansky syndrome are genetic females; they develop normally in adolescence and have all of the usual feminine attributes, except they suffer from amenorrhea and infertility. A karyotype should be obtained from all patients with vaginal agenesis to rule out the rare instances in which vaginal agenesis represents the effects of testicular activity, thus indicating that this individual is a male pseudohermaphrodite.

Creation of a satisfactory vagina is the objective in treatment of vaginal agenesis, and several techniques are available. An exploratory laparotomy is rarely indicated in these patients; the creation of a vagina should be deferred until the girl is contemplating sexual activity. The nonoperative creation of a vagina, first described by Frank and modified by Ingram, is relatively risk-free but requires motivation and patient cooperation.[22,23] The region that the vagina should occupy is a potential space filled with comparatively loose connective tissue, which is capable of considerable indentation and attenuation. In this method, the patient is given a series of dilators of graduated widths and lengths and is taught how to place them against the vaginal dimple and how to apply constant pressure. This maneuver is repeated three times daily for 20 to 30 minutes, using wider and longer dilators. The procedure takes a few months to complete. If it fails, a surgical correction may be required. A popular method is the McIndoe procedure, which involves the creation of a cavity between the urethra and bladder anteriorly and the perineal body and rectum posteriorly by surgical dissection. The newly created cavity is then lined by a split-thickness skin graft overlying a plastic or soft silicone mold.[24] Further dilation may be required to prevent scarring and narrowing of the vagina. An alternative procedure is the Williams vulvovaginoplasty, which uses the labia majora to construct a coital pouch.[25]

PARTIAL VAGINAL AGENESIS. Partial vaginal agenesis denotes the absence of a large portion of the vaginal plate, usually the distal part. The lower vagina is replaced by a soft mass of tissue. The cause of this uncommon anomaly is unknown. Partial vaginal agenesis may be diagnosed when the lower vagina is missing but sonographic examination demonstrates the presence of a cervix and

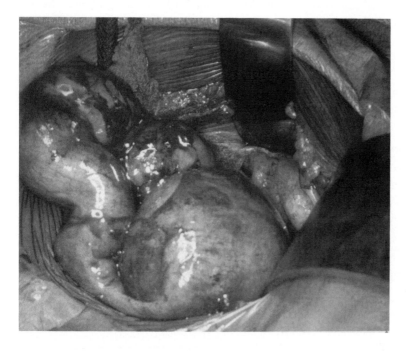

Figure 2–14. A rudimentary, noncommunicating uterine horn. Note the hematosalpinx caused by retrograde menstruation.

uterus. If the uterus has developed normally, the upper part of the vagina fills with blood when menstruation begins. The symptoms are similar to those associated with an imperforate hymen after the menarche. Vulvar inspection reveals findings identical with those of vaginal agenesis but rectoabdominal palpation reveals a large, boggy pelvic mass.

Although it is impossible to specify a routine for management of such patients, obstruction to menstrual flow must be corrected. In some, drainage of the uterus may be achieved through a reconstructed vagina. In others, particularly when the uterus is rudimentary, consideration may be given to performing a hysterectomy (Fig. 2-14).

ANDROGEN INSENSITIVITY. Another condition in which patients present with amenorrhea and adequate breast development is one of the complete forms of androgen insensitivity. These patients are genetic males, in whom the testes developed normally and produce adequate amounts of androgens. End-organ tissues (eg, sexual hair, genitalia) are not responsive to androgens and as a result, the patients do not virilize in utero or at puberty. In utero, the fetus develops along female lines but the müllerian ducts regress under the influence of the müllerian-inhibiting substance. The newborn infant appears to be a normal female because the external genitalia appear normal. The vagina is absent but the diagnosis is rarely made during childhood. During puberty, adequate breast development is often present, secondary to the small amounts of unopposed estrogen produced by the testes. Pubic and axillary hair are scant and often missing (Fig. 2-15). Only a short or blind vaginal pouch is present, and the patient presents with complaints of primary amenorrhea. The testes are often palpable in the inguinal canals. Once pubertal development is complete, surgical extirpation of the gonads and reconstruction of the vagina is necessary.

PREGNANCY. Lastly, the possibility that an adolescent may become pregnant before she menstruates is highly unlikely but must be borne in mind when considering the causes of delayed menarche in these patients.

Patients With Inadequate Secondary Sexual Development

HYPOTHALAMIC OR PITUITARY FAILURE. Both reversible and irreversible etiologies for delayed puberty secondary to lack of pubertal maturation of the hypothalamus and pituitary have been described. The onset of puberty depends on an ill-defined stage of maturity, which is reflected in skel-

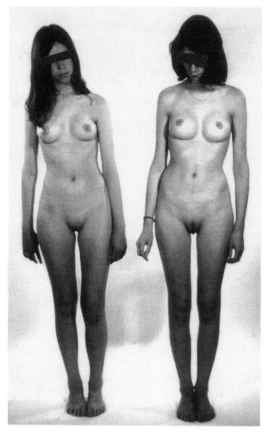

Figure 2–15. Sisters with androgen insensitivity syndrome (Courtesy of Professor Sir John Dewhurst, from Huffman JW, Dewhurst CJ, Capraro VJ: The gynecology of childhood and adolescence, 2nd ed. Philadelphia, WB Saunders, 1981, with permission.)

etal age. Maturation is partly determined by genetic factors but also depends on environmental factors. Thus, the chronologic age of puberty varies considerably from person to person. The statistical limits of normal variation of a defined population indicates that by definition, 2.5% of all normal adolescents would develop later than what is defined as normal. This group has been labeled "late bloomers" or girls with constitutional delay. The lack of signs of puberty (including the pubertal growth spurt) often concerns the patient when her adolescent friends have secondary sexual features and the characteristic increase in height.

The diagnosis is made by excluding other causes of delayed sexual maturation. The GnRH challenge test differentiates constitutional delay from similar conditions associated with a deficiency of gonadotropin-releasing hormone (GnRH). Reassurance is the only necessary treatment but the patient must be kept under observation until she begins normal menstrual cycles. Occasionally, an adolescent requires hormonal replacement therapy because of the emotional distress caused by her condition and the associated infantile appearance.

Isolated deficiency of GnRH, often associated with intracranial anomalies and anosmia (Kallmann's syndrome), is uncommon. Every patient suspected of having the syndrome should be tested for sense of smell because many have only a minor degree of anosmia. All of these patients fail to develop secondary sexual features, and blood levels of gonadotropins are low. After a GnRH challenge, a rise in gonadotropin levels is noted. Estrogen therapy is used to initiate and later sustain sexual development. Induction of ovulation with Pergonal or GnRH is necessary when fertility is desired.

A pituitary or parasellar tumor, particularly craniopharyngioma or pituitary adenoma, must be considered in the evaluation of a patient with delayed sexual maturation. Craniopharyngiomas are rapidly growing tumors that often develop in late childhood, whereas pituitary adenomas, although slow-growing, may become symptomatic during puberty and interfere with sexual maturation.

An occult pituitary prolactinoma in adolescents with unexplained delayed sexual maturation must also be ruled out. Indeed, serum prolactin levels should be measured yearly in patients with unexplained delayed sexual maturation.

Weight loss due to severe dieting, marked protein deficiency, and fat loss without notable loss of muscle (often seen in athletes) may also delay or suppress hypothalamic–pituitary maturation. Additionally, heroin addiction may cause amenorrhea but its effect on sexual maturation has not been documented.

GONADAL FAILURE. The largest number of patients with delayed sexual development fall into this category. Lack of gonadal function most frequently occurs as a result of primary ovarian failure, which results in an elevation of gonadotropins. Most present with delayed puberty, having ovarian failure secondary to privation of X chromosome material and important ovarian-determinant genes.

Two intact X chromosomes are usually necessary for normal ovary structure and function. Chromosomal abnormalities that may be associated with failure of ovarian development include loss of all of one X chromosome, deletion of part of one X chromosome, or transverse division at the centromere rather than longitudinal division, leading to isochromosome formation. Mosaicism with two or more cell lines, one containing an abnormal X chromosome, is probably more common than nonmosaic abnormalities.[26]

Failure of sexual maturation is due to loss of the ovarian-determinant gene that induces ovary formation. Somatic abnormalities with gonadal dysgenesis may be the result of the deletion of genetic material carried with the lost portion of the X chromosome. As a result, some patients with gonadal dysgenesis have only failure of sexual maturation, whereas others exhibit the complete phenotype of Turner's syndrome (Fig. 2-16).

Adolescents with ovarian failure present with undeveloped breasts, little or no pubic hair, an atrophic vaginal smear, and elevated gonadotropin levels. When X chromosome material is missing, somatic anomalies may also be present. The classic features of Turner's syndrome are well-recognized: short stature, absent or minimal secondary sexual development, neck webbing, and coarctation of the aorta.[26] In all patients with gonadal failure, chromosomal analysis should be undertaken to help define its nature. Replacement hormone therapy, given in a cyclic manner, is the treatment of choice. When a Y chromosome complement or derivative is discovered, gonadectomy is indicated because of the possibility of neoplastic changes in the retained gonad.[27,28]

Some patients may have ovarian failure with normal sex chromosomes (46,XX). In these patients, ovarian failure may be secondary to etiologies other than privation of X chromosome material. An autosomal recessive form of ovarian failure has been determined in some families.[29] Other etiologies of follicular depletion include chemotherapy; irradiation; infections (eg, mumps); infiltrative disease processes of the ovary (eg, tuberculosis); autoimmune diseases; and other known environmental agents. Submicroscopic X chromosome deletions in an ovarian-determinant region may result in ovarian failure, however, similar to that found in patients with Turner's syndrome.

The resistant ovary syndrome is characterized by delayed menarche or primary amenorrhea; a 46,XX karyotype; high follicle-stimulating hormone (FSH) levels; and ovaries that, despite apparently normal follicle apparatus, do not respond to endogenous gonadotropins. It is assumed that the absence of follicular receptors for gonadotropins is responsible for ovarian failure in these patients. These individuals have normally developed secondary sexual characteristics, which contrasts with other adolescents who have delayed sexual maturation, high FSH levels, and a normal chromosome constitution. Estrogen-replacement therapy should be initiated to prevent long-term com-

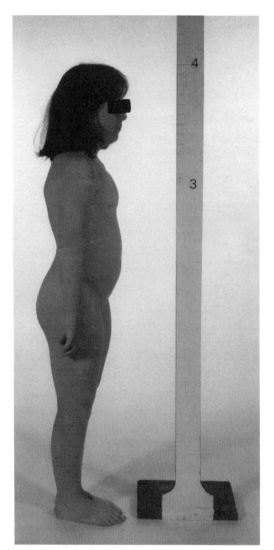

Figure 2–16. Short stature and absent secondary sexual development in a patient with 45X gonadal dysgenesis. (Courtesy of Professor Sir John Dewhurst, Huffman JW, Dewhurst CJ, Capraro VJ: The gynecology of childhood and adolescence, 2nd ed. Philadelphia, WB Saunders, 1981, with permission.)

plications (eg, vaginal dryness and osteoporosis). Pregnancies have been reported in some patients treated with Pergonal or after discontinuation of estrogen therapy.[30]

DELAYED PUBERTY WITH THE DEVELOP-MENT OF HETEROSEXUAL FEATURES. Virilization at puberty is the result of elevated androgens from adrenal or gonadal sources. These may be the result of an enzyme deficiency (eg, late-onset congenital adrenal hyperplasia) or a neoplasm (eg,

Leydig cell tumor). A small group of these patients are male pseudohermaphrodites (ie, adolescents who are being reared as girls, have female external genitalia, intra-abdominal or ectopic malfunctioning testes, and a normal 46,XY chromosomal constitution). This may be the result of mutation within the testis-determining region found in the Y chromosome.

Evaluation of the Patient With Delayed Sexual Development

Determination of gonadal function for categorization into hypogonadal or eugonadal groups can be accomplished by obtaining a medical history and performing a physical examination.

Historical information should center around previous growth and pubertal development. Linear and velocity growth charts as well as a pubertal development chart clarify previous growth patterns and are useful in subsequent follow-up. Knowledge of previous medical disorders may immediately identify the cause of aberrant puberty.

Physical examination must include height, weight, and a search for somatic anomalies. Staging of pubertal development by Tanner criteria is most important in determination of gonadal function. Presence of breast development signifies prior gonadal function. A vaginal smear for cytohormonal evaluation can determine whether the gonad is continuing to produce estrogen. Pelvic and rectal examinations identify patients with an obstructed outflow tract and patients with congenital absence of the vagina and uterus. Further confirmation of patients with Rokitansky sequence depends on a karyotype to identify normal 46,XX complement and a pelvic sonogram to confirm uterine absence and ovarian presence.

Absence of pubic hair suggests androgen insensitivity syndrome. Karyotype analysis identifies 46,XY individuals with testicular feminization syndrome. Patients with complete pubertal development, evidence of continued estrogen production, and normal müllerian systems probably have inappropriate positive feedback and therefore, chronic anovulation. Progesterone challenge in such patients is helpful; a withdrawal bleed signifies a normal müllerian system and continued estrogen production.

When breast development is minimal, the usual diagnosis is hypogonadism. Serum gonadotropin assays are performed for further elucidation; elevated FSH levels suggest gonadal failure. Other endocrine profiles should be obtained if hypothyroidism, congenital adrenal hyperplasia, or Cushing's syndrome is suspected. Karyotype analysis is necessary in all patients with gonadal failure. The presence of a Y chromosome in either group dictates gonadal extirpation.

Low FSH levels suggest an interference with hypothalamic–pituitary maturation and gonadotropin release. Skull films and prolactin assays must be obtained in all patients to rule out the more serious irreversible causes such as pituitary tumors. Appropriate endocrine evaluation identifies the occasional patient with hypothyroidism or congenital adrenal hyperplasia and the rare patient with Cushing's syndrome. Diagnosis of Kallmann's syndrome is suspected in hypogonadotropic patients who have associated anosmia but it is confirmed only after GnRH challenge tests are performed. The presumed diagnosis of physiologic delay is made by exclusion of all other causes and by the typical gonadotropin-release patterns after GnRH challenge.

COMMON DISORDERS

Abnormal Uterine Bleeding

Excessive or irregular bleeding from the vagina is a common disorder of menstrual function. Although few patients have an organic lesion that causes the bleeding, most suffer from dysfunctional uterine bleeding (DUB), a condition defined as abnormal bleeding from the uterine endometrium that is unrelated to anatomic lesions of the genital tract. It is caused by a hormonal imbalance due to derangements in the interactions along the hypothalamic–pituitary–ovarian axis. Dysfunctional uterine bleeding is only a symptom; before therapy is instituted, the more serious causes of genital bleeding in the adolescent age group should be ruled out (Table 2-2).

There are two types of DUB. The first, which is found in almost all cases in the adolescent age group, is caused by anovulation, resulting in a total lack of progesterone. Dysfunctional uterine bleeding in these patients is due to prolonged and unopposed estrogen stimulation of the endometrium, which leads to proliferation and eventually hyperplasia of the endometrium. The second type of DUB, relatively rare in this age group, is caused by a shortened or prolonged life span of the corpus luteum. In this instance, premenstrual and postmenstrual spotting occur as a result of a disturbance in the relative ratio of progesterone to estrogen.

Anovulatory uterine bleeding tends to follow one of several patterns, and the specific pattern encountered depends on the duration and intensity of

Table 2–2
Differential Diagnosis of Dysfunctional Uterine Bleeding

Pregnancy complications
    Abortion
    Ectopic pregnancy
    Trophoblastic disease
Benign and malignant neoplasms of the genital tract
    Endometrial polyp
    Cervical polyp
    Vaginal adenosis
    Vaginal carcinoma
    Cervical carcinoma
    Granulosa–theca cell tumors
    Endometriosis
    Leiomyoma
Genital tract infection
    Vaginitis
    Cervicitis
    Vaginal foreign body
    Intrauterine contraceptive device
    Salpingo-oophoritis
Endocrinopathies
    Polycystic ovary disease
    Hyperprolactinemia
    Hypothyroidism
    Hyperthyroidism
Administration of drugs or hormones
Trauma
Coagulation disorders
    Idiopathic thrombocytopenic purpura
    von Willebrand's disease
Chronic systemic illness
    Liver cirrhosis
    Renal failure

estrogen stimulation of the endometrium. In the presence of continual high levels of estrogen, continued endometrial proliferation occurs. When estrogen levels become insufficient to support further endometrial growth or to maintain endometrial integrity, desquamation and bleeding occur. The menstrual cycles are usually longer than the average span for ovulatory cycles, and the bleeding is often heavy. In the presence of continual low circulating levels of estrogen, endometrial growth extends for a longer period, with a greater interval of amenorrhea between successive menstrual periods. The bleeding may be heavy and prolonged. In the presence of fluctuating levels of estrogens, there is an increase in the frequency of bleeding episodes. The patient often has more than one bleeding episode each month. With each decline in circulating estrogen levels, endometrial integrity is compromised and bleeding ensues.[31]

The diagnosis of DUB is based on history, general physical examination, pelvic examination, and rarely, on selected laboratory tests. Diagnosis requires exclusion of the organic causes of abnormal vaginal bleeding. In a typical teenager with DUB, the history reveals irregular periods since menarche, with a heavy flow that lasts several days or even weeks. Generally, the physical examination is normal. A Pap smear is obtained at the time of the pelvic examination. It is often useful to obtain a simple vaginal smear for cytology (maturation index). Although there is no typical anovulatory pattern, a progesterone-dominated maturation index is consistent with an ovulatory cycle and might therefore suggest a diagnosis other than dysfunctional bleeding (eg, pregnancy). To complete the evaluation of a patient with presumed DUB, the following tests should be included: pregnancy test, urinalysis, complete blood count, serum prolactin level, and in selected cases, thyroid function tests. Although endometrial biopsy is often performed in adult patients, these are seldom necessary in a teenager.

The possibility of an underlying coagulation disorder in the adolescent patient with perimenarcheal menorrhagia needs to be considered. Idiopathic thrombocytopenia purpura and von Willebrand's disease are the most common. A careful medical history is recommended, with specific questioning as to episodes of easy bruising, epistaxis, gingival bleeding, and family history. A thorough physical examination, blood smear, and coagulation screen should be performed routinely in any patient with severe menorrhagia or prolonged episodes of dysfunctional bleeding. The coagulation screen should include prothrombin time, partial thromboplastin time, phase platelet count, and bleeding time. This relatively simple screen will effectively rule out all but the rare hematologic disorders. These tests should be performed before transfusion and administration of hormones.[32]

A simple classification based on hemoglobin concentration is required for effective clinical management (Table 2-3). Those who have a hemoglobin level greater than 12 g/dL are considered to have a mild disturbance (group I); those having between 10 and 12 g/dL have a moderate abnormality (group II); and those with hemoglobin level of less than 10 g/dL are considered to have a severe problem (group III). In group I, reassurance and explanation are necessary, with an ongoing review of the patient's progress at regular intervals. The patient is

Table 2–3

Hemoglobin Classification for Management of Dysfunctional Uterine Bleeding

Hgb > 12 g%

Reassurance

Menstrual calendar

Iron supplement

Periodic reevaluation

Hgb 10–12 g%

Reassurance and explanation

Menstrual calendar

Iron supplement

Cyclic progestin therapy or oral contraceptive pills

Reevaluation in 6 months

Hgb < 10 g%

No active bleeding
  Explanation
  Transfusion/iron supplement
  Oral contraceptive pills
  Reevaluation in 6–12 months

Acute hemorrhage
  Transfusion
  Fluid replacement therapy
  Hormonal hemostasis (IV Premarin)
  Intensive progestin therapy
  Dilation and curettage when hormonal hemostasis fails
  Oral contraceptive pills for 6–12 months

given a menstrual calendar and encouraged to have a daily dietary iron supplement.[33] Most patients spontaneously convert to normal menstrual cycles within 1 or 2 years. In group II, the bleeding is severe enough to warrant action. One may choose to use oral contraceptive pills (OCP) for a short time. The pill reverses the effects of estrogens and prevents further endometrial proliferation. The use of OCPs should be considered in all sexually active girls. The other alternative, to be considered for girls who are not sexually active, is to institute intermittent progestin therapy, using medroxyprogesterone acetate (Provera), 10 mg daily for 5 to 7 days every 25 to 30 days. This is an excellent cycle regulator because it allows spontaneous menses to occur between treatment cycles and prevents chronic unopposed estrogen stimulation of the endometrium. In group III, the bleeding episodes are severe, and some patients require emergency hospital management. Patients who are bleeding heavily or become hypotensive require transfusions and fluid replacement. Associated pathology, specifically complications of pregnancy and coagulopathy, must be excluded. In one series, 20% of all adolescent patients requiring hospitalization for DUB were found to suffer from a coagulation disorder.[32] Regardless of the cause, the bleeding may be controlled in most patients by the administration of estrogens or sometimes progestins. In a few rare instances, when primary medical management has failed, dilation and curettage may be required. Initial hormonal hemostasis may be achieved by the administration of conjugated estrogens (Premarin), 20 to 25 mg intravenously every 4 hours for a maximum of six doses. It is usually unnecessary to continue the parenteral estrogen therapy beyond 24 hours.[34] Continued bleeding beyond this time is an indication for diagnostic dilation and curettage. Concurrently, a highly progestational OCP (ie, Ovral) is given. An initial loading dose of two tablets is followed by one tablet twice daily for seven days, and then one tablet p.o. daily for 6 to 9 months. Despite the dosage, this regimen is well tolerated and antiemetics are seldom required.

After this intense hormone therapy, 6 months of cyclic therapy with conventional combined OCPs is undertaken. It is expected that the withdrawal flow will be reasonable and regular and that each successive cycle will be accompanied by a progressive reduction in endometrial height. After 6 months, the patient is reassessed. If she is sexually active, continued treatment with OCP is required. Otherwise, the patient may be allowed to menstruate without medication. Careful follow-up is undertaken to assess the timing and duration of menses, with the aid of a menstrual calendar, and to treat any relapses that may occur. If the anovulatory pattern recurs, medroxyprogesterone acetate (Provera) is used as described for group II patients. By adhering to this medical protocol of initial hormonal hemostasis, followed by cyclic regulation of menses and continuous long-term observation, unnecessary dilation and curettage may be avoided and surgical management may be reserved for the small percentage of patients who fail to respond to conservative measures.

Generally, adolescent menstrual problems are viewed with optimism and 50% of adolescents with DUB return to a regular menstrual pattern within 4 years after menarche. If anovulation persists longer than 4 years, however, the chance of recovery is low. The risks of exposure to continued unopposed estrogen stimulation must then be considered.[35]

Dysmenorrhea

Dysmenorrhea affects almost half of all female adolescents today and is probably the most frequently encountered gynecologic disorder. The term dysmenorrhea is derived from the Greek language and although it means difficult monthly flow, it is commonly used to refer to painful menstruation. Dysmenorrhea is classified as primary or secondary. Primary dysmenorrhea has no detectable pelvic pathology, whereas in secondary dysmenorrhea, the pain is the result of an existing pelvic disease.

Primary Dysmenorrhea

Adolescent dysmenorrhea often begins shortly after menarche (within 6 to 12 months) and coincides with the onset of ovulatory cycles. The patient complains of colicky pain that begins several hours before or just at the onset of menstrual flow. The pain usually begins in the mid-pelvis and radiates to the back and sometimes to the legs. The pain is most severe during the first day of menstruation but may last for two or three days. In more than half the patients, the pain is accompanied by other systemic signs which include nausea and vomiting, fatigue, diarrhea, headaches, and irritability. In rare instances, syncope attacks have been reported. Patients with primary dysmenorrhea report diminishing symptoms with increasing age. In some, the pain may disappear after the first childbirth.

The diagnosis of primary dysmenorrhea is made by its clinical features and the onset of pain at or shortly after menarche. The pain begins shortly before or immediately after menstruation and disappears completely within 2 or 3 days. The pain is crampy in nature, and pelvic examination is normal.

It is well accepted that in many women with primary dysmenorrhea, the production and release of endometrial prostaglandins give rise to abnormal uterine activity and that this abnormal activity is perceived by the patient as discomfort or pain. It has been shown that the intensity of abnormal uterine activity is related to the amount of prostaglandins released into the menstrual flow from the degenerating decidua. Prostaglandin levels are highest during the first 48 hours of menstruation. In addition to uterine hyperactivity, prostaglandins may give rise to pain by directly affecting nerve endings.[36]

Both OCPs and prostaglandin inhibitors were found to be highly effective in the treatment of dysmenorrhea. The use of OCPs was found to be effective in at least 90% of women with primary dysmenorrhea. The OCPs suppress endometrial proliferation, resulting in an endocrine environment similar to that of the early proliferative phase of the menstrual cycle, when prostaglandin levels are lowest. An OCP is the drug of choice for sexually active teens who also need contraception.[36]

Prostaglandin inhibitors are used mainly in young patients who do not need contraception. It is the drug of choice for the treatment of primary dysmenorrhea because the pills are taken only during the first 2 or 3 days of the menstrual cycle. The medication either inhibits cyclic endoperoxide synthesis or acts through the cyclic endoperoxide cleavage enzyme system. As a result, endometrial prostaglandin synthesis is suppressed, restoring normal uterine activity and providing relief from menstrual cramps.[36]

Secondary Dysmenorrhea

In patients with secondary dysmenorrhea, the pain is the result of an existing pelvic pathology. Often, the pain does not begin shortly after menarche but instead begins years later. At times there is a history of congenital malformations or previous pelvic inflammatory disease. Although early onset of pain often suggests that the patient has primary dysmenorrhea, it is well accepted that in some patients endometriosis may occur soon after the onset of menarche.[37] If the patient fails to respond to medical therapy, she should be further evaluated to exclude pelvic pathology. Diagnostic laparoscopy is indicated to establish the diagnosis of endometriosis.[37] The treatment for secondary dysmenorrhea is directed toward the underlying pelvic disorder.

REFERENCES

1. Grunberger W, Fisch LF: Pediatric gynecological outpatient department. A report on 600 patients. Wien Klin Wochenschr 94:614, 1982
2. Muram D: Pediatric and adolescent gynecology. In Pernol ML, DeCherney AH, Pernoll ML (eds): Current gynecologic and obstetric diagnosis and treatment, 8th ed, pp 633. Norwalk, CT, Appelton & Lange, 1994
3. Dewhurst Sir J: Lichen sclerosus of the vulva in childhood. Pediatr Adolesc Gynecol 1:149, 1983
4. Redmond CA, Cowell CA, Krafchik BR: Genital lichen sclerosus in prepubertal girls. Pediatr Adolesc Gynecol 1:177, 1988
5. Ben-Ami T, Boichis H, Hertz M: Fused labia. Clinical and radiological findings. Pediatr Radiol 7:33, 1978
6. Huffman JW, Dewhurst CJ, Capraro VJ: The gynecology of childhood and adolescence, 2nd ed. Philadelphia, WB Saunders, 1981
7. Berkowitz CD, Elvik SL, Logan MK: Labial fusion in prepubescent girls: a marker for sexual abuse? Am J Obstet Gynecol 156:16, 1987
8. Muram D: Labial adhesions: a possible marker of sexual abuse (Letter). JAMA 259:352, 1988
9. Stovall TG, Muram D: Urinary retention secondary to labial adhesions. Adolesc Pediatr Gynecol 1:203, 1988
10. Muram D, Elias S: The treatment of labial adhesions in prepubertal girls. Surgical Forum 34:464, 1988
11. Mercer LJ, Mueller CM, Hajj SN: Medical treatment of urethral prolapse. Adolesc Pediatr Gynecol 1:182, 1988
12. Muram D: Vaginal bleeding in children and adolescents. Obstet Gynecol Clin North Am 17:389, 1990
13. Velcek FT, Kugaczewski JT, Klotz DH, Kottmeier PK: Surgical therapy for urethral prolapse in young girls. Adolesc Pediatr Gynecol 2:230, 1989
14. Dewhurst Sir J: Botryoid sarcoma of the cervix and vagina in children. In Studd J (ed): Progress in obstetrics and gynecology, vol 3, pp 151. Edinburgh, Churchill Livingstone, 1983
15. Muram D: Genital tract trauma in pre-pubertal children. Pediatr Ann 15:616, 1986
16. Kaplowitz PB, Cockrell JL, Young RB: Premature adrenarche. Clinical and diagnostic features. Clin Pediatr 25:28, 1986
17. Muram D, Dewhurst Sir J, Grant DB: Premature menarche: a follow-up study. Arch Dis Child 58:142, 1983
18. Muram D, Grant DB, Dewhurst Sir J: Precocious puberty: a follow-up study. Arch Dis Child 59:77, 1984
19. Simpson JL, Golbus MS, Martin AO, Sarto GE: Genetics in obstetrics and gynecology. Orlando, FL, Grune & Stratton 1982
20. Shulman LP, Elias S: Developmental abnormalities of the female reproductive tract: pathogenesis and nosology. Adolesc Pediatr Gynecol 1:230, 1988
21. Griffin JE, Edwards C, Madden JD, Harrod MJ, Wilson JD: Congenital absence of the vagina. The Mayer-Rokitansky-Kuster-Hauser syndrome. Ann Intern Med 85:224, 1976
22. Frank R: Formation of artificial vagina without operation. Am J Obstet Gynecol 35:1053, 1938
23. Ingram JM: The bicycle seat stool in the treatment of vaginal agenesis and stenosis: a preliminary report. Am J Obstet Gynecol 140:867, 1981
24. McIndoe AH, Banister JB: An operation for the cure of congenital absence of the vagina. J Obstet Gynecol Br Emp 45:490, 1938
25. Williams EA: Congenital absence of the vagina. A simple operation for its relief. J Obstet Gynecol Br Commonw 71:511, 1964
26. Simpson JL: Disorders of sexual differentiation: etiology and clinical delineation. New York, Academic Press, 1976
27. Simpson JL, Photopulos G: The relationship of neoplasia to disorders of abnormal sexual differentiation. Birth Defects 12(1):15, 1976
28. Talerman A: Germ cell tumors of the ovary. In

Blaustein A (ed): Pathology of the female genital tract. New York, Springer-Verlag, 1977

29. Dewhurst Sir J: Female puberty and its abnormalities. Edinburgh, Churchill Livingstone, 1984

30. Muram D, Jolly EE: Pregnancy and gonadal dysgenesis. J Obstet Gynecol 3:87, 1982

31. Yen SSC, Jaffe RB: Reproductive endocrinology, 2nd ed. Philadelphia, WB Saunders, 1986

32. Claessens EA, Cowell CA: Acute adolescent menorrhagia. Am J Obstet Gynecol 139:277, 1977

33. Arvidsson B, Ekenved G, Rybo G, Sölvell: Iron prophylaxis in menorrhagia. Acta Obstet Gynecol Scand 60:157, 1981

34. DeVore GR, Owens O, Kase N: Use of intravenous Premarin in the treatment of dysfunctional bleeding—a double-blind randomized control study. Obstet Gynecol 59:285, 1982

35. Southam AL, Richart RM: The prognosis for adolescents with menstrual abnormality. Am J Obstet Gynecol 94:637, 1966

36. Smith RP: Primary dysmenorrhea and the adolescent patient. Adolesc Pediatr Gynecol 1:23, 1988

37. Goldstein DP, deCholnoky C, Emans SJ: Adolescent endometriosis. J Adolesc Health Care 1:37, 1980

Ambulatory Gynecology, Second Edition,
edited by David H. Nichols and Patrick J. Sweeney.
J. B. Lippincott Company, Philadelphia, © 1995.

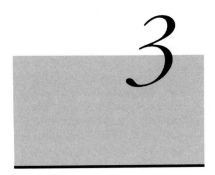

Genetic Counseling

Jeffrey S. Dungan and Sherman Elias

Genetics has become an integral part of modern obstetric and gynecologic practice. This chapter considers the basic principles underlying genetic counseling in addition to commonly encountered clinical situations. Some sections of this chapter are adapted from previous works by the authors.[1,2]

In 1974, the American Society of Human Genetics defined genetic counseling as:

> . . . a communication process which deals with the problems associated with the occurrence, or risk of occurrence, of a genetic disorder in a family. This process involves an attempt by one or more appropriately trained persons to help the individual or the family to (1) comprehend the medical facts, including the diagnosis, the probable course of the disorder and the available management; (2) appreciate the way heredity contributes to the disorder and the risk of recurrence in specified relatives; (3) understand the options for dealing with the risk of recurrence; (4) choose the course of action which seems appropriate to them in view of their risk and their family goals and act in accordance with that decision; and (5) make the best possible adjustment to the disorder in an affected family member and/or to the risk of recurrence of that disorder.[3]

The principles underlying genetic counseling are similar to those of counseling for other medical conditions. Accurate elicitation of information, lucid communication, sympathetic listening, and avoidance of judgments are paramount. Persons providing genetic counseling must have accurate genetic and medical knowledge and be able to communicate this information in terms that are readily comprehensible by patients.

PRINCIPLES OF HUMAN GENETICS

Phenotypic variation may be considered in terms of four broad etiologic categories:

1. Chromosomal (numeric or structural) abnormalities

2. Single-gene (mendelian) inheritance
3. Polygenic–multifactorial inheritance
4. Environmental (teratogenic) factors

Each of these categories are discussed, with examples relevant to the obstetrician–gynecologist.

Chromosomal Abnormalities

The incidence of chromosomal abnormalities in liveborn infants is about 0.5%.[4] There are hundreds of syndromes associated with chromosomal abnormalities. A few of the most common are discussed here.

Numeric Abnormalities

In humans, the expected number of chromosomes in the haploid gamete is 23 (n) and in the diploid cell is 46 (2n). Any number of chromosomes that is not an exact multiple of *n* is termed *aneuploid*. The addition of a single chromosome to a diploid cell (2n + 1) is a *trisomy*. If a single chromosome is missing from a diploid cell, *monosomy* exists. Trisomies and monosomies result primarily from nondisjunction (ie, failure of paired chromosomes to disjoin during mitosis or meiosis). Trisomies for nearly all the chromosomes have been reported in abortuses. The three most common autosomal trisomies observed in newborns involve chromosomes 21, 18, and 13.

TRISOMY 21. Trisomy 21 (Down syndrome) is the most frequent autosomal chromosome syndrome, with an incidence of about one in 800 liveborn infants.[5] Characteristic features include brachycephaly, upward-slanting palpebral fissures, epicanthal folds, protruding tongue, and small low-set ears. At birth, these infants are generally hypotonic and have an average birthweight somewhat below the population mean. Other features include Brushfield spots (speckled rings around the periphery of the iris); broad, short fingers; clinodactyly; and a single flexion crease on the fifth digit. The so-called "simian crease," a single palmar crease extending the width of the palm, is not pathognomonic, being present in only about 30% of individuals with Down syndrome and in 5% of normal individuals. Common internal anomalies include cardiac defects and duodenal atresia.[6]

Individuals with Down syndrome who survive beyond infancy exhibit varying degrees of mental retardation. The mean IQ is around 50, with a range of about 25 to 70. Although males with Down syndrome are generally sterile, females with this condition have been known to reproduce. About 30% of offspring of females with Down syndrome are also trisomic.

Trisomy 21 is found in about 95% of Down syndrome, with the extra chromosome generally being of maternal origin.[7] The relation between advanced maternal age and the increased risk for producing a child with Down syndrome is discussed later.

About 3% to 5% of Down syndrome cases are due to translocations, generally involving chromosomes 14 and 21. Among those cases due to a translocation, about 75% occur de novo and the remainder are inherited.[8] For this reason, it is essential that the chromosome makeup of a child with Down syndrome be determined to allow accurate counseling of recurrence risks. For women younger than age 29 years, the empiric recurrence risk for a trisomic fetus when a previous child has trisomy 21 is about 1%.[9,10] For women older than that, the recurrence risk is probably about the same as that based on age alone.

When a child with Down syndrome has a translocation as the etiology, it is crucial to determine the parents' chromosome complements. For example, if the mother is a carrier of a balanced translocation, involving chromosomes 14 and 21, the recurrence risk is in the range of 10% to 15%.[6] If the father is a carrier of a 14/21 balanced translocation, the recurrence risk is on the order of 1% to 2%.[11]

TRISOMY 18. Trisomy 18 occurs with a frequency of about one in 8000 live births and as with other nondisjunctional events, the risk is higher with advanced maternal age. Distinctive phenotypic features include microcephaly, short palpebral fissures, prominent occiput, receding mandible, low-set malformed ears, overlapping fingers (V over IV and II over III), "rocker-bottom" feet, severe growth retardation, heart defects, renal malformations, and numerous other anomalies. About 50% develop fetal distress in labor. Postnatal survival is rare; most infants die within 2 to 3 months. Survivors are severely mentally retarded.

After the birth of a child with trisomy 18, the recurrence risk for either trisomy 18 or a different trisomy is about 1% to 2%.

TRISOMY 13. This syndrome, due to trisomy 13, occurs with a frequency of about one per 10,000 live births. It is a generally lethal condition, with most infants dying within the first 3 months of life. Those who do survive into childhood have profound mental retardation. Characteristic phenotypic features include cleft lip and palate; eye abnormalities (cyclopia, microphthalmia, anophthalmia); holoprosencephaly or other brain malformations; heart malformations; scalp defects; and numerous other anomalies. Recurrence risks are similar for the previously mentioned trisomies: 1% to 2% for this or other chromosomal abnormalities.

45,X. 45,X (Turner syndrome) is the only nonmosaic monosomy that may result in a live birth, with an incidence of about one per 5000 live female births. The chromosome defect is lack of either an X or Y chromosome, resulting in monosomy X, or 45,X. Because monosomy X is present in 10% of all first-trimester abortuses, it can be calculated that more than 99% of 45,X conceptuses end in early pregnancy loss.[6] Clinical features in these phenotypic females include sexual infantilism, short stature (less than 150 cm), webbed neck, primary amenorrhea, streak gonads, shield chest, cardiac anomalies, and renal anomalies. Most 45,X patients have normal intelligence but any given patient has a slightly higher probability of being mentally retarded than a genetically normal individual (ie, 46,XX).[12] Patients with 45,X have an unusual cognitive defect in that they have an inability to appreciate the comparative shape of objects (space-form blindness).

The lack of development of secondary sexual characteristics is due to gonadal dysgenesis, leaving these patients with streak ovaries. Thus, there are few or no oocytes, leading to a hypoestrogenic state and sterility. 45,X females comprise about 40% of gonadal dysgenesis ascertained by gynecologists.[4]

In contrast to trisomies, there is no correlation between advanced maternal age and the risk of offspring with 45,X. Additionally, the recurrence risk for a couple with a previous child affected with 45,X is no higher than the baseline population risk.

47,XXY. Klinefelter syndrome is the name given to the spectrum of phenotypic abnormalities that occurs in the presence of two or more X chromosomes and one or more Y chromosomes—the most common genotype being 47,XXY. The incidence is about one per 1000 liveborn males.

Adult males with 47,XXY display the following features: small, firm testes; azoospermia; gynecomastia; scant facial and pubic hair; small penis; decreased testosterone levels; and a tall "eunuchoid" body habitus. These individuals generally appear normal at birth and develop the associated findings only after puberty.[13] Patients with 47,XXY genotypes are also more likely to be mentally retarded or socially maladjusted than 46,XY males but the exact risk is unknown. Klinefelter syndrome patients with more than two X chromosomes are invariably mentally retarded.

There is the same correlation with advanced maternal age as with other nondisjunctional events but recurrence risks for younger mothers are unknown.

Structural Abnormalities

Numerous minor structural variations exist in the human genome (polymorphisms), which are not associated with any phenotypic abnormalities. Major changes in chromosome structure may have serious consequences, however, particularly those changes involving an excess or lack of the normal amount of chromosomal content.

A chromosomal *deletion* involves loss of a portion of a chromosome, either from one of the ends (terminal deletion) or from within the chromosome (interstitial deletion). The fragment is lost in subsequent cell divisions because there is no centromere (acentric). Autosomal deletions lead either to embryonic death or severe phenotype abnormalities. Sex chromosome deletions have also been reported and generally have less serious phenotypic consequences.

The most common syndrome caused by a chromosomal deletion is the cri du chat syndrome, which was described in 1963 and so-called because of the distinctive cat-like mewing of the affected newborns.[14] The chromosomal abnormality is a deleted portion of the short arm of chromosome 5 (5p−). The reported incidence is about one per 45,000 infants but the frequency in mentally retarded, institutionalized individuals is about 1.5 per 1000.[15] In addition to the characteristic cry, these individuals have severe mental retardation (average IQ is 20), microcephaly, hypertelorism, and other malformations.

Duplications involve an additional piece of a chromosome inserted into the individual's genome. Pure duplications are rare, however; most exist in combination with a deletion. Another term for duplications (not in combination with any other structural defect) is partial trisomy. Such complements generally occur de novo but may be the result of a chromosomal abnormality in the parent called an *inversion*, which is due to unequal crossing-over during meiosis.[16]

A *ring chromosome* occurs when the end of each chromosome arm has been deleted and the broken arms reunite in a ring formation. All human chromosomes have been reported to be involved.[17] There is a great deal of phenotypic variability in individuals with ring chromosomes. The formation of the ring necessarily involves deletion of the two ends (telomeres) of the chromosome. Presumably, the phenotypic effect depends on the size of these deletions.

Inversions occur when a segment of a chromosome undergoes breakage at two points and then is reinserted back into the chromosome in a reversed direction. If the inversion occurs outside the centromere, it is termed paracentric; if the centromere is included in the inverted segment, it is termed pericentric. Pericentric inversions are more common than paracentric. The clinical significance of inversions is that during meiosis, chromosomes with inverted segments may undergo unequal crossing-over, leading to chromosomal deletions and duplications.

Translocations involve exchange of chromosomal segments between two nonhomologous chromosomes. If there is no net loss or gain of genetic material, the translocation is said to be *balanced.*

Generally, individuals carrying a balanced translocation chromosome display no phenotypic effects. A *reciprocal translocation* involves rearrangement between two or more chromosomes but not the centromeres. The incidence of this type of translocation in newborns is about one per 1000.[5] A *Robertsonian translocation* occurs when there is centromeric fusion between two of the acrocentric chromosomes (13,14,15,21, or 22); that is, exchange of entire chromosome arms, leaving the individual with 45 chromosomes (one of these being the double chromosome). The incidence of robertsonian translocations in newborns is about 1 per 1000.[5]

Clinically, the most important robertsonian translocation involves chromosomes 14 and 21. As mentioned earlier, about 2% to 3% of individuals with Down syndrome are a result of this translocation. In couples wherein one of the parents is a carrier of this translocation, one would theoretically expect a 33% risk for Down syndrome (Fig. 3-1).

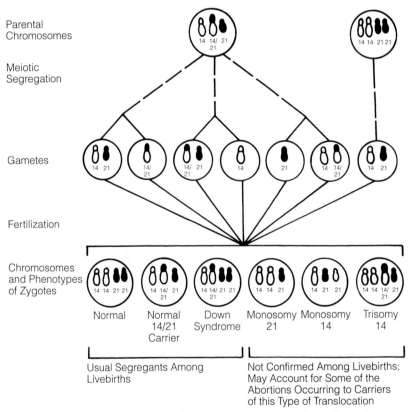

Figure 3–1. Segregation of possible gametes and progeny of an individual heterozygous for a robertsonian translocation between chromosomes 14 and 21. Three of the six possible gametes are incompatible with life. See text for details. (Gerbie AB, Simpson JL: Antenatal diagnosis of genetic disorders. Postgrad Med 59(6):129, 1976. Used with permission.)

Empiric data, however, demonstrate a risk of about 15% for fetal Down syndrome when the mother is the carrier and about 1% to 2% when the father is the carrier.[18]

For non-robertsonian balanced translocation carriers, the overall empiric risk for producing an offspring with an unbalanced chromosome complement is about 11%.[18] The precise risk, however, for any given translocation carrier depends on how that carrier was detected (ascertainment bias). If a family history of unbalanced progeny led to the detection of the balanced translocation in one of the parents, the risk of a liveborn with an unbalanced complement would probably be higher than that of a couple ascertained because of repeated early pregnancy losses. Presumably, the unbalanced embryos from this latter couple are not viable; therefore, a pregnancy results either in embryonic death or a genetically normal offspring.

Mendelian Inheritance

Chromosomes exist in pairs; therefore, genes likewise exist in pairs on *homologous* chromosomes. It is more correct to state it is *alleles*, or alternate forms of a gene, that exist in pairs. Alleles occupy the same geographic location (locus) on each member of a homologous pair of chromosomes. If a pair of alleles at a given locus are identical, the individual is *homozygous* for that allele. If the alleles are dissimilar, the individual is said to be *heterozygous*. When an allele is expressed only in a homozygous individual, that trait is said to be *recessive*. A trait is *dominant* when it is expressed in a heterozygous individual. These types of inheritance patterns are termed "mendelian" after Gregor Mendel, who delineated them in 1865.

The situation is somewhat different for loci on the X chromosome. Because a recessive allele on the X chromosome is expressed by all males carrying it, these males are called *hemizygous*. Figure 3-2 contains pedigree charts that demonstrate the various mendelian inheritance patterns.

Diseases produced by a single mutant gene (either dominantly or recessively inherited) are uncommon, with an incidence of one in 10,000 to 50,000 births. Although individually rare, mendelian disorders in aggregate cause abnormalities in about 1% of liveborns.[6]

Autosomal Dominant Inheritance

A dominant allele is one that produces an effect even if the other (homologous) allele is normal. An individual carrying a mutant autosomal dominant allele has a 50% risk of transmitting that allele to offspring. Males and females are affected in equal ratios. Table 3-1 lists selected common autosomal dominant disorders.

Some autosomal dominant traits do not display these ideal characteristics, however. Two important terms are used with reference to these types of traits. *Penetrance* refers to the ability of a gene to be expressed (ie, an all or none phenomenon). When all individuals carrying the gene show its

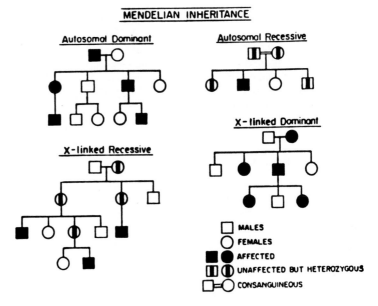

Figure 3–2. Patterns of familial transmission expected of autosomal dominant, autosomal recessive, X-linked recessive, and X-linked dominant traits. (Elias S, Annas GJ: Reproductive genetics and the law, p 27. Chicago, Year Book Medical Publishers, 1987. Used with permission.)

Table 3–1
Common Autosomal Dominant Disorders

Huntington chorea

Marfan syndrome

Neurofibromatosis

Achondroplasia

Familial hypercholesterolemia

Hereditary spherocytosis

Cleft lip with lip pits

Acute intermittent porphyria

von Willebrand disease

Adult-type polycystic kidney disease

Tuberous sclerosis

Myotonic dystrophy

Craniofacial dysostosis (Crouzon disease)

Hyperbilirubinemia I (Gilbert disease)

Noonan syndrome

Idiopathic hypertrophic subaortic stenosis

Mandibulofacial dysostosis (Treacher Collins syndrome)

Peroneal muscular dystrophy (Charcot–Marie–Tooth disease)

Polyposis of the colon (intestinal polyposis I)

Waardenburg syndrome

Hand-foot-uterus syndrome

Table 3–2
Common Autosomal Recessive Disorders

Cystic fibrosis

Sickle cell anemia

Tay-Sachs disease

Phenylketonuria

β-Thalassemia

α-Thalassemia

Albinism (various forms)

Adrenogenital syndrome (various forms)

α_1-Antitrypsin deficiency

Homocystinuria

Friedreich's ataxia

Galactosemia

Glycogen storage disease (various forms)

Hepatocellular degeneration (Wilson disease)

Laurence–Moon–Biedl syndrome

Methemoglobinemia

Meckel syndrome

manifestations, there is complete penetrance. If a person carries the gene but has no manifestations, the gene has incomplete penetrance.

Expressivity refers to the degree to which a mutant gene is expressed (ie, mild to severe gradation). Variable expression may occur not only between families but also among affected members of a single family. Incomplete penetrance and variable expressivity are properties of autosomal dominant traits that may make genetic counseling problematic. No methods exist to predict the severity of most conditions that display such variation in their manifestations.

Autosomal Recessive Inheritance

An autosomal recessive trait is expressed only when an individual carries both of the appropriate alleles (homozygous recessive). Generally, heterozygous individuals are clinically normal, although in some rare instances, these carriers may show mild manifestations of the disorder. Table 3-2 lists selected common autosomal recessive diseases.

These recessive alleles are inherited singly from each heterozygous (carrier) parent. Each child of carrier parents has a 25% chance of receiving both mutant alleles and being affected (homozygous). The risk of a child receiving only one of these mutant genes—thus making him or her a carrier—is 50%. The remaining 25% of offspring will be homozygous normal. These ratios of the distribution of alleles in offspring of heterozygous parents are useful when counseling siblings of affected individuals about their risk for being a carrier of that recessive trait. Because the individual in question is not affected, this leaves three possible genotypes (AA, Aa, aA), each being of equal likelihood. Two of these possible genotypes include one copy of the mutant allele, thus creating a two in three chance of an unaffected individual being a carrier.

A feature of autosomal recessive inheritance is that affected individuals are more likely to have parents who are related (consanguineous) and thus share more alleles. The more rare the mutant gene in the population, the more likely it is the parents are related.

The mathematic relation between the frequencies of homozygotes and heterozygotes is expressed by the Hardy-Weinberg equilibrium. For purposes of discussion, assume A is the normal allele, with a frequency in the population of p. The mutant allele is a and appears with a frequency q.

Because the frequencies of the two alleles must equal 1, we may write $p + q = 1$. Applying the binomial expansion, we get $p^2 + 2pq + q^2 = 1$. In this equation, p^2 equals the frequency of *AA* homozygous individuals, $2pq$ equals the frequency of heterozygous (*Aa*) individuals, and q^2 is the frequency of *aa* homozygous individuals.

When the frequency of a mutant allele (q) is rare, the frequency of the normal allele (p) is close to 1 and the carrier frequency ($2pq$) is also larger than the frequency of homozygous individuals with the mutant trait (q^2). Therefore, most of the genetic "load" for this trait is carried by heterozygous individuals.

This information may also be used when counseling couples regarding their risk for having a child with a recessive condition that is present in some other family member. Suppose a disease exists in the population with a frequency (q^2) of one per 6400 and one member of the couple being counseled has a sib with this condition. The individual with an affected family member has a risk of two in three for being a carrier. The risk for the other member of the couple can be determined from the Hardy–Weinberg equation: q^2 is 1/6400, q is 1/80, and p is $1 - 1/80$ (or 79/80, nearly 1); thus, the carrier frequency ($2pq$) is $2 \times 1 \times 1/80$, or 1/40. Taken altogether, this couple's risk for having an affected offspring is $2/3 \times 1/40 \times 1/4$, or one in 240.

X-Linked Inheritance

There are two forms of X-linked disease: dominant and recessive. There are few X-linked dominant conditions, vitamin D–resistant rickets being an example. The more clinically relevant conditions are those inherited in an X-linked recessive pattern. Table 3-3 lists selected common diseases inherited in this fashion.

Because males have only one X chromosome (hemizygous), they express any mutant alleles located on the X chromosome. These alleles are inherited from the phenotypically normal but heterozygous mother. Each son of a carrier female has a 50% chance of being affected and each daughter has a 50% chance of being a carrier. These diseases are readily recognized in pedigrees because only males are affected, and disease transmission never occurs from an affected male. Unaffected males do not carry the mutant gene on their X chromosomes and hence do not transmit the gene to their offspring. Individuals may have an X-linked disease but have no other affected family members. When this occurs, there is a one in three chance that the gene

Table 3–3
Common X-Linked Recessive Disorders

Hemophilia A (factor VIII deficiency)

Hemophilia B (factor IX deficiency)

Duchenne or Becker muscular dystrophy

Glucose-6-phosphate dehydrogenase deficiency

Agammaglobulinemia (Bruton disease)

Androgen insensitivity syndrome

Diffuse angiokeratoma (Fabry disease)

Anhidrotic ectodermal dysplasia

X-linked hydrocephalus (aqueductal stenosis)

Chronic granulomatous disease

Lesch–Nyhan disease

Menkes' kinky hair syndrome

Hunter syndrome

Wiskott–Aldrich syndrome

Cutis hyperelastosis

Color blindness

Diabetes insipidus (X-linked forms)

Hypospadias–dysphagia syndrome (G syndrome)

was not transmitted but was the result of a new mutation.[1]

Polygenic–Multifactorial Inheritance

Numerous traits exist that appear to be familial but do not fit mendelian inheritance patterns and are not associated with a chromosomal abnormality. A model used to explain these patterns is that of polygenic–multifactorial inheritance. Table 3-4 lists selected examples of such conditions.

These traits generally have recurrence risks of 2% to 5%. The most plausible explanation for this observation is that the trait is influenced by multiple genes (polygenic). This concept assumes many nonallelic genes, each contributing a small effect, cumulatively determining the phenotype. The presence of several genes contributing to one trait produces a continuous-frequency distribution curve with respect to not only the distribution of genes but to the degree of phenotypic expression. In some instances, an environmental influence plays a role in determining the phenotype (multifactorial).

To more easily understand the concept of polygenic–multifactorial inheritance as it relates to disease states, it is useful to assume an individual

Table 3–4
Common Polygenic–Multifactorial Disorders

Cleft lip/palate

Neural tube defects

Congenital hip dislocation

Congenital aganglionic megacolon (Hirschsprung's disease)

Pyloric stenosis

Peptic ulcer disease

Congenital heart defects (most forms)

Hypertension

Talipes equinovarus (clubfoot)

Scoliosis

Hydrocephalus (most forms)

Aseptic necrosis of the femoral epiphysis (Legg–Perthes disease)

Endometriosis

Müllerian fusion anomalies

possesses an underlying graded predisposition, or *liability*, that is related to the causation of a disorder. The expression of the trait, or disease, is manifest only when the total liability, genetic and environmental, exceeds a *threshold* (Fig. 3-3).

Important aspects of the polygenic–multifactorial model are (1) recurrence risk increases as the number of affected first-degree relatives (parents, sibs, offspring) increases; (2) when a sex difference in the population incidence of a disease state exists, the relatives of the less frequently affected sex are more frequently affected; and (3) the more severe a malformation, the higher the recurrence risk.

Teratogenesis

A complete discussion of the principles underlying teratogenesis is beyond the scope of this chapter but a few basics, as they relate to genetic counseling, are discussed. The most important factors that govern teratogenicity are the specificity of the agent, exposure time during embryonic or fetal development, genotype of the mother and the conceptus, dosage, and concurrent exposure to other agents.

Certain embryonic tissues have a greater sensitivity to a specific teratogen. The various mechanisms by which these agents can exert their influence include (1) mutation; (2) chromosomal nondisjunction and breakage; (3) interference with cell division; or (4) alteration of any of the many factors involved in cell and tissue function, including nucleic acids, enzymes, and cell transport mechanisms.[19]

Susceptibility to teratogenic agents varies with the developmental stage at the time of exposure. Some generalizations can be made, however. Teratogenic exposure during the first 2 weeks of embryonic life either are lethal or survivors generally display no increase in phenotypic abnormalities; this has been termed the "all or nothing" phenomenon.[20] The most vulnerable time during embryogenesis for production of structural abnormalities is during organogenesis (middle to late first trimester and early second trimester). After the fourth month of pregnancy, embryonic development primarily involves growth in size and differentiation of specialized tissues. A teratogenic exposure at this time may affect the overall growth of the embryo or the size of a specific organ but usually does not produce

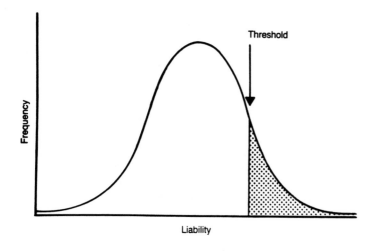

Figure 3–3. Schematic model of polygenic–multifactorial inheritance, demonstrating a "threshold" of genetic liability, beyond which an abnormality is expressed.

a visible malformation, with the possible exception of gonadal and brain tissues.

Susceptibility to teratogens depends on the genotype of the embryo or fetus because various genetic determinants play a role in the processes by which an agent exerts its effects. A good example of this concept is the variation among individuals in response to different drugs, a field of study known as pharmacogenetics.

Generally, manifestations of abnormal development increase in frequency and degree as dosage of the agent increases. At any given time, an embryo or fetus may respond to a teratogen in one of three ways, depending on the dosage level: at a low dosage, there may be no effect; at an intermediate dosage, a pattern of organ-specific malformations may result; at a high dosage, the embryo or fetus may be killed. For a list of teratogenic agents and their effects, the reader is referred to appropriate sources.[21,22]

INDICATIONS FOR GENETIC COUNSELING

Several of the more common indications for genetic counseling, especially as they relate to prenatal diagnosis, are listed in Table 3-5.

The most common indication for genetic counseling and prenatal diagnosis is advanced maternal age, the impetus for about 85% of the women tested. The relation between advanced maternal age and increased incidence of offspring with chromosomal abnormalities, primarily trisomies, has been known for many years. The biologic explanation for this phenomenon, however, has not been established with certainty.

The overall incidence of trisomy 21 is about one in 800 births. Starting at about age 30, however, the risk increases substantially (Table 3-6). Additionally, trisomy 21 is not the only chromosomal abnor-

Table 3-5
Common Indications for Genetic Counseling

1. Advanced maternal age (≥ 35 years old at estimated delivery date)
2. Previous child with a chromosomal disorder
3. Parent with a chromosome abnormality
4. Recurrent spontaneous abortions
5. Family history of mental retardation
6. Known or suspected hereditary disease
7. Teratogen exposure
8. Previous child with a congenital abnormality

Table 3-6
Risk of Having a Live-born Child With Down Syndrome or Any Chromosomal Abnormality by Maternal Age

Maternal Age	Risk	Total Risk of Chromosome Abnormality
20	1/1667	1/526*
21	1/1667	1/526*
22	1/1429	1/500*
23	1/1429	1/500*
24	1/1250	1/476*
25	1/1250	1/476*
26	1/1176	1/476*
27	1/1111	1/455*
28	1/1053	1/435*
29	1/1000	1/417*
30	1/952	1/384*
31	1/909	1/384*
32	1/769	1/323*
33	1/625	1/286
34	1/500	1/238
35	1/385	1/192
36	1/294	1/156
37	1/227	1/127
38	1/175	1/102
39	1/137	1/83
40	1/106	1/66
41	1/82	1/53
42	1/64	1/42
43	1/50	1/33
44	1/38	1/26
45	1/30	1/21
46	1/23	1/16
47	1/18	1/13
48	1/14	1/10
49	1/11	1/8

*47,XXX excluded (data not available).

Data modified from Hook EB: Rates of chromosome abnormalities at different maternal ages. Obstet Gynecol 58:282, 1981 and Hook EB, Cross PK, Schreinemachers DM: Chromosomal abnormality rates at amniocentesis and in live-born infants. JAMA 249:2034, 1983

mality that increases with maternal age. Other autosomal trisomies and X chromosome polysomies also demonstrate a relation to increased maternal age. The frequency of chromosomal abnormalities detected at the time of second-trimester prenatal diagnosis is higher than the frequency of such abnormalities among liveborn infants; at 16 to 18 weeks, this prevalence is about 50% higher. This discrepancy is likely explained by the disproportionate number of chromosomally abnormal fetuses that abort spontaneously between 16 weeks and term.

A strict definition of "advanced maternal age" is not appropriate. It is commonly accepted practice in the United States, however, to counsel all women who will be age 35 or older at the expected date of delivery concerning their risk of producing a child with a chromosomal abnormality and the availability of prenatal diagnosis. Flexibility is desirable when confronted with inquiries from women younger than 35 years of age.

Prenatal diagnostic studies are offered to couples who have had a prior pregnancy affected with a chromosomal disorder. The increased risk in such couples has been attributed to (1) parental mosaicism; (2) a structural chromosome rearrangement; (3) a mendelian gene, producing a higher rate of nondisjunction; or (4) exogenous factors.[10] This increased risk is most striking for women under 30; the risk for a chromosomally abnormal fetus after having a child with a noninherited chromosome abnormality is between 10 and 20 times the population risk for Down syndrome for mothers of the same age. As a general rule, these patients should be counseled that the recurrence risk is about 1%. For older women, the risk is probably not elevated beyond their risk based on age alone. Nevertheless, we believe that all couples who have had a previous offspring with a chromosome abnormality should be counseled about prenatal diagnosis.

Parental chromosomal abnormalities may be either structural or numeric. Generally, individuals carrying any imbalance of chromosomal material, particularly a deficiency, have serious phenotypic abnormalities and rarely reproduce. However, persons with balanced (reciprocal) translocations (ie, no leftover segments) are phenotypically normal but carry a significant risk for producing genetically unbalanced offspring.

Structural abnormalities of chromosomes, particularly translocations, are accepted as one explanation for recurrent spontaneous abortions. About 1% to 2% of couples experiencing recurrent losses are found to have a translocation carried by one of the partners.[23] Although this percentage is relatively low, the evaluation of a couple with recurrent pregnancy loss should include cytogenetic studies.

A family history of mental retardation needs to be investigated because a significant proportion may be due to a mendelian disorder, chromosomal imbalance, or an environmental cause that may be amenable to intervention. An important cause of heritable mental retardation is the fragile X syndrome. This X-linked disorder has an estimated prevalence of one to 1000 males and is implicated in 6% to 10% of mentally retarded males. In addition to mental retardation, these males also display macro-orchidism (enlarged testes) and less frequently, prognathism (forward-projecting jaw), prominent supraorbital ridges, and large ears. The molecular events surrounding this uniquely inherited condition have been elucidated, although some details remain unclear.[24,25] Nonetheless, prenatal diagnosis is available with greater accuracy than before.[26]

The list of mendelian disorders that are detectable in utero by DNA analysis of amniotic fluid cells or chorionic villi grows steadily. Table 3-7 lists selected mendelian disorders amenable to prenatal diagnosis. Physicians who are not geneticists cannot be expected to be informed on all aspects of prenatal diagnosis of these disorders. It is incumbent on the primary physician to obtain appropriate consultation when a question arises concerning the availability of prenatal diagnosis of any given disorder.

Some disorders result from the cumulative effects of several genes (polygenic) and their interactions with environmental factors (multifactorial).

Table 3–7

*Mendelian Disorders Detectable In Utero With Prenatal Diagnostic Techniques**

Sickle cell anemia

Cystic fibrosis

Tay-Sachs disease

Duchenne or Becker muscular dystrophy

21-Hydroxylase deficiency

Phenylketonuria

Factor VIII deficiency

α-Thalassemia

β-Thalassemia

Neurofibromatosis

Spinal muscular atrophy

α_1-Antitrypsin deficiency

Lesch–Nyhan disease

Ornithine transcarbamylase deficiency

Huntington disease

Fragile X syndrome

---

*Failure of a disorder to appear in this table does not necessarily imply that prenatal diagnosis is not available.

As discussed earlier, the likelihood of recurrence is generally 2% to 5%. Prenatal diagnosis is available for many of these conditions using ultrasound (eg, hydrocephalus), fetal echocardiography (congenital heart defects), or amniocentesis (neural tube defects), depending on the particular disease entity.

Finally, although exposure to a teratogenic agent is not a genetic abnormality per se, some couples seek genetic counseling because of concern regarding potential harm to a pregnancy from such exposure. In our environment, pregnant women and those contemplating pregnancy are inevitably exposed to scores of agents that are potential teratogens. A major problem is determining the level of risk or safety of such exposures. How then should the physician approach counseling patients about possible teratogenicity? The first step is gathering information that is as complete as possible through a careful literature search. The counseling session should be performed in a sympathetic manner so that the patient is not unduly alarmed or burdened by guilt. Most questions involve agents of either low-level risk or unknown risk. Couples must be provided with a careful explanation of general principles of teratology, the 2% to 3% background level of birth defects in the general population, and the possibility of individual susceptibility of a fetus to any specific agent. The period of development during which the conceptus is exposed should also be considered.

Some patients have been exposed to agents that are recognized as having a significant teratogenic potential. Examples of such agents include the drugs isotretinoin (Accutane), warfarin (Coumadin), and valproic acid (Depakote). These couples frequently inquire about prenatal diagnosis and should be informed that amniocentesis or chorionic villus sampling (CVS) for chromosomal analysis is not specifically informative for this category of birth defects. Amniocentesis to determine the level of α-fetoprotein may be diagnostically useful in certain exposures. For example, the incidence of neural tube defects is about 1% to 2% in fetuses exposed to valproic acid in the first trimester. Additionally, ultrasonography may detect some anatomic defects; however, a negative study does not necessarily mean that the fetus has not been adversely affected.

OBTAINING A GENETIC HISTORY

All obstetrician–gynecologists must attempt to determine whether a couple or anyone in their families has a heritable disorder. Some obstetricians find it helpful to use a questionnaire, such as that recommended by the American College of Obstetricians and Gynecologists (Fig. 3-4).

It is necessary to ask about the health status of first-degree relatives (sibs, parents, offspring); second-degree relatives (uncles, aunts, nephews, nieces, and grandparents); and third-degree relatives (first cousins). Specifically, such abnormal reproductive outcomes as spontaneous abortions, stillbirths, and anomalous liveborn infants should be recorded. If there is a history of such a problem, counseling may either prove simple or may require formal genetic consultation.

In addition to the considerations of advanced maternal age, the offspring of fathers in the fifth and sixth decades of life are at increased risk for new dominant mutations. Unfortunately, these are generally not amenable to prenatal diagnosis.

Ethnic origin should be recorded. Ashkenazic Jews are at increased risk for offspring with Tay-Sachs disease and therefore should be screened to determine heterozygote frequency. We offer screening to all Jewish couples because some of these couples are uncertain whether they are of Ashkenazic or Sephardic descent. Routine heterozygote screening should also be offered for sickle cell anemia in African Americans, β-thalassemia in Italians and Greeks, and α-thalassemia in Southeast Asians and Filipino. The reader is referred elsewhere for details concerning genetic-carrier screening.[27]

The ability to relate good genetic advice requires certainty of diagnosis; even the best counseling cannot compensate for an inaccurate diagnosis. Although this point seems obvious, its importance cannot be overstated. Even if the diagnosis seems obvious, confirmation is always obligatory. One should not accept a patient's word nor even accept a diagnosis made by a physician who is not highly knowledgeable about the condition. Medical records should be obtained and carefully reviewed. If possible, the anomalous individual should be examined. If the affected relative is still alive, appropriate laboratory work may include cytogenetic studies, DNA analysis, or biochemical analysis of blood, urine, or cultured cells.

ESSENTIALS OF A COUNSELING SESSION

Communication

In counseling, one should use terms that are easily understood by the patients yet avoid a patronizing attitude. Writing out unfamiliar words and using

Sample Prenatal Genetic Screen*

Name_____ Patient#_____ Date_____

1. Will you be 35 years or older when the baby is due?   Yes_____ No_____
2. Have you, the baby's father, or anyone in either of your families ever had any of the following disorders?   Yes_____ No_____
   - Down syndrome (mongolism)   Yes_____ No_____
   - Other chromosomal abnormality   Yes_____ No_____
   - Neural tube defect, ie, spina bifida (meningomyelocele or open spine), anencephaly   Yes_____ No_____
   - Hemophilia   Yes_____ No_____
   - Muscular dystrophy   Yes_____ No_____
   - Cystic fibrosis   Yes_____ No_____
   If yes, indicate the relationship of the affected person to you or to the baby's father: _____
3. Do you or the baby's father have a birth defect?   Yes_____ No_____
   If yes, who has the defect and what is it?_____
4. In any previous marriages, have you or the baby's father had a child, born dead or alive, with a birth defect not listed in question 2 above?   Yes_____ No_____
   If yes, what was the defect and who had it?   _____
5. Do you or the baby's father have any close relatives with mental retardation?   Yes_____ No_____
   If yes, indicate the relationship of the affected person to you or to the baby's father: _____
   Indicate the cause, if known: _____
6. Do you, the baby's father, or a close relative in either of your families have a birth defect, any familial disorder, or a chromosomal abnormality not listed above?   Yes_____ No_____
   If yes, indicate the condition and the relationship of the affected person to you or to the baby's father: _____
   _____

7. In any previous marriages, have you or the baby's father had a stillborn child or three or more first-trimester spontaneous pregnancy losses?   Yes_____ No_____
   Have either of you had a chromosomal study?   Yes_____ No_____
   If yes, indicate who and the results: _____
   _____

8. If you or the baby's father are of Jewish ancestry, have either of you been screened for Tay–Sachs disease?   Yes_____ No_____
   If yes, indicate who and the results: _____
   _____

9. If you or the baby's father are black, have either of you been screened for sickle cell trait?   Yes_____ No_____
   If yes, indicate who and the results: _____
   _____

10. If you or the baby's father are of Italian, Greek, or Mediterranean background, have either of you been tested for β-thalassemia?   Yes_____ No_____
    If yes, indicate who and the results: _____
    _____

11. If you or the baby's father are of Philippine or Southeast Asian ancestry, have either of you been tested for α-thalassemia?   Yes_____ No_____
    If yes, indicate who and the results: _____
    _____

12. Excluding iron and vitamins, have you taken any medications or recreational drugs since being pregnant or since your last menstrual period? (include nonprescription drugs.)   Yes_____ No_____
    If yes, give name of medication and time taken during pregnancy:_____

*Any patient replying "YES" to questions should be offered appropriate counseling. If the patient declines further counseling or testing, this should be noted in the chart. Given that genetics is a field in a state of flux, alterations or updates to this form will be required periodically.

Figure 3–4.   Sample prenatal questionnaire for genetic disorders. (American College of Obstetricians and Gynecologists: Antenatal diagnosis of genetic disorders. ACOG Technical Bulletin 108. Washington, DC, 1987. Used with permission.)

diagrams to reinforce important concepts is helpful. Repetition is generally necessary to ensure the couple comprehends what is being presented.

Preprinted forms describing common problems such as advanced maternal age have the advantage of emphasizing that a couple's problem is not unique. Written information in the form of letters or brochures can serve as a useful permanent record, allaying misunderstanding and helping the couple to communicate with relatives.

Nondirective Counseling

The most widely used and promoted method of genetic counseling is called nondirective genetic counseling. The counselor makes clear from the onset that the process is educational and no decisions will be made for those being counseled. The counselor should provide information but avoid dictating (directing) a particular course of action. Completely nondirective counseling is probably impossible, however. Counselors invariably interject their own biases by either verbal or nonverbal messages. As difficult as it is, one should endeavor to avoid letting the counselor's value system impinge on the right of a family to autonomy and self-determination.

Psychological and Social Considerations

The proper time to initiate genetic counseling depends on the genetic problem. After the birth of an abnormal child, the parents may be shocked, bewildered, grieved, frustrated, frightened, or angry. Counseling at this point is best directed toward explaining the nature of the disorder, including the prognosis; providing answers to questions; and offering emotional support. This initial stage is usually not appropriate for detailing recurrence risks and the availability of prenatal diagnosis; they should be made aware that this information will be available later.

Psychological Defenses and Coping

Psychological defenses underlie all genetic counseling sessions and, if not appreciated, may hinder the entire counseling session. As an example, anx-

iety is low in couples counseled for advanced maternal age or for an abnormality in a distant relative. When the anxiety level remains low, comprehension of the information is generally not impaired. Couples who have experienced a stillborn infant, an anomalous child, or multiple pregnancy losses are inevitably more anxious and their ability to retain information is thus diminished.

Couples experiencing abnormal pregnancy outcomes display the same identifiable sequential grief reactions that occur after the death of a loved one: denial, anger, guilt, depression, and finally, resolution.

An additional concern for the genetic counselor is that of parental guilt. It is natural for parents to search for exogenous factors that might have caused an abnormal outcome. In the process of that search, guilt or even a tendency to blame the spouse may arise. Fortunately, most couples can be assured that nothing could have prevented an abnormal pregnancy.

TECHNIQUES FOR PRENATAL DIAGNOSIS

The ability to diagnose hereditary conditions in the fetus has had a profound effect on the practice of obstetrics as well as having enabled couples to make informed decisions regarding pregnancy management.

This section discusses the two primary invasive modalities of obtaining cells or tissue for genetic analysis of the fetus.

Amniocentesis

Genetic amniocentesis is best performed around 15 to 16 weeks gestation, at which time the ratio of viable to nonviable cells is the greatest. Additionally, the uterus is readily accessible by an abdominal approach and a sufficient volume of amniotic fluid can be removed safely. "Early amniocentesis," performed during the late first trimester, is being investigated; however, safety at this gestation is not universally accepted.[28,29]

An ultrasound examination should be performed before amniocentesis to (1) detect multiple gestation; (2) document fetal viability; (3) confirm gestational age; (4) localize the placenta; (5) determine fetal position; (6) select the optimal pocket of amniotic fluid for sampling; (7) detect obvious fetal malformations; and (8) detect uterine or adnexal abnormalities.[30] The umbilical cord and insertion site should be identified and avoided if possible.

Genetic amniocentesis may be performed in an outpatient facility. After selection of the needle-insertion site, the maternal abdomen is cleansed with an antiseptic (eg, povidone–iodine solution) and draped. Under direct ultrasound guidance, a 20- or 22-gauge spinal needle with stylet is then directed into the amniotic cavity, with the needle being visualized during the entire procedure. The stylet is removed, a 10-mL syringe is attached and a few milliliters of amniotic fluid withdrawn and discarded. These first milliliters of fluid theoretically contain maternal cells collected on passage of the needle. Twenty to 30 mL of amniotic fluid are then aspirated into sterile, disposable syringes. The needle is then removed and fetal cardiac activity observed with ultrasound. The patient may be discharged after brief observation, with instructions to report any fluid loss or bleeding through her vagina, persistent uterine cramping, or fever. No strict limitations are placed on maternal activity, with the exception of strenuous exercise and coitus for a day. If the patient is Rh-negative (and unsensitized), we give Rh-immune globulin after the amniocentesis unless the father can be documented to be Rh-negative as well.

The risks of this procedure can be divided into those affecting the fetus and those affecting the mother. Maternal risks are extremely low. Intra-amniotic infection has been reported to occur in about one in 1000 cases. This usually leads to fetal loss and only rarely causes a serious problem for the mother.

Potential fetal risks include spontaneous abortion, needle-related injuries, placental separation, premature labor, and injuries due to amniotic membrane disruption (amniotic bands). Numerous large-scale studies have documented the safety of this procedure, with the following conclusions: (1) the *increased* risk of fetal loss after amniocentesis is about 0.5% over the background rate, (2) the maternal risk appears to be minimal, (3) the risk for fetal injury is minute, and (4) the fetal risk of a small needle mark is low.[30,31]

Chorionic Villus Sampling

Chorionic villus sampling was designed to permit prenatal diagnosis at an earlier gestational age (ie, 10 to 12 weeks). The primary advantage of this procedure is that if an abnormality is detected and the patient elects to terminate the pregnancy, an abortion can be performed with less maternal risk, expense, and psychological stress compared with a late second-trimester abortion. Both chorionic villi and amniotic fluid cells offer the same information

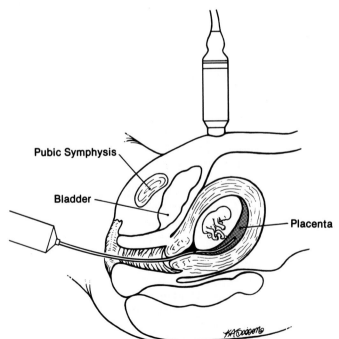

Pubic Symphysis

Bladder

Placenta

Figure 3–5. Transcervical chorionic villus sampling. (Elias S, Simpson JL: Techniques and safety of genetic amniocentesis and chorionic villus sampling. In Sabbagha RA [ed]: Diagnostic ultrasound in ob/gyn, 3rd ed, p 120. Philadelphia, JB Lippincott, 1994. Used with permission.)

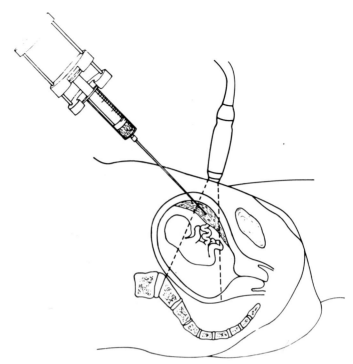

Figure 3–6. Transabdominal chorionic villus sampling. (Simpson JL, Elias S: Prenatal diagnosis of genetic disorders. In Creasy RK, Resnik R [eds]: Maternal-fetal medicine: principles and practice, 2nd ed, p 86. Philadelphia, WB Saunders, 1989. Used with permission.)

regarding chromosome and DNA status; however, α-fetoprotein (used to detect fetal neural tube defects) cannot be assayed with chorionic villi.

Chorionic villus sampling is generally performed using either a transcervical or transabdominal approach.[6] Transcervical CVS is performed with a sterile flexible plastic catheter inserted under ultrasound guidance into the placenta (Fig. 3-5). A removable stylet or obturator is contained within the plastic catheter for insertion and removed before aspiration of the villi. Once the catheter has been placed and the obturator removed, 10 to 25 mg of villi are aspirated with a syringe containing a small amount of culture media. Verification of specimen adequacy should be made immediately after the procedure. A second pass into the placenta may be required to obtain an adequate sample size.

Transabdominal CVS may be performed if the placenta is accessible to this approach (Fig. 3-6). Concurrent ultrasound guidance is used to direct a 19- or 20-gauge spinal needle into the placenta; the stylet is removed and a syringe containing a small volume of culture media is used to aspirate the villi. A breast cyst–aspirator device works well for this purpose.

Chorionic villus sampling compares favorably with amniocentesis with regard to safety and accuracy.[32,33] The procedure-related pregnancy loss rate

is not statistically higher than that associated with traditional amniocentesis. Recently, concern has been raised regarding an association of limb reduction defects in fetuses whose mothers underwent CVS.[34] This purported risk, however, has yet to be adequately quantified.[35]

REFERENCES

1. Elias S, Annas GJ: Reproductive genetics and the law. Chicago, Year Book Medical Publishers, 1987
2. Simpson JL, Elias S: Prenatal diagnosis of genetic disorders. In Creasy RK, Resnik R (eds): Maternal-fetal medicine: principles and practice, 2nd ed, p 78. Phildelphia, WB Saunders, 1989
3. Fraser FC: Genetic counseling. Am J Hum Genet 26:636, 1974
4. Evans HJ: Chromosome anomalies among livebirths. J Med Genet 14:309, 1977
5. Hook EB, Hamerton JL: The frequency of chromosome abnormalities detected in consecutive newborn studies—differences between studies—results by sex and by severity of phenotypic involvement. In Hook EB, Porter IH (eds): Population cytogenetic studies in humans, p 63. San Diego, CA, Academic Press, 1977
6. Simpson JL: Genetic counseling and prenatal diagnosis. In Gabbe SG, Niebyl JR, Simpson JL (eds): Obstetrics: normal and problem pregnancies, 2nd ed, p 269. New York, Churchill Livingstone, 1991

7. Antonarakis SE: Parental origin of the extra chromosome in trisomy 21 as indicated by analysis of DNA polymorphisms. N Engl J Med 324:872, 1991

8. Wright SW, Day RW, Müller H, et al: Frequency of trisomy and translocation in Down's syndrome. J Pediatr 70:420, 1967

9. Mikkelsen M: Down syndrome: current stage of cytogenetic epidemiology. In Bonne-Tamir B, Cohen T, Goodman RM (eds): Human genetics: medical aspects, p 297. New York, Alan R. Liss, 1982

10. Stene J, Stene E, Mikkelsen M: Risk for chromosome abnormality at amniocentesis following a child with a non-inherited chromosome aberration: a European collaborative study on prenatal diagnosis, 1981. Prenat Diagn 4:81, 1984

11. Lister TJ, Frota-Pessoa O: Recurrence risks for Down syndrome. Hum Genet 55:203, 1980

12. Garron DC, Vander Stoep LR: Personality and intelligence in Turner's syndrome. Arch Gen Psychiatry 21:339, 1969

13. Leonard MF, Landy G, Ruddle FH, et al: Early development of children with abnormalities of the sex chromosomes: a prospective study. Pediatrics 54:208, 1974

14. Lejeune J, Lafourcade J, Berger R, et al: Trois cas de deletion partielle du bras court d'un chromosome 5. CR Seances Acad Sci 257:3098, 1963

15. Niebuhr E: The cri du chat syndrome. Hum Genet 44:227, 1978

16. Simpson JL: Genetics. CREOG basic science monograph in obstetrics and gynecology, p 27. Washington, DC, Council on Resident Education in Obstetrics and Gynecology, 1986

17. Therman E: Structurally abnormal human autosomes. In Human chromosomes—structure, behavior, effects, 2nd ed, p 219. New York, Springer-Verlag, 1986

18. Boue A, Gallano P: A collaborative study of the segregation of inherited chromosome structural rearrangement in 1356 prenatal diagnoses. Prenat Diagn 4:45, 1984

19. Wilson JG: Environment and birth defects. New York, Academic Press, 1973

20. Wilson JG, Fraser FC: Handbook of teratology: general principles and etiology, vol 1. New York, Plenum Press, 1977

21. Shepard TH (ed): Catalog of teratogenic agents. Baltimore, Johns Hopkins University Press, 1986

22. Reproductive Toxicology Center: ReproTox database. Washington, DC, Reproductive Toxicology Center

23. Simpson JL, Meyers CM, Martin AO, et al: Translocations are infrequent among couples having repeated spontaneous abortions but no other abnormal pregnancies. Fertil Steril 51:811, 1989

24. Oberle I, Rousseau F, Heitz D, et al: Instability of a 550-base pair DNA segment and abnormal methylation in fragile X syndrome. Science 252:1097, 1991

25. Verkerk AJMH, Pieretti M, Sutcliffe JS, et al: Identification of a gene (FMR-1) containing a CGG repeat coincident with a breakpoint cluster region exhibiting length variation in fragile X syndrome. Cell 65:905, 1991

26. Rousseau F, Heitz D, Biancalana V, et al: Direct diagnosis by DNA analysis of the fragile X syndrome of mental retardation. N Engl J Med 325: 1673, 1991

27. Elias S, Simpson JL: Genetic screening. In Simpson JL, Elias S (eds): Essentials of prenatal diagnosis, p 15. New York, Churchill Livingstone, 1993

28. Elejalde BR, Elejalde MM, Acuna JM: Prospective study of amniocentesis performed between weeks 9 and 16 gestation: its feasibility, risks, complications and use in prenatal diagnosis. Am J Med Genet 35:188, 1990

29. Verp MS, Simpson JL: Amniocentesis for prenatal diagnosis. In Filkins K, Russo J (eds): Human prenatal diagnosis, 2nd ed, p 305. New York Marcel Dekker, 1990

30. Elias S, Simpson JL: Amniocentesis. In Milunsky A (ed): Genetic disorders and the fetus: diagnosis, prevention, and treatment. 3rd ed, p 33. Baltimore, Johns Hopkins University Press, 1992

31. NICHD National Registry for Amniocentesis Study Group: Midtrimester amniocentesis for prenatal diagnosis: safety and accuracy. JAMA 236:1471, 1976

32. Rhoads GG, Jackson LG, Schlesselman SE, et al: The safety and efficacy of chorionic villus sampling for early prenatal diagnosis of cytogenetic abnormalities. N Engl J Med 320:609, 1989

33. Canadian CVS Group: Multicentre randomized clinical trial of chorion villus sampling and amniocentesis. Lancet 1:1, 1989

34. Firth HV, Boyd PA, Chamberlain P, et al: Severe limb abnormalities after chorion villus sampling at 56–66 days' gestation. Lancet 337:762, 1991

35. Jackson L, Wapner R, Barr-Jackson M: Chorionic villus sampling (CVS) is not associated with an increased incidence of limb reduction defects. Am J Hum Genet 53:A94, 1993

Ambulatory Gynecology, Second Edition, edited by David H. Nichols and Patrick J. Sweeney. J. B. Lippincott Company, Philadelphia, © 1995.

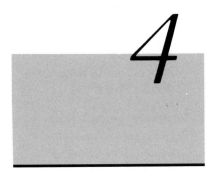

Menstrual Abnormalities

M. Yusoff Dawood

Menstrual abnormalities are the most common reason women consult their physician or gynecologist. Because of the common assumption that menstruation should have begun by the teenage years, occur cyclically at regular intervals, and last only a few days, deviations tend to produce concern on the part of the patient. The four principal groups of menstrual abnormalities seen in ambulatory gynecology are:

1. Premature menarche
2. Amenorrhea (absence of menstruation)
3. Dysfunctional uterine bleeding
4. Menorrhagia

The symptoms of menstrual abnormalities are either frequent or infrequent menstruation, heavy or light menstruation, no menstruation, or a combination of two or more of these symptoms. The approach to these common menstrual problems by many practitioners has often been empiric therapy based on symptoms; with so-called "heavy flow," the patient may ultimately undergo a hysterectomy

or some other surgical extirpation of the reproductive organs. Such an approach often belies the need to have a clear grasp of the physiologic basis of regular menstrual cycles, with orderly controlled bleeding during menstruation. Although it is true that some of the mechanisms regulating or disrupting this highly orchestrated cyclic event have not been fully uncovered, considerable information is available to form the basis for an informed rational approach to the successful management of menstrual abnormalities.

PREMATURE MENARCHE OR PUBERTY

In premature menarche, secondary sexual characteristics (pubic and axillary hair, breast development) and onset of the first menstrual flow (menarche) occurs early, by 8 years of age. Premature or precocious puberty is discussed in detail in Chapter 2 and therefore is not covered in this chapter.

AMENORRHEA

Amenorrhea is the absence of menstruation. *Primary amenorrhea* is absence of menarche by 16 years of age in girls who have never menstruated.[1] *Secondary amenorrhea* is absence of menstruation for three cycle lengths or more in women who have previously menstruated.[1] Although a delay of menstruation by a week or more may become amenorrhea, as in the case of pregnancy, the above definitions have been employed from a standpoint of investigations involving more than just a pregnancy test to rule out this common physiologic condition.

Amenorrhea is a symptom, not a disease. Amenorrhea indicates either (1) a failure of the hypothalamic–pituitary–gonadal axis to induce menstruation, or (2) the absence or obstruction of the end organs (uterus, vagina). The mechanism or hormone affected at the different levels of the hypothalamic–pituitary–ovarian–uterine–vaginal axes that may result in disruption of the normal cyclic ovarian events is outlined in Table 4-1.

In patients with primary amenorrhea, 40% to 50% have sex chromosome disorders, 25% to 40% have disturbances of hypothalamic–pituitary–ovarian function, and the rest have systemic, nutritional, or psychological disorders, including many of those associated with secondary amenorrhea.[1]

Differential Diagnosis of Amenorrhea

Primary Amenorrhea

With primary amenorrhea, the differential diagnosis includes the following.

UTEROVAGINAL DISORDERS.   About 20% of patients with primary amenorrhea have a congenital müllerian duct anomaly of some type. These anomalies include absent or hypoplastic uterus, imperforate hymen, transverse vaginal septum, and absence of the vagina.

Table 4–1
Etiology of Amenorrhea

Level	Cause	Hormone Affected
Hypothalamus	Psychosomatic factors Obesity Brain tumor, cyst, toxic or traumatic damage	GnRH
Pituitary	Nutritional, chronic disease Excessive exercise Pituitary tumors or hypofunction Medication (antihistamines, psychotropic agents) Adrenal tumors or hyperplasia Thyroid disorders	FSH, LH, Prolactin
Ovary	Polycystic ovary disease, hyperthecosis syndrome Gonadal dysgenesis, congenital absence Bilateral oophorectomy Premature menopause Thyroid disorders Hormone-producing ovarian tumors	Estrogen, progesterone, androgens
Uterus	Congenital absence or hypoplasia Iatrogenic (surgery, irradiation) Uterine disease (endometritis, Asherman's syndrome)	No hormone affected Endometrial response and bleeding absent
Vagina	Imperforate hymen Transverse vaginal septum Iatrogenic (surgery, chemicals)	If uterus is functional, menses occur but do not flow out

OVARIAN DISORDERS. Causes of primary amenorrhea having ovarian origin include primary gonadal disorder, congenital absence of the ovaries, and hypogonadotropic hypogonadism. Primary gonadal disorder encompasses gonadal dysgenesis, testicular feminization syndrome, and androgen insensitivity syndrome. About 40% to 50% of externally apparent females who have primary amenorrhea have a sex chromosome disorder. Of these, 75% have Turner's syndrome (46, XO chromosome karyotype) or mosaic forms of gonadal dysgenesis; the other 25% have a 46, XY chromosome karyotype and either the testicular feminization syndrome or less frequently, pure gonadal dysgenesis, mixed gonadal dysgenesis, or dysgenetic male pseudohermaphroditism. Hypogonadotropic hypogonadism, presenting with primary amenorrhea, is usually associated with anosmia (probably of central nervous system origin) and is referred to as Kallmann's syndrome, although the original syndrome was described in males with hypogonadotropic hypogonadism and anosmia. Because the hypogonadism responds to clomiphene citrate or gonadotropin therapy, there is likely a hypothalamic dysfunction, with a gonadotropin-releasing–hormone (GnRH) defect.

HYPOTHALAMIC DISORDERS. Disorders at the hypothalamic level that produce primary amenorrhea include (1) generalized hypothalamic defect, with deficiency of thyrotropic-stimulating hormone (TSH), adrenocorticotropic hormone (ACTH), and GnRH; and (2) isolated gonadotropin deficiency (low to absent luteinizing hormone [LH], FSH, and estradiol), with normal TSH, ACTH and growth hormone secretion. The defect in isolated gonadotropin deficiency is again due to a hypothalamic lack of GnRH due to lack of the gene for GnRH.

PITUITARY DISORDERS. Pituitary insufficiency may produce primary amenorrhea through hypogonadotropic hypogonadism. Unlike other forms of hypogonadotropic hypogonadism, patients with pituitary insufficiency are pituitary dwarfs.

OTHER DISORDERS. Any of the disorders that can produce secondary amenorrhea can also produce primary amenorrhea if they occur before menarche and are uncorrected.

Secondary Amenorrhea

Differential diagnosis of secondary amenorrhea includes the following.

PHYSIOLOGIC CHANGES.

1. Pregnancy, which is still the most common cause of secondary amenorrhea in premenopausal females
2. Postpartum states, if menstruation does not return within 18 months after delivery; this condition usually responds to cyclic estrogen–progesterone therapy; Sheehan's syndrome or postpartum pituitary necrosis or the Chiari–Frommel syndrome, consisting of amenorrhea and galactorrhea, should be ruled out
3. Menopause, if menopausal symptoms such as hot flashes, mood changes, anxiety, tiredness, and depression are evident; elevated FSH and LH levels combined with subnormal estradiol levels are diagnostic

HYPOTHALAMIC–PITUITARY DISORDERS. Hypothalamic-pituitary disorders associated with secondary amenorrhea include Sheehan's syndrome (pituitary failure due to pituitary necrosis); Simmond's disease; tumors (adenomas, cysts) of the pituitary gland, stalk or suprasellar space; and Chiari–Frommel syndrome and related amenorrhea–galactorrhea disorders. Major psychosis, emotional shock, stress, pseudocyesis, anorexia nervosa, and organic brain disease can cause amenorrhea through their effect at the pituitary or hypothalamic level. With anorexia nervosa, the hypothalamic–pituitary endocrine function regresses to an infantile level; hypogonadotropic hypogonadism associated with emaciation results from this eating disorder.

EXERCISE. Excessive exercise is associated with disruption of menstrual function, leading to menstrual irregularity, oligo-ovulation, and eventually, chronic anovulation and amenorrhea. Competitive female athletes and women with excessively strenuous and stressful activity (such as ballet dancing) have a high incidence of amenorrhea or oligoamenorrhea. Weight loss and inadequate body fat (below the critical 22% of body weight)[2] are important factors in the development of secondary amenorrhea. Not unlike anorexia nervosa, the initial loss of weight and body fat produced by exercise induces amenorrhea through hypothalamic dysfunction. In addition, competitive athletics and ballet dancing may produce added psychological stress factors, which act through the hypothalamus to disrupt regular cycling.

OVARIAN DISORDERS. Ovarian dysfunction causes anovulatory cycles, with either oligomenorrhea or amenorrhea. Other ovarian disorders that may cause amenorrhea include polycystic ovarian disease; hyperthecosis; premature ovarian failure (premature menopause); hormone-producing ovarian neoplasms such as granulosa cell, theca cell, hilar cell, and lipoid cell tumors; arrhenoblastoma; and severe pelvic inflammatory disease or bilateral ovarian destruction after mumps oophoritis.

ADRENAL DISORDERS.   Adrenogenital syndrome and related disorders, Cushing's disease, and Addison's disease often cause secondary amenorrhea.

THYROID DISORDERS.   Both hyperthyroidism and hypothyroidism may produce amenorrhea. Hyperthyroidism is more apt to produce irregular heavy menstruation initially, whereas hypothyroidism usually induces oligomenorrhea and then amenorrhea.

METABOLIC AND NUTRITIONAL DISORDERS. Severe malnutrition, marked obesity, and diabetes mellitus may lead to anovulation and amenorrhea.

CHRONIC DISEASE.   Chronic disease, such as tuberculosis, nephritis, and rheumatoid arthritis, is often accompanied by secondary amenorrhea. Artificial causes of secondary amenorrhea need to be considered or ruled out. These include hysterectomy with or without bilateral salpingo-oophorectomy, radiation therapy, excessively traumatic curettage, severe endometritis, and Asherman's syndrome (intrauterine adhesions).

Evaluation and Work-Up

Primary Amenorrhea

By definition, the diagnosis of primary amenorrhea is made if there is no spontaneous menstruation by the age of 16 years but the diagnostic work-up should be performed earlier—certainly by the age of 15 years—if the patient (1) has no breast development (absence of secondary sexual characteristics); or (2) has not menstruated within 2 years of thelarche and development of other secondary sexual characteristics.

A clinical approach based on the absence or presence of a uterus and whether there is breast development provides a sound and focused diagnostic work-up for primary amenorrhea. Breast development indicates a strong likelihood of exposure to adequate endogenous estrogen, reflecting probably adequate ovarian estrogen output at thelarche. Absence of breast development reflects low endogenous estrogen output due to failure or dysfunction of the hypothalamic–pituitary–ovarian axis at any level. The presence of a uterus, with no anatomic obstruction of the outflow tract, militates against congenital müllerian tract anomalies as a cause of the amenorrhea. Absence of a uterus suggests testicular feminization syndrome, congenital absence of the uterus, or enzyme deficiency (17,20-desmolase, 17-hydroxylase). A systematic approach to the investigation of patients with primary amenorrhea is outlined in Figure 4-1.

Secondary Amenorrhea

Certain aspects of the history are particularly important for evaluation of a woman with secondary amenorrhea.

1. Sudden weight changes (gain or loss)
2. Stress factors (eg, bereavement, loss, job-related pressures, educational pressures)
3. Geographic change (eg, moves across time zones)
4. Radiation exposure or treatment, medication or drug intake (psychotropic drugs such as the tricyclic antidepressants, haloperidol, estrogens, androgens, corticosteroids, phenothiazine compounds)
5. Family history of premature menopause
6. Presence of galactorrhea
7. Excessive cigarette smoking (causes early menopause)
8. Excessive exercise (running, jogging, ballet dancing)

During the physical examination, attention should be especially directed to the following:

1. Breast development (Tanner staging) and presence of galactorrhea (spontaneous or expressible)
2. Any change in voice
3. The presence of a receding hairline
4. Body dimensions and habitus
5. Distribution and extent of terminal androgen-stimulated body hair (moustache area, face, between the breasts, pubic hair distribution)
6. External and internal genitalia, especially for effects of androgens (clitoromegaly) and estrogens

Pregnancy must be ruled out, using a reliable, sensitive pregnancy test initially. Having ruled out pregnancy, further laboratory or ancillary tests are performed, as outlined for the work-up of secondary amenorrhea in Figure 4-2.

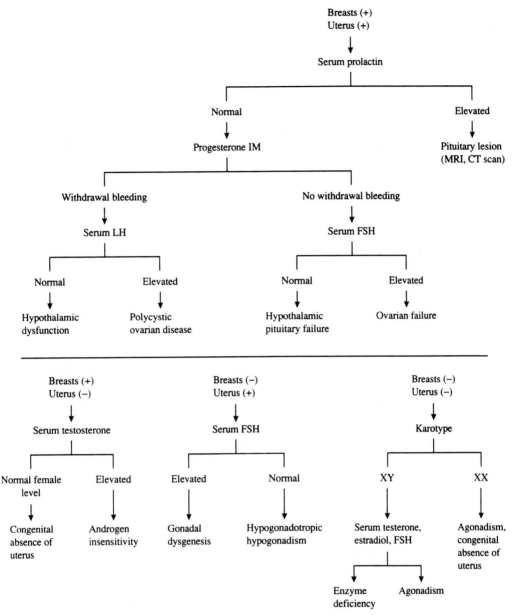

Figure 4–1. Algorithm for work-up of patients with primary amenorrhea based on the presence (+) or absence (−) of the uterus and breast development. (Dawood MY: Disorders of anovulatory cycles. In Clarke-Pearson DL, Dawood MY [eds]: Green's gynecology, 4th ed, p 216. Boston, Little, Brown, 1990.)

Therapy for Amenorrhea

Amenorrhea is purely a symptom. Therefore, proper therapy should be directed to the specific underlying cause as soon as the diagnosis is established. For most problems due to chronic anovulation secondary to a disturbance of the hypothalamic–pitu-

itary–ovarian axis, the therapy depends on short- and long-term plans for childbearing.

When Not Infertile

If infertility is not the immediate concern of the patient, treatment may still be necessary because prolonged anovulation (especially that accompanied

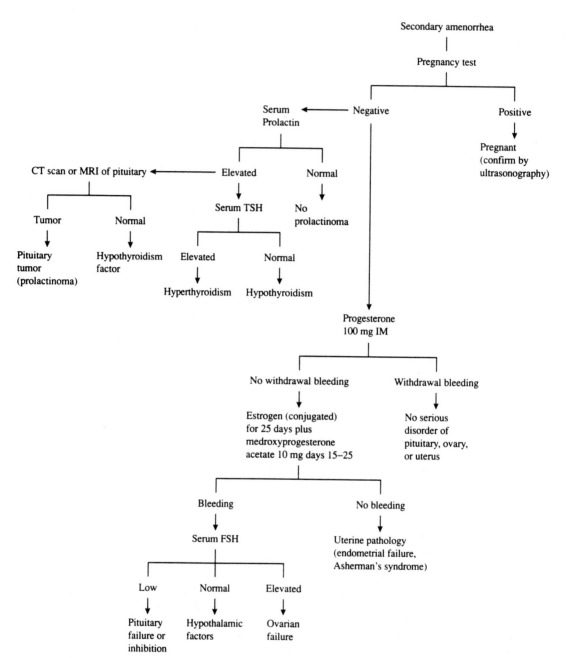

Figure 4–2. Algorithm for work-up of patients with secondary amenorrhea. This systematic approach is based on secondary amenorrhea with no other positive features detected in the history and physical examination. In the presence of special or specific features (eg, hirsutism, symptoms or signs of hypothyroidism) in the history or examination, appropriate work-up and investigations for those abnormalities should also be performed. (Dawood MY: Disorders of anovulatory cycles. In Clarke-Pearson DL, Dawood MY [eds]: Green's gynecology, 4th ed, p 217. Boston, Little, Brown, 1990.)

by hypoestrogenemia) adversely affects trabecular bone mass (leading to osteoporosis) and may adversely affect cardiovascular status. All patients with amenorrhea who are not interested in getting pregnant must be advised about the risk of pregnancy that may result from unanticipated ovulation, which may occur at any time even without treatment.

After ruling out pregnancy, withdrawal bleeding can be induced with a single course of progestin or a cyclic course of estrogen–progestin. After withdrawal bleeding, the patient may be given an oral contraceptive for up to 6 months or longer if she chooses to use this as a method of contraception. At the end of 6 months or when she is ready to attempt pregnancy, the oral contraceptive may be discontinued and the ensuing cycle monitored for normal ovulation with a basal body temperature chart. Oral contraceptives do not adversely affect bone mass and may actually result in up to 1% gain in bone per year of use.[3,4]

An alternative to oral contraceptives is cyclic estrogen–progesterone therapy. If the patient has adequate estrogen levels (more than 70 pg/mL), cyclic progesterone therapy for 4 to 6 months or intermittent cyclic progesterone therapy (oral or by injection) once every 3 months after ruling out pregnancy is a reasonable practical alternative approach.

Another form of cyclic estrogen–progesterone therapy is one of the regimes employed for hormone-replacement therapy.[5] This is indicated in amenorrheic women who are hypoestrogenic, those with premature ovarian failure, or those who have exercise-induced amenorrhea. A good regimen is to give conjugated estrogens (1.25 mg daily) from days 1 through 25 of each month, with 10 mg medroxyprogesterone acetate added from days 14 through 25. If there are intolerable side effects using 10 mg medroxyprogesterone acetate (eg, mood swings, depression, bloating, mastalgia, and excessive water retention), the dose may be reduced to 5 mg.

For patients who have hyperprolactinemia not due to hypothyroidism and even in the absence of a demonstrable pituitary adenoma, therapy with bromocriptine (a dopamine agonist) is needed. Bromocriptine given orally, 1.25 mg daily, is increased and maintained at 2.5 mg daily after a week. The prolactin level is evaluated 3 to 4 weeks after starting therapy; if it is still elevated, the bromocriptine may be gradually increased by 2.5 mg to 5 mg, up to a maximum of 10 mg. Most patients require a daily maintenance dose of only 2.5 to 5 mg. If nausea or vomiting becomes a problematic side effect

and does not subside, the bromocriptine may be administered intravaginally in the dose given orally. Treatment is usually for 6 months, and basal body temperature may be recorded to determine when ovulatory cycles resume. Patients should be counseled about the risk of pregnancy and the need for the use of an effective form of barrier contraception (condom, diaphragm, Today vaginal contraceptive sponge, spermicide) because ovulation will ensue. At the end of 6 months, treatment is stopped and the patient's cycles are monitored for resumption of spontaneous ovulatory cycles. Hyperprolactinemia warrants treatment because this condition is often associated with hypoestrogenism; women with hyperprolactinemia have been reported to have reduced bone mass and accelerated bone loss.[6]

In the Presence of Infertility

If the patient is infertile and chronic anovulation is due to a disturbance in the hypothalamic–pituitary–ovarian axis, medical induction of ovulation is indicated. Five agents used for induction of ovulation are (1) bromocriptine; (2) clomiphene citrate (CC); (3) human menopausal gonadotropin (hMG); (4) human follicle-stimulating hormone (hFSH); and (5) gonadotropin-releasing hormone.

BROMOCRIPTINE. The ergot derivatives bromocriptine and lergotrile mesylate are dopamine-receptor agonists, which activate postsynaptic dopamine receptors in the hypothalamus and pituitary, thereby acting similar to prolactin-inhibiting factor to bring about suppression of prolactin secretion by the pituitary lactotropes.

Both compounds may be used for induction of ovulation in women with hyperprolactinemia with or without a microprolactinoma but not for hyperprolactinemia secondary to hypothyroidism. Neither of these compounds has any value for ovulation induction in normoprolactinemic females, even if they are anovulatory. To avoid the common and sometimes intolerable side effects of nausea and vomiting, it is best to start bromocriptine at the lowest possible dose, 1.25 mg (half a tablet) once a day (at bedtime) for a week, then increase the dosage to 2.5 mg once a day for another week and increase it again thereafter to 2.5 mg twice a day. The usual dose of bromocriptine is 2.5 mg twice a day. Daily basal body temperature charts should be kept and coitus should be timed to coincide with a rise in body temperature or when the urine LH indicates a preovulatory surge. The bromocriptine may be discontinued a couple of days after a definite shift in basal body temperature or other evidence of ovulation occurs. Alternatively, bromocriptine medication is continued for another 2 weeks after ovulation and is discontinued if there is no menses, at which time a serum pregnancy test is indicated.

In selected patients with hyperprolactinemia, bromocriptine induces ovulation successfully in 80% of cases, with good pregnancy rates and no significantly increased incidence of multiple gestations. Similarly, the incidence of congenital anomalies in the fetuses arising from successful ovulation induction is similar to that of pregnancies resulting from spontaneous ovulation.

Side effects include nausea, vomiting, symptomatic hypotension (often postural), and muscle aches and pains. Pulmonary infiltrates, pleural effusion, and thickening of the pleura have been noted with long-term therapy, albeit rarely. Bromocriptine should not be used in patients who have uncontrolled hypertension, a history of toxemia of pregnancy, or sensitivity to ergot alkaloids.

CLOMIPHENE CITRATE.   Closely related to chlorotrianisene and diethylstilbestrol, clomiphene citrate (CC) has estrogenic and anti-estrogenic properties. It is a racemic mixture composed of en-clomiphene and zu-clomiphene. Clomiphene citrate binds to pituitary and hypothalamic estrogen receptors and prevents their replenishment. Thus, the positive feedback of a rising estrogen level on LH surge is prevented and the pituitary is allowed to continue to secrete both FSH and LH, which in turn stimulates ovarian folliculogenesis. Given appropriately (dose and timing), CC is capable of inducing ovulation in 70% to 80% of cases of anovulation, including hypothalamic amenorrhea and polycystic ovary syndrome. Clomiphene citrate is only effective if the hypothalamus and gonadotropes are intact and functional. Therefore, CC cannot be used in women with amenorrhea if the pituitary has been irradiated, surgically transected, destroyed, or sufficiently infarcted, as in Sheehan's syndrome.

The usual starting dose is 50 mg daily for 5 days, beginning on day five, although it could be started on day 3 for controlled ovarian hyperstimulation to recruit more follicles (and therefore oocytes) for intrauterine insemination, in vitro fertilization, or gamete intrafallopian transfer. If the patient is sensitive to CC, the daily starting dose may be reduced to 25 mg (half a tablet). If ovulation occurs, the dose is maintained and given for three cycles. The dose is increased by 50 mg daily if pregnancy does not occur after three ovulatory cycles, up to a maximum dose of 200 mg daily.

Ovulation occurs 3 to 9 days after the last dose of CC, usually on day 15 or 16, but can be from days 12 through 18. Coitus daily or at least every other day is encouraged during this preovulatory phase. Alternatively, the patient can perform her own urinary LH self-testing with available kits (Ovuquick, Ovugen) to determine the day of her preovulatory LH surge and have intercourse that day and the following day. If pregnancy does not occur, human chorionic gonadotropin (hCG; 5000 IU) may be added to the CC treatment on days 15 and 17 or as determined by transvaginal sonography that the lead follicle is preovulatory and measuring 20 mm or more. This addition of hCG improves the pregnancy rates slightly. The untreated cycle after CC treatment may be fertile, and pregnancies are reported to ensue during that cycle.

With CC treatment, pregnancy occurs in 35% to 40% of those who ovulated. If there is poor cervical mucous due to the antiestrogenic effect of CC, estrogens (conjugated estrogens, 0.3 mg; or diethylstilbestrol, 0.1 mg) given daily from days 10 through 14 of the cycle may improve mucous quality; intrauterine insemination may be performed the day after the urinary LH surge.

Side effects of CC include nausea; vomiting; hot flashes; headache; disturbances of vision, such as spots in the eye and blurring; multiple pregnancy; and ovarian hyperstimulation of varying degrees (10% to 20%). The rate of multiple pregnancy is about five- to eightfold higher than in unstimulated cycles, with twin pregnancies occurring in about one of 15 pregnancies (compared with a twinning rate of one in 90 pregnancies, normally). It is beyond the scope of this chapter to detail the management of ovarian hyperstimulation but practitioners who give CC must be prepared to recognize and detect ovarian hyperstimulation and manage such patients, including those who may require hospitalization. Alternatively, such therapy should be referred to trained reproductive endocrinologists who are familiar with it.

There is no direct evidence showing a dose-dependent risk of developing severe hyperstimulation syndrome with CC. When ovarian hyperstimulation occurs, the only change may be slight enlargement of the ovary, with multiple follicles. In contrast, it may be as extreme as severe massive ovarian multicystic enlargement extending up to the umbilicus, accompanied by hemorrhage; torsion of the ovary; ascites; pleural effusion or pulmonary edema; hydrothorax; contraction of the circulating plasma volume due to fluid shift into the third space, with consequent hypercoagulability and intravascular coagulation.

HUMAN MENOPAUSAL GONADOTROPIN AND HUMAN FOLLICLE-STIMULATING HORMONES.

If CC therapy does not successfully produce a pregnancy, use of hMG or hFSH is indicated. Eight-five percent of all CC-induced conceptions occur in the first three ovulatory cycles; fewer than 5% of pregnancies occur after six or more cycles.[7] Therefore, amenorrheic or anovulatory patients who have had four to six CC-induced ovulatory cycles should be considered for treatment with hMG or hFSH. Other indicators for use of hFSH or hMG in women with anovulatory cycles include hypothalamic amenorrhea with low FSH and LH levels, Sheehan's syndrome, or any condition (surgery, irradiation, infarction, trauma) that has destroyed the pituitary gland. Human follicle-stimulating hormone is similar to hMG except that the LH in hMG has been removed and thus has only follicle-stimulating hormone (FSH). Human follicle-stimulating hormone is used similar to hMG but is probably best limited to (1) ovulation induction in patients with polycystic ovaries who have elevated LH levels, or (2) situations calling for multiple recruitment of follicles, in which hFSH alone is probably required in the early stages of induction (corresponding to the early follicle-recruitment phase of the cycle). Pure FSH, produced by recombinant molecular genetic technology, is being evaluated and should offer another source of gonadotropin for clinical therapy.

Human menopausal gonadotropin therapy is initiated on either day 3, for controlled multiple follicular recruitment, or day 5, for in vivo induction of ovulation. If there is no menstruation, withdrawal bleeding is induced with either progesterone or progestin therapy (if the patient has adequate endogenous estrogens) or estrogen–progesterone therapy (if the patient is hypoestrogenic after confirmation that she is not pregnant). Given as a daily intramuscular injection, each ampule of hMG usually contains 75 IU of FSH and 75 IU of LH, whereas each ampule of hFSH usually contains 75 IU of FSH. A double-dose vial is also available. Induction of ovulation with gonadotropins is best left to the reproductive endocrinologists or to those gynecologists who are familiar with the protocols, prescribe the therapy frequently and regularly, and have the facilities to monitor patients daily, including weekends. A baseline serum estradiol level is measured and the ovarian response is monitored with a combination of serum estradiol and vaginal ultrasonography to determine the number and size of the follicles. After the first 4 to 5 days of hMG therapy, the dose is titrated daily (based on the patient's individual ovarian response) to avoid hyperstimulation and delays due to poor response. For in vivo

ovulation, a follicle size of 20 to 24 mm after 5 days of successive increases in the serum estradiol level (by at least 50% each day) is the goal. To trigger ovulation, 5000 IU of hCG are then given and may be repeated 48 hours later. The couple should have coitus every day over this 3- to 4-day period. Serum progesterone may be measured during the mid-luteal phase to confirm that ovulation has occurred.

Ovulation is produced using hMG in 80% to 90% of cases, and cumulative pregnancy rates of 60% to 65% have been achieved. Human menopausal gonadotropin treatment produces higher pregnancy rates in women with amenorrhea than in women with oligomenorrhea.

Disadvantages of hMG-induced ovulation include the high cost of medication and treatment, the need for daily injections, frequent physician visits, daily monitoring, and increased incidence of multiple pregnancies and ovarian hyperstimulation syndrome. The rate of multiple births may be as high as 15% to 30% but can be kept low with good monitoring and experienced and skillful use of the medication. The risk of ovarian hyperstimulation syndrome is also higher than with CC and occurs in 15% to 20% of patients. The critical features of ovarian hyperstimulation syndrome are similar to those described when it occurs with CC treatment. Clinical manifestation of ovarian hyperstimulation occurs about 3 to 5 days after the first dose of hCG is given, and the condition runs its course over the next 7 to 10 days. Thus ovarian hyperstimulation syndrome can be avoided by withholding the hCG whenever there is monitoring evidence to indicate ovarian hyperresponse.

GONADOTROPIN-RELEASING HORMONE. A decapeptide secreted by the hypothalamus to induce secretion of FSH and LH, GnRH is particularly useful and effective for inducing ovulation in patients with hypothalamic amenorrhea if the pituitary is functional.[8] Such patients usually have low or subnormal levels of serum FSH and LH. Gonadotropin-releasing hormone must be given subcutaneously in pulses every 90 minutes through an automatic programmable pump, which delivers the pulses at a dose and frequency that can be set and adjusted based on the patient's response. The pulses of GnRH are given on a continuing basis until follicular growth reaches a maximum of at least 20 mm (preferably 24 mm), at which time hCG 5000 IU is administered intramuscularly to trigger ovulation. Thus, the patient has the pump and medication with her around the clock during the therapy.

Ovarian response to GnRH is monitored by using serum estradiol levels and vaginal ultrasound of the ovaries, similar to that used for hMG but not as frequently. The risk of ovarian hyperstimulation with GnRH is less than with hMG. Although the incidence of multiple pregnancies is slightly higher than with spontaneous pregnancies, it is lower than with hMG-induced ovulation. Gonadotropin-releasing hormone is also less expensive than hMG.

Common Amenorrhea–Oligomenorrhea Syndromes

Polycystic Ovary Syndrome

Polycystic ovaries or polycystic ovary syndrome are a common cause of oligoamenorrhea and probably the most common cause of dysfunctional uterine bleeding. In its extreme form, polycystic ovary syndrome is represented by the classic description from Stein and Leventhal in a group of women who had bilateral pale, smooth, markedly enlarged polycystic ovaries, with varying combinations of amenorrhea, infertility, obesity, and hirsutism. Polycystic ovary syndrome is a broader clinical entity, however, with varying intensity of these clinical changes, depending on when the patient presents herself.

Typically, the patient is young (in her twenties or thirties) and presents with a history of irregular anovulatory cycles after normal menarche. Either oligomenorrhea or secondary amenorrhea then follows. Ten to fifteen percent of these patients have menorrhagia, with episodes of prolonged and somewhat profuse bleeding alternating with intervals of amenorrhea. Many such patients tend to be obese, which compounds the chronic anovulation and heavy uterine bleeding through increased production of estrone. Hirsutism is present in 50% to 60% of patients but virilization is rare. Infertility is a common accompaniment and may be the patient's primary complaint.

PATHOLOGY.   The ovaries are usually bilaterally and symmetrically enlarged to varying degrees—up to five times their normal size. The surface of the ovary is smooth, pearly white in appearance, with markedly thickened capsule and hyperthecosis. Many small follicular cysts, usually 5 to 10 mm in diameter and at various stages of atresia, are present in the subcapsular area. Corpora lutea or albicantia are absent except in occasional cases.

PATHOGENESIS.   Evidence indicates constant elevated tonic secretion of pituitary LH, presumably through the increased production of estrone in patients with polycystic ovaries. Although FSH stimulates folliculogenesis, the developing follicles undergo developmental arrest and atresia because of the elevated tonic LH levels and the increased androgen production by the ovaries. Androstenedione production by the ovarian stroma is increased, leading to increased ovary and peripheral aromatization to produce estrone. Testosterone production is also increased by the LH stimulation of the ovaries. Therefore, hirsutism is often seen in these patients. The irregular follicular development and its consequent irregular estradiol production combined with the increased estrone production stimulate the endometrium to proliferate, resulting in irregular uterine bleeding and menorrhagia. If untreated, women with polycystic ovaries are at increased risk for the development of endometrial hyperplasia and eventually, endometrial carcinoma. Inhibin production by the ovaries is believed to be increased and therefore FSH levels may decrease. Thus, the serum LH to FSH ratio increases to more than 2:1 in well-established cases without the absolute levels of the gonadotropins being elevated.

In spite of the above, the primary defect in polycystic ovary syndrome has not been clearly identified and established. It is unclear whether the defect is at the hypothalamic–pituitary level and compounded by the increased estrone through its positive LH feedback or at the ovarian level, compounded by the sustained and elevated tonic pituitary LH levels. It has even been hypothesized that there may be enzymatic defects in the ovaries or adrenal glands.

DIAGNOSIS.   The clinical diagnosis is readily made from the clinical features of menstrual abnormalities, chronic anovulation, infertility, hirsutism, obesity, and gross bilateral ovarian enlargement. Pelvic examination may be difficult because of obesity, however, and not all features may be present. Transvaginal ultrasonography is useful and can be confirmatory. The enlarged ovaries, with subcapsular cysts, are characteristic in appearance. Serum FSH and LH are useful and can be diagnostic. In classic established cases, LH levels are elevated and LH to FSH ratio is often increased to 2:1 or more. Serum prolactin and thyroid studies are warranted, as in the work-up of amenorrhea. Daily basal body temperature recordings, luteal phase or late cycle progesterone levels, endometrial biopsy, and urine LH self-testing for LH surge are helpful to determine whether the patient is ovulating. Patients who have hirsutism should have serum androgens and appropriate work-up for hirsutism (see Chapter 11 for a more detailed discussion of hirsutism). In the presence of infertility and bilaterally enlarged ovaries, laparoscopy may be considered and ovary biopsy performed, depending on intraoperative findings.

MANAGEMENT. Management of polycystic ovary disease is governed by the primary need or complaint of the patient. Regulation of menstrual disturbance and prevention of endometrial hyperplasia can be undertaken with the oral contraceptive pill, as described for dysfunctional uterine bleeding. If infertility is the main concern, medical induction of ovulation is performed. Surgical wedge resection of the ovaries and laser ovary drilling should be required rarely and reserved only for those in whom medical therapy has truly failed to induce ovulation or arrest hirsutism. If hirsutism is the primary complaint, oral contraceptives, spironolactone, or the antiandrogen cyproterone acetate may be used (see Chapter 11).

Amenorrhea–Galactorrhea

Galactorrhea is the excretion of milky fluid from the breast, as occurs during lactation. It may be spontaneous or on expression during examination or handling of the breast. Amenorrhea, when accompanied by galactorrhea, usually is due to inappropriate hypersecretion of prolactin, either by (1) a prolactin-secreting tumor of the pituitary, or (2) a hypothalamic–pituitary disturbance, causing deficiency of prolactin-inhibiting factor, which in women is dopamine or a dopamine-like substance. Excessive prolactin is responsible for the galactorrhea and indirectly for the amenorrhea or oligomenorrhea. Use of certain medications such as psychotropic agents (tricyclic antidepressants, haloperidol); antihistamines; rauwolfia alkaloids (reserpine); and phenothiazines (chlorpromazine) for an extended time can produce amenorrhea–galactorrhea. Withdrawal of oral contraceptive pills may also produce galactorrhea–amenorrhea due to oversuppression of the hypothalamic–pituitary axis in a few cases. In normal postpartum women, amenorrhea and galactorrhea constitute the Chiari–Frommel syndrome. In the presence of a prolactinoma (prolactin-secreting pituitary tumor) in a nonpregnant woman, amenorrhea and galactorrhea constitute the Forbes–Albright syndrome. The Ahumada–Argonz–del Castillo syndrome consists of amenorrhea and galactorrhea in the absence of pregnancy or a pituitary adenoma.

Clinically, the woman presents with amenorrhea (occasionally oligoamenorrhea) and milky breast discharge (galactorrhea), which is usually chronic (lasting months or years) and spontaneous but sometimes only on gentle expression. Often, there is accompanying hypoestrogenism, with atrophic vagina and endometrium. The diagnosis is confirmed by elevated levels of serum prolactin, normal or reduced levels of serum pituitary gonadotropins (FSH and LH), and hypoestrogenemia. Thyroid dysfunction, especially hypothyroidism, should be ruled out with an initial screening with serum TSH. Depending on elevation of the serum prolactin level and presence or absence of visual field restriction, magnetic resonance imaging or CT scanning of the pituitary or cone-down view of the sella turcica is performed to determine the presence or absence of a detectable pituitary or rarely, a hypothalamic tumor (see Fig. 4-2).

Spontaneous recovery or resolution of amenorrhea–galactorrhea is rare. Specific therapy is directed toward suppression of the hyperprolactinemia that not only induces the galactorrhea but also antagonizes the action of pituitary gonadotropins on the ovary and therefore, follicular recruitment and ovulatory cycles. The ergot alkaloid bromocriptine, which is a dopamine agonist, and several new long-acting similar ergot alkaloids inhibit prolactin secretion, restore euprolactinemia, establish ovulatory cycles and menstruation, and slowly eliminate or reduce the galactorrhea.

If there is a pituitary tumor and it is 10 mm or larger, it is a macroadenoma. A microadenoma is smaller than 10 mm. With a microadenoma, the patient can be allowed to become pregnant, with little risk of complications during pregnancy. Macroadenomas require shrinkage in size (usually medically but sometimes surgically) before attempting pregnancy because of significant pituitary-related complications (infarction, visual field compression, headaches). If bromocriptine is unsuccessful in inducing ovulation and conception, prolactin secretion can be suppressed with bromocriptine or other prolactin-inhibiting ergot alkaloids; ovulation induction may be achieved with either clomiphene citrate, hMG, hFSH, or a combination of these.

Menstrual Abnormalities With Hirsutism

Hirsutism, the presence of excess body hair in women, often presents with menstrual disturbances and is a common gynecologic endocrine disorder. Hirsutism is discussed in detail in Chapter 11. The underlying cause of the hirsutism is usually also the etiology of the accompanying menstrual disruption. Initially, and when exposed to short durations of hyperandrogenemia, the menstrual abnormality is irregular vaginal bleeding that tends to be light but could also be heavy if there is estrogen dominance, as in the obese hirsute female. With prolonged duration of elevated androgen levels, oligoamenorrhea and eventually amenorrhea result. With sustained elevated androgen levels, virilization is clinically apparent, evidenced by clitoromegaly, receding hairline in the front and the temples or frontal baldness, increased muscularity and muscle strength, and deep voice or change in the voice pitch. Patients with hirsutism are frequently also obese because the level of bound testosterone in the circulation is reduced and inversely proportional to the body weight once this exceeds the ideal body weight.

DIFFERENTIAL DIAGNOSIS. Differential diagnosis of menstrual abnormalities with hirsutism should include the following.

IDIOPATHIC CAUSES. Idiopathic causes that are congenital, familial, racial should be excluded. (Normal ovulatory menses with mildly elevated or normal plasma testosterone are found in several of these patients.) The hirsutism is probably due to a familial tendency to excessive androgen sensitivity of the hair follicles and sebaceous glands at certain times, especially during puberty, menopause, or pregnancy. Alternatively, increased local metabolism of testosterone to other androgens occurs at the hair follicles, with subsequent uptake.

ADRENAL DISEASE. Adrenal disease should be ruled out, including (1) mild congenital hyperplasia, which may go unrecognized until primary amenorrhea and hirsutism with virilization appear; (2) adrenal tumors (adenoma or carcinoma) or hyperplasia: acquired adrenogenital syndrome; (3) Cushing's disease (hyperplasia or tumor); and (4) mild hyperplasia, with a syndrome resembling Stein–Leventhal syndrome.

OVARIAN DISORDERS. The most common cause of female hirsutism is ovarian disorders. Ovarian causes include polycystic ovary syndrome, ovarian hyperthecosis, and androgen-producing ovarian tumors such as arrhenoblastomas (Sertoli–Leydig cell tumors); hilus cell (pure Leydig cell) tumors or hyperplasia; adrenal rest (lipoid cell) tumors; and gynandroblastomas (mixed granulosa–theca cell and Sertoli–Leydig cell tumors).

PITUITARY DISORDERS. These include nonfunctioning tumors and cysts, with pituitary destruction, acromegaly (eosinophilic adenoma), and Cushing's disease (basophilic adenoma).

MISCELLANEOUS DISORDERS. These include postmenopausal hirsutism; androgen therapy; diphenylhydantoin (Dilantin) therapy (some epileptic patients); and Morgagni–Stewart–Morel syndrome (hyperostosis frontalis interna, obesity, mental retardation, and hirsutism of unknown cause; diabetes mellitus, thyroid dysfunction, menstrual disorders, and hypertension are often present also; there is usually no demonstrable disease in either the pituitary or the hypothalamus despite the many similarities to acromegaly and Cushing's disease; androgen levels are usually normal).

Investigation and Treatment

Investigation and management of hirsutism is discussed in detail in Chapter 11.

DYSFUNCTIONAL UTERINE BLEEDING

Dysfunctional uterine bleeding is any irregular, anovulatory uterine bleeding not associated with an anatomic lesion or other detectable organic cause.[9,10] Although the literature refers to studies that include ovulatory dysfunctional uterine bleeding, the term is best restricted to the above definition. Although many acyclic menstrual bleeding disorders are accompanied by short intervals of amenorrhea or involve oligomenorrhea, the most prominent clinical feature is the appearance sooner or later of excessive bleeding—too frequent, too heavy, or too prolonged. Thus, the spectrum of bleeding patterns spans several types, including polymenorrhea (periods occurring at intervals of less than 21 days); hypermenorrhea (periods lasting longer than 7 to 10 days); metrorrhagia (bleeding between periods either light, normal, or heavy); and menometrorrhagia (heavy irregular bleeding). Regular cycles with longer than 30-day intervals are not classified as dysfunctional uterine bleeding because many women have normal cycles occurring once every 30 to 35 days. Thus, oligoamenorrhea (irregular and infrequent cycles occurring at intervals of more than 35 days, interspersed with intervals of amenorrhea) is considered dysfunctional but oligomenorrhea (regular cycles occurring at intervals of more than 35 days) is not.

Incidence and Prevalence

Dysfunctional uterine bleeding is responsible for the largest single group of clinical problems seen by the gynecologist. Estimates indicate that 10% to 15% of all gynecologic patients present with dysfunctional uterine bleeding. Most commonly, it occurs in adolescents, followed by those in the premenopausal age group. The common occurrence of dysfunctional uterine bleeding during adolescence is due to the prevalence of anovulatory cycles in this age group. About 55% to 82% of cycles are anovulatory during the first 2 years after menarche, declining to 30% to 55% of cycles 2 to 4 years after menarche and only 0% to 22% of cycles 4 to 5 years postmenarche.[11]

Etiology and Associated Conditions

In a small percentage of women, the anovulatory cycles and irregular uterine bleeding are due to a more fundamental endocrine disorder, such as those listed below.

1. Thyroid disease, such as hyperthyroidism or hypothyroidism; hyperthyroidism usually disrupts menstrual cycles by inducing irregular heavy vaginal bleeding; although hypothyroidism may eventually present with progressive oligomenorrhea and then amenorrhea, early hypothyroidism has a high association with menorrhagia; 15 out of 67 apparent euthyroid menorrhagic women had laboratory evidence of early hypothyroidism[12]
2. Adrenal disease, such as hyperplasia and benign or malignant tumors
3. Pituitary disease, such as pituitary failure or neoplasms
4. Diabetes mellitus, with its generalized metabolic and steroid hormonal disturbances; may present with either the dysfunctional uterine bleeding, which may be secondary to endometrial hyperplasia or endometrial carcinoma in what may otherwise be a palpably normal size uterus

Dysfunctional uterine bleeding may be associated with a specific primary ovary lesion. The principal ovary disorders encountered are:

1. Stein–Leventhal syndrome; ovary hyperthecosis
2. Functioning ovary tumors; arrhenoblastoma, granulosa or theca cell tumors, hilus cell tumors
3. Chronic pelvic inflammatory disease (or more rarely, extensive pelvic endometriosis), in which there are severe pathologic changes in the ovaries leading to disturbances of follicular function

All the above endocrinopathies or conditions may lead to a disturbance in the normal pituitary–ovarian axis, causing anovulation and irregular cycles characterized by amenorrhea, oligomenorrhea, or dysfunctional uterine bleeding.

Other generalized metabolic disturbances also seem to predispose to the development of an anovulatory type of menstrual function. These include marked obesity (even in the absence of diabetes or thyroid disease); severe malnutrition (for example anorexia nervosa syndrome); and chronic, debilitating, systemic disease such as tuberculosis. In obese patients, there is increased extraovarian production of estrogens from androgens in the adipose tissues, often giving rise to elevated tonic LH secretion and therefore anovulation. With severe malnutrition and in anorexia nervosa patients, pituitary gonadotropin function and secretion revert to a more infantile form, thereby leading to anovulation. With these conditions, the major therapeutic effort should be directed at the underlying systemic abnormality. Treatment aimed at restoring ovulatory cycles can be of considerable symptomatic value but should not be attempted until the underlying cause has been corrected.

In the absence of underlying disease, dysfunctional uterine bleeding often resolves spontaneously and is nearly always temporary if properly managed. There are often certain background contributing or precipitating factors, however. These factors include transient acute physical or psychic stress, moderate or severe fluctuations in body weight, and chronic physical, mental, or emotional fatigue. Temporary emotional influences leading to menstrual irregularities and even hypothalamic amenorrhea are commonly seen among women in the first year of college or high school. Emotional upsets such as family illness or death, marital discord, problems with children, pressures of outside activities, and social or occupational personality clashes are seen in those in the prime of reproductive life presenting with dysfunctional uterine bleeding. Febrile illness can lead to delayed or missed periods, followed by dysfunctional uterine bleeding. Prolonged administration of certain tranquilizers and psychotropic agents could also produce anovulatory cycles with menstrual irregularities. Excessive exercise can initially produce dysfunctional uterine bleeding; with progressive intensity and duration of the exercise, amenorrhea results. Interestingly, there is a seasonal variation, with episodes of dysfunctional uterine bleeding or anovulatory cycles with short intervals of amenorrhea being more common during July and August.

Finally, dysfunctional uterine bleeding is more common at the beginning and at the end of the reproductive years (ie, during adolescence and the premenopausal phases) because of the apparently more unstable cycles as the ovary initiates and terminates its life-long activity. The cycles appear to be more vulnerable to disruptive influences early and late in life.

Pathophysiology

Dysfunctional uterine bleeding is precipitated by endometrial exposure to an imbalance of ovarian steroid hormones due to anovulation, exogenous administration, or an imbalance of prostaglandin production.

Steroid Hormones

The pathophysiologic basis for dysfunctional uterine bleeding and the pattern of abnormal bleeding can be readily explained by endometrial exposure to an imbalance between estrogen and progesterone or the duration of exposure. Basically, it is due to too much or too little estrogen, too much or too little progesterone, or a nonphysiologic combination of these (Table 4-2). In most occurrences of noniatrogenically induced dysfunctional uterine bleeding, excessive estrogen or insufficient progesterone is the endocrine basis of the irregular bleeding. If the endometrium is exposed to low levels of estrogens over a short time, the bleeding is intermittent spotting that may be prolonged but usually light because of poor or little proliferative development of the endometrium. In contrast, sustained normal or high levels of estrogen inevitably lead to intervals of amenorrhea, followed by acute profuse uterine bleeding (Fig. 4-3). Both situations are instances of estrogen breakthrough bleeding. Progesterone breakthrough bleeding occurs when the progesterone to estrogen ratio is unfavorably high, such as that found in women given long-acting contraceptive implants of progestins such as norethindrone (Norplant) or depo-medroxyprogesterone acetate. There is ovarian inhibition, resulting in normal but low levels of estrogen, with a high sustained level of progestin continuously providing the antiestrogenic effect on the endometrium. Thus, the endometrium is poorly developed and intermittent light bleeding of variable duration occurs when the progestin levels fluctuate or decline. Finally, insufficient progesterone leads to progesterone withdrawal bleeding, classically seen in the normal regular ovulatory cycle and manifest as regular menstrual flow. If, however, the corpus luteum is artificially removed (surgically or pharmacologically) or after the discontinuation of progestin, bleeding ensues. If the corpus luteum has a short life-span, bleeding begins earlier than anticipated. If luteolysis is erratic in onset and course, spotting occurs for several days before the onset of actual flow. Given this endocrine pathophysiologic basis, the clinical features of the menstrual abnormality and uterine bleeding pattern, interpreted against the history and clinical findings, enable the clinician to draw some basic conclusions about the patient's estrogen–progesterone milieu.

Table 4–2
Pathophysiologic Mechanisms of Dysfunctional Uterine Bleeding

Steroid Hormone Abnormality	Clinical Examples
Excess Estrogen	Obesity Polycystic ovary disease Most dysfunctional uterine bleeding, 25–40 years of age
Insufficient Estrogen	Low-dose oral contraceptive Hypogonadism Some perimenopausal dysfunctional uterine bleeding
Excess Progesterone	Use of Norplant, Depo-Provera Persistent corpus luteum Progesterone withdrawal bleeding
Insufficient Progesterone	Chronic anovulation Oligo-ovulation

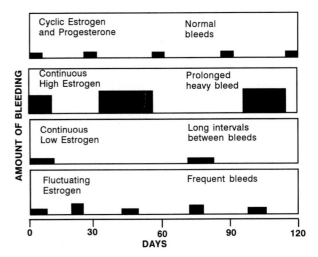

Figure 4–3. Schematic representation of relation between estrogen exposure and the pattern and amount of menstrual bleeding in women with dysfunctional uterine bleeding mediated by estrogen breakthrough. Each solid rectangle represents a bleeding episode, with the height or width (*y axis*) of the rectangle representing the amount of bleeding and the length (*x axis*) of the rectangle representing the duration (days) of bleeding.

Abnormal Prostaglandins

Abnormalities in uterine prostaglandin production or uterine prostaglandin receptors may be the pathophysiologic mechanism or mechanisms for menorrhagia and ovulatory dysfunctional uterine bleeding when there is no anatomic intrauterine abnormality.[13-18] The stable metabolite of prostacyclin, 6-keto-prostaglandin F_1, is significantly elevated in women with menorrhagia.[13] Endometrial prostacyclin production is enhanced by co-incubation with myometrium in women with menorrhagia.[13] Prostacyclin is vasodilatory, relaxes uterine smooth muscle, and inhibits platelet aggregation. Thus, excessive prostacyclin can prolong uterine bleeding and produce menorrhagia.

When given intrauterine, prostaglandin E_2 relaxes the uterus. The ratio of prostaglandins F_2 to E_2 is inversely correlated with the volume of menorrhagia, reflecting increased endometrial prostaglandin E_2 production. In addition, significantly increased prostaglandin E_2 receptors are present in some uteri from menorrhagic women.[17] Therefore, increased endometrial prostaglandin E_2 combined with increased sensitivity (by increased uterine receptors) and increased uterine prostacyclin may explain the pathophysiology of menorrhagia or ovulatory dysfunctional uterine bleeding in some women.

Clinical Diagnosis

A careful and accurate history should always suggest the probability that abnormal vaginal bleeding is dysfunctional uterine bleeding. The various clinical manifestations of the anovulatory type of ovarian function include (1) a premature or delayed period that is then prolonged; and (2) oligomenorrhea or polymenorrhea, with the episodes of bleeding irregular in duration, followed by the onset of continuous bleeding that may vary in amount from day to day. Although highly variable in amount, the bleeding is at sometime or another profuse but invariably painless.

Possible factors precipitating the change from a previously normal, regular menstrual pattern may be uncovered in the history. Finally, the general physical survey and pelvic examination usually reveal no evidence of an underlying endocrine or metabolic disorder and no sign of local pelvic disease. The presence of incidental but asymptomatic local pelvic disease must be carefully evaluated and integrated with the overall clinical picture to arrive at a correct explanation for the abnormal bleeding.

Differential Diagnosis

It is important to exclude the following causes of genital tract bleeding when dealing with dysfunctional uterine bleeding.

Pregnancy

Pregnancy, including ectopic pregnancy, threatened abortion, incomplete abortion, missed abortion, or gestational trophoblastic disease should be ruled out. In all these situations, there may be varying intensities of vaginal bleeding, occurring after intervals of amenorrhea or delayed menses.

Organic Gynecologic Disease

Organic gynecologic disease must be excluded, including endometrial cancer, cervical cancer, uterine leiomyomas, uterine polyps, adenomyosis, polycystic ovary syndrome, vaginitis, cervicitis, endometritis, or salpingitis. An endometrial curettage that reveals secretory endometrium may be a clue to a primary uterine disease as the cause of the bleeding.

Systemic Disease

The presence of systemic disease, especially hypothyroidism, hyperthyroidism, and liver disease must be excluded.

Iatrogenic Causes

Iatrogenic causes such as use of estrogens, oral contraceptives, intrauterine contraceptive devices, corticosteroids, androgens, anabolic agents, hypothalamic depressants, anticholinergic drugs, digitalis, and anticoagulants must be ruled out.

Blood Dyscrasia

Blood dyscrasia, particularly idiopathic thrombocytopenic purpura, von Willebrand's disease, anemia, and leukemia must be excluded. A complete blood count and platelet count with a peripheral blood smear would be useful. Easy bruising, menorrhagia, and even significant mid-cycle hemorrhage are common initial manifestations of von Willebrand's disease. This coagulopathy is characterized by a prolonged bleeding time, a reduced level of factor VIII, a capillary defect, and probably deficient platelet adhesiveness. The diagnosis can be made from an accurate history (the condition is an autosomal dominant hereditary disorder) and a simple test of bleeding time. This avoids diagnostic curettage, which may provoke even more excessive bleeding. Bleeding can be readily arrested by intravenous transfusion of plasma or factor VIII preparations and platelet transfusions, if necessary.

Trauma

The patient should be examined for trauma, such as that from sexual assault or a foreign body. An accurate history should suggest trauma as a cause. The patient may be fearful or reluctant to discuss details, however, particularly if the injury is a result of domestic violence. Physicians must be skillful in asking questions in nonthreatening and nonjudgmental tones. A pelvic examination generally is diagnostic. In pediatric and young adolescent patients, the examination may be difficult and an examination under anesthesia may become necessary.

Differential Diagnosis by Age

Because anovulatory uterine bleeding is most common at the extremes of reproductive life (pubertal and perimenopausal years) and other likely causes of abnormal uterine bleeding vary according to age, the age of the patient can be helpful in narrowing the probable causes of the bleeding.

Adolescence

Most abnormal bleeding is due to anovulation because of inactivity of the hypothalamic–pituitary–ovarian axis, which is trying to become established and is therefore dysfunctional uterine bleeding.

Prime Childbearing Years

Pregnancy, endometritis, iatrogenic causes, cervical, ovary or vaginal disease, adrenal disease, and hepatic disease are common. Severe stress may be the cause of dysfunctional uterine bleeding in this age group and should be investigated.

Premenopause

Both proliferative and secretory endometrium may cause dysfunctional uterine bleeding. Endometrial atrophy, endometrial polyps, submucous myomas, or malignancy is more likely to occur.

Investigations

Always rule out a pregnancy, especially the possibility of an ectopic pregnancy, before proceeding. A qualitative test for hCG with one of the newer sensitive kits, employing a specific antibody against hCG-β, suffices for diagnosis of pregnancy. For determination of viability of the pregnancy or if an ectopic pregnancy is suspected, a quantitative hCG assay, employing the antiserum against hCG-β, and ultrasonography are required. In addition, all patients should have (1) a Pap smear (if one has not been done within the last year); (2) a complete blood count, including platelets, to determine whether the patient is anemic or thrombocytopenic; (3) a bleeding time to screen for a coagulopathy; and (4) urine for glucose to screen for diabetes.

Further work-up of patients with dysfunctional uterine bleeding can be guided by the patient's age group because of the prevalence of other causes of abnormal vaginal bleeding. Generally, patients can be divided into three groups and the work-up largely tailored, using any specific hallmarks in the history, the character of the bleeding, or the physical findings.

Adolescents and Women in the Early Twenties

A detailed history and a careful, complete pelvic–rectal examination are generally sufficient to exclude other conditions and confirm a clinical diagnosis of dysfunctional uterine bleeding. Thyroid function studies are frequently indicated because thyroid dysfunction is relatively more frequent in this age group. There is also a 22.4% incidence of early hypothyroidism in apparently euthyroid menorrhagic women.[12] A complete endocrine survey is indicated if there are symptoms suggestive of a basic underlying disorder or if there is poor or no response to adequate therapy. Blood dyscrasia and abnormal bleeding tendencies should be ruled out in this age group before doing a curettage or endometrial biopsy. The possibility of polycystic ovary syndrome should be entertained and serum FSH and LH assays combined with a pelvic sonogram may be useful. Curettage or endometrial biopsy is rarely necessary for either diagnostic or therapeutic purposes.

Women Aged 25 to 40 Years

The most important conditions to be ruled out in this age group are disorders of early pregnancy. The importance of pregnancy testing has been mentioned. Rapid quantitative hCG-β assays combined with transvaginal sonography has reduced the need for laparoscopy in most cases; however, in acute situations, laparoscopy may still be necessary. Curettage is occasionally needed to exclude submucous fibroids or endometrial polyps or to control excessive bleeding if response to conservative management is not satisfactory. Pelvic malignant disease must also be excluded by thorough examination, cytologic studies, and appropriate biopsies, if indicated.

Thyroid-function studies should be considered in this age group because they are relatively inexpensive and noninvasive. Nonthyroid endocrine disorders or blood dyscrasias seldom manifest for the first time in this age group unless the history or physical findings are suggestive.

Premenopausal and Menopausal Women

The same general principles of work-up apply to these women but curettage is almost always necessary to ensure ruling out endometrial or endocervical cancer. It is necessary to perform a complete sampling of the uterine cavity and not just a small endometrial biopsy at one site because malignancies or hyperplasia can be missed with such limited sampling. Thyroid-function studies should be performed because thyroid dysfunction is not uncommon in these age groups.

In all age groups, if the patient is obese, complete endometrial sampling by curettage of one sort or another is necessary to rule out endometrial hyperplasia or carcinoma; there is often excessive extraglandular peripheral estrogen production in such women. Curettage can be readily performed as an office procedure, using a small-bore (2 to 4 mm) plastic suction curette attached to a suction pump or large-volume syringe, with controlled gentle suction. To reduce discomfort, a nonsteroidal anti-inflammatory drug (NSAID) such as ibuprofen, 400 to 800 mg, or sodium naproxen, 550 mg, may be given 30 to 60 minutes before beginning the procedure.

Management and Treatment of Acute Bleeding Episodes

Dysfunctional uterine bleeding is sometimes heavy. Not infrequently, an acute episode of profuse hemorrhage, with a fall in hemoglobin and blood volume, occurs and may necessitate transfusion. Prompt arrest of bleeding is indicated. The most rapidly effective means of achieving control is curettage; however, this is not useful if the bleeding has been profuse and prolonged because all or most of the endometrium has already been shed. The patient should be admitted to the hospital for treatment if the bleeding is sufficient to require transfusion.

If immediate curettage is contraindicated or inadvisable, short-term intensive hormone therapy should arrest excessive dysfunctional uterine bleeding. In this setting, estrogens are usually more rapid than progestins, especially when most of the endometrium has been shed with prolonged and profuse hemorrhage. Estrogen may be given intravenously (conjugated estrogens, 20 mg) or orally (conjugated estrogens, 2.5 mg; micronized estradiol, 3 to 6 mg) every 2 hours until bleeding stops or is reduced considerably.[19] A maintenance dose should be continued for 20 to 25 days and progesterone added during the last 2 weeks so that a more normal secretory endometrium is developed and withdrawal bleeding follows. Cyclic estrogen–progesterone therapy is then advisable for another 3 to 4 months. Perhaps an even simpler alternative when the oral medication route is feasible is the use of one of the combination oral-contraceptive agents. One tablet, two to four times daily, is given to arrest the hemorrhage and allow a more normal withdrawal menstrual flow to follow. Thereafter, cyclic oral contraceptive therapy is given for 3 or 4 months to reduce the chance of recurrent dysfunctional bleeding.

If curettage is necessary, 40% to 60% of cases resume normal ovulatory cycles without further treatment. Premenopausal patients may be provided with sufficiently long remission to carry them into the menopause.

If a fundamental endocrine disorder (eg, thyroid dysfunction, polycystic ovary disease, or diabetes mellitus) is the underlying basis of the dysfunctional uterine bleeding, treatment should be directed to the underlying cause. Nevertheless, initial symptomatic control of the anovulatory bleeding may be necessary. Specific treatment of dysfunctional uterine bleeding is either by medical therapy or by surgery. Dysfunctional uterine bleeding is usually temporary and correctable in most cases and the anovulatory cycles completely reversible by simple treatment. Thus, medical therapy often corrects the abnormal bleeding and restores ovulatory cycles. If medical therapy or acute bleeding cannot be satisfactorily controlled, surgery becomes necessary. Even with some surgical therapy, such as endometrial ablation, preoperative preparation with hormonal treatment is required.

General Measures

Reassurance and a thorough explanation of the mechanisms involved in dysfunctional uterine bleeding are critical to the proper management of these patients. Body weight may have to be regulated toward ideal body weight to avoid obesity or inadequate body fat.

Medical Treatment

Anovulatory cycles are characterized by a lack of a progestational effect in the endometrium, resulting in proliferative or hyperplastic (occasionally atrophic) changes and subsequent irregular shedding. Therapeutic regimens therefore aim to supply progesterone to the endometrium to promote its maturation and ultimately control the shedding. If the patient has had continuous prolonged heavy bleeding when first seen, her endometrium is likely to be atrophic; in such cases, estrogen therapy should be initiated because there is little or no endometrium to be transformed by progesterone. Specific hormone regimens for dysfunctional uterine bleeding that may be employed are given below.

SINGLE COURSE OF PROGESTERONE. A single course of progesterone is useful if the bleeding is of short duration (one or two cycles) in women with little or no history of previous irregularities. Intramuscular injection of progesterone in oil (short-acting), 25 to 50 mg, or one of the more potent long-acting progestational preparations such as hydroxyprogesterone caproate (Delalutin), 250 mg, can be conveniently given (Table 4-3). The bleeding usually stops within a few days of the injection as the endometrium undergoes progestational changes. An artificially produced "normal period" or with-

Table 4–3
Progestin Therapy for Dysfunctional Uterine Bleeding

Regimen	Indication	Progestins
Single-Course	Short bleeding (1–2 cycles), 25–40 years of age, no previous irregularities	Progesterone IM, 50–150 mg, × 1 dose Delalutin IM, 250 mg, × 1 dose Norethindrone acetate, orally, 5–10 mg, × 12–14 days Dydrogesterone, orally, 10–20 mg, × 12–14 days Medroxyprogesterone acetate, orally, 10 mg, × 12–14 days
Multiple-Cycle Course	Failed single course Prolonged dysfunctional bleeding Excessive prolonged flow but minimal irregularity	Same as above, initially; then start treatment orally on days 14–25, × 12 days, × 3–4 cycles

drawal flow follows a few days to as long as 1 or 2 weeks later. This form of therapy is sometimes referred to as "medical curettage." The patient should be warned that during the first 48 hours of this "normal period," the flow may be excessive because of the varying degrees of endometrial overproliferation before the administration of progesterone. She should be reassured that the flow thereafter will be more normal and ordinarily will cease within the usual 5 to 7 days.

An alternative to the progestin injection is a course of oral progestins using norethindrone acetate (5 to 10 mg) or dydrogesterone (10 to 20 mg), each given daily for 10 to 14 days. A single course of progestin therapy causes return of ovulatory function in the ensuing cycles in about 85% of patients when the dysfunctional bleeding is an isolated event. Other progestins that may be given orally for a course of treatment include the 19-nor steroid compounds (norethindrone, norethisterone, levonorgesterol, nomegesterol acetate), the 17-hydroxyprogesterone compounds (medroxyprogesterone acetate, 17-hydroxyprogesterone caproate, megesterol acetate), and dydrogesterone, which is 6-dehydroretroprogesterone. Dydrogesterone is structurally related to natural progesterone but is more than 30 times as potent pharmacologically, does not inhibit ovulation, and has no thermogenic or androgenic effects.

Therapy with progestin should be started during the second half of the cycle so as to allow initial endometrial proliferation and subsequent secretory transformation by the progestin. During an acute bleeding episode, progestin is given immediately.

CYCLIC PROGESTERONE THERAPY. Cyclic progesterone therapy is required in patients who fail to respond to a single course of progesterone, if the bleeding irregularities are of considerable duration, if the "menses" remain fairly regular but there is increasing menorrhagia, or if curettage was needed to control the original bleeding episode but anovulatory cycles promptly recur. To simulate closely the normal progestational phase and secretory transformation of the endometrium, the progestin should be given in the second half of the cycle, beginning on the eleventh or thirteenth day of the cycle and continued for 12 to 14 days. Upon completing the progestin on day 25, menstruation or bleeding can be anticipated within 3 to 5 days. Initially, the bleeding may start a little later (ie, 5 days or more after stopping the medication), thus giving what appears to be a cycle of 30 days or longer. With successive cycles of therapy, the cycles begin to regress progressively toward 28 to 30 days. Any of the oral progestins in the dosage described for single-course therapy (medroxyprogesterone, 10 mg daily and up to 10 mg three times a day; norethisterone acetate, 5 to 10 mg daily and up to 5 mg three times a day) will suffice. Cyclic therapy should continue for three to four consecutive cycles and then be discontinued. There is a marked reduction in blood loss and duration of bleeding in the first cycle of treatment, with further diminution in subsequent cycles (Fig. 4-4).[20]

Return to spontaneous, normal ovarian function and ovulatory cycles occurs in most patients after completing cyclic progestin therapy. The precise mechanism reinstating the ovulatory cycles is not

Figure 4–4. Mean (± standard deviation) blood loss before and during cycles of treatment with a progestin on days 12–25 (14 days) of each cycle for dysfunctional uterine bleeding. The number in the rectangle with each mean blood loss bar represents the duration of bleeding for that treatment cycle. (Data from Fraser IS: Treatment of ovulatory and anovulatory dysfunctional uterine bleeding with oral progestogens. Aust NZ J Obstet Gynaecol 30:353, 1990.)

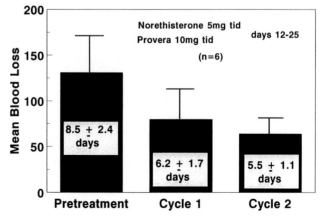

understood but presumably the normal estrogen–progesterone balance helps to reestablish the normal reciprocity between the pituitary and the ovary, leading to restoration of normal folliculogenesis, ovulation, and corpus luteum formation and function. If a satisfactory response is not obtained, further investigation is required to rule out other endocrine disturbances or local (intrauterine) organic causes.

CYCLIC ESTROGEN–PROGESTERONE THERAPY.   In some patients, especially adolescents and premenopausal women, cyclic estrogen–progesterone treatment is necessary because of deficiencies in both hormones. The endometrial biopsies usually reveal atrophic or early proliferative endometrium.

Estrogen, such as conjugated estrogen (Premarin, 1.25 mg) or micronized estradiol (Estrace, 2 mg) is given orally once or twice daily beginning on day one for 25 days, with a progestin added from days 13 through 25, when both hormones are stopped. Bleeding usually follows 2 to 5 days later. This cyclic estrogen–progestin therapy is repeated for three to four cycles, beginning again with the first day of the onset of withdrawal bleeding. After completion of a 3- to 4-month course of therapy, ovulatory cycles are generally reestablished.

An alternative to cyclic estrogen–progesterone therapy is the use of an oral contraceptive that contains both estrogen and progestin. It is started on day one and continued for 21 days. If there is still breakthrough bleeding, the dose may be increased to one tablet twice a day.

OTHER MEDICAL THERAPIES.   In addition to estrogens and progestins, several other hormonal and nonhormonal medications are effective for controlling excessive bleeding or menorrhagia in women with dysfunctional uterine bleeding. Other hormonal medications include danazol and gonadotropin-releasing hormone agonist (leuprolide acetate, nafarelin, buserelin, goserelin), which are suitable for patients who do not wish to conceive or for preoperative preparation to induce endometrial thinning before endometrial ablation. Nonsteroidal anti-inflammatory drugs that inhibit excessive prostanoid production by the uterus are the only nonhormonal medications that have been shown to be effective in controlling heavy menstrual blood loss. Nonsteroidal anti-inflammatory drugs are more likely to be effective when the dysfunctional bleeding is associated with ovulatory cycles. These therapies (danazol, GnRH agonist,

NSAIDs) are discussed in the section of this chapter on menorrhagia.

Surgical Treatment

Three types of surgery—dilation and curettage, endometrial ablation, and hysterectomy—have been employed for management of dysfunctional uterine bleeding or menorrhagia.

DILATION AND CURETTAGE.   Dilation and curettage is diagnostic and can also be therapeutic. The basis for curettage being therapeutic has never been satisfactorily explained. Additionally, curettage is a useful adjunct when the endometrium has not been thoroughly and completely shed and when it is desirable to strip the endometrium to the basalis layer before initiating hormone therapy.

ENDOMETRIAL ABLATION.   If adequate curettage and attempts to control refractory dysfunctional uterine bleeding by the above supplemental hormone therapies are unsuccessful, hysteroscopic endometrial ablation or ultimately hysterectomy may be necessary.

HYSTERECTOMY.   Hysterectomy is obviously a "last resort" and is indicated only if all other medical and surgical therapies have truly failed and the bleeding is excessive.

MENORRHAGIA

Menorrhagia is heavy menstrual flow in a normal ovulatory cycle. By strict definition, the cycles are usually regular but menorrhagia is also sometimes loosely used to refer to heavy menstrual flow in irregular cycles. Thus, menorrhagia is also used to indicate heavy menstrual flow in patients with dysfunctional uterine bleeding or ovulatory dysfunctional uterine bleeding when the cycles may be regular but the bleeding is heavy.

Normal menstrual blood loss is usually about 20 to 80 mL. A blood loss of more than 80 mL per menstrual flow is considered heavy and constitutes menorrhagia.[21] In some studies, menorrhagia is defined as a loss of more than 50 mL.

The diagnosis of menorrhagia requires objective measurement of the amount of blood loss. Perceptions of heavy menstrual bleeding and the clinical diagnosis of menorrhagia based on the patient's history are inaccurate in almost 40% of cases.[22,23] Although subjective assessments of blood loss, the duration of menstruation, and the number of tampons and napkins used reflect relative changes in the amount of blood loss from what the patient normally experiences, they are not accurate in determining whether the bleeding constitutes menorrhagia.[24] The most frequently used objective method of blood loss is the alkaline hematin method, involving extraction of used tampons or pads with 5% sodium hydroxide and subsequent optical density measurement.[25] A more clinical and practical approach is estimation of blood by asking the patient to indicate on a pictorial chart the number of pads or tampons used and the extent to which each is soaked (Fig. 4-5). This method has been shown to have a significant correlation with the measured amount of menstrual blood loss.[26]

Causes and Differential Diagnosis

The causes of menorrhagia are similar to those given for dysfunctional uterine bleeding. When there is no anatomic pathologic cause in the uterus or reproductive tract for the bleeding, the diagnosis of unexplained, essential, or idiopathic menorrhagia has been employed. Unexplained or idiopathic menorrhagia is also loosely used to refer to heavy or ovulatory dysfunctional uterine bleeding. Common organic causes of menorrhagia worthy of mention are uterine fibroids, uterine polyps, intrauterine device–induced or associated menorrhagia, adenomyosis, bleeding disorders, and hypothyroidism. In most of these situations, the cycles are ovulatory. Sterilization has also often been cited as a cause of menorrhagia.

Fibroids are probably the most frequent accompanying pathology in menorrhagia but may not necessarily be the cause of the menorrhagia, especially if they are small or if exclusively subserosal or only partially intramural. As many as 20% of patients with menorrhagia eventually are shown to have fibroids.[27] Leiomyosarcoma should be considered if the menorrhagia does not respond to treatment or there is rapid, progressive growth of the uterine mass.

In patients using the intrauterine device, menorrhagia is a frequent accompaniment after its insertion.[17] When an intrauterine device is the basis of the menorrhagia, it is usually obvious from the history and the device or its tail is visible on speculum examination.

Adenomyosis usually presents with menorrhagia, dysmenorrhea, a dull dragging discomfort in the pelvis. The uterus may be of normal size or uniformly enlarged, either minimally or up to 10 to 14 weeks gestation size and often boggy on bimanual examination. Occurring usually in the woman who is in her 30s, adenomyosis is often misdiagnosed as uterine myoma until the specimen is examined microscopically. In a series of 2616 consecutive hysterectomies, 16% were noted to have adenomyosis, and abnormal uterine bleeding was the most common symptom.[28] Often, adenomyosis is present with fibroids. Hysteroscopic diagnosis and biopsy

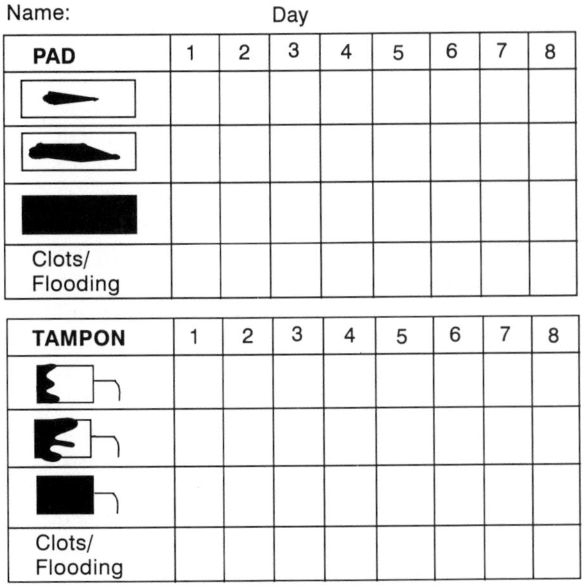

Figure 4–5. Pictorial blood loss–assessment chart, evaluating menstrual blood loss. This chart has diagrams depicting **light, moderate,** and **heavy** soiling of either tampons (*lower panel*) or sanitary pads (*upper panel*). A mark is made in each appropriate box at the time each tampon or pad is discarded. For each box charted, the pads or tampons are counted in groups of five. Passage of clots (the size was equated to that of coins) and episodes of flooding are also recorded. A score of 1 is given for lightly stained tampon or pad, 5 for moderately soiled tampon or pad, 10 for heavily soiled tampon, and 20 for heavily soiled pad. A score of 100 or more is diagnostic for menorrhagia, with a sensitivity of 86% and specificity of 89% when recorded by the patient and 86% and 81%, respectively, if scored by the gynecologist. (Modified from Higham JM, O'Brien PMS, Shaw RW: Assessment of menstrual blood using a pictorial chart. Br J Obstet Gynaecol 97:734, 1990.)

as well as ultrasound may offer more reliable pre-operative diagnosis.[29,30]

Bleeding disorders, including the use of anticoagulants, are correctable causes of menorrhagia and dysfunctional uterine bleeding.

Although sterilization has often been regarded as a cause of menorrhagia, there is little objective data to support this belief. On the contrary, studies with objective measurements of blood loss have found no difference in menstrual blood loss before and after tubal ligation and between different methods of tubal ligation.[31,32]

Although some researchers report an association between endometriosis and menorrhagia, others found that the incidence of menorrhagia, menstrual irregularity, and premenstrual spotting were similar in women with endometriosis compared to those without endometriosis.[27,33]

Pathophysiology

When there is no underlying anatomic pathology to explain the heavy bleeding, the condition is called essential or unexplained menorrhagia. Unexplained menorrhagia is probably due to a locally enhanced fibrinolysis or a shift in prostanoid production toward the vasodilatory, uterine-relaxing, and platelet anti-aggregatory prostanoids such as prostaglandin E_2 and prostacyclin.[13-16,34] Increased prostaglandin E_2 and prostacyclin produce vasodilation and uterine muscle relaxation, leading to prolonged bleeding. Poor compression of the bleeding vessels combined with the platelet anti-aggregatory effect of the increased prostacyclin add to a slowdown in the clotting process. Additionally, uterine prostaglandin E_2 receptors are increased in patients with menorrhagia, thereby greatly enhancing the uterine sensitivity to prostaglandin E_2 and further accentuating vasodilation and uterine relaxation.[18] Hemostasis is limited in the endometrium of women with menorrhagia. Fragile plugs are formed, with large protrusion into the extravascular space, or there are decreased hemostatic plugs due to increased vascular defects.[35,36] The hemostatic plugs are often recanalized, reflecting increased fibrinolysis.

When an intrauterine device is inserted, there is increased macrophage infiltration into the endometrium, followed by increased abnormal amounts of prostanoids.[17,37-39] Whether the prostanoids are largely produced by the endometrium, the macrophages, or both remains unknown but the increased prostanoids cause uterine relaxation, vasodilation, and inhibition of platelet aggregation and combine with enhanced fibrinolytic activity to provide the framework for menorrhagia. A schematic representation of the mechanism leading to increased bleeding is outlined in Figure 4-6. Although it is claimed that the copper-impregnated intrauterine device reduces the antifibrinolytic activity, prostaglandin production appears to be increased.[40] The progesterone-medicated intrauterine device (Progestasert) does not increase the uterine prostaglandin release, however, and actually reduces blood loss and causes less dysmenorrhea.[41] Intrauterine devices laden with NSAIDs, antifibrinolytic agents, or the progestin levonorgesterol are being evaluated and appear promising for control of intrauterine device–induced menorrhagia.[40]

Evaluation and Investigations

The evaluation and work-up of menorrhagia is in many ways similar to that of dysfunctional uterine bleeding. Once early pregnancy disorders have been considered, a dilation and complete curettage is essential to rule out other intrauterine pathology. A complete blood count including platelet count and coagulation studies should be obtained. If an intrauterine device is present and the uterus was normal before its insertion, curettage is usually not necessary early in the investigation.

Transvaginal Ultrasonography

Transvaginal ultrasonography may be readily performed in the office. Uterine myomas, polycystic ovaries, and uterine polyps can be identified. If the

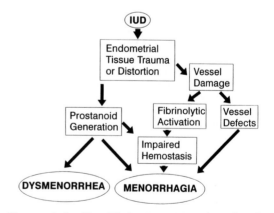

Figure 4–6. Simplified schematic outline for the mechanism of menorrhagia and dysmenorrhea in women using the nonmedicated or copper-laden intrauterine contraceptive device (Dawood MY: Nonsteroidal anti-inflammatory drugs and reproduction. Am J Obstet Gynecol 169:1255, 1993.)

uterine cavity contains blood and clots, however, intrauterine lesions such as polyps can be more difficult to define. Adenomyosis can often be identified by the characteristic arborization pattern spreading into the myometrial wall, and intrauterine devices can be localized.[29] For more details on ultrasonographic appearances of intrauterine and uterine pathology, please see Chapter 21.

Transvaginal ultrasonography can be helpful in evaluating the thickness of the endometrium before and after medical therapy or endometrial ablation.[42] The endometrium should be thinner after danazol therapy to facilitate endometrial resection. After endometrial resection, if the patient continues to bleed but there is minimum endometrium, conservative therapy is employed; if the endometrium is unchanged, repeat resection may be performed; if there is irregular endometrial cavity or fibroid, a hysterectomy should be considered. Sonography can also detect complications after endometrial ablation. In a study of women who had transvaginal sonography performed after endometrial ablation, seven of 16 were symptomatic; two were found to have hematometra, four had islands of functional endometrial tissue in combination with hematometra, and one had a nonviable pregnancy.[43]

Hysteroscopy

Hysteroscopy has become an increasingly useful tool for detecting intrauterine lesions and can be performed in the office setting. It allows a more directed biopsy of an abnormal or bleeding site within the uterine cavity and therefore provides a more specific histologic diagnosis. Details of hysteroscopy are given in Chapter 22.

The value of direct visualization of the endometrial cavity in women with menorrhagia is underscored by the high percentage of visible uterine pathology detected on hysteroscopy. Of 182 women with menorrhagia submitted to hysteroscopy, 49% had an abnormal finding.[27] The incidence of an abnormal finding increased with the severity of the menorrhagia: 25% of those with a blood loss of less than 60 mL had abnormal findings, compared with 56% of those with moderate menorrhagia (60 to 120 mL blood loss) and 64% of those with severe menorrhagia (more than 120 mL blood loss).

Hysteroscopic visualization with biopsy appears to be a valuable diagnostic tool in the work-up of patients with menorrhagia. In the absence of any pathology in the endometrial cavity, hysteroscopic biopsy of the myometrium allows for diagnosis of adenomyosis and selection of appropriate surgical therapy. In 50 patients with menorrhagia and hysteroscopically normal-appearing endometrial cavities, 66% had significant adenomyosis greater than 1 mm in depth.[30] There was significant correlation between the depth of adenomyosis and the severity of menorrhagia; thus, minimal adenomyosis could probably be treated with GnRH-agonist therapy or endometrial ablation, whereas deeply implanted adenomyosis may require hysterectomy.

Hysteroscopy with endometrial sampling has 98% sensitivity, compared with 65% for curettage, but both procedures have 100% specificity.[44] Although hysteroscopy with endometrial sampling is more accurate in 9.1% and less accurate than blind dilation and curettage in only 0.5%, the missed pathology usually consists of benign conditions such as endometrial polyps and uterine fibroids.[44,45] In addition, most cases of menorrhagia or dysfunctional uterine bleeding resolve with medical therapy. For these reasons, hysteroscopy is probably best used in patients who have poor or no response to medical therapy, persistent abnormal bleeding, visible polyps at the cervix, or a suspicion of uterine fibroids. Thus, an important value of diagnostic hysteroscopy is its potential to prevent unnecessary hysterectomy when medical therapy is unsuccessful.

Laparoscopy

Laparoscopy is usually not required for the work-up of menorrhagia or dysfunctional uterine bleeding. If, however, the woman is infertile and desires to conceive or if there are symptoms such as dysmenorrhea, pelvic pain, or dyspareunia, laparoscopy should be considered and may be combined with hysteroscopy. In a study of 117 women with dysfunctional uterine bleeding and menorrhagia who had laparoscopy *and* hysteroscopy, 37 had uterine myomas and 45 were found to have endometriosis, which would otherwise not have been detected—albeit 28 had only mild endometriosis.[27] The incidence of endometriosis was greatest in women with moderately heavy menstrual blood loss (60 to 120 mL).

Treatment

If an organic cause or a bleeding disorder is found, the menorrhagia is usually correctable by treating the underlying problem. If there is no specific organic lesion or cause identified, initial treatment is medical, reserving surgical interventions for those cases in which medical therapy is unsuccessful or there is uncontrollable menorrhagia.

Medical Therapy

The medications effective in reducing menstrual blood flow include sex steroid hormone (oral contraceptives, progestins); prostaglandin synthetase inhibitors; antifibrinolytics (eg, tranexamic acid and ε-aminocaproic acid); androgen derivatives (eg, danazol, gestrinone); and GnRH agonists.

SEX STEROID HORMONE. Therapy with oral contraceptives, estrogens, and progestins can control bleeding due to dysfunctional uterine bleeding. The same principles, medications, and dose regimens apply for management of menorrhagia. Hormone therapy induces endometrial atrophy and therefore reduces menstrual blood loss.

Oral contraceptives or continuous progestin therapies are effective for menorrhagia. Progestin therapy may be given orally and continuously throughout each cycle for 21 or 25 days, followed by a rest of 3 to 7 days, or can be given cyclically in the second half of the cycle. The intrauterine device medicated with progesterone (Progestasert) or levonorgestrel (Levonova) may also be used to reduce menstrual blood loss in patients with menorrhagia.[41,46] This is a more invasive way of administering the medication, however, and has the added complications of the intrauterine device and its insertion.

PROSTAGLANDIN SYNTHETASE INHIBITORS. Because imbalance of uterine prostanoid production and secretion may be the underlying pathophysiology of dysfunctional uterine bleeding or menorrhagia, NSAIDs that inhibit cyclo-oxygenase and therefore prostaglandin (including prostaglandins E_2 and F_2 and prostacyclin) biosynthesis may be used to reduce the bleeding. Nonsteroidal anti-inflammatory drugs that are effective in reducing uterine blood loss include mefenamic acid, 500 mg, three times daily;[47-55] flurbiprofen, 100 mg, twice daily for 5 days;[56,57] meclofenamate sodium, 100 mg, three times daily;[58] and naproxen sodium, 550 mg loading dose, followed by 275 mg twice a day.[49] In addition, because there are increased uterine prostaglandin E_2 receptors, selection of an NSAID that also acts as a prostaglandin antagonist (such as mefenamic acid) may achieve optimum results in reducing blood loss. Nonsteroidal anti-inflammatory drugs are usually effective (and therefore better employed) in therapy of unexplained or idiopathic menorrhagia or for ovulatory dysfunctional uterine bleeding. An average reduction of 20% to 40% in blood loss from the pretreatment loss may be expected.[52,54,57,58] Nonsteroidal anti-inflammatory drugs appear to be particularly effective in correcting menorrhagia that is induced by intrauterine devices. Mefenamic acid, ibuprofen, and naproxen are effective for this indication and should be given for the number of days that heavy menstrual flow occurs.[47,59-61] Nonsteroidal anti-inflammatory drugs should not be given to patients with gastric ulcers, renal and hepatic dysfunctions, or allergies to aspirin or aspirin-like drugs. Nonsteroidal anti-inflammatory drugs are not effective in reducing menstrual blood loss from menorrhagia that is caused by fibroids.[61] Aspirin does not reduce menorrhagia, even in doses of 3000 mg daily.[62]

ANTIFIBRINOLYTICS. The antifibrinolytics ethamsylate and tranexamic acid have been evaluated for treatment of dysfunctional uterine bleeding and for menorrhagia.[54,57] There is a significant reduction in blood loss with both tranexamic acid or ethamsylate. Generally, the reduction in blood loss is greater with antifibrinolytic therapy than with NSAIDs but side effects are more common with the former than with the latter. The dose of tranexamic acid used for treating menorrhagia and dysfunctional uterine bleeding is 1.5 g three times daily for 3 days, followed by 1 g twice daily for another 2 days. An average of 40% reduction from pretreatment blood loss can be expected with tranexamic acid or ethamysylate.[54,57] Antifibrinolytics reduce menstrual blood loss in menorrhagia induced by the intrauterine contraceptive device and are also effective in some cases of uterine fibroids.

Side effects of antifibrinolytics include nausea, dizziness, and diarrhea and less frequently intracranial venous or arterial thrombosis, thus limiting their practical usefulness.[63] Therefore, antifibrinolytics should not be used in patients who have a history or family history of thromboembolic events, subarachnoid hemorrhage, or deficiency of proteins S, C, or antithrombin III.

DANAZOL. Danazol, an isoxazole derivative of 17α-ethinyl testosterone, is an impeded form of testosterone that is readily absorbed from the gastrointestinal tract and metabolized in the liver to mostly inactive metabolites.[64] Proved to be effective in medically ablating both eutopic and heterotopic endometrium in the management of patients with endometriosis, danazol is effective in the medical management of menorrhagia by reducing blood loss and improving symptoms.[65,66] The dose of danazol for reducing menstrual blood loss is 200 mg daily, which is less than the 600- to 800-mg daily dose used for treatment of endometriosis. Danazol, 200 mg daily, significantly reduces menstrual blood loss within a month, with further reductions after 2 months if the maintenance dose is also 200 mg daily after the first month.[67] The response is more variable if the maintenance dose is reduced to 50 or 100 mg. Although androgen-related side effects such as acne, oily skin, weight gain, muscle aches, and hot flushes may occur, they are less intense and less frequent with the lower doses. Additionally, the patient should be counseled about preventive steps, such as reducing acne and oily skin by washing with soap and water regularly, reducing weight gain by attention to diet, and reducing muscle aches and cramps with extra calcium or quinine-based tonic water.

Gestrinone, another androgen-derived antiprogesterone–antiestrogen steroid effective for suppressing endometriosis, is also effective in reducing blood loss in women with menorrhagia.[68] The dose is 1.25 or 2.5 mg orally, twice a week, but the medication is not available for clinical use in the United States and studies are needed.

GONADOTROPIN-RELEASING HORMONE AGONISTS. By creating hypogonadotropic hypogonadism through down-regulation of pituitary GnRH receptors, GnRH-agonist therapy induces amenorrhea and is an effective treatment for menorrhagia and dysfunctional uterine bleeding.[69] Such treatment and the accompanying amenorrhea are particularly useful in patients with heavy bleeding and anemia who may not be suitable for or do not want surgical therapy. The anemia can be corrected with appropriate hematinics, whereas blood loss is eliminated with the amenorrhea. Because of the undesirable hypoestrogenic side effects (causing hot flushes, vaginal dryness, and bone loss), cyclic hormone-replacement therapy may be added to GnRH-agonist therapy to overcome these side effects and produce controlled cyclic bleeding. Hormone-replacement therapy is usually associated with small menstrual blood loss. Therapy with GnRH agonist combined with hormone replacement corrects menstrual blood loss in patients with menorrhagia and those with dysfunctional uterine bleeding.[70,71] The dose of GnRH agonist employed is similar to that used for treatment of endometriosis; nafarelin acetate, 400 to 800 mg a day intranasally; buserelin, 1200 mg a day intranasally, or 0.1 mg subcutaneously daily; leuprolide acetate, 0.2 mg subcutaneously daily; depot leuprolide acetate, 3.75 mg intramuscularly once a month; or goserelin, 3.6 mg subcutaneously once a month. Treatment is usually for 3 months but may be extended to 4 months. Hormone-replacement therapy may be administered with conjugated estrogen in a daily dose of 1.25 mg orally, days 1 through 25, and me-droxyprogesterone, 10 mg daily from days 14 through 25. Because the monthly cost of this therapy is currently about $400, it cannot be recommended as a routine first-line medical therapy when equally effective and less expensive alternatives are available. Therefore, GnRH-agonist therapy should be reserved for those who do not respond to other medical management and do not want or are not hematologically fit for surgery. It is noteworthy that after administration of GnRH agonist, there is initial stimulation of the pituitary gonadotropes, and gonadotropins are increased, resulting in ovarian stimulation. Thus, it cannot be expected to arrest heavy bleeding during the first week of GnRH agonist treatment, and management of the acute bleeding episode requires specific medical therapy described earlier.

Gonadotropin-releasing–hormone agonists may be used alone to produce endometrial atrophy, secondary to the induced hypogondatropic hypoestrogenism, for preoperative preparation of patients with menorrhagia who are undergoing endometrial ablation.[72-74] Preoperative treatment for 6 weeks is usually adequate but up to 3 months may be needed in some cases.

Surgical Treatment

Although possibly therapeutic in dysfunctional uterine bleeding, curettage is only a diagnostic procedure in women with menorrhagia. Surgical treatment of menorrhagia is either by hysterectomy or by a hysteroscopic procedure. Because many of the medical therapies for menorrhagia are effective and there is overdiagnosis of menorrhagia based on perceived heavy menstrual flow, surgical treatment is best limited to cases not controlled by medical management or for those with life-threatening hemorrhage.

HYSTEROSCOPIC SURGERY. Two types of hysteroscopic surgery are employed for managing menorrhagia: resection of uterine myomas and endometrial ablation.

HYSTEROSCOPIC RESECTION OF LEIOMYOMA. In menorrhagia due to submucous uterine fibroids, the intrauterine portion of the myoma is resected (shaved off) or intrauterine pedunculated myomas are transected at the base or pedicle via the cervix through the hysteroscope. This requires distension of the uterine cavity and is usually performed as outpatient surgery. Such resection of uterine fibroids is ideally reserved for only the pedunculated or solitary myoma that is submucous or largely protruding into the uterine cavity. The procedure spares a laparotomy, reduces or eliminates postoperative pelvic adhesions, reduces blood loss, may enhance the chances of a successful pregnancy, and reduces recovery time. Selection of suitable cases is critical to avoid complications and increase the chance of a successful outcome. Patients with intramural leiomyomas or multiple myomas are best treated by more aggressive approaches for complete multiple myomectomies. For hysteroscopic resection of submucous myomas, preoperative treatment with a GnRH agonist for 6 to 12 weeks is recommended to induce endometrial atrophy and reduce myoma size.

ENDOMETRIAL ABLATION.   Endometrial ablation has been increasingly advocated and performed for treatment of menorrhagia. Advanced as a less invasive surgical procedure, with therefore less morbidity and mortality and shorter recovery time, hysteroscopic endometrial ablation was initially employed to control menorrhagia arising from a bleeding diathesis, especially that secondary to chemotherapy, wherein the patients are not suitable for hysterectomy and control of uterine blood loss is mandatory for continued chemotherapy. Overenthusiasm for the procedure has reached such proportions that it is sometimes being employed as a first-line therapy in place of cheaper noninvasive medical management or as an unnecessary intermediate step for patients who are fit and suitable for either abdominal or vaginal hysterectomy (laparoscopic-assisted or otherwise).

Hysteroscopic endometrial ablation can be performed using either laser photovaporization, usually with the Nd:YAG laser; transcervical endometrial resection with the resectoscope; or electrocoagulation with the "rollerball."[75–79] All these methods require uterine cavity distension and flushing of the uterine cavity with fluid media. The technique can be performed as an outpatient procedure. Besides other complications such as uterine perforation, infection, retention of endometrial glands, and hematometra, excessive fluid absorption is a particular and important hazard. For further details on hysteroscopy, see Chapter 22. Preoperative preparation with either a GnRH agonist for 6 weeks or danazol for 2 to 6 weeks is often needed to produce endometrial atrophy before the endometrial ablation procedure and is continued for several weeks postoperatively.[72–75]

In a 3-year observation multicenter study of 859 women with menorrhagia treated with Nd:YAG laser ablation, 0.4 % had transient fluid overload, 0.4% had infection, and 0.3% had uterine perfora-

tion.[77] Mean operating time was 24 minutes and hospital stay was 24 hours. Of 479 patients who had at least 6 months follow-up, 60% had complete amenorrhea, 32% had continuing but satisfactorily reduced menstrual bleeding, and 8% had no improvement after the first treatment.[77] Two thirds of those with no improvement after the first surgery had improvement after the second ablation. Eventually, 3% required hysterectomy.

With the rollerball endometrial ablation for treatment of menorrhagia, a 1-year follow-up study of 77 women found that 25% were amenorrheic, 29% had staining only, 30% had light periods, 10% had "normal" periods, and 6% had unchanged menstrual bleeding.[79] Five patients (6.5%) underwent a second ablation and three subsequently had hysterectomy. In 18 women, objective measurement of blood loss showed a remarkable reduction from a mean of 104 mL to 1.7 mL 6 months after the ablation.

Thus, endometrial ablation can reduce menstrual blood loss significantly but there is a failure rate of at least 6% to 10% in experienced hands. Although endometrial ablation may spare a hysterectomy, it is doubtful that fertility is always preserved because amenorrhea is an outcome in many women. Intrauterine adhesions and Asherman's syndrome occurs in some of these amenorrheic women. Therefore, endometrial ablation is a less desirable choice than hormone or medical therapy in those women for whom fertility retention and enhancement are important considerations.

Economic comparison between endometrial resection and abdominal hysterectomy in the United Kingdom reveals that endometrial ablation has significant cost savings over abdominal hysterectomy at 2 weeks but not at 4 months after surgery.[80] Because a subgroup of women undergoing endometrial resection requires retreatment—and some even hysterectomy—the long-term costs and benefits between these two types of surgery for menorrhagia may not be different and warrant further systematic evaluation.

A new approach to endometrial ablation using radiofrequency heating is being tested. Without need for hysteroscopy, a capacitively coupled probe is inserted into the uterine cavity and the endometrium (down to the basalis layer) is heated at a power level of 550 W to 50° to 55°C for 20 minutes while the rest of the pelvic contents remain at normal body temperature.[81] Initial success rates are 84%, with 31% becoming amenorrheic and 53% having significant reduction in menstrual bleeding.[81] The advantage appears to be in (1) not requiring the hysteroscope and the necessary endoscopic skills, and (2) the avoidance of potentially toxic effects from flushing and distending the uterus with fluid.

HYSTERECTOMY. Indications for hysterectomy in the surgical treatment of menorrhagia include failed medical therapy, failed endometrial ablation, a patient whose childbearing is completed and who is fit to withstand major surgery, or a patient whose bleeding is excessive and life-threatening. If it can be properly accomplished, a vaginal approach is preferable because postoperative pain is less and recovery is quicker. To accomplish this, a laparoscope-assisted vaginal hysterectomy may be considered in some cases that would otherwise require an abdominal approach.

In a randomized controlled trial that compared 99 women undergoing endometrial resection with 97 women undergoing abdominal hysterectomy for treatment of menorrhagia, significantly more patients were in favor of hysterectomy 4 months after surgery, despite endometrial resection being associated with less morbidity in the short term.[82] It should be noted that a 10% failure rate was already observed with this short follow-up, even when the endometrial resection was considered to be complete.

REFERENCES

1. Dawood MY: Disorders of anovulatory cycles. In Clarke-Pearson DL, Dawood MY (eds): Green's gynecology: essentials of clinical practice, 4th ed, p 195. Boston, Little, Brown, 1990
2. Frisch RE: Food intake: fatness and reproductive ability. In Vigersky RA (ed): Anorexia nervosa, p 149. New York, Raven Press, 1977
3. Lindsay R, Johne J, Kanders B: The effect of oral contraceptive use on vertebral bone mass in pre- and post-menopausal women. Contraception 34: 333, 1986
4. Kleerekoper M, Brienza RS, Schultz LR, Johnson CC: Oral contraceptive may protect against low bone mass. Arch Intern Med 151:1971, 1991
5. Dawood MY, Tidey GF: Menopause. Curr Probl Obstet Gynecol Fertil 16:169, 1993
6. Biller BM, Baum HB, Rosenthal DI, Saxe VC, Charpie PM, Klibanski A: Progressive trabecular osteopenia in women with hyperprolactinemic amenorrhea. J Clin Endocrinol Metab 75:692, 1992
7. Gysler M, March CM, Mishell DR, Bailey EJ: A decade's experience with an individualized clomiphene treatment regimen including its effect on the postcoital test. Fertil Steril 37:161, 1982
8. Lunenfeld B, Vardimon D, Blankstein J: Induction of ovulation with GnRH. In Behrman SJ, Kistner RW, Patton GW (eds): Progress in infertility, 3rd ed, p 513. Boston, Little, Brown, 1988
9. American College of Obstetricians and Gynecologists: Dysfunctional uterine bleeding. American College of Obstetricians and Gynecologists Technical Bulletin 134:1, 1989
10. Dawood MY: Current approaches to dysfunctional uterine bleeding. Diagnosis 5:138, 1983
11. McDonald PG, Ganett P: Dysfunctional uterine bleeding in the adolescent. In Barron BN, Belisle BS (eds): Adolescent gynecology and sexuality. New York, Masson Publishing, 1982
12. Wilansky DL, Greisman B: Early hypothyroidism in patients with menorrhagia. Am J Obstet Gynecol 160:673, 1989
13. Smith SK, Abel MH, Kelly RW, Baird DT: A role of prostacyclin (PGI_2) in excessive menstrual bleeding. Lancet 1:522, 1981
14. Smith SK, Abel MH, Kelly RW, Baird DT: Prostaglandin synthesis in the endometrium of women with ovular dysfunctional uterine bleeding. Br J Obstet Gynaecol 88:434, 1981
15. Rees MC: Human menstruation and eicosanoids. Reprod Fertil Dev 2:467, 1990
16. Rees MCP, Anderson ABM, Demers LM, Turnbull AC: Endometrial and myometrial prostaglandin release during the menstrual cycle in relation to menstrual blood loss. J Clin Endocrinol Metab 58:813, 1984
17. Dawood MY: Nonsteroidal antiinflammatory drugs and human reproduction. Am J Obstet Gynecol 169: 1255, 1993
18. Adelantado JM, Rees MC, Lopez-Bernal A, Turnbull AC: Increased uterine prostablandine E receptors in menorrhagic women. Br J Obstet Gynaecol 95:162, 1988
19. DeVore GR, Owens O, Kase N: Use of intravenous premarin in the treatment of dysfunctional uterine bleeding—a double-blind randomized control study. Obstet Gynecol 59:255, 1982
20. Fraser IS: Treatment of ovulatory and anovulatory dysfunctional uterine bleeding with oral progestogens. Aust NZ J Obstet Gynaecol 30:353, 1990
21. Hallberg I, Nilsson L: Menstrual blood loss—a population study. Acta Obstet Gynaecol Scand 45: 320, 1966
22. Haynes PJ, Hodgson H, Anderson ABM, Turnbull AC: Measurement of menstrual blood loss in patients complaining of menorrhagia. Br J Obstet Gynaecol 84:763, 1977
23. Rees MCP, Chimbira TH, Anderson ABM, Turnbull AC: Menstrual blood loss: measurement and clinical correlates. Research and Clinical Forums 4:69, 1982
24. Chimbira TH, Anderson ABM, Turnbull AC: Relation between menstrual blood loss and patient's subjective assessment of loss, duration of bleeding, number of sanitary towels used, uterine weight and endometrial surface area. Br J Obstet Gynaecol 87:603, 1980
25. van Eijkeren MA, Scholten PC, Christiaens GCML, Alsbach GPJ, Haspels AA. The alkaline hematin method for measuring blood loss: a modification and its clinical use in menorrhagia. Eur J Obstet Gynecol Reprod Biol 22:365, 1986
26. Higham JM, O'Brien PM, Shaw RW: Assessment of menstrual blood loss using a pictorial chart. Br J Obstet Gynaecol 97:736, 1990

27. Fraser IS: Hysteroscopy and laparoscopy in women with menorrhagia. Am J Obstet Gynecol 165:1264, 1990

28. Raju GC, Naraynsingh V, Woo J, Jankey N: Adenomyosis uteri: a study of 416 cases. Aust NZ J Obstet Gynecol 28:72, 1988

29. Fedele L, Bianchi S, Dorta M, Arcaini L, Zanotti F, Carinelli S: Transvaginal ultrasonography in the diagnosis of diffuse adenomyosis. Fertil Steril 58: 94, 1992

30. McCausland AM: Hysterscopic myometrial biopsy: its use in diagnosing adenomyosis and its clinical application. Am J Obstet Gynecol 166:1619, 1992

31. Kasonde JM, Bonnar J: Aminocaproic acid and menstrual loss in women using intrauterine devices. Br Med J 4:17, 1975

32. Sahwi S, Toppozada M, Kamel M, Anwar MY, Ismail AA: Changes in menstrual blood loss after four methods of female tubal sterilization. Contraception 40:387, 1989

33. Mahmood TA, Templeton AA, Thomson L, Fraser C: Menstrual symptoms in women with pelvic endometriosis. Br J Obstet Gynaecol 98:558, 1991

34. Rybo G: Plasminogen activators in the endometrium. Acta Obstet Gynaecol Scand 45:411, 1966

35. van Eijkeren MA, Christiaens GCML, Genze JH, Haspels AA, Sixma AA: Morphology of menstrual hemostasis in essential menorrhagia. Lab Invest 64:284, 1991

36. Hourihan HM, Sheppard BL, Bonnar J: The morphologic characteristics of menstrual hemostasis in patients with unexplained menorrhagia. Int J Gynecol Pathol 8:221, 1989

37. Chandhuri G: Release of prostaglandins by IUD. Prostaglandins 3:773, 1973

38. Saksena SK, Harper MJK: Prostaglandin-mediated action of intrauterine devices: F-prostaglandins in the uterine horns of pregnant rabbits with unilateral intrauterine devices. Fertil Steril 25:121, 1974

39. Hillier K, Kasonde JM: Prostaglandin E and F contraceptives in human endometrium after insertion of intrauterine contraceptive device. Lancet 1:15, 1976

40. Toppazada M: Treatment of increased menstrual blood loss in IUD users. Contraception 36:145, 1987

41. Scholten PC, Christiaens GCML, Haspel AA: Intrauterine steroid contraception. Wien Med Wochenschr 137:497, 1987

42. Khastgir G, Mascarenhas LJ, Shaxted EJ: The role of transvaginal ultrasonography in preoperative case selection and post-operative follow-up of endometrial resection. Br J Radiol 66:600, 1993

43. Perella RR, McLucas B, Ragavendra N, Tessler FN, Schiller UL, Grant EG: Sonographic findings after surgical ablation of the endometrium. Am J Roentgenol 159:1239, 1992

44. Loffer FD: Hysteroscopy with selective endometrial sampling compared with D&C for abnormal uterine bleeding: the value of negative hysteroscopic view. Obstet Gynecol 73:16, 1989

45. Brooks PG, Serden SP: Hysteroscopic findings after unsuccessful dilatation and curettage for abnormal uterine bleeding. Am J Obstet Gynecol 158:1354, 198°

46. Andersson JK, Rybo G: Levonorgestrel-releasing intrauterine device in the treatment of menorrhagia. Br J Obstet Gynaecol 97:690, 1990

47. Anderson ABM, Haynes PJ, Guillebaud J, Turnbull AC: Reduction of menstrual blood-loss by prostaglandin-synthetase inhibitors. Lancet 1:774, 1976

48. Jakubowicz DL, Wood C: The use of the prostaglandin synthetase inhibitor mefenamic acid in the treatment of menorrhagia. Aust NZ J Obstet Gynaecol 18:135, 1978

49. Hall P, Maclachlan N, Thorn N, Nudd MWE, Taylor CG, Garrioch DB: Control of menorrhagia by the cyclo-oxygenase inhibitors naproxen sodium and mefenamic acid. Br J Obstet Gynaecol 94:554, 1987

50. Fraser IS, Pearce C, Sherman RP, Elliott PM, McIlveen J, Markham R: Efficacy of mefenamic acid in patients with a complaint of menorrhagia. Obstet Gynecol 58:543, 1981

51. Cameron IT, Haining R, Lumsden MA, Thomas VR, Smith SK: The effects of mefenamic acid and norethisterone on measured menstrual blood loss. Obstet Gynecol 76:85, 1990

52. van Eijkeren MA, Christiaens GCML, Genze HJ, Haspels AA, Sixma JJ: Effects of mefenamic acid on menstrual hemostasis in essential menorrhagia. Am J Obstet Gynecol 166:1419, 1992

53. van Eijkeren MA, Christiaens GC, Scholten PC, Sixma JJ: Menorrhagia. Current drug treatment concepts. Drugs 43:201, 1992

54. Chamberlain G, Freeman R, Price F, Kennedy A, Green D, Eve L: A comparative study of ethamsylate and mefenamic acid in dysfunctional uterine bleeding. Br J Obstet Gynaecol 98:707, 1991

55. Fraser IS, McCarron G: Randomized trial of 2 hormonal and 2 prostaglandin-inhibiting agents in women with a complaint of menorrhagia. Aust NZ J Obstet Gynaecol 31:66, 1991

56. Andersch B, Milsom I, Rybo G: An objective evaluation of flurbiprofen and tranexamic acid in the treatment of idiopathic menorrhagia. Acta Obstet Gynaecol Scand 67:645, 1988

57. Milsom I, Andersson K, Andersch B, Rybo G: A comparison of flurbiprofen, tranexamic acid, and a levonorgestrel-releasing intrauterine contraceptive device in the treatment of idiopathic menorrhagia. Am J Obstet Gynecol 164:879, 1991

58. Vargas JM, Campeau JD, Mishell DR Jr: Treatment of menorrhagia with meclofenamate sodium. Am J Obstet Gynecol 157:944, 1987

59. Roy S, Shaw ST: Role of prostaglandins in IUD-associated uterine bleeding—effects of a prostaglandin synthetase inhibitor (ibuprofen). Obstet Gynecol 58:101, 1981

60. Makarainen L, Ylikorkala O: Primary and myoma-associated menorrhagia: Role of prostaglandins and the effect of ibuprofen. Br J Obstet Gynaecol 93:974, 1986

61. Ylikorkala O, Pekonen F: Naproxen reduces idiopathic but not fibromyoma-induced menorrhagia. Obstet Gynecol 68:10, 1986

62. Pedron N, Lozano M, Gallegos AJ: The effect of acetylsalicylic acid on menstrual blood loss in women with IUDs. Contraception 36:295, 1987

63. Achirron A, Gornish M, Melamed E: Cerebral si-

nus thrombosis as potential hazard in antifibrinolytic treatment in menorrhagia. Stroke 21:817, 1990

64. Dawood MY: Considerations in selecting appropriate medical therapy for endometriosis. Int J Gynecol Obstet 40:529, 1993

65. Lamb MP: Danazol in menorrhagia: a double blind placebo controlled trial. J Obstet Gynecol 7:212, 1987

66. Bonduelle M, Walker JJ, Calder AA: A comparative study of danazol and norethisterone in dysfunctional uterine bleeding presenting as menorrhagia. Postgrad Med J 67:833, 1991

67. Need JA, Forbes KL, Milazzo L, McKenzie E: Danazol in the treatment of menorrhagia: the effect of a 1 month induction dose (200 mg) and 2 month's maintenance therapy (200 mg, 100 mg, 50 mg or placebo). Aust NZ J Obstet Gynaecol 32:346, 1992

68. Turnbull AC, Rees MCP: Gestrinone in the treatment of menorrhagia. Br J Obstet Gynaecol 97:713, 1990

69. Shaw RW, Fraser HM: Use of a superactive luteinizing hormone releasing hormone (LHRH) agonist in the treatment of menorrhagia. Br J Obstet Gynaecol 91:913, 1984

70. Fedorkow DM, Corenblum B, Shaffer EA: The use of a gonadotropin-releasing analog and transdermal estrogen to preserve fertility in a woman with menorrhagia. Fertil Steril 52:512, 1989

71. Thomas EJ, Okuda KJ, Thomas NM: The combination of a depot gonadotrophin releasing hormone agonist and cyclical hormone replacement therapy for dysfunctional uterine bleeding. Br J Obstet Gynaecol 98:1155, 1991

72. Brooks PG, Serden SP, Davos I: Hormonal inhibition of the endometrium for resectoscopic endometrial ablation. Am J Obstet Gynecol 164:1601, 1991

73. Petrucco OM, Fraser IS: The potential for the use of GnRH agonists for treatment of dysfunctional uterine bleeding. Br J Obstet Gynaecol 99:34, 1992

74. Perino A, Chianchiano N, Petronio M, Cittadini E: Role of leuprolide acetate depot in hysteroscopic surgery: a controlled study. Fertil Steril 59:507, 1993

75. Goldrath MH, Fuller TA, Segal S: Laser photovaporization of endometrium for the treatment of menorrhagia. Am J Obstet Gynecol 140:14, 1981

76. Goldfarb HA: A review of 35 endometrial ablations using the Nd-YAG laser for recurrent menometrorrhagia. Obstet Gynecol 76:833, 1990

77. Garry R, Erian J, Grochmal SA: A multicenter collaborative study into the treatment of menorrhagia by Nd-YAG laser ablation of the endometrium. Br J Obstet Gynaecol 98:357, 1991

78. DeCherney AH, Diamond MP, Lavy G, Polan ML: Endometrial ablation for intractable uterine bleeding: hysteroscopic resection. Obstet Gynecol 70:668, 1987

79. Fraser IS, Angsuwathana S, Mahmoud F, Yezerski S: Short and medium term outcomes after rollerball endometrium ablation for menorrhagia. Med J Aust 158:454, 1993

80. Sculpher MJ, Bryan S, Dwyer N, Hutton J, Stirrat GM: An economic evaluation of transvaginal endometrial resection versus abdominal hysterectomy for the treatment of menorrhagia. Br J Obstet Gynaecol 100:244, 1993

81. Prior MV, Phipps JH, Roberts T, Lewis BU, Hand JW, Field SB: Treatment of menorrhagia by radiofrequency heating. Int J Hyperthermia 7:213, 1991

82. Dwyer N, Hutton J, Stirrat GM: Randomized controlled trial comparing endometrial resection with abdominal hysterectomy for the surgical treatment of menorrhagia. Br J Obstet Gynaecol 100:237, 1993

Ambulatory Gynecology, Second Edition,
edited by David H. Nichols and Patrick J. Sweeney.
J. B. Lippincott Company, Philadelphia, © 1995.

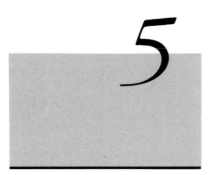

Noninfectious Diseases of the Vulva

J. Donald Woodruff and David C. Foster

HISTOLOGY

Knowledge of the histology of an area contributes to an understanding of the disease processes that affect that area. Because the vulva is of ectodermal origin, the histopathologic alterations are similar to those seen on skin elsewhere. Conversely, they are different from those of the cervix and upper genital canal. Consequently, attempts to correlate the clinicopathology of disease in the paramesonephric system with vulvar lesions often lead to inaccurate evaluation and treatment. The epithelium of the vulva is stratified squamous. Keratinization is present on the labia majora; the labia minora, although similarly stratified, demonstrate less keratinization, except under chronically irritative conditions. The underlying appendages of the labia majora are similar to those seen in the skin elsewhere (Color Fig. 5-1). The basal epithelial layer of the labia—in contrast to that of the cervix—is irregular, with "pegs" dipping into the underlying stroma. The latter is divided into (1) the papillary dermis (immediately below the papillae or rete ridges); (2) the subjacent reticular dermis; and (3) the deepest layer, subcutaneous adipose tissue. These zones are of patho-

logic significance in identifying the depth of invasion, particularly of melanoma. Accentuation of the rete pegs (acanthosis) is a hallmark of chronic dermatitis and the hyperplastic dystrophies.

In the subepithelial tissues, a variety of glands may be recognized. On the labia majora, there are (1) the classic sebaceous glands, secreting along the hair follicles, (2) the common eccrine sweat gland, providing moisture for the skin, and (3) the unique apocrine glands. The latter are found in specific areas—namely, the axillae, the perianal zone, the external genitalia, and the breasts—and begin to secrete at menarche and continue cyclically in the female throughout the menstrual years. These glands may be occluded or infected and thereby produce major problems. They are absent for the most part on the labia minora, as are hair follicles. The labia minora, however, have an abundant number of sebaceous glands that secrete directly onto the skin. The importance of these glands in the identification of certain physiologic and pathologic processes is discussed later.

The vascular supply of the vulva comes primarily from the pudendal vessels, entering the area just above and lateral to the fourchette. Branches extend inferiorly to the anal orifice (the hemorrhoidal vessels) and anteriorly to the clitoris. A small supply comes from the pampiniform plexus along the inguinal canal. The nerve supply is primarily from the pudendal nerve and the ilioinguinal and genitofemoral nerves.

There are specialized glands at the introitus or vestibule (Color Fig. 5-2). The orifice of the major (Bartholin's) gland (corresponding to Cowper's gland in the male urethra) lies just above and lateral to the fourchette. The minor vestibular glands, corresponding to male Littre's glands, have their orifices immediately lateral to the hymenal ring. Infection of the latter may produce dyspareunia as a result of constriction of the outlet due to edema and scarring of the hymeneal ring. The major gland is commonly infected, with the resultant abscess formation producing severe, acute local pain.

TRAUMA

The common causes of trauma in the first 2 decades of life are those associated with direct injury incurred by a fall astride a rigid structure such as the bar of a bicycle or a fence railing. To these traumas must be added sexual molestations, which most commonly occur in teenagers and women in their 20s.

The local trauma produced by a fall astride a bicycle bar usually results in a hematoma (Color Fig. 5-3). The patient should be examined thoroughly because hemorrhage may be active at the time of initial examination and may extend deep into the ischiorectal fossa in addition to the lower abdominal wall. Fascial planes determine the extent of the bleeding. If the bleeding is active, the period of convalescence may be reduced by simple incision and ligation of the vessel, with drainage of the accumulated blood. Knowledge of the vulvar blood supply is mandatory if such a procedure is to be performed. Because the pudendal vessels are primarily involved, the incision should be at the site where they enter the vulva, just above and lateral to the fourchette. Occasionally, the vessels that accompany the round ligament may be the source of the bleeding; in women, unlike men, these vessels are small in comparison with the pudendal vasculature.

If the hematoma is large, it may impinge on the urethra, causing urinary retention. Such a complication is best treated with an indwelling catheter. If this is necessary, antibiotics or chemotherapeutic agents such as trimethoprim plus sulfamethoxazole may be used to avoid urinary tract infection. Most vulvar hematomas should be treated conservatively, using local ice packs rather than heat. The addition of cool compresses (with Burow's solution of aluminum acetate) reduces the swelling. Bed rest and sedation for a short time are indicated. It is generally unnecessary to employ antibiotics routinely unless the patient has a fever above 100°F. All patients with extravasation of blood into the tissues have some local response to the irritation in the form of a low-grade fever.

The trauma of sexual molestation or overly vigorous sexual activity usually consists of lacerations in the vagina and at the fourchette. Occasionally, the injury extends into the rectum or bladder. The injury should be identified promptly and repaired at the time of the initial evaluation. The urethra is rarely involved but catheterization may be necessary if surgery to the vulva and rectum is indicated. Appropriate antibiotic therapy must be instituted, particularly if there has been bowel injury. Finally, the psychosexual aspects of the problem must be addressed if recurrences are to be avoided.

A form of "ritual" trauma can be found in some emigres from areas of northern Africa who have undergone female circumcision. The extensiveness of these procedures may vary from partial loss of the prepuce to complete loss of prepuce, labia minora, and labia majora. Such procedures have been performed without specific medical indications; with education, the number of such procedures is declining.

Rarely, injury may result from an attempt to insert a foreign body into the vagina. For example, Coke bottles and small glass jars have been found occluding the entire vagina. They may be removed easily, particularly if the vagina is adequate and the glass is firm; however, if such a procedure is not simple, the patient should be anesthetized to minimize any additional trauma due to the procedure. Major lacerations may occur on insertion or withdrawal of the foreign body. Such injuries must be identified immediately to control bleeding and allow primary closure. In most instances of a foreign body in the vagina, the patient is inebriated, psychologically disturbed, or involved in a psychosexual aberration. The one exception to this is the pediatric patient. An accurate history and careful follow-up are mandatory in these cases.

INFLAMMATORY DISEASE

The dermatitides and the dermatoses primarily affect the labia majora. Dermatosis includes a wide variety of local diseases and dermatitis and thus is not a specific disorder.[1] The common afflictions are reactive or contact in origin, previously known as eczema or atopic dermatitis; nevertheless, essentially all varieties of dermatitis have been described on the vulva and careful evaluation of the patient for other foci and a complete history are essential if an accurate diagnosis is to be made.

Reactive Dermatitis

Reactive lesions are due to a wide variety of local agents, such as those used for local hygiene (sprays and lotions); cleansing agents (detergents or strong soaps); colored or perfumed toilet paper; tight-fitting, nonabsorbent underclothing and slacks; bubble bath; and bath oils (Color Fig. 5-4). Local anesthetic agents are often prescribed for such lesions; unfortunately, they may magnify the problem as a result of the patient's sensitivity to the agent or the base in which it is dispensed.

An adjacent vaginitis may also be a cause of reactive dermatitis. Many irritating discharges produce reactive alterations. Thus, it is imperative that areas adjacent to the lesion be examined, so that appropriate therapy may be instituted. The watery vaginal discharge often seen in women of postmenopausal age is commonly due to a thin, irritated vaginal mucosa. The cause of the local or systemic irritation should be recognized and eliminated. Therapy for the symptom commonly consists of a topical fluorinated corticosteroid. The patient should avoid prolonged use of topical corticosteroids in order to prevent fibrosis of the underlying dermis. The adjacent vagina should also be treated with a topical estrogen. A minimal amount of estrogen inserted into the vagina two to three times a month is usually sufficient to maintain the tissues in good condition and eliminate the possibility of other estrogen-induced alterations such as endometrial proliferation.

Because of a relative deficiency of estrogen receptors on the vulva and vestibule, estrogen is not effective for the treatment of vulvar and vestibular lesions.[2]

Despite symptoms commonly localized to the vulva, patients commonly state that they have "chronic vaginitis." This condition is relatively rare except among prepubertal or postmenopausal patients. The symptom of pruritus, associated with the initial episode of vaginitis, is interpreted by patients as an indication of a recurrent vaginal infection. Similarly, the physician may interpret recurrent or persistent pruritus as an indication of adjacent vaginal infection and may continue to give the patient a multiplicity of intravaginal agents when the problem is actually a dermatitis. Thus, it is imperative not to make a "telephone diagnosis" and institute inappropriate therapy; not only does this not improve the symptoms, it is also psychologically destructive because the patient's symptoms continue to persist.

A chronic irritating discharge from the vagina in a prepubertal child should alert the physician to the possibility of a foreign body. Children are frequently diagnosed as having chronic dermatitis without the cause of the irritation being thoroughly investigated. A bloody, watery discharge in the child should be evaluated accurately because it may be a harbinger of the rare but aggressive vaginal tumor, sarcoma botryoides. On most occasions, a thorough washing of the vagina by saline solution introduced through a soft rubber catheter demonstrates the presence of the foreign material. Vaginoscopy or cystoscopy (used vaginally) may be considered if the symptoms persist.

Chronic Dermatitis

Chronic vulvar dermatitis is extremely common, as is its acute counterpart. The vulva is exposed constantly to a variety of local irritants such as clothing, vulvar secretions, urine (particularly in the patient with incontinence or fistula), fecal contamination, menstrual effluvium, and secretions from the specialized glands. The thickening and hyperkeratosis associated with chronic dermatitis may prevent absorption of the local medications used effectively in the treatment of acute dermatitis. The fluorinated hydrocortisones are still the initial treatment of choice but because of malabsorption may not be as effective as in acute dermatitis. Other approaches must therefore be considered. The superficial excoriation associated with chronic irritation may allow the ingress of various infective agents, which over time may produce irreversible histopathologic changes. As a result of hyperkeratosis, the skin surface become gray or grayish-white in color and thus resembles the so-called leukoplakia (Color Fig. 5-5).

If the application of topical steroids is effective for a few hours, triamcinolone acetonide may be injected subcutaneously (1 mL equals 10 mg per GG), with effect lasting longer than 1 year.[3]

The term leukoplakia has been so poorly used over the years that it should be eliminated as a specific diagnosis for vulvar disease. It basically means

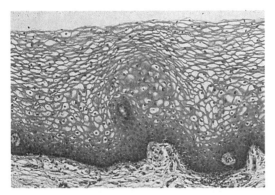

Color Figure 5–1.

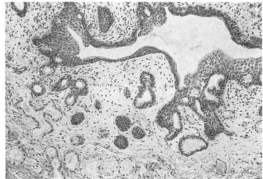

Color Figure 5–2.

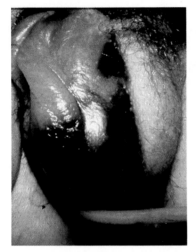

Color Figure 5–3.

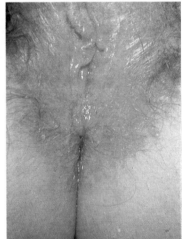

Color Figure 5–4.

Color Figure 5–1.   Normal stratified squamous epithelium of the vulva.

Color Figure 5–2.   Microscopic example of Bartholin's duct and glands.

Color Figure 5–3.   Example of labial trauma with developing hematoma.

Color Figure 5–4.   Erythema seen in acute vulvitis.

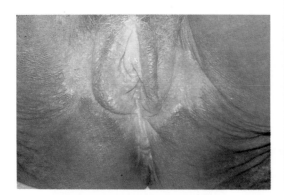

Color Figure 5–5.

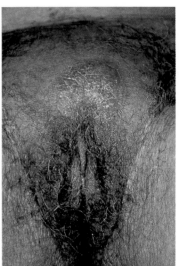

Color Figure 5–6.

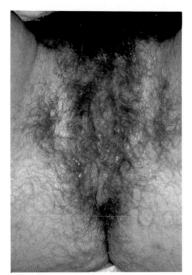

Color Figure 5–7.

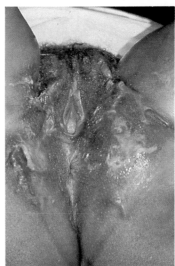

Color Figure 5–8.

Color Figure 5–5. Skin changes associated with chronic vulvitis.

Color Figure 5–6. Sharply demarcated foci seen in tinea cruris.

Color Figure 5–7. Vulvar involvement with psoriasis.

Color Figure 5–8. Multiple draining sinuses of hidradenitis suppurativa.

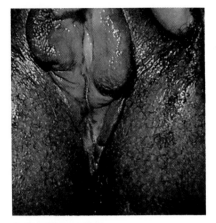

Color Figure 5–9.

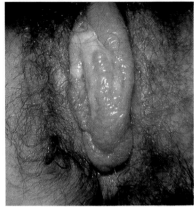

Color Figure 5–10.

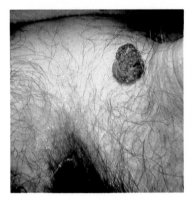

Color Figure 5–11.

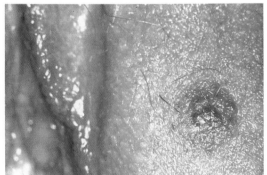

Color Figure 5–12.

Color Figure 5–9.   Inflammation and lymphedema found in Crohn's disease.

Color Figure 5–10.   Decubitus ulcer of the vulva in a hemiplegic patient.

Color Figure 5–11.   Pigmented and raised lesion of seborrheic keratosis.

Color Figure 5–12.   Lentigo of the vulva.

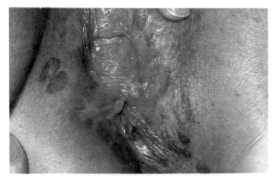

Color Figure 5–13.

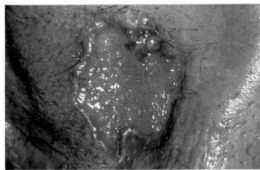

Color Figure 5–14.

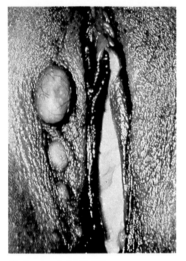

Color Figure 5–15.

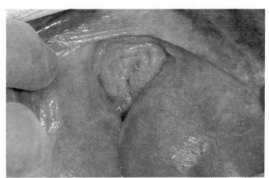

Color Figure 5–16.

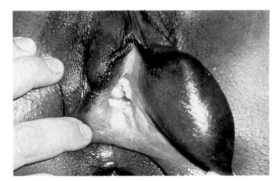

Color Figure 5–17.

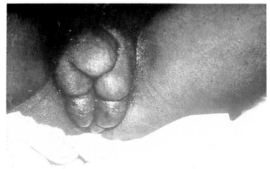

Color Figure 5–18.

Color Figure 5–13. Pigmented lesion of carcinoma-in-situ of the vulva (VIN).

Color Figure 5–14. Erosive appearance of basal cell carcinoma of the vulva.

Color Figure 5–15. Multiple epidermal inclusion cysts.

Color Figure 5–16. Cyst of the Bartholin's gland.

Color Figure 5–17. Hydrocele of the vulva.

Color Figure 5–18. Vulvar edema in pregnancy.

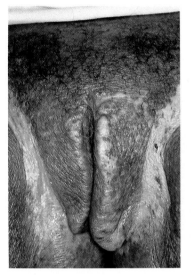

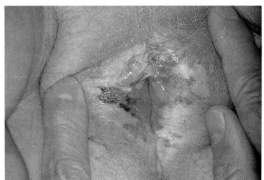

Color Figure 5–19.

Color Figure 5–20.

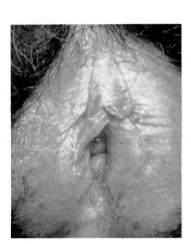

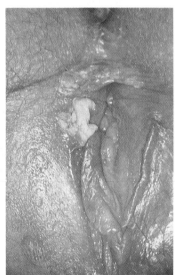

Color Figure 5–21.

Color Figure 5–22.

Color Figure 5–19. Leukoderma of the vulva arising in irritative focus of the vulva.

Color Figure 5–20. Lichen sclerosus of the vulva demonstrating scarring and superficial ecchymosis.

Color Figure 5–21. Mixed dystrophy of the vulva.

Color Figure 5–22. Abnormal coloration indicating an area (VIN) which should be biopsied.

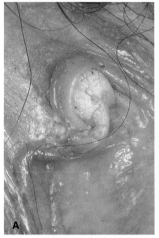

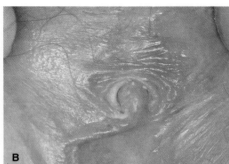

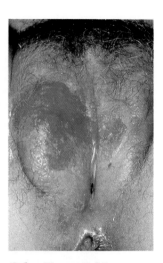

Color Figure 5–23.

Color Figure 5–24.

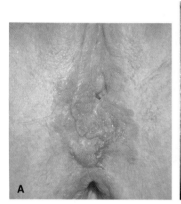

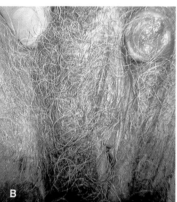

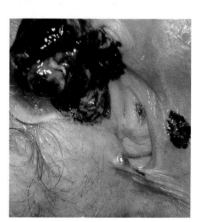

Color Figure 5–25.

Color Figure 5–26.

Color Figure 5–23. (**A**) VIN of the clitoris. (**B**) Clitoris after 6-week course of interferon.

Color Figure 5–24. Brick-red coloration of Paget's disease of the vulva.

Color Figure 5–25. (**A**) One presentation of invasive carcinoma of the vulva. (**B**) Variation of a presentation of invasive carcinoma of the vulva.

Color Figure 5–26. Malignant melanoma of the vulva.

only "white patch," and any lesion that is hyperkeratotic becomes white, whether it is due to chronic dermatitis or invasive cancer. Although the term was initially applied to lesions in the buccal mucous membranes, it was subsequently used to describe many white lesions of the vulva—most commonly chronic dermatitis, lichen sclerosus, and similar benign hyperkeratotic lesions. As a result, many unnecessary vulvectomies were performed because the lesions were thought to be premalignant. The term has since been eliminated by the International Society for the Study of Vulvar Disease (ISSVD) in favor of a more specific designation, "the dystrophies."

Biopsy of chronically irritated tissues should be performed, with concentration on ulcerative, erythematous, pigmented, or elevated white lesions. The latter classically show hyperkeratosis, acanthosis (elongation of the rete pegs), and a chronic inflammatory infiltrate. Atypical proliferation, demonstrated by the presence of increased mitotic activity or abnormal maturation, is absent. Thus, there is no malignant potential. Nevertheless, it seems possible that over a period of many years, the chronic irritation may convert a benign into a premalignant process as a result of metabolic disturbances produced by the fingernail. Thus, it is of importance that the symptoms be eliminated and the extent of the histologic abnormality be assessed accurately.

Because of the marked hyperkeratosis seen in many types of chronic dermatitis, the topical application of fluorinated hydrocortisones may be unsuccessful in alleviating pruritus. The steroid may alternatively be injected subcutaneously (intralesionally), by which route it becomes available to the underlying tissue (specifically, the nerve endings). Triamcinolone acetonide, 30 mg (3 mL), can be injected into an area of about 12 cm.[3] The agent is rubbed in thoroughly so that it is dispersed into the tissues. This approach alleviates the pruritus in about 80% to 90% of cases, with relief lasting for 1 year. If the "scratch–itch reflex" is broken, the relief may last even longer.

Occasionally, the above approach is unsuccessful and other measures must be taken. Injection of alcohol in the area produces relief in recalcitrant cases. This procedure necessitates general anesthesia and hospitalization for 24 hours. There is a recognized surgical risk of sloughing of the vulvar skin with inadvertent deep injection of absolute alcohol. Furthermore, the patient routinely complains of numbness and swelling in the area for about 3 to 4 weeks thereafter. Nevertheless, alcohol injection almost routinely eliminates vulvar pruritus for at least 6 months to 1 year and occasionally, permanently. Finally, if the above procedures fail, denervation as suggested by Mering is worthy of consideration.[3a] The procedure is extensive, consisting of a long incision severing the nerves that lead into the vulva from the level of the clitoris to the fourchette. The recovery period is long and hospitalization is usually required for at least 2 to 3 days. The procedure is effective, however, and usually eliminates the symptoms for a period of 3 or more years.

Other Inflammatory Lesions

Seborrhea or seborrheic dermatitis (dandruff) is frequent on the vulva and usually appears on the mons and above the prepuce. Because these areas are sometimes poorly studied, the lesions may not be identified easily. It is therefore important to ask the patient to identify specifically the area in which the symptoms are present. Treatment basically consists of elimination of the itch, which may be most easily accomplished by the use of the fluorinated hydrocortisones. In recalcitrant cases, treatments for dandruff at other sites such as selenium sulfide may be employed.

A more extreme form of seborrheic dermatitis is seen in obese diabetics. The lesions, know as intertrigo or intertriginous dermatitis, classically appear as thickening and cracking of the skin in the crural and intralabial folds. Because the vulva of the diabetic is always irritated and commonly erythematous, additional cracking and splitting of the tissues make the pruritus more of a problem than usual. The area must be kept dry, an almost impossible feat. A combination of cornstarch and baby powder is probably the most effective preparation to accomplish the drying. As noted, biopsy is important to ensure that the chronic irritation has not produced abnormal, sometimes irreversible, histologic changes in the tissue. The diabetes must be kept under as satisfactory control as possible.

Lichen Planus

This painful erosive condition of unknown etiology affects the mouth with a lacy-appearing white plaque and the vulva with a violaceous plaque and labial fusion at later stages. The diagnosis can be confirmed by immunofluorescence directed toward the fibrillar fibrin deposition along the basement membrane of affected tissue (Fig. 5-1). Topical flu-

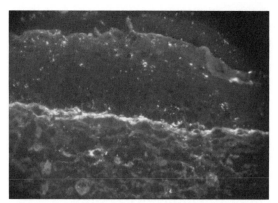

Figure 5–1.   Immunofluorescence of basement membrane seen in lichen planus.

orinated or subcutaneous corticosteroids continue to be the treatment of choice. Successful therapeutic trials with topical cyclosporine have recently been reported.[4]

Tinea

Tinea (cruris or versicolor) is occasionally seen in the vulvar and perianal areas. Similar foci may be found at other sites, particularly the feet. The lesion is characterized by slightly elevated, sharply demarcated erythematous foci, with accentuated skin markings (lichenification; Color Fig. 5-6). The associated pruritus is intense. Diagnosis can be made by the examination of scraped material under the microscope. The fungi can usually be identified readily. The lesion grossly, however, is so specific that laboratory tests are often unnecessary. Tinea versicolor is occasionally seen on the vulva, although its most common site is between the breasts. The term versicolor refers to the fact that coloration does vary but classically, the lesion is brownish and scaly. Routinely, tinea versicolor is asymptomatic. Clotrimazole is the most commonly suggested therapy for tinea cruris. Tolnaftate, haloprogin, and miconazole nitrate are also effective agents.

Psoriasis

Psoriasis, common elsewhere on the body, is rarely seen on the vulva. Skin lesions are characterized by irregular, multifocal patches having an erythematous background and elevated silver scales. The extragenital tissues demonstrate linear excoriation (accentuation of the skin markings or lichenification). Such classic appearances are found on raised dry skin surfaces. The moisture of the vulvar lesion disrupts the scales, making the resultant dermatitis diffusely erythematous and nonspecific in appearance (Color Fig. 5-7). Thus, to make the appropriate diagnosis, it is important to appreciate the difference between the lesions seen on the vulva and their counterparts elsewhere on the body.

It is known that a hereditary factor is involved in psoriasis. Nevertheless, this factor has not been helpful in the management of psoriasis-associated pruritus. Topical hydrocortisone is helpful but it is often necessary to resort to more astringent medications.

Phototherapy with or without adjunctive retinoid therapy has been effective in other areas of the body.[5] Due to the difficulty of getting phototherapy to the area of the vulva, such treatment for vulvar psoriasis is less effective.

Hidradenitis

Hidradenitis is an inflammation in the specialized apocrine glands seen on the vulva, in the perianal area, and in the axillae. Although the breast is a modified apocrine gland, the dramatic clinical features are rarely seen in the breast.

Because these specialized glands secrete cyclically, the disease commonly flares up premenstrually. Consequently, oral contraceptives (which reduce secretions in the apocrine system during the progestational phase of the cycle) may be helpful in the treatment of the lesions. Nevertheless, in patients with chronic suppurative hidradenitis, such agents are of little assistance, although they may be used as adjunctive forms of therapy.

Classically, patients with extensive inflammatory disease (hidradenitis suppurativa) have draining sinuses in the vulva, mons, and adjacent perineum (Color Fig. 5-8). Although conservative therapy (antibiotics, local heat) may be tried, it is commonly necessary to debride the area because of the intercommunication of the sinus tracts. When performing such procedures, it is important to remember that the prepuce and labia minora rarely contain apocrine glands and thus can usually be spared. Excision of infected intercommunicating sinuses, leaving "bridges" of normal intervening tissue, is the therapy of choice. This prevents, to a degree, the extensive scarring and distortion that may follow vulvectomy. Antibiotics are to be used as indicated, although such agents alone are not curative because of the deep-seated nature of the infection.

Fox–Fordyce Disease

Fox–Fordyce disease is a pruritic affliction characterized by small, sometimes almost imperceptible maculopapular lesions involving the labia majora, mons, and perianal areas. The process is primarily due to occlusion of the apocrine glands, without major degrees of inflammatory reaction. Consequently, oral contraceptives, which reduce the secretion in the glands, are the treatment of choice. In certain cases, however, the severe pruritus is recalcitrant and the fluorinated hydrocortisones may be helpful, either topically or subcutaneously. Finally, on rare occasions some type of nerve block, such as alcohol injection or the Mering procedure, may be necessary to control the symptoms.[3a]

Crohn's Disease

Crohn's disease in the perianal area of the female is common. It is estimated that about 25% of patients with gastrointestinal Crohn's disease demonstrate some abnormality in the perianal area, usually draining sinus or fistulas. Rarely, the local lesions may be present without any demonstration of intestinal involvement. The classic features are draining sinuses in the posterior fourchette and perianal areas, linear excoriations in these areas, and lymphedema (Color Fig. 5-9). It is important to make an accurate diagnosis to institute the appropriate therapy. Incision or excision of draining sinuses without preoperative therapy simply produces additional problems. Furthermore, surgery without preoperative therapy for the lesions in the anal orifice may result in total breakdown of the septum, with loss of sphincter control. Biopsy often identifies an inflammatory reaction, with noncaseating granulomas. Patients should be investigated for the presence of intestinal Crohn's disease and should be treated medically before undergoing surgery. The appropriate medications are systemic cortisone and metronidazole. Approximately 20 mg/day of prednisone plus 20 mg/kg per day of metronidazole in divided doses for 1 month to 6 weeks before surgery reduces the possibility of complications. Medication should be continued for at least 2 to 3 months postoperatively, although the dosage of prednisone may be reduced. Follow-up is man-

datory, and most physicians continue a maintenance dose of prednisone indefinitely.

Systemic Disease

Diabetes classically demonstrates itself in the vulvar area as a diffuse, pruritic, erythematous lesion. In the chronic phase, the usual hyperkeratosis appears with the associated grayish-white change.

ULCERATIVE LESIONS

Many of the lesions already discussed, including the granulomatous diseases, Crohn's disease, and traumatic lesions, appear initially as ulcers. Certain ulcers do not fall into any of these categories, however.

Tuberculosis

Tuberculosis is an inflammatory process that is rare in the vulvar area. Nevertheless, it should be considered as a potential cause of the recalcitrant inflammatory ulcerations. Ulcerations are frequently seen in the vagina or at the outlet rather than in the vulvar skin. Thorough physical examination commonly reveals the presence of pulmonary disease. The diagnosis is confirmed locally by biopsy and the subsequent finding of the classic tubercles. Treatment is similar to that for pulmonary tuberculosis.

Behçet's Disease

Behçet's disease is relatively nonspecific in its initial appearance. Nevertheless, the presence of similar ulcerations on the buccal mucous membrane (Fig. 5-2) and the occasional involvement of the eye (iridocyclitis) help establish the diagnosis.

The lesions are sharply marginated, with a grayish-white necrotic center. The disease is characterized by spontaneous remissions and recurrences. Patients often give a history of intermittent ulcerations over a period of many years. The lesions are generally asymptomatic; however, they may be locally destructive. Ophthalmologic infections are the most serious, possibly leading to blindness and in some cases infection of the central nervous system, which usually results in death. Patients often develop recurrent arthritis, with the usual accompa-

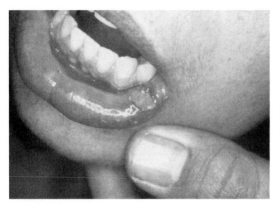

Figure 5–2. Oral mucosal ulcer in Behçet's disease.

nying disability. The presentation may not necessarily include all criteria for inclusion into a diagnostic category of incomplete Behçet's disease. Such presentations often lack uveitis and iritis.[6] Biopsy of the lesions often reveals dramatic vasculitis, suggesting that the disease is of the autoimmune variety. Consequently, systemic cortisone is the treatment of choice. Some investigators believe that the lesions of Behçet's disease are of viral origin but virus has not been identified in the tissue of any patient. In isolated instances, oral contraceptive therapy has been used with temporary results; however, because the disease is prone to spontaneous remission, all therapies must be viewed with skepticism.

Aphthous Ulcers

Aphthous ulcers are common in the vulva but are usually superficial and relatively asymptomatic. They may be the result of trauma to the vulvar skin (eg, from rough protective pads used during menstruation) and can be treated by local applications of silver nitrate. More serious disease should be ruled out before this diagnosis is reached, particularly if the lesion is nonhealing or associated with lymphadenitis.

Ecthyma

Ecthyma is a proliferative infectious lesion that simulates condylomata lata but is probably a variety of folliculitis. Darkfield microscopic studies and serology should performed to eliminate syphilis as the causative agent.

Lipschütz Ulcer

The original description of this poorly identified lesion may well have been that of an aphthous ulcer; however, larger and more destructive lesions (particularly that known as esthiomene) were also included in the category. Esthiomene was a "wastebasket" term often used to refer to malignancy but primarily associated with lymphogranuloma. Because of lack of specificity of the concept and the sophisticated techniques available for diagnosis, the category "Lipschütz ulcer" should be eliminated.

Other Ulcerative Lesions

Several other varieties of ulceration may occur in the vulva. The patient with psychiatric problems, particularly those related to sexual aberrations, may have factitious (self-induced) lesions. This cause must be considered if all other possible causes of the problem have been carefully eliminated. Occasionally, the diagnosis can only be made by admission of the patient to the hospital and careful observation of her habits. Decubitus ulcers, although rare, may occasionally be seen in patients with some major disturbance of blood supply to the lower extremities and adjacent area (Color Fig. 5-10). A new ulcerative process has been recognized in women with acquired immunodeficiency syndrome. These ulcers appear erosive, often result in rectovaginal fistulae, and defy surgical correction. Both etiology and effective therapy remain unclear. There is one report, however, of successful treatment with zidovudine.[7]

Finally, pemphigus, Darier's disease, and Hailey-Hailey disease have been noted on the vulva. Biopsy, which is mandatory for all ulcerative lesions, often demonstrates the presence of acantholysis. In this condition, the superficial epithelium is divorced from the basal layer and small cells with dark nuclei and perinuclear halo (corps ronds) are recognized in this zone of separation. Histologic diagnosis can be aided through the use of immunofluorescence.[8] These lesions are extremely difficult to treat and may require surgery. The significance of an inherited disease must always be kept in mind and the family carefully investigated.

BENIGN TUMORS

Benign Solid Tumors

Tumors that occur elsewhere on the skin may also be found on the vulva. In most instances, the lesions are asymptomatic and are noted by the patient only as a lump or bump. Although the clinician is usually convinced that the lesion is benign, a positive diagnosis commonly cannot be established unless the lesion is removed and subjected to histopathologic interpretation. Such biopsies relieve the patient's anxieties regarding the nature of the lump and establish an accurate diagnosis.

Acrochordon

A fibroepithelial polyp is recognized as a soft, fleshy, pedunculated lesion, generally causing no symptoms (Fig. 5-3). If the patient is concerned about its presence, the lesion should be removed. Generally, excision can be accomplished easily with the patient under local infiltrative anesthesia. If there is any discoloration or thickening at the

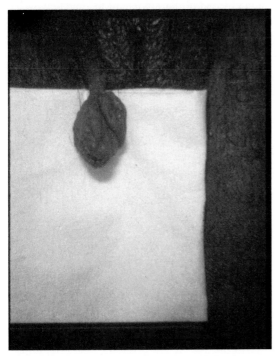

Figure 5–3. Example of a fibroepithelial polyp (acrochordon).

base of the lesion, it is wise to excise the lesion widely and orient the specimen properly in fixative so that an accurate diagnosis can be made.

Seborrheic Keratosis

Seborrheic keratosis is a common brownish lesion, generally seen on the trunk and back. It is asymptomatic and frequently can be evulsed by scratching or other trauma. On the vulva and adjacent areas, the lesions may become deeply pigmented and grossly suggest melanoma (Color Fig. 5-11). If there is any question to the diagnosis, the lesions should be removed for histopathologic study. The classic picture is that of a lesion elevated above the adjacent normal epithelium, demonstrating marked epithelial proliferation with keratotic foci or "horn cysts." The latter are simply inclusions of keratin that lie above the base of the lesion, demonstrating that the lesion is superficial to the normal surface. Because these lesions have no malignant potential, additional therapy is unnecessary.

Pigmented Lesions

Pigmented alterations on the vulvar skin represent a tremendously varied group of histopathologic lesions—from simple lentigines, which simulate a freckle, to malignant melanoma.

Lentigines, amelanotic spots, appear similar to the freckle (Color Fig. 5-12). Nevertheless, lesions of a similar nature may be carcinoma in situ (Color Fig. 5-13). The focal pigmented lesions do not demonstrate any gross alterations that would differentiate one from the other. Consequently, biopsy is mandatory for differentiation of malignant and potentially malignant lesions.

The slightly elevated melanotic lesion should always undergo biopsy. Whereas a flat alteration found in lentigines appears benign because it does not alter the architecture of the vulva, an elevated lesion is always suspect and must be removed with a wide margin. An "ABCD rule" has been described as criteria raising suspicion of the presence of a melanoma. These criteria include: *A*symmetry of the lesion, irregular *B*order, variegated *C*olor, and *D*iameter greater than 6 mm (larger than a pencil eraser).[9]

Microscopically, alterations vary from the intradermal nevus to changes that show junction activity. The latter may reveal both intradermal and junction components. It was previously thought that the compound nevus, which demonstrates junction activity, had some malignant potential. Although junction alterations are occasionally seen in malignant melanoma, such activity is not diagnostic of a malignant melanoma or potentially malignant lesion.

As mentioned, seborrheic keratosis is a great masquerader. Its lesions are frequently almost black, simulating melanoma. Interestingly, the pigmentation in such lesions is more common on the vulva than elsewhere on the skin.

Finally, tumors demonstrating atypical proliferation vary from atypical melanocytic hyperplasia to malignant melanoma. Biopsy is mandatory if appropriate therapy is to be instituted. In the International Association of Gynecologic Pathologists (IAGP) terminology, the term melanoma in situ is used for the pathologic finding of atypical melanocytic hyperplasia. This is unfortunate terminology because of the less aggressive behavior of this lesion.

Hidradenoma

A confusing lesion rarely more than 1 to 1.5 cm in diameter, hidradenoma classically appears in the interlabial sulcus. Occasionally, these lesions are extruded spontaneously through the duct to lie detached on the surface. They are easily removed by simple excision and often "pop out," having an apparently well-defined capsule. In spite of their benign gross appearance, the histopathology may be confusing, characterized by a complex papillary–adenomatous pattern, suggestively aggressive. Nevertheless, mitoses are absent. The surface epithelium comprises two cell types: a flattened cuboidal basal layer and a superficial large ovoid cell with brilliant eosinophilic cytoplasm. The latter, the classic element that is "decapitated," is composed largely of lipid. Occasionally, there is also a flattened subepithelial layer, the so-called myoepithelial cell. In spite of their intricate pattern, these lesions are benign and need no postoperative therapy. Rarely, a case of hidradenocarcinoma has been reported but this lesion is poorly documented. Most adenomatous malignancies in the vulva are metastatic cancers, usually from an endometrial primary lesion. Hidradenomas are routinely solitary lesions, although multiple nodules have been recognized occasionally, particularly near the anal orifice. It is suggested that hidradenomas do not occur in blacks but exceptions to this rule have occasionally been recorded.

Accessory Breast Tissue

Because the vulva is in the "milk line," breast tissue may be recognized both in the vulva and in the lower abdomen along the inguinal canal. These extramammary foci may enlarge with pregnancy; excision is unnecessary and even contraindicated. Any operation on the vulva during pregnancy is hazardous because of potentially excessive bleeding. On biopsy, the breast tissue can be readily identified histopathologically. During pregnancy, it may lactate. At least seven carcinomas of the breast have been diagnosed in the inguinal and upper vulvar regions.

Vascular Lesions

Congenital hemangiomata may appear in children on the vulva and other areas of the body such as the head, neck, back, and lower extremities. If a local lesion is recognized, the child should be investigated for other foci. The latter usually appear in the second or third month of life and may be extensive. Surgery should be avoided because excessive bleeding may occur, with resultant disfiguring scars. The lesions almost routinely regress spontaneously and rarely need treatment. Liquid nitrogen or "carbon dioxide snow" may be applied to the area in minute quantities. Because the resultant slough may produce bleeding, a temporizing approach is recommended.

Hemangiomas may appear in persons of any age. The small, reddish lesion, or cherry hemangioma, is brilliantly red and usually flat. It needs no therapy. In the postmenopausal patient, keratin may appear on the surface of the hemangioma, so that it appears white with a red background. The lesion is then known as keratohemagioma and usually can be readily identified because of its reddish base with the "white cap."[10] Unless there is a question as to whether it is a pigmented tumor, excision is unnecessary. Conversely, it can be easily fulgurated if bleeding takes place.

Finally, numerous small reddish elevations may develop, usually on both labia. These lesions are most common in women of postmenopausal age. They are termed hemangiomas but actually represent small varicosities. They may be the cause of postmenopausal bleeding if the patient rubs her labia too vigorously after bathing. If a patient is having postmenopausal bleeding, the presence of these little varicosities is not sufficient to eliminate the necessity for thorough study of the entire genital canal and adjacent areas.

During the menstrual years, varicosities may be dramatic and are almost routinely unilateral. The classic varicocele, which is prevalent in the male, is unusual in the female. Therapy is surgical; the entire lesion must be excised, with careful ligation of the major vascular supply. Most varicoceles in the male arise from obstruction to the vasculature of the pampiniform plexus originating in the inguinal canal. Similar lesions in the female are most commonly of pudendal vascular origin. An appreciation of the difference between the major blood supplies to the perineum in the male and the female is necessary for adequate treatment of the lesion.

Fibromyoma and Lipoma

Fibromyoma and lipoma are found on the vulva and elsewhere on the body. Grossly, it is essentially impossible to differentiate one from the other. They may both reach a massive size and become pedunculated, in which case they should be excised to eliminate discomfort. Small lesions that interrupt the normal architecture but are asymptomatic need no therapy. As noted, if there is doubt as to the diagnosis, the lesion must be removed.

The dermatofibroma, usually a small subcutaneous nodule, is a variant of the fibromyoma group. Its vascularity has led to an alternative diagnosis of "sclerosing hemangioma." This lesion has no malignant potential, the histopathology being its only confusing feature.

Neurofibromatosis (von Recklinghausen's disease) may also be seen on the vulva. The widespread nature of fibromatosis and its association with other abnormalities such as the cafe au lait spots must be appreciated.

Pyogenic Granuloma

Pyogenic granuloma is a slightly elevated grayish-white lesion suggestive of a chronically infected nodule. Because of its ambiguous gross appearance, the lesion must be removed. The superficial surface is denuded and the edges of the apparent ulceration demonstrate proliferation of the epithelium, "pseudoepitheliomatous hyperplasia." Such alterations are simply reflections of the body's at-

tempt at repair and not symptoms of malignant alterations. The numerous small vessels seen with the inflammatory infiltrate are reminiscent of the granulation tissue seen in many chronic irritative processes. Nevertheless, the remarkable vascular pattern in the underlying tissue demonstrates that the lesion is not granulomatous in nature, suggesting instead that it is a hemangioma. These lesions are benign but may be confusing because of the unusual nature of the histopathologic alterations.

Granular Cell Myoblastoma

The granular cell myoblastoma is rarely seen on the vulva. The most common site is the nasopharyngeal region, particularly the tongue. The lesions do not present with a classic gross appearance but usually are thought to be subcutaneous fibrofatty nodules. Excision is complicated by the locally infiltrative nature of the lesions. Wide excision is difficult because the margins cannot be easily delineated.

Although the reaction of the overlying epithelium is suggestive of early malignancy, this pseudoepitheliomatous hyperplasia is actually purely a reaction to the subepithelial tumor. Large cells with multiple eosinophilic granules, identified as "myoblasts," infiltrate the adjacent tissue. Such lesions arise from the nerve sheath, however, and should therefore be termed schwannomas. They are benign but locally infiltrative and prone to recur because of the lack of a specific capsule. They are occasionally associated with lesions of a similar nature elsewhere in the body. The latter are demonstrations of multifocal, not metastatic, disease.

Other Benign Appendage Tumors

A variety of benign lesions arise in the underlying epithelium. The syringoma is probably not a true tumor but the result of blockage in the duct of the eccrine sweat glands. Multiple foci are routinely present. The small lesions are manifest histopathologically by slightly dilated eccrine sweat glands with comma-like tails.

Basal Cell Epithelioma or Carcinoma

Basal cell carcinoma can be discussed under the heading of benign or malignant tumors (Color Fig. 5-14). Its name implies that it has the potential not only for local invasion but eventually for metastasis. Nevertheless, these "rodent ulcers" rarely metastasize. Although they extend into the underlying dermis and occasionally involve the regional lymph nodes, they do not metastasize beyond the local area.

The classic appearance is that of a well-defined lesion with rolled edges and a superficially ulcerative center. Actually, the surface epithelium is intact in the central portion but spreads into the underlying tissue. The infiltration is irregular, the basal layer is intact, and the monotonous basal cells are regularly "palisaded" at the periphery of the leading edge. Mitoses may be seen but are characteristic of those present in the active basal layer. Occasionally, keratotic foci appear in the center of the nests of basal cells, making the lesion a keratotic basal cell carcinoma.

Regardless of their various features, all basal cell lesions have the same excellent prognosis. Local excision is the treatment of choice. Radiation therapy has been curative in other areas of the body such as the face and neck but should not be used on the vulva because of adverse, often long-term irritative reactions.

A variant on the basal cell carcinoma is the trichoepithelioma. This lesion simulates the basal cell carcinoma in that it is usually small with a punched-out center. Histopathologically, it may arise from the surface epithelium. More commonly, it arises from the basal cells of the hair follicle, in which case it suggest invasive cancer; however, as are all basal cell carcinomas, the lesion is only locally invasive and not metastasizing.

CYSTIC TUMORS

Epidermal Inclusion Cyst

The epidermal inclusion cyst was previously termed sebaceous cyst because of the malodorous greasy material that sometimes exudes from the orifice or on incision, from the nodule. This material usually represents desquamated epithelial cells, which line the cysts. Occasionally, the infiltration of this irritative material into the adjacent tissue produces a foreign-body giant cell reaction. This reaction associated with the greasy contents is probably the justification for the term sebaceous cyst (Color Fig. 5-15).

Such cysts are extremely common on the vulva and usually appear as multiple small subcutaneous nodules. Because the surface of the cysts is intact, there is rarely justification for excision. Nevertheless, the nodules occasionally are recurrently infected and irritating, thus requiring either excision or incision with drainage. Silver nitrate cauterization of the cavity may reduce recurrences of individual lesions; however, the condition is so common that elimination of the problem is almost impossible. Reassurance that the lumps are benign is of major importance to the patient's well-being.

Mucous Cyst

Mucous cysts are commonly seen on the inner surfaces of the labia minora at the introitus and may also be recognized just beyond the hymenal ring as either single or multiple nodules. They are termed dysontogenetic; however, they probably represent blocked minor vestibular glands. The lining is usually multilayered (transitional), thus simulating that seen in Bartholin's gland. This multilayered epithelium superficially suggests a squamous or epidermoid lesion.

Because the epithelium at the introitus is a result of the separation of the cloaca by the urorectal fold, it is not unusual to find mucous epithelium in the introital area. The physician should appreciate the genesis of the cysts and not misconstrue the transitional epithelium as premalignant because of its apparent loss of stratification.

BARTHOLIN'S DUCT ABSCESS AND CYSTS

The Bartholin's gland, entering the introitus just above the fourchette at the vaginal outlet, may be dilated as a result of chronic infection or cyst formation. It was previously suggested that most Bartholin's gland abscesses and residual chronic infection are of gonorrheal origin; however, this is not the case. Cultures of infected material reveal the presence of the gonococcus in 25% to 30% of cases, and culture usually reveals a mixed bacterial flora.

The treatment of these abscesses is incision and drainage. There is no justification for the use of a catheter at this stage of the disease; unimpeded drainage is a more important treatment. Furthermore, the injection of antibiotic into the abscess is painful and unrewarding. Marsupialization is indicated for the residual cyst if one develops, although more commonly, resolution is complete. Cysts usually arise from occlusion of the duct by surgery or scarring (Color Fig. 5-16).

Ductal occlusion used to be accomplished by surgical incision and suture of the duct lining to the epithelium at the vaginal outlet, with the patient under general anesthesia. The most appropriate therapy is as follows. After infiltration with local anesthetic, a tiny incision is made at the introitus near the region of the natural orifice of the gland (the introitus, not the skin) and a Word catheter is inserted. The deflated bulb is then distended with 2 to 3 mL of saline and the nipple inserted into the vagina. There is essentially no discomfort to the procedure, which leaves no residual foreign body. The catheter should stay in place for 3 or more weeks, after which it can be deflated and removed. By this time, the opening has been epithelialized and there is little chance for recurrence of the cystic enlargement. Any surgical approach to Bartholin's duct should be made by an incision at the introitus, not on the skin; fenestration resulting from skin incisions may be psychologically if not physically traumatic.

HYDROCELE, HERNIA, AND CYSTS OF THE CANAL OF NUCK

Cystic lesions appearing in the labium majus, either near the external inguinal ring or in the mid-vulva, commonly represent fluid accumulations along the extension of the peritoneal sac through the inguinal ligament into the vulva. Because the peritoneal investment of the round ligament is continuous with the peritoneum of the abdominal cavity, an inguinal hernia may be manifest by swelling and discomfort in the inguinal canal, not in the vulva. Nevertheless, swelling in the labium majus near the point of insertion of the round ligament may indicate the presence of bowel. Such lesions should be evaluated accurately by careful palpation with the patient standing and coughing before any surgery is contemplated. Usually, the sac contains only fluid, or a cystic tumor. Bowel in the sac, however, may be injured if the possibility of its presence is not considered. Furthermore, incision and drainage of a hydrocele misdiagnosed as a Bartholin's duct cyst leads only to recurrence of the condition. Accurate diagnosis is imperative.[11] If bowel is not present, the cyst (hydrocele) should be opened, the peritoneal lining excised, and the closure carried to the region of the external ring (Color Fig. 5-17).

ENDOMETRIOSIS

Endometriosis may occur in the inguinal canal and thus extend into the labium majus, following the course of the peritoneum along the round ligament. Mostly, however, endometrioid lesions occur near the introitus in association with the implantation of endometrium (eg, after incision or excision of a Bartholin's duct cyst).[12] The paramesonephric structures extend in the vagina to the introitus. Assuming that much endometriosis arises as a result of irritation by desquamated endometrium (as seen in the ovary and pelvis), any irritation by trauma or surgery at the introitus during menstruation may result in the development of endometriotic foci. Regardless of the origin of endometriosis, excision is the treatment of choice. Recurrences may be treated hormonally after the diagnosis is established.

EDEMA

Edema of the vulva is associated with a variety of physiologic and pathologic conditions. Diffuse asymptomatic swelling of the vulva during pregnancy is not uncommon (Color Fig. 5-18). This is magnified if the patient has any local inflammatory disease such as herpes. If breast tissue is present, the edema may be more dramatic due to lactation. As stated, any surgery on the vulva should be avoided during pregnancy; instead, conservative therapy for the swelling (eg, Burow's solution compresses) should be used.

Occlusion of the lymphatics by malignant disease often produces edema. Occlusion may be unilateral or bilateral, depending on whether the neoplastic involvement is intra-abdominal or inguinal.

Similarly, blockage of the lymphatics by other agents often result in marked edema. The condition is most commonly seen in climates in which filariasis is prevalent. These enlargements are generally asymptomatic, although they may present problems during pregnancy or if associated with inflammatory disease.[13]

Patients with Crohn's disease often develop only local distortion and edema; it is thus important to do a thorough general examination in addition to investigating the genitalia. Other systemic diseases such as multiple sclerosis and severe anemia may also affect local circulation. Obstruction to lymph–vascular drainage of the vulva has other potential causes, and each case must be evaluated on its own merits. A general physical examination and thorough history are essential to an appropriate interpretation of vulvar abnormalities.

VULVAR DYSTROPHIES

Before the term dystrophy was used to designate lesions demonstrating atypical epithelia patterns in the vulva, many of these cellular distortions were called leukoplakia. This term was first applied to lesions of the buccal mucous membranes more than a century ago. Since then, almost any white patch on the vulva has been given this nondescript diagnosis. These lesions are classified in Table 5-1. It is obvious from this widely diverse group of pathologic entities that leukoplakia does not describe any specific lesion. The term should be discarded in favor of more specific categories based on specific therapy required.

Absence of Pigment

The term vitiligo has been applied to lesions in which there is congenital absence of pigment. For the most part, these atypicalities develop at menarche and thus appear to be related to the concomitant activity of the pituitary gonadotropins and the melanin-stimulating hormone, which is also produced by the anterior pituitary. Conversely, leukoderma is a term describing lesions associated with an acquired lack of pigment. In certain irritative conditions, melanocytes may be unable to perform normally because of an underlying inflammatory reaction, and thus the epithelium cannot respond adequately (Color Fig. 5-19). In the congenital condition, it appears that the melanocytes are present in

Table 5–1
White Lesions of the Vulva

Absence of Pigment
　Leukoderma
　Vitiligo
Hyperkeratotic Conditions
　Inflammatory
　Benign tumors
　Lichen sclerosus
　Epithelial hyperplasia
　Carcinoma in situ
　Carcinoma

Table 5–2
1975 International Society for the Study of Vulvar Disease Classification of Dystrophic Vulvar Conditions

Hyperplastic Dystrophy
　Typical (without cellular atypia)
　Atypical (mild, moderate, or marked)
Lichen Sclerosus (et atrophicus)
Mixed Dystrophy
　Without atypia
　Atypical (mild, moderate, or marked)

From Kaufman RH: Vulvar dystrophies. ACOG Tech Bull 139:1, 1990

normal numbers but that there is a deficiency in the enzyme system.

Regardless of the mechanism behind lack of pigment, these conditions have no malignant potential and need no treatment except elimination of the commonly associated pruritus.

Hyperkeratotic Condition

The hyperkeratotic conditions, as listed above, may vary from simple chronic dermatitis to invasive cancer. Biopsy is mandatory to identify the benign or malignant nature of the lesion. All keratotic lesions are white or grayish-white from the absorption of fluid into the overlying keratin. Conversely, parakeratosis (incomplete keratinization) produces a red or reddish-brown appearance.

In 1975, the ISSVD adopted the term "dystrophy of the vulva" and divided the dystrophic conditions into those listed in Table 5-2.[14]

Although the classification has been widely accepted and has promoted comparative studies between researchers, criticism of the classification has also developed. The inclusion of atypical, presumably neoplastic lesions in a classification of nonneoplastic lesions was thought to be misleading. Many believed that the classification "mixed dystrophy" was commonly lichen sclerosis with reactive epithelial hyperplasia. Finally, the classification "hyperplastic dystrophy" was thought to represent variants of the established dermatologic disorder, lichen simplex chronicus. Because of these criticisms of the 1975 classification, the ISSVD revised the classification in 1987, as shown in Table 5-3.[14]

Squamous cell hyperplasia

Lichen sclerosis

Other dermatoses (consists of a large mixed group of disorders including lichen planus and psoriasis)

From Kaufman RH: Vulvar dystrophies. ACOG Tech Bull 139:1–5, 1990

Dystrophy is not a specific term. It means only "abnormal nutrition" and thus does not identify a degree of histopathologic abnormality that may or may not lead to the development of neoplasia. Its purpose is to avoid terms that have been arbitrarily associated with the development of malignancies. The clinician should recognize that treatment and follow-up are imperative.

Typical hyperplastic dystrophy is usually characterized by hyperkeratosis, elongation and blunting of the rete pegs (acanthosis), and essentially normal maturation of the proliferate epithelium, with associated underlying inflammatory infiltrate. Thus, the classic picture is one of chronic dermatitis with hyperkeratosis (previously called leukoplakia). It may be present in any age group. After confirmation of the diagnosis by biopsy, lesions are treated symptomatically by administration of topical or intralesional fluorinated hydrocortisone to eliminate pruritus.

Atypical hyperplasia is characterized by the following two basic alterations. The first is proliferation of the basal and parabasal cells with occasional mitosis, more than is seen in normal maturation. This change may extend throughout the entire surface epithelium, under which circumstance it is similar to and should be identified as carcinoma in situ. The second and possibly more ominous pattern is characterized by atypical maturation at the rete tips. Keratinized cells in the basal layer show intraepithelial "pearl" formation. Because malignant lesions arising on the vulva are usually squamous cell carcinomas, this keratinizing atypia may be the first evidence of early invasion. Under such circumstances, selective, wide local excision or simple vulvectomy is the treatment of choice; however, neither of these procedures eliminates the possibility of recurrence in the adjacent skin. Most of these lesions develop in patients 50 years old or older. Careful follow-up is of importance because patients are at risk for vulvar cancer.

Lichen sclerosus, often designated lichen sclerosus et atrophicus, may be seen in any age group, although it is most common in postmenopausal patients (Color Fig. 5-20). Grossly, the lesions are characterized by a thin white surface (cigarette paper or parchment skin) and loss of normal architecture, often associated with disappearance of the labia minora, constriction of the vaginal outlet (kraurosis), and superficial ecchymoses. In the early stages of development, particularly during the menstrual years, the lesions may be asymptomatic. Nevertheless, in the postmenopausal patient, itching and irritation are prevalent and superficial excoriations often develop. Biopsy is imperative in such cases.

Histopathologically, lichen sclerosus is characterized by a mild to moderate degree of hyperkeratosis; thinning of the epithelium with loss of the rete pegs; homogenization of the subepithelial layer (a generally acellular zone, often with dilated vascular channels); and inflammatory infiltrate beneath of the subepithelial layer. Keratin frequently plugs the superficial invaginations (eg, hair follicles or sebaceous glands).

The term et atrophicus indicates that the epithelium is wasting or degenerative. Metabolic studies in our laboratory, using tritiated thymidine and acridine orange fluorescence, demonstrate that the epithelium is actually more active than normal.

It is important to confirm the diagnosis by biopsy, often at multiple foci, specifically those with marked keratin (whitish) deposits or ulcerations.

Treatment of lichen sclerosus lesions consists primarily of 2% testosterone cream in a unibase or stearin–lanolin base applied topically to the vulva at least twice a day for a period of up to 3 months. The patient should be made aware that it is necessary to continue the treatment for at least this long and possibly forever because discontinuation of the treatment often results in recurrence of the lesions and their symptoms. The patient should also know that the associated itching must be treated with topical fluorinated hydrocortisone because testosterone is not antipruritic. The agent must be rubbed vigorously until absorbed by the tissue.

Testosterone is not recommended for the premenarchal patient.

Enlargement of the clitoris (which occurs in about 20% of patients on long-term testosterone) and occasional facial hair growth preclude such therapy in the young patient. The best approach to the problem in young patients is treatment of symptoms by the occasional use of fluorinated hydrocortisones and the elimination of local irritants. The family must be reassured that lichen sclerosus is simply a local change, without significant social or pathologic potential. Occasionally, it may be necessary to administer a topical 2% progesterone preparation in aquaphor.[15] This agent is effective in prepubertal patients and may even be employed in other age groups if testosterone is unsuccessful or the patient has a local reaction to it. Adverse reactions are commonly due not to the testosterone but to the base in which it is prepared. Although some authors suggest that alterations in the premenarchal girl regress at the time of menarche, this is true only about half the time.

The mixed dystrophies are a combination of lichen sclerosus and hyperplasia (Color Fig. 5-21). Biopsies are important to rule out neoplastic change, and therapy depends on the symptoms and the biopsy findings. Occasionally, wide local excision is necessary, particularly if there are atypical proliferative changes or constriction of the outlet, with dyspareunia. Otherwise, the patient is treated symptomatically and followed-up carefully with repeat biopsies when indicated by a change in coloration or architecture.

The dystrophies have malignant potential. Because they were most commonly known as leukoplakia (a premalignant lesion), the dystrophies were thought to be the common precursors of invasive cancer. It is widely recognized, however, that lichen sclerosus rarely results in invasive cancer. Similarly, most of the hyperplastic dystrophies can be treated by wide excision and careful biopsy, with elimination of pruritus. Nevertheless, patients should be subjected to constant and careful follow-up every 6 to 9 months, depending on the extent of the dystrophy and the control of the symptoms. Vulvectomy is rarely necessary for patients with mixed dystrophy. Finally, atypical hyperplastic dystrophy with keratinization at the rete tips is the most significant premalignant change. This should be managed with excision and careful follow-up.

VULVAR INTRAEPITHELIAL NEOPLASIA

Vulvar intraepithelial neoplasia (VIN or in situ carcinoma) presents problems to the clinician, pathologist, and oncologist. Whereas 40 years ago such lesions were relatively unknown entities, they are more common than invasive cancer in many clinics.[16] Terminology confused the issue because of a myriad of designations such as Bowen's disease, erythroplasia of Queyrat, bowenoid papulosis, and atypical pigmentation. All of these lesions are incorporated under the heading VIN because there are commonly multiple histopathologic patterns within the same lesion. Particularly in the young patient, they pursue a proliferative recurrent pattern but rarely invade, metastasize, or result in death. The incidence is increasing and the average age of occurrence is in the late third and early fourth decades of life. Patients in the seventh, eighth, and ninth decades are not exempt, however, nor is the teenager.

The classification in Table 5-4 attempts to clarify some of the ambiguous categories encountered in the past. Paget's disease is included as a separate entity. Although it is commonly an intraepithelial lesion on the vulva, it is biologically different from carcinoma in situ and thus demands special attention.

Table 5–4
Classification of Vulvar Carcinoma In Situ

Gross Appearance	Epithelial Changes	Common Term
Red lesion with white island	Abnormal maturation, with individual cell keratinization, corps ronds, chromatin fragmentation	Bowen's disease
Diffuse or patchy erythematous lesion	Proliferation of basal cells, with loss of normal surface maturation	Erythroplasia of Queyrat
Brown to brownish-black patches	Loss of normal maturation, with pigment in cells at all layers	Pigmented vulvar intraepithelial neoplasia
Brick-red patches	Presence of Paget's cells	Paget's disease

In spite of the strong evidence that human papillomavirus (HPV) may be the primary etiologic agent in cervical intraepithelial neoplasia (CIN), the evidence for VIN is not as clear. More than 60 types of HPV have been isolated in lower genital tract infections. Human papillomavirus types 6 and 11 comprise more than 90% of condylomata acuminata and low-grade VIN lesions, whereas types 16 and 18 are found in more than 90% of high-grade lesions. The association of HPV subtypes is variable in proportion in various reported studies. Kaufman and coworkers report type 6 or 11 in 26%, types 16, 18, and 31 in 37%, and a mixture of types in 11% of cases of VIN III, using in situ hybridization.[17] In contrast, Buscema and coworkers report finding HPV DNA in 81% of condylomata, 84% of VIN III, and 58% of invasive carcinomas of the vulva, using Southern Blot hybridization.[18] The invasive potential of VIN is not clearly established, whereas it is known that a significant proportion of untreated CIN progresses to invasive cancer. A review of invasive vulvar carcinoma in our laboratory found that typical and atypical hyperplastic dystrophy were more commonly found adjacent to invasive vulvar malignancy than was vulvar carcinoma in situ (VIN III), which is seen in 20% to 30% of cases. This raises the question whether the progression to invasive vulvar malignancy is commonly analogous to the progression in cervical neoplasia. The untreated case of vulvar dystrophy may progress to cancer over time. Thus, all patients with dystrophic alterations should be treated for the common symptom (eg, pruritus) and a biopsy should be taken if specific foci of atypicality develop, identified by the presence of firm cartilaginous areas of nonhealing superficial ulcerations.

Symptoms

The common symptom of in situ vulvar carcinoma (and of most vulvar lesions) is pruritus. Nevertheless, patients are often also aware of a local abnormality such as a lump or white patch. In about 25% to 30% of cases, the lesions are asymptomatic and are found only on careful follow-up examination of patients with a history of regional neoplasia.

Diagnosis of vulvar carcinoma in situ depends on careful inspection of the entire genital tract. The clinician should remember that vulvar in situ neoplasms are associated with cervical neoplasm 20% to 30% of the time. Any gross atypicality—white, red, atypically pigmented, warty, or any mixture of the above—should undergo biopsy. Staining with the Collins test (1% toluidine blue, followed in 3 minutes by 1% to 2% acetic acid) may identify abnormal areas. Toluidine blue is a nuclear stain; if the lesions are red, the nuclei are usually exposed (as in parakeratosis) and absorb the dye. Even abnormally proliferating epithelium in the white (hyperkeratotic) lesion may demonstrate some degree of bluish stain. There are many false-negative and false-positive results; for example, any area that is ulcerated or excoriated may appear positive because of exposed nuclei at the base of the lesion. Nevertheless, any area showing uptake of the blue dye should attract the clinician's attention and biopsy instrument.

Colposcopy is not as helpful in demonstrating vulvar neoplasia as it is in identifying abnormal cellular activity in the cervix and vagina; however, red lesions commonly reveal the familiar atypical vascular patterns. Similarly, cytologic smears rarely yield atypical cells unless scraping is sufficiently abrasive to produce elements from deep cellular components. The relative inadequacy of cytology and colposcopy calls for biopsy of any lesion. The 6-mm Keyes dermatologic punch is recommended for the procedure.

When tissue is removed, the pathologist must be given adequate clinical information regarding the gross pattern of the condition, associated lesions in the area, and the age of the patient. Finally, the tissue fragments should be accurately placed in fixative so that tangential cuts, which often result in incorrect interpretation, may be avoided. The tissue may be placed on a fragment of filter paper or paper toweling, with the epithelial surface up so that the pathologist may embed the specimen accurately in paraffin. Knife biopsies are not recommended in this procedure; the specimen is often sliced from the surface and only the superficial layers are obtained. If the patient is anesthetized for removal of abnormal foci, the scalpel is the instrument of choice, and accurate orientation is important.

The microscopic pathology of vulvar carcinoma in situ is variable and as noted in the Table 5-4, each of the categories may demonstrate a different pattern of cellular atypicality. There may even be variation from area to area in the same lesion. Frequently, there is hyperkeratosis in the white lesion, with elongation of the rete pegs and nuclear atypicalities extending through the epithelium. The formation of "epithelial pearls" in the deep layers of the epithelium is of particular significance in ectodermal lesions because squamous cell keratinizing carcinoma is the common vulvar malignancy. Parakeratosis, with abnormal proliferation of the basal cells, may also be noted, particularly in pigmented lesions. Careful evaluation usually demonstrates the presence of pigment, not only in the basal layer but also in the superficial layers. This may be due to the rapid proliferation of the epithelial elements that carry the pigment from the basal layer throughout the epithelium.

All suspicious lesions must be evaluated carefully and undergo biopsy frequently (Color Fig. 5-22). Given the frequency of multifocal disease, multiple biopsies should be taken from all suspicious areas and identified carefully in separate bottles of fixative for referral to the pathologist. The incidence of in situ neoplasia in many laboratories exceeds that of invasive cancer. The ratio of in situ carcinoma to invasive carcinoma at the Johns Hopkins University is about 3:2.

Treatment

The treatment of vulvar carcinoma in situ must be individualized. The lesion may regress spontaneously, as documented by Friedrich (personal communication) in his study of multiple foci of in situ carcinoma of the vulva during pregnancy. Biopsy of one lesion revealed the classic histopathologic picture of carcinoma in situ. In the follow-up postpartum period, spontaneous regression of the remaining foci occurred in all cases. This sequence of events is similar to that seen in many patients with condylomata acuminata followed-up over a period of years. Other studies suggest that lesions developing in persons in their 20s rarely progress to invasive cancer. Several characteristics of the disease support this thesis.

First, as is true for most other invasive carcinomas, carcinoma of the vulva is generally a single-cell phenomenon. If this is true for the in situ vulvar lesions, either they do not represent true malignancy or all but one regress and progression to invasion develops in the single remaining focus. The latter sequence of events seems unlikely. Second, the average age of patients with invasive cancer of the vulva is 60 to 65 years. If the lesions seen in patients in their 20s are precursors, an interval of about 30 years must be expected before development of the invasive phase of the disease. This interval seems unrealistically long if our knowledge of cervical neoplasia is accurate. Nevertheless, it must be granted that vulvar and cervical neoplasms

differ strikingly, both histologically and biologically. Third, many lesions either disappear or appear to regress spontaneously. More cases of this latter phenomenon must be evaluated, however.

Wide local excision is the treatment of choice for solitary or multifocal lesions that can be removed without marked distortion of the vulva. A variety of other techniques have been proposed for the treatment of vulvar carcinoma in situ, particularly the multifocal variety. Cryosurgery is not a widely accepted therapy, although in some cases it is sufficient to destroy small foci. Electrocoagulation has also been used but is not recommended. Reports of laser therapy suggest a high degree of success. All of these ablative techniques entail local discomfort, regardless of the alleged lack of reactions. They also have the disadvantage of destroying tissue before it is adequately evaluated. Finally, recurrences are not uncommon, regardless of the therapeutic method used.

Vulvectomy is to be criticized, especially in young patients. This procedure not only destroys the architecture of the vulva but is also psychologically traumatic. The skinning vulvectomy has been proposed as an alternative but it just adds the trauma of healing of the donor site to the trauma of healing of the vulva. Furthermore, it leaves the adjacent skin still at risk and is therefore unwarranted. Regardless of the therapy that is chosen, the patient should be followed-up carefully and should avoid local irritants and infectious processes. Any suspicious lesions should undergo biopsy.

Topical chemotherapeutic agents have been used but neither 5-fluorouracil nor bleomycin is associated with a major degree of success. Furthermore, the local reaction is severe in many instances. Consequently, neither of these agents is recommended. Finally, immunotherapy in the form of sensitization of the patient to dinitrochlorobenzene (a nonspecific chemical) and subsequent local use of the agent has proved successful, particularly in patients with pigmented lesions, which are refractory to most forms of local therapy except ablation.[19]

Treatment of VIN with interferon can offer an effective alternative to surgery, particularly in areas of the vulva where wide local excision would be unacceptable, such as VIN of the clitoris (Color Fig. 5-23*A* and *B*). Interferon alpha is a naturally occurring protein having antiviral, antiproliferative, and immune-enhancing properties. Recommended intralesional treatment entails intralesional injection of 250,000 IU (0.05 mL) twice weekly for 8 weeks.

Injection is best given late in the day to permit most of the debilitating flu-like symptoms to occur at night. Flu-like symptoms were reported in 30% of patients after the first injection. Other severe symptoms include back pain, insomnia, and sensitivity to allergens.

Several lesions have been implicated as possible precursors of vulvar carcinoma. A chief precursor is HPV infection, characterized by the condylomatous change and the atypical hyperplastic dystrophies, which are characterized by generally thickened grayish-white plaques, often traversed by linear excoriations. Toki and coworkers have correlated clinical, virologic, and pathologic examination of more than 60 cases of VIN III and invasive vulvar carcinoma and have developed a pathologic classification of warty VIN, basaloid VIN, and squamous hyperplasia as precursor lesions and warty carcinoma, basaloid carcinoma, and typical squamous cell carcinoma as the corresponding cancers.[20] Using polymerase chain reaction, they found that warty or basaloid VIN III and the associated vulvar carcinomas (warty and basaloid carcinomas) typically contained HPV genome; these lesions occurred in younger women (mean age, 54 years for basaloid and 47 years for warty carcinoma). Conversely, the typical squamous cell carcinoma of the vulva occurred in older women (mean age, 77 years) and seldom contained HPV genome. The epithelium adjacent to the squamous cell carcinoma on older women often showed atypical hyperplastic dystrophy. It should be added that the association of HPV infection combined with environmental factors may increase risk of vulvar cancer even further. Brinton and coworkers report a case–control study of patients with pathologically defined VIN III. Relative risk significantly increased to more than 15-fold if the patient had a history of condyloma.[21] This risk increased to 35-fold when the history of smoking and condyloma were both present. Of additional importance is the symptom of chronic pruritus and the epithelial alterations associated with the scratch–itch cycle. Indeed, the fingernail may be one of the most malignant agents. It is of major importance that the local lesions be excised widely if recurrences in the perineal area are to be avoided.

Multifocal Disease

Multifocal disease in the lower genital canal has been a well-recognized entity for the past 30 years. Studies demonstrate that about 30% of patients with vulvar neoplasia in situ have lesions in the cervix, either in situ or invasive. Rarely, a lesion is found in the vagina.

Recognition of these multicentric lesions is of major significance, from both an etiologic and a therapeutic point of view. If such lesions go unrecognized, they may continue to proliferate, with development of more serious disease.

The possible geneses of multifocal disease include the following. First, multicentric lesions are evidence that a local carcinogenic agent is affecting various sites. It is possible that the proliferating agent is affecting the areas at risk, primarily the squamocolumnar junction of the cervix and irritative foci on the vulva. Although not proved, papillomavirus and herpesvirus seem to be the most logical candidates for the local irritant. Second, multifocal disease may simply represent inadequate excision of in situ disease, such as that of the cervix that has extended into the vagina. This phenomenon is known as cancerization. Third, it is possible that the treatment used to eliminate one lesion may produce irritation in an adjacent area and thus produce a second tumor. This has been observed in patients irradiated for carcinoma of the cervix who later developed lesions in the vagina or vulva.

In view of the above, it is of major importance to study the entire area at risk. This includes the perianal zone, which has occasionally been the site of development of invasive disease in cases of previously treated vulvar carcinoma in situ.

PAGET'S DISEASE

Vulvar Paget's disease, a variety of extramammary Paget's disease occurring primarily in persons in their 50s and 60s, develops in apocrine-gland–bearing areas of the body. As a result, the lesions may be seen on the breast (modified apocrine gland), the vulva, the perianal area, and rarely, the axilla.

Primary symptoms are burning and pruritus. Occasionally, the patient notices a change in coloration. Neither bleeding nor a nodule or mass has been recognized in association with Paget's disease.

Grossly, the lesions are fiery red with white patches, involving multifocal areas of the vulva (Color Fig. 5-24). There may be occasional swelling, although this is usually seen in the later stages of the disease. Thorough inspection of the perianal area and the breasts is important in the recognition of multifocal disease—not only locally, but at other areas at risk. The breast is the most common site for Paget's disease.

Histopathologically, the Paget's cell is seen initially just above the basal layer, which suggests that it originates from the undifferentiated embryonal stratum germinativa.[22] The large pale cells are occasionally arranged in a gland-like pattern. Commonly, the entire surface epithelium is involved, with individual or small groups of the classic large pale cell. These cells are periodic-acid–Schiff- and mucicarmine-positive, which clearly differentiates them from the cells of the amelanotic melanoma. The appendages are also involved in about 75% to 80% of the cases. The condition is then termed Paget's disease with gland involvement but the prognosis remains the same.

Lesions on the vulva remain largely intraepithelial, although recurrences are frequent. Progression from intraepithelial to invasive Paget's disease appears to be rare. Nevertheless, patients should be followed-up carefully and biopsies taken of new areas of involvement. Rarely, an underlying adenocarcinoma in the apocrine system has been recognized in the removed tissue. Mostly, the histopathologic signs of malignancy have been those noted with many in situ cancers: the breaking through of the so-called basement membrane, with extension into the underlying tissue by the Paget's disease, and undifferentiated epithelial cells in the basal layer. Metabolic studies demonstrate that these undifferentiated epithelial cells are more active than Paget's cells. There is no difference in gross appearance or the individual histopathology between invasive and intraepithelial lesions.

Because the tumor in Paget's disease arises from the apocrine type of cell (in the glands or in the surface) and because it is classically multifocal, the area containing apocrine glands must be removed. Thus, simple vulvectomy is the treatment of choice. It seems possible that the labia minora and clitoris could be saved because they rarely contain apocrine glands. Nevertheless, patients are generally in their 50s and 60s and thus do not find the procedure as psychologically traumatic as do younger patients with carcinoma in situ.

Vulvectomy with regional node dissection is the treatment of choice for invasive tumors, whether they are in the apocrine glands or simply extend from the surface epithelium. Postoperative irradiation has been used in most cases with lymph node involvement. Nevertheless, the prognosis is poor.

Recurrences of vulvar Paget's disease are common, and patients must thus be followed-up carefully. Topical 5-fluorouracil has been used for recurrences, with some reports of success. Radiation therapy to the local area is contraindicated. Patients should be followed-up and evaluated carefully because of the possibility of multifocal involvement of the apocrine system. Despite the performance of wide local excision of recurrences, additional foci commonly reappear.

EARLY INVASIVE CANCER

Early invasive (microinvasive) cancer is a poorly defined condition. In about 300 cases reported in the literature, the measurement of the depth of invasion varies, with some investigators using the surface and others the basal layer. There is a tendency to adopt the basal layer as the more appropriate gauge because the depth of the rete pegs varies widely from case to case. The possibility of the development of invasive cancer has been demonstrated by several cases, in which widespread invasive disease developed shortly after inadequate therapy for microinvasive disease of less than 5 mm and even less than 3 mm.

Because of the difficulties encountered in the interpretation of microinvasive cancer and the unfortunate results of inadequate treatment, our laboratory has adopted the approach of measuring the depth of invasion from the basal layer of the deepest rete peg. Lesions that involve only the interpapillary ridges are considered microinvasive. The extent beyond the rete peg is then identified in millimeters. Patients with microinvasive cancer (ie, involvement of only the interpapillary ridges) are treated by either wide local excision or simple vulvectomy. There have been no recurrences in this group.

Among patients with lesions extending only 1 mm or less below the deepest rete peg, there have been two deaths.[23] One of the latter occurred in an 83-year-old patient 6 years after she had undergone vulvectomy. Local growth of lesions was treated only by excision and radiation, and the patient succumbed in 6 years to hemorrhage. The second patient was in her 70s when she developed widespread metastatic disease. She died 6 years postsurgery.

There were three deaths in the group with 2 to 4 mm of invasion. Two of these were due to widespread disease developing 15 and 30 months after vulvectomy. The third patient who died had been inadequately treated because of severe reaction of the pelvic and vulvar tissue to irradiation for cervical cancer. Of the five deaths that occurred in both of these groups, four occurred in patients older than the age of 70. Age often indicates long-standing irritation and must be considered to be an at-risk factor.

Each case of early invasive cancer must be evaluated carefully. Multiple sections should be made. With unilateral invasion between 3 and 5 mm, it would seem wise to perform a vulvectomy and sample the ipsilateral nodes; however, this depends to a great extent on the condition of the patient. Further studies are necessary to determine the most appropriate therapy for each case. In addition, the following questions should be asked:

Is the cell type of prognostic importance?
Is the definition of lymph–vascular invasion adequate at these superficial levels? If so, what is the significance?
Is the pattern of invasion a spray pattern or a pattern of confluence?
Is the size of the tumor of major importance?
Is the age of the patient significant?
Is the position of the tumor significant?

As the above and other questions are more adequately answered, we may be able to determine and predict those cases that can be treated by node sampling or even node dissection. Until then, every effort must be made to evaluate each case individually and treat the patient accordingly.

CHANGES ADJACENT TO INVASIVE CANCER

The working hypothesis on cervical neoplasia suggests that there is a continuum of histologic changes from CIN I, II, or III to invasive cervical cancer. The finding of in situ disease adjacent to invasive cancer suggests that the former precedes the latter.

In contrast, in invasive vulvar cancer, such a continuum is demonstrated. In about 30% to 40% of cases, in situ neoplasia is found adjacent to the invasive cancer. Other changes, however, particularly the hyperplastic dystrophies, seem more significant. Lichen sclerosus, long thought to be a precursor of cancer, appears to have little significance in the stages of development of the malignancy.

A few cases have been followed-up from preinvasive disease to invasive cancer. The most significant alteration that has preceded invasive cancer is marked atypical hyperplastic dystrophy, in which

keratin pearls are seen in the rete tips. This alteration is most frequently seen in patients in their 60s and 70s, the common age for the development of invasive cancer.

INVASIVE CARCINOMA

Invasive carcinoma of the vulva is a squamous cell, not an epidermoid, lesion. It comprises about 5% of all primary malignancies arising in the female genital canal and 92% to 95% of all vulvar malignancies found in postmenopausal patients. Most persons who develop invasive carcinoma are in the seventh decade of life; however, about 5% to 10% are between the ages of 25 and 60. It has been suggested by molecular techniques of in situ hybridization and polymerase chain reaction that squamous cell carcinoma occurring in the older woman may be less likely to be associated with human papillomavirus.[20] The symptoms are those classic for most vulvar diseases: pruritus, pain, bleeding, and lump (tumor). Other symptoms depend on extension of the lesion into the urethra, rectum, vagina, or deeper tissues.

The diagnosis is made by biopsy. Any suspicious lesion, particularly of the chronic irritative variety, should undergo biopsy.

The gross appearance of the lesion may be ulcerative or proliferative (Color Fig. 5-25A and B). Whereas in situ cancer is commonly multicentric, invasive lesions are most frequently unifocal, except the extensive disease involving much of the external genitalia. Invasive carcinoma is most frequently found in the labium minus, although any area may be involved, including the clitoris and the fourchette.

Histopathologically, 75% of the lesions of invasive carcinoma are of the mature variety and 25% are less well differentiated. It is not uncommon to find both histopathologic alterations in the same lesion at various sites or even immediately adjacent to another.

The classic treatment is radical vulvectomy with regional node dissection. The status of regional lymph nodes is highly significant in predicting outcome.[24] There is little enthusiasm for extraperitoneal node removal, for which the 5- and 10-year survival rates are extremely low if deep nodes are involved. It may be considered reasonable to irradiate the deep nodes if the superficial nodes were positive, given the age of most patients. Tumor variables that are predictive of node metastasis include presence of vascular invasion, clinical stage, tumor thickness or depth of invasion, and amount of keratin within the tumor.[25] It is suggested that for unilateral lesions not involving the clitoris, vagina, urethra, or fourchette, ipsilateral node removal may be sufficient. More work needs to be done in this area.

The results of therapy indicate that in patients without regional lymph node involvement, the 5-year survival is about 90%; in patients with invaded regional nodes, the survival rate drops to 30% to 40%. Local recurrences are not common and reexcision often results in long-term cure. Tumor variables that are predictive of reduced local recurrence include surgical margin greater than 8 mm, depth of invasion less than 9.1 mm, tumor thickness less than 10 mm, less than 10 mitoses per 10 high-power fields, lack of an infiltrative growth pattern, lack of lymph vascular invasion, and low degree of tumor keratinization.[26] Radiation therapy is not indicated for local lesions, primary or recurrent. There appears to be no difference in survival rate between the histologic varieties.

The contemporary International Federation of Obstetrics and Gynecology classification, based on the TNM (*t*umor, *n*ode, *m*etastasis) nomenclature, is complex and confusing and needs to be reevaluated. For example, patients with extensive local invasion and patients with extrapelvic disease may be classified as having stage IV disease. In our experience, squamous cell carcinoma of the vulva appears to be a locally invasive disease that can be satisfactorily treated by extensive operative procedures. In patients who also have extrapelvic disease, however, the 5-year survival rate is essentially nil.

OTHER MALIGNANCIES

Verrucous Carcinoma

Verrucous carcinoma is locally invasive and commonly recurrent. Extensive wide local excision is the treatment of choice. Irradiation of the locally invasive disease often results in the subsequent development of invasive cancer, and this is to be avoided. Regional lymph nodes are not involved and thus node dissection is unnecessary. As the result of frequent recurrences, more extensive surgery (eg, exenterative procedures) is occasionally necessary; however, such surgery should be avoided if possible.

Basal Cell Carcinoma

Basal cell carcinoma of the vulva, as it is elsewhere, is superficially invasive. Wide local excision is the treatment of choice.

Malignant Melanoma

Malignant melanoma may be of the spreading or nodular variety (Color Fig. 5-26). It comprises about 2% to 3% of all melanomas arising in the human body and thus is probably no more common on the vulva than elsewhere. It usually arises on the labia minora and occurs in persons of all age groups. Biopsy of all suspicious lesions is mandatory, and follow-up therapy must be instituted promptly if there is any question about the interpretation of the pathology. The prognosis is based largely on the level of involvement. Levels I and II are intraepithelial (invasion into the interpupillary ridges). Such lesions need only wide local excision. The commonly used classification for defining the most appropriate therapy for the individual case is the modified Breslow proposal (Table 5-5).[26a]

Melanomas may be multifocal. Invasion below the epidermis should be treated by vulvectomy and node dissection. The survival rate for patients with lesions involving the underlying fat is about 10% to 20%, regardless of treatment. Adjunctive medications have not been helpful, although DTIC has been used along with local irradiation.

Bartholin's Gland Cancer

Three varieties of malignancy may develop in the region of the Bartholin's gland. A classic squamous cell carcinoma may originate at the orifice of the gland from the stratified epithelium of the introitus. This is actually a tumor—not of Bartholin's gland but of the native squamous epithelium.[27] A second malignancy may develop in the duct of the gland. This transitional malignancy is similar histopathologically to that arising in the bladder. It has a poor prognosis despite surgery or irradiation.

A third and most classic malignancy of Bartholin's gland develops in the region of the glandular portion. Known as adenoid cystic carcinoma, it is similar histopathologically to the disease of the same name arising in the salivary glands. It extends locally and metastasizes late. Metastasis is classically to the lung. The treatment is wide and deep

Table 5-5
Treatment of Malignant Melanoma (Modified Breslow Proposal)

Tumor Depth	Therapy
0.75 mm	Wide local excision, 2-cm margin; no lymphadenectomy
0.76–1.49 mm	Wide local excision, 3–4-cm margin; elective lymph node sampling
1.5–4.0 mm	Wide local excision, 3–4-cm margin; elective lymph node dissection

From Breslow A, Macht SD: Optimal size of resection margin for the cutaneous melanoma. Surg Gynecol Obstet 145:691, 1977

local excision, often involving the rectum and the ischiorectal fossa. Regional nodes are rarely involved; thus, radical vulvectomy with lymph node dissection is not indicated. For tumors arising in the salivary glands and elsewhere (eg, the neck), recurrences are common and patients must be followed-up carefully and treated by wide excision. Radiation therapy has not been helpful in treatment of such lesions.

Metastatic Cancer

Metastatic carcinoma in the vulva is commonly secondary to cancer in the endometrium. Thus, if adenocarcinoma is recognized in the biopsy of vulvar lesions, the immediate response should be to investigate the uterus or, if it has been removed, to determine the reason for hysterectomy.

Malignancies arising in the cervix, vagina, and rectum may directly involve the vulva, which must therefore be investigated thoroughly and the type of neoplasm evaluated for the most likely primary site.

SUMMARY

For institution of appropriate therapy in inflammatory disease, an accurate diagnosis is of obvious importance. The following features of history and physical examination are mandatory:

1. Past history—previous illnesses, particularly infectious disease (specifically, the sexually transmitted variety) and therapies; social history (partners and contraceptive measures); parity and pregnancy outcome; surgeries; age at menopause, and therapies

2. Careful physical examination to identify dermatologic lesions elsewhere and systemic disease (eg, diabetes)
3. Gross appearance of vulva and its lesions—correlate to other skin lesions
4. Pathology—interpretation and adequacy thereof
5. Discussion—physician and patient relative to diagnosis; terminology; significance of pathology; proposed therapies; necessity for careful follow-up

REFERENCES

1. McKay M: Vulvar dermatoses; common problems in dermatological and gynecological practice. Br J Clin Pathol 71(Suppl):5, 1990
2. Mosney DS, Brito F, Bender HG: Immunohistochemical investigations of estrogen receptors in normal and neoplastic squamous epithelium of the vulva. J Reprod Med 35:1005, 1990
3. Kelly RA, Foster DC, Woodruff JD: Subcutaneous use of triamcinolone acetonide in chronic vulvar pruritus. Am J Obstet Gynecol 169:568, 1993
3a. Mering JH: A surgical approach to intractable pruritis vulvae. Am J Obstet Gynecol 67:619, 1952
4. Iest J, Boer J: Combined treatment of psoriasis with acitretin and UVB phototherapy compared with acitretin alone and UVB alone. Br J Dermatol 120:665, 1989
5. Borrego L, Ruiz-Rodriguez R, de Fructos JO, Sebastian FV, Diez LI: Vulvar lichen planus treated with topical cyclosporine (Letter). Arch Dermatol 125:794, 1993
6. Morgan ED, Laszlo JD, Stumpf PG: Incomplete Behçet's syndrome in the differential diagnosis of genital ulceration and postcoital bleeding, a case report. J Reprod Med 33:844, 1990
7. Covino JM, McCormack WM: Vulvar ulcer of unknown etiology in a human immunodeficiency virus-infected woman: response to treatment with zidovudine. Am J Obstet Gynecol 163:116, 1990
8. Marren P, Wojnarowska F, Venning V, Wilson C,

Nayar M: Vulvar involvement in autoimmune bullous diseases. J Reprod Med 38:101, 1993

9. Koh HK: Cutaneous melanoma. N Engl J Med 325:171, 1991

10. Cohen PR, Young AW, Tovell HMM: Angiokeratoma of the vulva: diagnosis and review of the literature. Obstet Gynecol Surv 44:339, 1989

11. McElfatrick RA, Condon WB: Hydrocele of the canal of Nuck, a report of two adult cases. Rocky Mount Med J 112, 1975

12. Pollack R, Gordon PH, Ferenczy A, Tulandi T: Perineal endometriosis, a case report. J Reprod Med 35:110, 1990

13. Morris LF, Rapini RP, Herbert AA, Katz AR: Massive labial edema in pregnancy. South Med J 83:846, 1990

14. Kaufman RH: Vulvar dystrophies. ACOG Tech Bull 139:1, 1990

15. Parks G, Growdon WA, Mason GD, Goldman L, Lebherz TB: Childhood anogenital lichen sclerosis, a case report. J Reprod Med 35:191, 1990

16. Sturgeon SR, Brinton LA, Devesa SS, Kurman RJ: In situ and invasive vulvar cancer incidence trends. Am J Obstet Gynecol 166:1482, 1992

17. Kaufman RH, Bornstein J, Adam E, Burek J, Tessin B, Alder-Storz K: Human papillomavirus and herpes simplex virus in vulvar squamous cell carcinoma in situ. Am J Obstet Gynecol 158:862, 1988

18. Buscema J, Naghashfar Z, Sawada E, Daniel R, Woodruff JD, Shah K: The predominance of human papillomavirus type 16 in vulvar neoplasia. Obstet Gynecol 71:601, 1988

19. Foster DC, Woodruff JD: The use of dinitrochlorobenzene in the treatment of vulvar carcinoma in situ. Gynecol Oncol 11:330, 1981

20. Toki T, Kurman RJ, Park JS, Kessis T, Daniel RW, Shah KV: Probable nonpapillomavirus etiology of squamous cell carcinoma of the vulva in older women: a clinicopathologic study using in-situ hybridization and polymerase chain reaction. Int J Gynecol Pathol 10:107, 1991

21. Brinton LA, Nasca PC, Mallin K, Baptiste M, Wilbanks GD, Richart R: Case-control study of cancer of the vulva. Obstet Gynecol 75:859, 1990

22. Neilson D, Woodruff JD: Electron microscopy in in-situ and invasive vulvar Paget's disease. Am J Obstet Gynecol 113:719, 1972

23. Buscema J, Stern JL, Woodruff JD: Early invasive carcinoma of the vulva. Am J Obstet Gynecol 140:563, 1981

24. Hopkins MP, Reid GC, Morley GW: The surgical management of recurrent squamous cell carcinoma of the vulva. Obstet Gynecol 1990, 75:1001, 1990

25. Binder SW, Huang I, Fu YS, Hacker NF, Berek JS: Risk factors for the development of lymph node metastasis in vulvar squamous cell carcinoma. Gynecol Oncol 37:9, 1990

26. Heaps JM, Fu YS, Montz FJ, Hacker NF, Berek JS: Surgical-pathologic variables predictive of local recurrence in squamous cell carcinoma of the vulva. Gynecol Oncol 38:309, 1990

26a. Breslow A, Macht SD: Optimal size of resection margin for the cutaneous melanoma. Surg Gynecol Obstet 145:691, 1977

27. Chamlin DL, Taylor HB: Primary cancer of Bartholin's gland. Obstet Gynecol 39:489, 1972

Ambulatory Gynecology, Second Edition,
edited by David H. Nichols and Patrick J. Sweeney.
J. B. Lippincott Company, Philadelphia, © 1995.

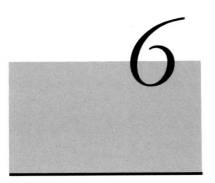

Inflammatory and Sexually Transmitted Diseases

Sebastian Faro

There are several sexually transmitted agents that can cause an infection that is associated with a significant inflammatory response. All organisms that cause sexually transmitted infections result in a local inflammatory response but some stimulate a broader response, including a systemic effect. The examining physician must realize that a variety of complaints may mimic other conditions but are actually infections caused by a sexually transmitted bacteria, virus, or protozoan. This chapter focuses on those sexually transmitted diseases (STDs) that are commonly seen by the physician who delivers care to women. Diagnosis and treatment of STDs is an important aspect of primary care of the female patient and should not be taken lightly. Improper evaluation and treatment may have significant effects on fertility, general well-being, social interaction, and personal financial stability.

PATIENT EVALUATION

History Taking

One of the most important initial aspects of the patient evaluation is to obtain a detailed history. The physician is often confronted with symptoms that suggest vaginitis. The patient may state that she has recurrent yeast infections or bacterial vaginosis or *Gardnerella vaginalis* vaginitis. The patient has already tried every medication available, has seen at least two physicians, spent a considerable amount of money, and is frustrated with her condition and the medical profession. The patient presents for another interview and examination and may lack confidence that her problem will be resolved. The mistake that may be made at this juncture is to perform a brief examination and prescribe a medication that she has already tried with no success.

Therefore, begin the session by taking a detailed history, asking significant and direct questions (Table 6-1). These questions should be presented in a manner that the patient can understand. The patient's past medical records should be obtained for review and documentation of all previous treatments and diagnoses. It is important to have the patient recall whether she or any of her partners has ever had any STD, such as condyloma. The viral STDs are particularly important because they can assume a latent existence within the host and may remain dormant for years. Often, the patient may manifest acute symptoms of *human papillomavirus* virus infection (HPV) years after the first

---

Table 6–1
Appropriate Questions to Ask of Patients Who Present With Signs or Symptoms of Infection

1. When did the symptoms first begin?
2. Exactly where are the symptoms located? (Often the assumption is made that the problem is located in the vagina. The examiner should ask if the symptoms are located on the labia or the entrance of the vagina or deep in the vagina.)
3. Describe the symptoms. Do you have pain, burning, itching, or a nondescript discomfort?
4. When are the symptoms present?
5. Are the symptoms aggravated by sexual intercourse?
6. How old were you when you had your first sexual intercourse?
7. How many sexual partners have you had to the present time?
8. Have you or any of your partners had an infection caused by *Neiserria gonorhoeae, Chlamydia trachomatis, Treponema pallidum,* herpes simplex, human papillomavirus, human immunodeficiency virus, hepatitis B virus?
9. Have you ever had a documented infection such as bacterial vaginosis, *Streptococcus agalactiae, Trichomonas vaginalis,* or *Candida albicans*?
10. Have you ever been treated with the following medications for a vaginal or pelvic infection: ceftriaxone, doxycycline, augmentin, azithromycin, or ofloxacin?
11. Have you ever been told that you had pelvic inflammatory disease?
12. Do you have intermenstrual spotting or bleeding?
13. Do you have postcoital bleeding?
14. Do you use birth control? If so, what method?
15. Do you and your partner or partners practice oral–genital sex? If yes, do either of you have a persistent sore throat or cough?

---

episode or exposure. It is important that this information be given to the patient because she likely will have assumed that she has recently contracted the disease.

Preparing the Patient for Examination

After completion of the history, the patient should be given an explanation of what will transpire during the examination. The examination should begin by first closely inspecting the external genital area for the presence of lesions and erythema. The lesion may be microscopic and the use of colposcope should be routinely employed. Table 6-2 describes the lesions associated with some of the STDs commonly seen in the United States. Patients often do not associate conditions of the vulva and vagina with systemic signs such as flu-like symptoms, yet it is not unusual for patients with the diseases listed in Table 6-2 (with the exception of HPV) to develop such symptoms. For this reason, it is important to determine whether such symptoms were present. This is important to assist in establishing a correct diagnosis. For example, in patients with herpes, the absence of such symptoms would suggest that this is a recurrent episode; in the case of syphilis, it suggests that this is the secondary stage.

The colposcope should be routinely employed in the examination of the vulva, introitus, vagina, and cervix. Many lesions that are due to herpesvirus and HPV often cannot be detected by gross examination, and magnification often reveals lesions that would otherwise remain undetected. Once a lesion is detected, it should be gently touched with a sterile cotton- or dacron-tipped applicator. If it proves tender or painful, the specimen should be placed in appropriate transport medium for the detection of herpesvirus. Raised or erythematous painful lesions should be painted with 5% acetic acid and examined colposcopically. If they become white, they should undergo biopsy. Before applying acetic acid, the vagina should be examined to determine whether healthy vaginal flora are present.

Vaginal Examination

The vaginal examination begins before inserting a speculum by noting whether there is a copious vaginal discharge exiting the vagina and if so, noting its color and odor. Before inserting the speculum, a gloved index finger should be inserted into the va-

Table 6–2
Vulvar Lesions Associated With Sexually Transmitted Diseases Commonly Seen in the United States

Disease	Lesion
Syphilis	Primary chancre: painless, solitary, base clean; erythematous and indurated; the border is raised and well-delineated Secondary syphilis: rash distributed over the soles of the feet and palms of the hands; rash is nonpruritic and maculopapular; another characteristic rash is the pustular, nodular eczema-like lesion, which may resemble acne; the anogenital condylomata lata Tertiary syphilis: gummata
Herpes simplex	Primary: ulcers—tend to be numerous and distributed over the vulva, may be pinpoint to large, very painful, associated bilateral inguinal painful lymphadenopathy Initial episode: usually few lesions, two to four Recurrent episodes: usually solitary
Chancroid	Ulcer: often referred to as dirty ulcer; the base is covered by a dirty-grayish necrotic exudate, painful; border is uneven, with undermined edges, bilateral inguinal lymphadenopathy
Human papillomavirus	Condylomata acuminatum: elevated, rough-appearing (pyriform or cauliflower-like); however, the lesions may be flat, smooth to papillary
Lymphogranuloma venereum	Primary: small papule or ulcer, painless Secondary: unilateral (occasionally bilateral) regional lymphadenitis; development of buboes; the inguinal femoral nodes are typically involved, creating the "groove sign"; esthiomene—labial lymphatics become edematous and develop draining sinuses

gina to determine the location and approximate depth of the cervix. This should be performed to prevent traumatizing the cervix, causing it to bleed, because the presence of blood alters the pH and obscures the microscopic examination of the vaginal discharge. The speculum can then be safely inserted. The vaginal epithelium should be inspected for the presence of petechial hemorrhages, ulceration, or projecting lesions. The discharge should be characterized according to the parameters listed in Table 6-3.

The presence of bacterial vaginosis (BV) or trichomoniasis is important because it suggests that the individual is sexually active and at risk for other STDs. Therefore, specimens should be obtained from the endocervix for the detection of *Neisseria gonorrhoeae* and *Chlamydia trachomatis*. The presence of petechial hemorrhages indicates that there is a localized inflammatory response. In such cases, the cervix also will be involved and may be

found to be tender on palpation and motion. The patient may also be found to have suprapubic tenderness, indicating the presence of cystitis due to either the presence of trichomonads or an accompanying organism. If uterine tenderness or adnexal tenderness is present, the presence of endometritis and salpingitis should be suspected.

Examination of the Cervix

After the examination of the vagina, attention should be focused on the cervix, attempting to characterize the squamous and endocervical epithelium. Herpetic lesions may appear as shallow ulcers or there may be necrosis associated with a copious clear, watery discharge. Human papillomavirus may be detected grossly by the presence of typical condylomatous lesions or flat white lesions. A Papanicolaou (Pap) smear should be obtained,

Table 6–3
Characteristics of Vaginal Discharge

Characteristic	Healthy	BV*	Trichomonas Species	Yeast
Color	White-gray	Other	Other	White
pH	3.8–4.2	>4.5	>4.5	<4.5†
Clue Cells	Absent	+	+	Absent
KOH Test	−	−	−	+
Whiff Test	−	+	−	−
Bacterial Morphotypes	Bacillary	Variety	Variety	Bacillary
Yeast	−	−	−	Hyphal forms, budding yeast

*BV, bacterial vaginosis.

†<4.5, yeast typically prefer more acidic conditions but may be found at higher pH values.

with specific instructions for the cytopathologist that you suspect herpes, HPV, or other infection. Appropriate specimens should be obtained for the detection of these STDs. After this has been completed, the cervix should be painted with 5% acetic acid to determine whether there are acetowhite areas, as well as evidence of dysplastic changes. Abnormal areas should undergo biopsy to confirm the diagnosis.

Attention should be returned to the vulva; erythematous areas should be gently palpated with a cotton-tipped applicator to determine areas of pain or tenderness. The area should be examined colposcopically and 5% acetic acid should be applied to the tissue. Areas that become white or have papillary structures, mosaicism, or increased vascularity should undergo biopsy.

Pelvic Examination

A bimanual examination is the final stage of the examination unless a mass is detected, in which case a pelvic ultrasound should be performed. The bimanual examination commences with detection of any significant areas of pain or tenderness to palpation, beginning with the introitus, continuing along the vaginal walls, and ending with palpation and motion of the cervix. The suprapubic area should be palpated to determine whether the bladder is tender, and the uterus should be gently examined to determine size, contour, symmetry, and

presence of pain or tenderness. The adnexa should be gently palpated to determine size, mobility, presence of a mass, and tenderness. A rectal examination should be performed to determine whether the cul-de-sac is free of masses and to ascertain whether there are any pelvic structures fixed to the cul-de-sac.

If there is a suspicion that pelvic pathology is present, a transvaginal and or abdominal ultrasound should be performed. This can be helpful in determining the presence of a mass, the nature of the mass, the anatomic location of the mass, and whether it is uni- or multiloculated. In addition, if fluid is present in the cul-de-sac, it may be aspirated and examined to attempt to establish a diagnosis (Table 6-4).

Differential Diagnosis

It is often difficult to establish a diagnosis of pelvic inflammatory disease (PID) because there are no physical findings or laboratory tests that are pathognomonic of PID. In studies addressing this issue, only two thirds of the patients with a clinical diagnosis of PID were actually found to have the disease when examined laparoscopically.[1-4] Specimens should be obtained for the culture of appropriate bacteria and viruses (Table 6-5).

Urine specimens should be obtained by the clean-catch method. If the patient has a significant discharge or is bleeding, a tampon may be inserted

Table 6–4
Value of Culdocentesis

Characteristic	Diagnosis	Additional Procedure
Blood	Ectopic pregnancy Ruptured hemorrhagic cyst Retrograde menstruation Endometriosis	Laparoscopy
Purulent fluid	Pelvic inflammatory disease Tubo-ovarian abscess Appendicitis Ruptured appendix Meckel's diverticulum abscess Diverticulitis	Ultrasound CT scan Laparoscopy Laporatomy
Serous fluid (cloudy)	Pancreatitis Cholecystitis	Amylase (serum and 2 hour urine determination) Ultrasound
Serous fluid (clear)	Normal	

in the vagina and instructions given on the appropriate technique to obtain a good urine specimen. A urine analysis and Gram stain should be obtained. The Gram stain provides an accurate interpretation of the presence of white blood cells and gram-positive or gram-negative bacteria. If bacteria are present, a culture may be performed. If pyuria is present but no bacteria are seen, the possibility of mycoplasmas or an inflamed structure lying against the bladder or ureter (eg, acute appendicitis, a Meckel's diverticulum, or an acute tubo-ovarian abscess).

Urethral specimens should be cultured if there is pyuria but no bacteriuria. The specimen should be obtained with a dacron urethral swab.

Endocervical specimens for the isolation of *C trachomatis* should be obtained with a dacron-tipped plastic-shafted swab. The specimen may be placed in transport media for culture or processed for antigen or DNA detection. Antigen- or DNA-

Table 6–5
Culture of Specimen in Evaluating Patients With Inflammation Associated with Sexually Transmitted Diseases

Site or Fluid	Organism to be Cultured
Urine	Uropathogens:
Urethra	*Neisseria gonorrhoeae, Chlamydia trachomatis, M hominis, U urealyticum.*
Skene's gland (purulent discharge)	*N gonorrhoeae, C trachomatis,* aerobes and anaerobes, *M hominis, U urealyticum*
Bartholin's gland (purulent discharge)	*N gonorrhoeae, C trachomatis,* aerobes and anaerobes, *M hominis, U urealyticum*
Cervix (endocervical canal)	*N gonorrhoeae, C trachomatis,* herpes simplex
Endometrium (biopsy)	*N gonorrhoeae, C trachomatis,* aerobes and anaerobes

detection methods are also available for gonorrhea in addition to culture. Culturing for herpes simplex virus (HSV) is easily accomplished with a rapid turnaround time (within 24 hours if the inoculum is high).

Endometrial cultures have proved to have a high correlation with the presence of PID.[5] Initially, the cervix should be cleansed with suitable disinfectant. An instrument such as a narrow-lumen uterine endometrial biopsy instrument should be used to obtain tissue. The tissue specimen should be divided so that part is sent for histologic study and the remainder used for the isolation of *N gonorrhoeae*, *C trachomatis*, *M hominis*, *U urealyticum*, and aerobic and anaerobic bacteria.

DIAGNOSIS AND MANAGEMENT

Syphilis

Syphilis has three basic stages, which are commonly referred to as primary, secondary, and tertiary. Primary syphilis is rarely diagnosed in women because the primary chancre is painless and may go unnoticed. Primary syphilis has an incubation period of 10 to 90 days, with an average time of appearance of the chancre being about 30 days. The chancre takes about 2 to 6 weeks to heal and is associated with inguinal lymphadenopathy.[6] In a study by Diaz-Mitoma and coworkers that examined genital ulcers, they found that the most common cause of nonvesicular genital ulcers was HSV.[7] In a study by Chapel and coworkers, using clinical criteria, only 78% of the cases could be accurately diagnosed.[8] As a rule, patients with primary syphilis do not manifest systemic signs of infection, and the inflammatory response is localized to the site of inoculation, which is the point where the chancre develops. Primary syphilis is usually diagnosed by microscopic darkfield examination. Serologic tests do not become positive until the late primary stage. The fluorescent antibody (FTA-ABS) test is the first serologic test to become positive. The Venereal Disease Research Laboratory (VDRL) and the rapid plasma reagin (RPR) tests become positive soon after the FTA-ABS converts to positive.

Secondary syphilis is divided into two stages: early and late latent disease. In the United States, early latent syphilis is defined as disease that has been present for less than 1 year (2 years in other countries). Late latent syphilis begins when the disease has been present for longer than 1 year. Secondary syphilis occurs 4 to 10 weeks after the appearance of the chancre and the patient develops systemic complaints that may resemble the flu (ie, elevated body temperature, malaise, arthralgia, and myalgia). Patients tend to develop a generalized lymphadenopathy. The patient may also develop pharyngitis, skin rash, patchy alopecia, hepatosplenomegaly, hepatitis, severe nocturnal headaches, photophobia, cranial nerve palsies that may result in deafness, optic neuritis, and papilledema. The most common lesions that occur in early secondary syphilis are the rash previously described and condylomata lata. The lesions of early secondary syphilis are infectious and therefore, the physician and other health care providers who come in contact with the patient should wear gloves and guard against being contaminated.

Tertiary syphilis may assume a variety of clinical presentations, depending on the duration of the illness, which develops anywhere from 15 to 30 years after the primary infection.[6,9] The inflammatory lesion of this stage of the disease is the gumma, which develops in the skin, subcutaneous tissue, or bone. The symptoms that develop depend on the location of the gumma (eg, pain is associated with bone lesions; jaundice or liver failure occurs when gumma form in the liver). Individuals with tertiary syphilis may develop cardiovascular complications, the most common being aortic aneurysm, aortic regurgitation, and coronary ostial stenosis.[10,11]

Involvement of the central nervous system (CNS) may occur at any stage of syphilis. The classic presentation of generalized paresis and tabes dorsalis is rarely seen today. It is not uncommon, however, to see patients with seizure activity or abnormal neuro-ophthalmologic findings.[12,13] Syphilitic meningitis, if it occurs, usually develops within the first 2 years after infection. The presentation is that of aseptic meningitis, with complaints of headache, mental confusion, nausea, vomiting, photophobia, or a stiff neck.[14,15] The patients tend to be afebrile but usually exhibit meningismus and often oculomotor or facial abnormalities. Penicillin treatment effects resolution of the disease within a few weeks.

Meningovascular neurosyphilis occurs within 5 to 10 years of infection in untreated or inappropriately treated individuals. These patients usually present with signs and symptoms of CNS vascular insufficiency.[13–15] The effects of meningovascular syphilis are not reversible.

Diagnosis

Treponema pallidum cannot be seen with light microscopy but can be readily detected using darkfield microscopy. This technique may be employed when there are chancres, condylomata lata, or mucous patches present. When obtaining specimens from oral lesions, however, care must be taken because there are treponemes present that are indigenous to the oral cavity. The appropriate method to obtain a specimen for darkfield microspopy is to first clean the surface of the lesion with sterile gauze and saline. This should allow the development of a serous exudate, which should be obtained and examined for treponemes. This provides rapid identification of *T pallidum* but care must be taken because (1) the organism cannot be differentiated from other commensal spirochetes; (2) the organism does not survive long outside the host, thus the examination must be performed rapidly; (3) the presence of red blood cells obscures the organism because the red blood cells themselves are highly refractile; and (4) if the patient has used a topical antibiotic, it may inhibit motility of the organism.[16] Another method is to use direct fluorescent antibody for *T pallidum*. Initially, fluorescein-tagged polyvalent anti–*T pallidum* globulin is used to identify the organism. This test has an advantage over the darkfield examination because the specimen can be fixed, transported, and is highly specific (100%) as well as sensitive (86%).[17]

The most widely used methods for the detection of syphilis are serologic, which fall into two basic categories: specific and nonspecific. The latter tests depend on the detection of a cholesterol–lecithin–cardiolipin antigen (reagin). This antigen cross-reacts with antibodies present in patients with syphilis. The two most widely used tests are the VDRL and the RPR. These tests are nonspecific but only used as a screening device. In individuals with primary syphilis, these tests become positive within 1 week of the appearance of the chancre. These tests have a false-negative rate that approaches 40% in individuals with primary syphilis.[18] Individuals with secondary syphilis almost always test positive. False-negative reactions may occur in individuals with extremely high antibody titers (prozone reaction), which can be overcome by diluting the serum. Patients adequately treated should be tested serially over a 12-month period and the RPR should revert to negative within 12 months. It is generally recommended that a repeat RPR be performed at 1, 3, 6, and 12 months after treatment. In some individuals, however, the RPR may remain positive at a low titer.[19–21] Individuals whose tests do not become negative should have a monthly RPR. After three monthly tests that have not shown a fourfold rise in titer, the test may be performed at 3, 6, and 12 months. These individuals may continue to have a fixed low titer (eg, 1 to 4 or

1 to 8). Titers that rise should be viewed as treatment failures or reinfections and treatment reinstituted.

All individuals who test positive to the RPR or VDRL and have no history of having had syphilis should have a confirmatory test. The specific tests are the fluorescent-treponemal antibody-absorbed test (FTA-ABS) and the microhemagglutination-*T pallidum* test (MHA-TP). The treponemal-specific tests usually become positive earlier than the RPR or VDRL but are more expensive and therefore not used for screening purposes. Individuals who have a positive FTA-ABS or MHA-TP usually remain positive, even after successful treatment. The one instance that the FTA-ABS or MHA-TP tests do serve a useful purpose is in the individual who is strongly suspected of having syphilis but has a nonreactive RPR. These individuals should be tested by the more specific and sensitive FTA-ABS or MHA-TP.[22]

Treatment

The most efficacious treatment for syphilis is penicillin. Alternative antibiotics such as erythromycin and tetracycline or doxycycline, although recommended, have not been tested sufficiently; therefore, patients treated with these agents should be monitored for relapse or recurrence.[23] Primary syphilis and disease that has been present for less than 1 year can be treated as outlined in Table 6-6.

Individuals treated with procaine penicillin or ceftriaxone for gonorrhea will also be cured of incubating syphilis. Patients treated with penicillin may experience a reaction that is characterized by myalgia, arthralgia, headache, fever, and hypotension. This reaction is known as the Jarisch–Herxheimer reaction and usually resolves within 24 hours. In pregnant patients, however, fetal deaths have occurred. Therefore, in treating pregnant patients with syphilis, it is best to monitor the fetus for 12 to 24 hours.

Late latent syphilis and syphilis that has been present for an unknown duration (including tertiary syphilis but excluding neurosyphilis) should be treated as outlined in Table 6-7.

Pregnant patients with documented syphilis should not be treated with erythromycin because it has not been proved to be effective and compliance is poor. Erythromycin is not well tolerated by pregnant patients because it causes significant gastrointestinal upset. Therefore, it is recommended that pregnant patients with documented syphilis who are allergic to penicillin should be desensitized.[24,25] Desensitization should be performed by experi-

Table 6–6
Treatment for Primary Syphilis of Less Than 1 Year Duration

	Regimen
Standard treatment	Benzathine penicillin, 1.2 million units, intramuscularly in each buttock
Patients allergic to penicillin	Doxycycline, 100 mg orally, twice daily for 14 days; or tetracycline, 500 mg orally, four times daily for 14 days
Pregnant patients	Erythromycin base, 500 mg four times daily for 14 days

enced physicians and precautions should be taken to manage anaphylaxis, should it occur.

Herpes Simplex

The herpesvirus family is made up of six DNA viruses: herpes types 1 and 2, cytomegalovirus, varicella-zoster, and the Epstein-Barr virus. The present discussion focuses on the herpes simplex types 1 and 2 viruses. These are probably the most common types among the world's population. Although both types cause genital lesions, type 2 is more frequently found to cause severe as well as recurrent infection.

The virus gains entrance to the host through microscopic or macroscopic breaks in the mucocutaneous tissue and eventually to the nucleus of nerve cells within sensory ganglia. The life cycle is perpetuated when the virus infects a mucocutaneous cell and replicates within the cell, causing cell death and thereby liberating the virus to infect adjacent cells. The virus can then elect to actively infect adjacent cells or migrate to neurons and become latent.[26,27] During the latent phase, the virus maintains an inactive posture, not having any symptomatic or asymptomatic effect on the nerve cell. It has been postulated that in about 1% of infected neurons, the viral gene is expressed.[28] This may explain why recurrent HSV episodes are extremely localized, even in patients who experience multiple recurrences.

Patients infected with HSV may either experience a primary (initial) or recurrent infection. Individuals who have not been exposed to the herpes virus and therefore have no antibodies are subject to a primary infection. The manifestation of the primary infection is characterized by numerous lesions, which begin as small vesicles or blisters. The lesions are preceded by systemic presentation, re-

Table 6–7
Treatment for Late Latent Syphilis and That of Unknown Duration

	Regimen
Standard treatment	Benzathine penicillin, 1.2 million units, intramuscularly in each buttock, weekly for 3 weeks
Penicillin-allergic patients	Doxycycline, 100 mg orally, twice daily for 28 days; or tetracycline, 500 mg orally, four times daily for 28 days
Neurosyphilis	Aqueous penicillin G, 12–24 million units/day intravenously, administered in divided doses of 2–4 million units every 4 hours; or procaine penicillin G, 2–4 million units/day, intramuscularly, with probenecid, 500 mg/day, orally, for a total of 14 days

sembling the flu. Although multi-organ infection is rare, it can occur. Therefore, it is important for the physician to perform a thorough examination to determine whether there is liver involvement (hepatitis) and or CNS involvement. The blisters that develop in conjunction with a primary attack usually are numerous and diffusely distributed over the vulva but may involve the vagina and cervix. Some patients may develop a herpetic cystitis and have extreme pain when urinating. Urine spilling over the vulvar lesions is also associated with pain. Patients experiencing a primary infection of the vulva usually develop significant vulval swelling and erythema.

Patients who have been previously exposed to HSV but have never had any symptoms and develop vulva lesions are experiencing an initial attack. This is usually characterized by the development of a few lesions. These individuals usually do not experience vulvar edema. Patients who are having recurrent herpetic outbreaks usually experience a prodrome, either localized pain or itching in the area where an ulcer will develop. There are usually 1 to 3 lesions and they tend to recur at the same location.

It is important to determine the viral type (ie, type 1 or 2) because it assists in determining the route of transmission and predicting chances of recurrences.[29,30] Patients infected with HSV-2 have about a 60% chance of recurrence, whereas those infected with HSV-1 have a 15% chance of recurrence.[30–32] It must also be understood by the physician and patient that most patients are unaware that they are infected and may not have symptomatic or frequent recurrences.[33,34] The risk of asymptomatic viral shedding from the vulva or cervix ranges from 0.4% to 1.3% per day.[35–38] This is extremely important because these patients are capable of transmitting the virus to their sexual partners or neonates if they are pregnant and deliver vaginally. Individuals who have no antibodies to HSV before infection tend to have severe primary or initial infections and symptomatic recurrences.[39,40] The knowledge that there are individuals who shed virus in the absence of lesions is important because they provide a perpetual pool of virus that is available for the transmission of the infection.

Obtaining antibodies in individuals who are suspected of having HSV is of limited value. Individuals who present with a primary attack should have an elevated IgM, thereby confirming this as their first episode. This does not alter the management of the patient. There is about a 50% DNA base-sequence homology between HSV-1 and HSV-2.

This homology between the two types causes patients who have HSV-1 labial infection to experience a less severe genital infection if they acquire HSV-2.[41,42] Although healthy patients develop a viremia with their first infection, they tend not to have systemic infection, whereas in the immunocompromised individual, disseminated disease is common. Thus, cellular immunity may be more important than humoral immunity.[28,35,36]

Diagnosis

Patients who present with genital ulcers may be a diagnostic dilemma because the etiology may be due to any one of several diseases (eg, syphilis, chancroid, lymphogranuloma venereum, granuloma inguinale, trauma, or Behçet's syndrome). Genital herpes, however, tends to have some unique characteristics: the primary episode typically is marked by numerous painful ulcers and vulvar edema; recurrent disease is marked by one to several ulcers that reoccur in the same area.

The diagnosis is established by obtaining specimens for culture. Although other etiologies should be considered, the physical symptoms and signs should guide the selection of diagnostic tests. It is important that when evaluating the patient for one STD, evidence of others should be sought. In this case, the patient should also be screened for gonorrhea, chlamydia, syphilis, human immunodeficiency virus, and hepatitis B. To obtain an appropriate specimen, a vesicle should be unroofed and the fluid cultured. Specimens obtained from fresh vesicles should yield virus in 90% of cases. Specimens obtained from crusted or healing lesions yield virus in about 40% of the specimens.[43] The appropriate technique is as follows: unroof a vesicle or pustule with a sterile needle, swab the ulcer with a sterile cotton-tipped applicator, and immerse it in viral-transport medium. If the specimen is not immediately processed, it should be refrigerated. If the specimen is not to be processed within 24 hours, it should be frozen at -70°C. If used to inoculate tissue culture, a cytopathic effect can be noticed within 24 hours if the inoculum is large.

The virus should be typed as to whether it is serotype 1 or 2 because this information can be used to give the patient a prognosis with regard to her rate of recurrence. Patients infected with HSV-2 have about a 60% chance of having recurrent episodes, whereas those infected with HSV-1 have a 15% recurrence rate.[44]

Serum antibody determinations do not alter the management of the patient's disease. It may, however, assist in determining whether the infection represents a primary or recurrent episode. Studies show that 50% of individuals with their first episode of herpes lack IgG antibodies to the herpes virus in the acute phase of the disease. Immune globulin G was found in the convalescent sera, however. This indicates that the infection was truly a primary episode. Twenty-five percent of patients with so-called primary infection have IgG antibodies to HSV-2, thus suggesting that these individuals had been previously exposed to the virus.[45] Thus, the combination of viral typing and serum antibody determination may prove helpful in the management of the patient. All patients who have genital ulcer disease should have a herpes culture performed to establish that it is indeed herpes. The patient should not be told that she has a STD until it has been confirmed. Telling an individual that she has an STD without confirming that one is present creates problems for the patient and her spouse or significant other. Treatment may have to be instituted before confirmation that an STD is present but this can be explained to the patient so that she understands the need for therapy. Patients with recurrent lesions who are suspected of having herpes and who have been told they have herpes without the diagnosis ever having been substantiated should have the lesions cultured. Recurrent herpetic lesions are usually more ephemeral than those seen with a primary or initial episode and should be cultured within 48 hours of their appearance. Often, the lesions are small and can be seen only with the aid of magnification. It is helpful to have the patient physically point to the area that is symptomatic. Sometimes the area of involvement may appear as a small abrasion, fissure, or an area of erythema.

Alternatives to viral culture are the Pap or Tzanck smears, immunofluorescence, immunoperoxidase staining, and enzyme-linked immunosorbent assay. All are less sensitive than culture but usually yield results more rapidly. These tests are not sensitive enough to be used on the patient who sheds virus in the asymptomatic state. These tests have a sensitivity in the 70% to 90% range; however, culture should be performed if time permits.

Treatment

Herpesvirus infection is not curable (ie, therapy is not available that eradicates the virus). Consequently, there is no place for surgery—specifically laser ablation or cryosurgery—in the management of the herpetic lesion. This is important to realize because the patient suspected of having vulvodynia

or vestibulitis or cervicitis should be evaluated for herpes before instituting therapy, especially destructive therapy.

The drug of choice in both the non- and immunocompromised patient is acyclovir. This antiviral agent is available in topical, oral, and intravenous forms.[46] Acyclovir has been used for the the the treatment of primary, disseminated, and recurrent herpes.

Acyclovir in its native form is inactive and must be phosphorylated to the triphosphate form to be active. The initial phosphorylation of acyclovir is accomplished using the HSV thymidine kinase. Thus, infected host cells are capable of initiating the phosphorylation process, whereas uninfected host cells have extremely limited capabilities to initiate phosphorylation of acyclovir. Once the initial phosporylation is complete, subsequent phosphorylations are accomplished by the host cell kinases. Resistance to acyclovir occurs when HSV strains become thymidine kinase deficient, thereby losing the ability to activate acyclovir.[47]

Acyclovir is a competitive inhibitor of deoxyguanosine triphosphate and inhibits viral DNA polymerase. A second mechanism of action is by chain termination. Acyclovir has no 3'-hydroxyl group; thus, when it is incorporated into viral DNA, no linkage can be formed with other nucleotides.[48]

Routes of administration depend on the severity of the infection. Topical therapy appears to be the least beneficial and probably has no real use, except perhaps for individuals with severe labial infection. Patients with severe genital infection associated with significant labial edema, urinary retention, and fever should be treated with intravenous acyclovir. These patients should be thoroughly examined to rule out the possibility of hepatic and CNS involvement. Intravenous administration should be as follows: 5 to 10 mg/kg every 8 hours, administered slowly and while maintaining the patient in a well-hydrated state.

It is important that the patient be given adequate intravenous fluids to prevent crystallization of the drug in the renal tubules and ureters. Patients with less severe primary or initial infection may be treated with oral acyclovir as follows: 200 mg orally, five times daily for 10 days.

I prefer not to prescribe maintenance therapy until the patient has experienced a recurrence. If the patient has had a recurrent herpetic infection, I will treat as follows: 200 mg orally, five times daily for 10 days; followed by 200 mg orally, three times daily for 30 days; followed by 200 mg orally, two times daily for 30 days; followed by 200 mg orally, once a day for 1 year.

Using this regimen has prevented patients from having recurrent episodes. This information has not been collected in a scientific or clinical study but the regimen has been in use for about 6 years, with excellent success. If this protocol is followed, the patients must understand that this is experimental and that they must keep themselves adequately hydrated.

Pelvic Inflammatory Disease

Pelvic inflammatory disease is actually a spectrum of disease that in this author's opinion begins with cervicitis and may progress to endometritis, salpingitis, pyosalpingx, and finally, tubo-ovarian abscess. If asymptomatic, left unattended, treated inappropriately, or not diagnosed correctly, this disease may lead to significant damage of the fallopian tubes, infertility, ectopic pregnancy, or chronic pelvic pain. Therefore, the most difficult aspect of this disease is in making the diagnosis. It is known that cervicitis and its related consequences are often asymptomatic, and PID of this type has been referred to as "silent PID."

It is estimated that there are 1 million office and emergency room visits a year for PID.[49] Unfortunately, every woman that is seen in the emergency room with a complaint of pelvic pain who has cervical, uterine, and adnexal tenderness on pelvic examination is likely to be diagnosed as having PID unless a pelvic mass is found. Patients with PID have an overall risk of 25% of becoming infertile.[50,51] The total costs related to the treatment of PID and its subsequent complications exceeded $4 billion in 1990.[52]

Microbiology

The bacteria most frequently associated with PID are *Neisseria gonorrhoeae* and *Chlamydia trachomatis*. It is not uncommon, however, to find both of these bacteria to be present simultaneously and on some occasions, neither may be present. On some occasions, other bacteria may be found in association with these two sexually transmitted bacteria; at times, other bacteria are found in the absence of the these two sexually transmitted bacteria (Table 6-8).

Polymicrobial PID in the absence of the gonococcal or chlamydial organisms is usually derived from the patient's own microflora. The endogenous

Table 6–8
Pelvic Inflammatory Disease Categories by Bacterial Etiology

Gonococcal pelvic inflammatory disease (PID)
Chlamydial PID
Gonococcal plus chlamydial PID
Gonococcal plus chlamydial plus polymicrobial PID
Nongonococcal, nonchlamydial, polymicrobial PID

microflora is made up of many different bacteria—gram-positive and gram-negative aerobes, facultative and obligate anaerobes. These bacteria can gain entrance to the upper genital tract by directly ascending through the endocervical canal to the uterine cavity and the fallopian tubes. The organisms of the lower genital tract may also gain entrance to the upper tract through sexual intercourse and instrumentation (eg, endometrial biopsy, hysterosalpingography, laparoscopy).

Diagnosis

There are no laboratory tests or physical findings that are pathognomonic of PID. Laparoscopy does not yield 100% assurance that patients will be identified as having PID. Therefore, it is critical that the physician have a high index of suspicion, which may be obtained from the patient's history. Again, the presence of a STD or contact with a sexual partner who has an STD should alert the physician to the possibilities of PID.

CERVICITIS. Patients with cervicitis do not usually present with overt symptoms; therefore, questions must be asked with regard to postcoital spotting, recent onset of dysparuenia, and dysuria. The pelvic examination can be extremely helpful in determining whether there is endocervical mucous present, whether the cervix bleeds easily when touched gently with a cotton- or dacron-tipped applicator, or if there is evidence of endocervical hypertrophy. The Pap smear may also be helpful in detecting evidence of inflammation or atypia.

Patients with endocervical mucous usually do not complain of an abnormal discharge. This can be detected by placing a cotton- or dacron-tipped applicator into the endocervical canal and rotating gently for 30 seconds. The applicator is withdrawn and examined for the presence of purulent mucus. The presence of 10 or more polymorphonuclear leukocytes on microscopic examination of the endocervical discharge correlates strongly with the presence of *C trachomatis*.[53,54] A study showed, however, that after successful treatment for chlamydial infection, 10 or more polymorphonuclear leukocytes could be found in the endocervical specimen.[55] A Gram stain may be helpful because it may reveal polymorphonuclear leukocytes and no bacteria, which would be suspicious but not conclusive of chlamydial infection. If the Gram stain revealed the presence of gram-negative intracellular diplococci, this would be suggestive but not conclusive of gonococcal infection. Treatment should not be withheld from patients whom the physician has strong clinical suspicion of having infection but confirmation of the disease should be obtained.

ENDOMETRITIS. Patients who develop intermenstrual spotting or bleeding should be viewed as possibly having endometritis. Unfortunately, many patients develop a vague lower abdominal pain, misinterpret it as menstrual cramps, and do not do anything but take ibuprofen. The patient who has intermenstrual spotting or breakthrough bleeding while taking oral contraceptive pills should be evaluated for PID or endometritis. This can be accomplished by performing an endometrial biopsy with an endometrial sampling device such as the Pipelle. The tissue sample should be divided into two equal portions—one to be sent for histologic evaluation and the other to be processed for the isolation of *N gonorrhoeae*, *C trachomatis*, aerobic, facultative, and obligate anaerobic bacteria.[56] The presence of plasma cells on the biopsy specimen is highly correlated with the existence of acute salpingitis. Another advantage of the biopsy specimen is that the tissue specimen can be transported in an anaerobic transport medium and used for the iso-

lation of all desired bacteria. Although culdocentesis may be useful in establishing a diagnosis, it is not a useful technique to obtain peritoneal fluid for culture of microorganisms. Transvaginal culdocentesis is likely to yield bacteria but these organisms are essentially contaminants obtained from the vagina during the procedure.[57,58] Neither the quality nor the validity of the specimen is improved by first cleansing the vagina with Betadine because it is virtually impossible to sterilize the vagina. Guidelines for obtaining specimens for culture in patients with PID are given in Table 6-9.

The diagnosis of PID is usually made on clinical grounds, using the criteria listed in Table 6-10. It must be noted, however, that the clinical parameters do not strongly correlate with the actual presence of PID. Often, the diagnosis is confused with other pathologic and nonpathologic conditions and therefore, it is advised that a list be constructed of differential diagnoses to aid the physician in evaluating and treatment of the patient (Table 6-11).

With such a long list of possible diagnoses (which still may be incomplete), it is no wonder that it is difficult to make a diagnosis of PID. Since it is not possible to perform laparoscopy on all patients suspected of having PID, the clinical parameters listed in Table 6-10 are intended to offer the clinician some guidelines in establishing the diagnosis. Often, it is difficult to perform an adequate pelvic examination; therefore, ultasonography may often be helpful in determining whether a mass is present.

The characteristics of the mass may be helpful in determining whether it is inflammatory. Typically, a mass that results from an acute or chronic inflammatory process is characterized by an irregular thick border. There is the appearance of an ir-

Table 6–9
Appropriate Sites for Culture in Patients With Pelvic Inflammatory Disease

Site	NG*	CT†	Aerobes	Facultative	Anaerobes
Endocervix	Yes	Yes	No	No	No
Endometrium (biopsy)	Yes	Yes	Yes	Yes	Yes
Peritoneal fluid (laparoscopy)	Yes	Yes	Yes	Yes	Yes
Fallopian tubes (laparoscopy)	Yes	Yes	Yes	Yes	Yes

*Neisseria gonorrhoeae
†Chlamydia trachomatis.

Table 6–10
Clinical Criteria for Diagnosing Pelvic Inflammatory Disease

ALL of the following must be present:
   Lower abdominal pain
   Cervical motion tenderness
   Adnexal tenderness
ONE of the following should be present:
   Temperature >38°C
   White blood cell count >10,500/μL or a left shift in the differential
   Purulent material obtained by culdocentesis
   Presence of a tender mass on bimanual pelvic examination
   Elevated erythrocyte sedimentation rate or C-reactive protein
   Isolation of *Neisseria gonorrhoeae* or *Chlamydia trachomatis* from the endocervix or endometrium
   Histologic evidence on endometrial biopsy of infection (e.g., presence of plasma cells)

regular mass, which indicates that bowel is adherent and is making up part of the mass. A benign mass may be cystic or solid, usually with a definitive border. If cystic, it may or may not have septations or internal echoes. Patients with a mass who have acute salpingitis usually do not have an abscess but an inflamed adnexa, with small and large

Table 6–11
Differential Diagnosis for Evaluating the Patient Suspected of Having Pelvic Inflammatory Disease

Appendicitis
Ectopic pregnancy
Endometriosis
Endometrioma
Torsion of an adnexa
Ureteral stone
Pyelonephritis
Ruptured ovarian cyst
Ruptured hemorrhagic ovary
Pancreatitis
Abscesses of Meckel's diverticulum
Ruptured tubo-ovarian abscess
Ruptured appendix
Ruptured Meckel's diverticula abscess
Ruptured diverticulitis

bowel adhering to the adnexa, creating a mass-like effect. A pyosalpinx appears ultrasonographically as an oblong cystic structure. On physical examination, it has findings consistent with peritonitis and cannot be differentiated from a tubo-ovarian abscess. Ultrasonography may be helpful in making this differentiation because the ovary can be frequently seen and typically measured and characterized. Tubo-ovarian abscesses can be uniloculated or multiloculated. Acute tubo-ovarian abscesses usually are uniloculated and thin walled, whereas those of relatively long standing are thick walled and often multiloculated. The presence of a mass, whether or not the patient presents acutely ill, requires that the physician create a differential diagnosis to effect appropriate management (Table 6-12).

Management

The management of the patient with acute inflammation of the pelvic organs must begin with establishing whether the patient has an infectious process. Once acute or chronic appendicitis has been ruled out, the decision must be made whether the patient has PID. In the absence of a definitive mass, if PID is highly suspect and there is no evidence of a surgical emergency, antibiotic therapy may be instituted (Table 6-13). In uncomplicated PID, antibiotic therapy should effect a marked improvement in the patient within 48 to 72 hours. Patients with signs of peritonitis, nausea, or elevated temperatures of more than 101°F or inability to tolerate oral liquids and solids should be hospitalized and receive intravenous antibiotics.

The use of doxycycline is required for the possible presence or coexistence of chlamydia. If the

Table 6–12
Differential Diagnosis of a Patient With Signs of Pelvic Infection and a Pelvic Mass

Appendicitis
Pyosalpinx
Tubo-ovarian abscess
Ovarian abscess
Torsion of an adnexa, with or without necrosis
Ruptured endometrioma
Ruptured hemorrhagic cyst
Infarcted and degenating mass (ovarian or leiomyomata)
Diverticulitis

Table 6–13
Intravenous Antibiotics for Treatment of Pelvic Inflammatory Disease

	Dose	Frequency
Cephalosporins*		
Cefotetan	2 g	q 12 hrs
Cefoxitin	2 g	q 6 hrs
Ceftizoxime	2 g	q 8 hrs
Penicillins		
Ampicillin/sulbactam (Unasyn)	3 g	q 6 hrs
Piperacillin/tazobactam (Zosyn)	3 g	q 6 hrs
Ticarcillin/clavulanate (Timentin)	3 g	q 6 hrs
Combinations of Antibiotic		
Clindamycin plus gentamicin	900 mg	q 8 hrs
	2 mg/kg loading dose; 1.5 mg/kg initial therapeutic dose (trough–peak levels to determine actual therapeutic dose)	

*All cephalosporins should receive additionally doxycycline, 100 mg, orally, q 12 hrs.

penicillins are used, doxycycline does not need to be added because these antibiotics are active against *Chlamydia trachomatis*.[59–63] If using combinations of antibiotics, it seem logical to select clindamycin plus gentamicin over metronidazole plus gentamicin because the former not only provides a broader spectrum of activity against aerobes and anaerobes but is also synergistic against *C trachomatis*. Clindamycin is active against *C trachomatis* and gentamicin is not but synergism has been demonstrated when the two are used together.[64] I prefer to reserve the use of clindamycin plus gentamicin for those patients who have pelvic inflammatory masses or abscesses. I also include ampicillin for its synergistic activity against enterococci. In treatment of uncomplicated salpingitis, I also prefer the use of the expanded-spectrum penicillins that contain a β-lactamase inhibitor because of the activity against enterococci and chlamydia.

Although it is difficult to establish that the enterococci are indeed pathogenic components in abscess development, these bacteria are abscessogenic when growing with *Escherichia coli* or *Previtella bivia*.[65] Because enterococci are commonly found as part of the endogenous vaginal and fecal flora, there is opportunity for these organisms to become part of the bacterial milieu of PID. In addition, individuals with advanced PID commonly are found to have the rectosigmoid colon involved in the inflammatory process. This bowel is often edematous, inflamed, and adherent to the adnexa as well as to the posterior aspect of the uterus. The inflammatory process involving the bowel creates microscopic breaks in the intestinal wall, thus allowing bacteria to migrate out of the bowel.

Patients who do not respond to treatment over a 48 to 72 hour period are either treatment failures or there has been an error in diagnosis. These individuals should be reevaluated by repeating their physical examination and obtaining new laboratory studies, such as a complete blood count with white blood cell differential, sedimentation rate or C-reactive protein, serum electrolytes, blood urea nitrogen, and creatinine levels. In addition, consideration should be given to performing a laparoscopy, which enables the physician to establish a correct diagnosis in most cases. If laparoscopy cannot be performed, a pelvic ultrasound or computed tomography scan may be used. If pelvic ultrasonography is to be depended on, it must be performed by a sonographer experienced in actually doing and reading pelvic ultrasonograms.

Patients who fail to respond to initial therapy and who are found at laparoscopy to have copious free pus in the peritoneal cavity may be treated by irrigating (through the laparoscope) the peritoneal cavity with copious amounts of sterile saline. This is continued until the aspirated fluid is clear and all the pelvic structures can be easily inspected. It is imperative that the appendix be brought into the field of examination along its entire length. If no mass or suspected abscess is found, the patient's antibiotic coverage may be broadened (eg, if the patient is on a cephalosporin or penicillin, these should be discontinued and clindamycin, ampicillin, and gentamicin administered in the proper dosages). If an abscess is found that is well delineated and that can easily be reached through the laparoscope, it may be drained and irrigated. A drain should be placed into the abscess cavity and exited through the abdominal wall. The drain should be attached to suction and sutured to the abdominal wall to prevent it from becoming prematurely dislodged. This is important because if infected contents remain and leak into the peritoneal cavity, recurrent abscesses will develop and the patient will be subjected to serious morbidity and perhaps mortality. Abscesses may be drained percutaneously but it is important to ensure that these masses are not malignant because early ovarian stage I disease could contaminate the entire peritoneal cavity, thereby changing the patient's prognosis.

Advanced PID is usually not amenable to laparoscopic management because there are usually diffuse adhesions of the small and large bowel, involving the peritoneal surfaces of the abdominal wall and pelvic organs. There is usually a significant degree of ileus, which makes laparoscopy more hazardous. Laparotomy is usually the best approach to ensure that complete surgical management can be performed. Initially, the abdomen should be entered with a vertical incision to permit complete exploration of the abdominal cavity. This becomes more critical if there is free purulent material in the peritoneal cavity. The abdominal cavity should be thoroughly explored, including the subdiaphragmatic area, subhepatic, and subsplenic areas. All adhesions must be lysed in order to run and inspect the entire bowel to prevent intraloop bowel abscesses from forming. If the omentum is significantly indurated and infected, a partial omentectomy is usually performed. Once all the adhesions have been taken down and the upper abdomen has been inspected, the bowel should be packed and the upper abdomen protected from contamination. Attention is turned to the pelvis. The exact surgical procedure depends on the nature and extent of disease and the patient's desires. It is critical that before surgery a detailed discussion be conducted with the patient, explaining the advantages and dis-

advantages of the various options. If the ovaries are not involved but there is a significant bilateral pyosalpinx and the patient desires to retain her reproductive capabilities, one of two routes may be taken. The conservative approach—drainage of the abscess, with retention of her reproductive organs—may require that she undergo a second laparotomy or if the initial procedure is successful may increase her risk for ectopic pregnancy or infertility. The alternative procedure would be removal of the fallopian tubes, making her a candidate for in vitro fertilization. Total abdominal hysterectomy with bilateral salpingectomy is indicated in severe cases. If the ovaries are involved, they should be removed; however, preservation of the ovaries should be attempted because these patients are usually young and total hormonal replacement is not possible.

Outpatient Management

It is not possible or necessary to admit all patients with PID to the hospital. If the patient's temperature is less than or equal to 101°F, if she is able to tolerate oral liquids and solids and does not have peritonitis or a mass, outpatient management is acceptable. When administering oral antibiotics for the outpatient treatment of PID, it is important to remember that the agents chosen should provide a broad spectrum of activity. The agents should be active against *N gonorrhoeae*, *C trachomatis*, gram-positive and gram-negative aerobes, and facultative and obligate anaerobes. This is not adequately achieved with ceftriaxone, 250 mg intramuscularly, given once, together with a 10-day course of doxycycline, 100 mg orally, twice a day. Table 6-14 lists oral agents that provide the required and desired activity against all bacteria that may be involved.

Table 6–14

Oral Antimicrobial Therapy for Outpatient Treatment of Pelvic Inflammatory Disease

Antimicrobial Agent	Dosage
Augmentin	500 mg, tid × 10 days
Clindamycin	300 mg, tid × 10 days
plus	
Ofloxacin	300 mg, bid × 10 days
Metronidazole	500 mg, tid × 10 days
plus	
Ofloxacin	300 mg, bid × 10 days

A second important aspect of the outpatient treatment of PID is the follow-up. All patients should be reevaluated within 72 hours to determine the effectiveness of treatment. Individuals who are not making progress may need to be hospitalized for reevaluation, intravenous antibiotics, and perhaps further diagnostic procedures.

Postoperative Management

Patients who undergo surgical exploration for PID usually have an ileus for several days. It is not uncommon to have a nasogastric tube in place during and after the operative procedure. The nasogastric tube should be placed on continuous intermittent suction. When bowel sounds have returned, rectal stimulants may be used to initiate the passage of flatus. Once the patient has active bowel sounds and is passing flatus, the nasogastric tube may be clamped for 1 hour; the clamp can then be released and suction resumed. If there is less than 100 mL of gastric fluid returned, the tube may be reclamped for 4 hours, then released. If there is less than 100 mL, the tube may be removed. This procedure reduces the possibility for aspiration if the patient cannot tolerate clamping and avoids the premature removal of the tube, necessitating its reinsertion. When the tube is removed, the patient may be placed on clear liquids for 24 hours. If this is tolerated, her diet may rapidly progress to a regular meal.

Patients with a drain in place are managed as follows:

1. Intraperitoneal drains are not exited through the incision but lateral to it and in the lowest place in the abdomen. The drain is attached to suction (eg, a Hemovac) and left in place until there is less than 30 mL of fluid accumulated in a 24-hour period.
2. Patients who have had a hysterectomy will have a large drain (mushroom collapsible drain) exiting through the vaginal cuff. This drain is also attached to a suction device and managed as described above.
3. Wound drains are placed if there has been intraperitoneal purulent material and the wound is closed primarily. These drains are usually placed subfascially and subcutaneously and do not exit through the incision but through separate stab wounds made for the drains. These drains are also attached to suction. Penrose drains are not used because they act as a wick, onto which fluid can move in two directions, carrying bacteria away from and to the wound.

All drains are managed in the same manner; before removing the drain serum or blood or fluid is aspirated through the drain and sent for Gram stain. If the Gram stain is negative, the drain is removed. If the Gram stain is positive, the drain is removed and antibiotic therapy is instituted (Table 6-15).

Patients receiving an aminoglycoside should have serum trough and peak levels determined to monitor adverse effects. This is also helpful in determining the ideal dose of aminoglycoside. Patients who are allergic to penicillin should be given vancomycin in addition to gentamicin. Again, the trough and peak levels of both antibiotics should be determined.

Once the patient has become afebrile for 72

Table 6–15
Antibiotic Management for Wound Infection

Gram Stain	Antibiotic	Dosage
Positive cocci	Piperacillin/tazobactam	3.375 g, IV, q 6 hrs
	Amoxicillin/sulbactam	3 g, IV, q 6 hrs
Negative bacilli	Cefoxitin	2 g, IV, q 6 hrs
	Ceftizoxime	2 g, IV, q 6 hrs
	Piperacillin/tazobactam	3.375 g, IV, q 6 hrs
Mixed	Piperacillin/tazobactam	3.375 g, IV, q 6 hrs
	Ticarcillin/clavulanic acid	3.1 g, IV, q 6 hrs
	Clindamycin	900 mg, IV, q 8 hrs
	plus	
	Gentamicin	2 mg/kg, IV, loading dose; 1.5 mg/kg maintenance dose, q 8 hrs

hours, intravenous antibiotic therapy can be discontinued and oral antimicrobial therapy started, using the same recommendations that were made for outpatient management of PID. The antibiotics should be continued for 14 days and the patient should be reevaluated within 72 to 96 hours after discharge and again, 14 to 20 days after discharge. Patients whose ovaries were not removed but were subject to considerable dissection of adhesion should be tested for adequate estrogen effect. If the patient's fallopian tubes were left in place, a hysterosalpingogram should be performed 3 months postoperatively. The hysterosalpingogram should be preceded by a thorough pelvic examination and ultrasound to rule out the presence of a mass, which may possibly be an abscess. A complete blood count with a white blood cell differential and sedimentation rate should be obtained. Endocervical specimens should be obtained for the detection of *N gonorrhoeae* and *C trachomatis*. The vagina should be checked for the presence of BV and trichomonads. If the evaluation does not reveal any abnormalities, the hysterosalpingogram can be performed. Patients who have had a bilateral oopherectomy should be seen quarterly to adjust their hormonal replacement therapy.

Patients who respond to treatment with antibiotics for the presence of tubo-ovarian abscesses but have a persistent mass should have an exploratory laparotomy to ensure that the mass is truly a residual sterile abscess. Transvaginal or transabdominal aspiration without knowing the exact etiology of the mass is not recommended. Many of these patients with a residual mass after antibiotic therapy complain of pain.

It is important to remember that patients with inflammatory disease secondary to an STD are most likely to be in the prime of their reproductive years. Therefore, every attempt should be made to preserve reproductive organs and ovarian function. The uterus is usually not involved, except for adherence on the serosal surface in cases of advanced disease.

REFERENCES

1. Jacobson L, Westrom L: Objectivized diagnosis of acute pelvic inflammatory disease: diagnostic and prognostic value of routine laparoscopy. Am J Obstet Gynecol 105:1088, 1969
2. Binstock M, Muzsnai D, Apodaca L, et al: Laparoscopy in the diagnosis and treatment of pelvic inflammatory disease: a review and discussion. Int J Fertil 31:341, 1986
3. Burchell HJ, Schoon MG: The value of laparoscopy in the diagnosis of acute pelvic inflammatory disease. S Afr Med J 72:197, 1987
4. Paavonen J, Teisala K, Heinonen PK, et al: Microbiological and histopathological findings in acute pelvic inflammatory disease. Br J Obstet Gynaecol 94:454, 1987
5. Heinonen PK, Teisala K, Punnonen R, Miettinen A, Lehtinen M, Paavonen J: Anatomic sites of upper genital tract infection. Obstet Gynecol 66:384, 1985
6. Gjestland T: The Oslo study of untreated syphilis. Acta Derm Venerol (Suppl) (Stockh) 35:34, 1955
7. Diaz-Mitoma F, Benningen G, Slutchuk M, et al: Etiology of non-vesicular genital ulcers in Winnipeg. Sex Transm Dis 14:33, 1987
8. Chapel TA, Brown WJ, Jeffries C, et al: How reliable is the morphological diagnosis of penile ulcerations. Sex Transm Dis 4:150, 1977
9. Clark EG, Danbolt N: The Oslo study of the neutral course of untreated syphilis: an epidemiologic investigation based on a restudy of the Boeck-Bruusgaard material. Med Clin North Am 48:613, 1964
10. Rockwell DH, Yobs AR, Moore MB: The Tuskegee study of untreated syphilis. Arch Intern Med 114:792, 1964
11. Pressler V, McNamara JJ: Thoracic aortic aneurysm. J Thorac Cardiovasc Surg 79:489, 1980
12. Hooshmand H, Escobar MR, Kopl SW: Neurosyphilis. A study of 241 patients. JAMA 219:726, 1972
13. Hotson JR: Modern neurosyphilis: a partially treated chronic mennigitis. West J Med 135:191, 1981
14. Meritt HH, Moore M: Acute syphilitic meningitis. Medicine 14:119, 1935
15. Simon RP: Neurosyphilis. Arch Neurol 42:606, 1985
16. Lukehart SA: Syphilis. In Wentworth BB (ed): Diagnostic procedures for bacterial infections, p 519. Am J Public Health, 1987
17. Daniels KC, Ferneyhough HS: Specific direct fluorescent antibody detection of *Treponema pallidum*. Health Lab Sci 14:164, 1977
18. Hutchinson CM, Hook EW: Syphilis in adults. In Martin DH (ed): Sexually transmitted diseases. Med Clin North Am 74:1389, 1990
19. Fiumara NJ: Treatment of early latent syphilis of less than a years duration: an evaluation of 275 cases. Sex Transm Dis 5:85, 1978
20. Fiumara NJ: treatment of secondary syphilis: an evaluation of 204 patients. Sex Transm Dis 4:96, 1977
21. Fiumara NJ: Treatment of seropositive primary syphilis: an evaluation of 196 patients. Sex Transm Dis 4:92, 1977
22. Rein MF, Banks GW, Logan LC, et al: Failure of the *Treponema pallidum* immobilization test to provide additional diagnostic information about contemporary sex. Sex Transm Dis 7:101, 1980
23. Schroeter AL, Lucas JB, Price EV, et al: Treatment for early syphilis and reactivity of serologic tests. JAMA 221:471, 1972
24. Ziaya PR, Hankins DV, Gilstrap LC, Halsey AB: Intravenous penicillin desensitization and treatment during pregnancy. JAMA 256:2651, 1986
25. Wendel GD, Stark BJ, Jamison RB, et al: Penicillin

allergy and desensitization in serious maternal/fetal infections. N Engl J Med 312:1229, 1985

26. Corey L, Spear LG: Infections with the herpes simplex viruses. Parts 1 and 2. N Engl J Med 314:686,749, 1986

27. Strauss SE: Clinical and biological differences between recurrent herpes simplex virus and varicella-zoster virus infections. JAMA 262:3455, 1959

28. Corey L, Adams HG, Brown ZA, et al: Genital herpes simplex virus infection: clinical manifestations, cause and complications. Ann Intern Med 98:958, 1983

29. Reeves WC, Corey L, Adams HG, et al: Risk of recurrence after first episodes genital herpes. Relation to HSV type and antibody response. N Engl J Med 805:315, 1981

30. Lafferty WE, Coombs RW, Benedetti J, et al: Recurrences after oral and genital herpes simplex virus infection. Influence of site of infections and viral type. N Engl J Med 316:1444, 1987

31. Mertz GJ, Schmidt O, Jourden IL, et al: Frequency of acquisition of first-episode genital infection with herpes simplex virus from symptomatic and asymptomatic source contacts. Sex Transm Dis 12:33, 1985

32. Prober CG, Hensleigh PA, Boucher FD, et al: Use of routine viral culture delivery to identify neonates exposed to herpes simplex virus. N Engl J Med 381:887, 1988

33. Douglas JM, Cutchlow C, Benedetti J, et al: A double blind study of oral acyclovir for suppression of recurrences of genital herpes simplex virus infection. N Engl J Med 310:1551, 1984

34. Mertz GJ, Ashley R, Burke RL, et al: Double blind placebo-controlled trial of a herpes simplex virus type 2 glycoprotein vaccine in persons at high risk for genital herpes infection. J Infect Dis 161:653, 1990

35. Meyers JD, Flournoy N, Thomas ED: Infection with herpes simplex virus and cell mediated immunity after marrow transplant. J Infect Dis 142:338, 1980

36. Quinan GV Jr, Masur H, Rook AH, et al: Herpesvirus infections in the acquired immune deficiency syndrome. JAMA 252:72, 1984

37. Brock BV, Selke S, Benedeti J, et al: Frequency of asymptomatic shedding of herpes simplex virus in women with genital herpes. JAMA 263:418, 1990

38. Prober CG, Sullender WM, Yasukawa LL, et al: Low risk of herpes simplex infections in neonates exposed to the virus at time of vaginal delivery to mothers with recurrent genital herpes simplex virus infection. N Engl J Med 316:240, 1987

39. Genital herpes infection, United States 1966 — 1984. MMWR 35:402, 1986

40. Mertz GJ: Herpes simplex virus. In Antiviral agents and viral diseases of man. New York, Raven Press, 1990

41. Wentworth BB, Alexander ER: Seroepidemiology of infection due to members of the herpesvirus group. Am J Epidemiol 94:496, 1971

42. Johnson RE, Nahamias AJ, Magden LS, et al: A seroepidemiologic survey of the prevalence of herpes simplex virus type 2 infection in the United States. N Engl J Med 315:796, 1986

43. Fife KH, Corey L: Herpes simplex virus. In

Holmes KK, Mirdh PA, Sparling PF, et al: Sexually transmitted diseases, p 941. New York, McGraw Hill, 1990

44. Goldstein LC, Corey L, McDougall JK, et al: Monoclonal antibodies to herpes simplex virus: use in antigenic typing and rapid diagnosis. J Infect Dis 147:829, 1983

45. Berstein DT, Lovett MA, Bryson YJ: Serologic analysis of first episode nonprimary genital herpes simplex virus infection: presence of type 2 antibody in acute samples. Am J Med 77:1055, 1984

46. Dorsky DI, Crumjeicker CS: Drugs five years later: acyclovir. Ann Intern Med 107:859, 1987

47. Erlich KS, Mills J, Chatis P, et al: Acyclovir resistant herpes simplex virus infection in patients with acquired immunodeficiency syndrome. N Engl J Med 320:293, 1989

48. Elcon GB: History, mechanism of action, spectrum and selectivity of nucleoside analogues. In Mills, Corey: Antiviral chemotherapy: new directions for clinical applications and research, p 118. New York, Elsevier, 1986

49. Rolfs RT, Galaid EI, Zaidi AA: Pelvic inflammatory disease: trends in hospitalization and office visits, 1979 through 1988. Am J Obstet Gynecol 166:983, 1992

50. Westrom L: Incidence, prevalence and trends of acute pelvic inflammatory disease and its consequences in industrialized countries. Am J Obstet Gynecol 138:880, 1980

51. Cates W Jr, Rolfs RT, Aral SO: Sexually transmitted diseases, pelvic inflammatory disease, and infertility: an epidemiologic update. Epidemiol Rev 12:199, 1990

52. Washington AE, Katz P: Cost of and payment source for pelvic inflammatory disease: trends and projections, 1983 through 2000. JAMA 266:2565, 1991

53. Brunham RC, Paavonen J, Stevens CE, et al: Mucopurulent cervicitis—the ignored counterpart in women of urethritis in men. N Engl J Med 311:1, 1984

54. Moscicki B, Schafer MA, Milstein SG, Irwin CE Jr, Schater J: The use and limitations of endocervical Gram stains and mucopurulent cervicitis as predictors of *Chlamydia trachomatis* in female adolescents. Am J Obstet Gynecol 157:65, 1987

55. Romanowski B, Talbot H, Stadnyk M, Kowalchuk P, Bowie WR: Minocycline compared with doxycycline in the treatment of nongonococcal urethritis and mucopurulent cervicitis. Ann Intern Med 119:16, 1993

56. Heinonen PK, Teisala K, Punnonen R, Miettinen A, Lehtinen M, Paavonen J: Anatomic sites of upper genital tract infection. Obstet Gynecol 66:384, 1985

57. Soper DE, Brockwell NJ, Dalton HP: False-positive cultures of the cul-de-sac associated with culdocentesis in patients undergoing elective laparoscopy. Obstet Gynecol 77:134, 1991

58. Soper DE, Brockwell NJ, Dalton HP: Microbial etiology of urban emergency department acute salpingitis: treatment with ofloxacin. Am J Obstet Gynecol 167:653, 1992

59. Bowie WR: In vitro activity of clavulanic acid, amoxicillin and ticarcillin against *Chlamydia trachomatis*. Antimicrob Agents Chemother 29:713, 1986

60. Martin DH, Pastorek JG, Faro S: In vitro and in vivo activity of parenterally adminstered beta-lactam antibiotics against *Chlamydia trachomatis*. Sex Transm Dis 13:81, 1986

61. Martens MG, Faro S: Beta-lactam antibiotics and *Chlamydia trachomatis*. Advances in Therapy 5:113, 1988

62. Mann MS, Faro S, Maccato ML, Kaufman R: Treatment of cervical chlamydial infection with amoxicillin/clavulanate potassium. Infectious Diseases in Obstetrics and Gynecology 1:104, 1993

63. Wolner-Hanssen P, Aavonen J, Kiviat N, et al: Ambulatory treatment of suspected pelvic inflammatory disease with Augmentin, with or without doxcycline. Obstet Gynecol 158:577, 1988

64. Pearlman MD, Faro S, Riddle GD, Tortolero G: In vitro synergy of clindamycin and aminoglycosides against *Chlamydia trachomatis*. Antimicrob Agents Chemother 34:1399, 1990

65. Martins MG, Faro S, Phillips LE, et al: Female genital tract abscess formation in the rat: use of pathogens including enterococci. J Reprod Med 38:719, 1993

Ambulatory Gynecology, Second Edition,
edited by David H. Nichols and Patrick J. Sweeney.
J. B. Lippincott Company, Philadelphia, © 1995.

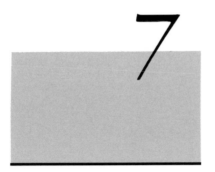

7

Human Immunodeficiency Virus and the Acquired Immunodeficiency Syndrome

Joseph G. Pastorek II

Now I saw a horse sickly green in color.
Its rider was named Death, and the nether world
was in his train. These four were given authority
over one quarter of the earth, to kill with sword
and famine and plague and the wild beasts of
the earth.

Revelation 6:8

In 1981, an unusual syndrome of immune deficiency leading to opportunistic infections and Kaposi's sarcoma, a rare malignancy, was reported in previously healthy homosexual men.[1-3] This condition was recognized to be the result of a deregulation of the cell-mediated immune system and was termed the acquired immunodeficiency syndrome (AIDS). The initial cases were described most commonly in male homosexuals, persons from Haiti, and hemophiliacs. The mortality at 2 years was 70%.[4] Acquired immunodeficiency syndrome was soon linked to a syndrome of chronic wasting and generalized lymphadenopathy, also in male homosexuals.[5] Later, heterosexual partners of AIDS patients were found to be affected, as were recipients of blood products collected from persons who later developed AIDS.[6]

Although multiple theories regarding the pathogenesis of this strange malady were offered (including such novel explanations as the immunologic effects of repeated exposure to allogeneic semen and cytomegalovirus),[7] it was ultimately decided that the disease was caused by infection with a human retrovirus called human T-lymphotropic virus type III (HTLV-III), now termed human immunodeficiency virus type 1 (HIV-1).[7-10] In the ensuing decade, the virus and the disease it causes have spread in an exponential manner (Fig. 7-1), to the horror of medical professionals and laymen.[11] Some have gone so far as to intimate that HIV and AIDS

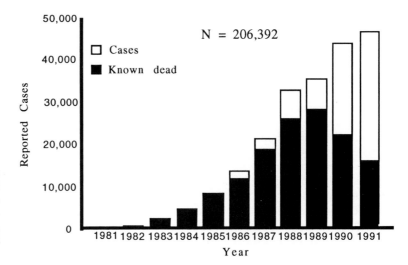

Figure 7–1. Reported cases and known deaths from AIDS United States, 1981–1991. (Centers for Disease Control: Summary of notifiable diseases, United States, 1991. MMWR 40[53]:15, 1991)

may be some ultimate manifestation of divine justice meted out on the population of the modern world for its poor husbandry of the global ecology or perhaps as a slap on the wrist to drive home the concept of the limitations of scientific prowess.[12] Whether or not one surmises that AIDS represents the beginning of the end of the world, there can be no argument that HIV and AIDS are the most studied disease states in modern medicine. Increasing amounts of research effort and research capital are being poured into the search for a cure, a vaccine, or another therapy. Judging from the profusion of manuscripts concerning HIV and AIDS published in the obstetric–gynecologic literature in the past decade, the obstetrician–gynecologist is not exempted from this medical single-mindedness.

PATHOPHYSIOLOGY

Human immunodeficiency virus type 1 (or HTLV-III), the retrovirus that causes AIDS, belongs to the family of human retroviruses (Table 7-1). Human T-lymphotropic virus type I has been recognized for more than a decade as a cause of adult T-cell leukemia and lymphoma, tropical spastic paraparesis, and possibly a few other disorders.[13,14] Human T-lymphotropic virus type II was discovered in association with hairy cell leukemia, although it was later found that most patients with hairy cell leukemia do not harbor the virus.[15,16] Human immunodeficiency virus type 1, or HTLV-III, was described in association with AIDS.[8–10] Finally, HIV-2 (HTLV-IV) causes a variety of AIDS commonly found in Africa that is not as severe as AIDS caused

by HIV-1; few cases have been described so far in the United States.[17]

Retroviruses are divided into three families. The oncoviruses are those that cause neoplastic change. This family includes HTLV-I and HTLV-II. The spumaviruses cause giant cell formation and vacuolation in the cytoplasm of some tissues, notably neural tissue, but no recognizable disease. The lentiviruses include both HIV-1 and HIV-2 and cause long-term infection such as AIDS, other wasting syndromes, pneumonia, and arthritis.[18]

Retroviruses are a remarkable group of RNA viruses that have the ability (by a DNA polymerase enzyme termed reverse transcriptase) to effect reverse transcription. That is, instead of following the normal pathway of transcription of cell DNA into RNA, these viruses (and this enzyme) cause new DNA to be transcribed in a reverse manner from

---

Table 7–1
Human Retroviruses and Resulting Disease

Virus	Disease
HTLV-1	Adult T-cell leukemia/lymphoma Tropical spastic paraparesis
HTLV-II	Hairy cell leukemia (doubtful)
HIV-1 (HTLV-III)	Acquired immunodeficiency syndrome
HIV-2 (HTLV-IV)	Acquired immunodeficiency syndrome (mainly Africa, less virulent than HIV-1)

the viral RNA. The new DNA is integrated into the host cell's genome and then conducts the cell machinery in the infected cell to the benefit of the infecting virus. The resultant infection is often not fatal to the host cell; chronic or permanent infection is therefore the rule.[19]

Human immunodeficiency virus type 1 gains access to its target cell through tropism for CD4 receptors, which are found on the surfaces of some human cells. Specific targets include CD4+ T cells (helper T cells), monocytes, macrophages, some fibroblasts, Langerhans' cells, and some central nervous system follicular dendritic and microglial cells. The initial step in infectious process is when the virus attaches to this surface receptor, attachment that is facilitated by a glycoprotein (gp120) on the viral outer envelope. Probably by fusion aided by a transmembrane glycoprotein, gp41, the virus is then internalized into the target cell, where the reverse transcription ultimately occurs. In the case of the helper T cell, infection is ultimately lytic and causes a progressive loss of these cells, which are instrumental in the maintenance of cell-mediated immunity. Infection of macrophages and monocytes is not generally lytic, so these cell types are not decimated, although they may serve as reservoirs for further viral spread. Thus, the lesion caused by HIV-1 may be thought of as a helper T-cell lymphopenia, at least partially. The clinical disease is primarily the result of the loss of cell-mediated immunity. Infectious diseases that are usually held at bay by the cellular immune system attack the immunologically debilitated patient, ultimately causing death. In addition, certain malignancies may be unleashed by the loss of this immunity.

CLINICAL DISEASE

Primary Human Immunodeficiency Virus Infection

Three to 6 weeks after initial exposure to and infection with HIV-1, 50% to 70% of individuals develop a mononucleosis-like syndrome associated with viremia; there may be an associated aseptic meningitis. Over the next 3 months or so, as virus is disseminated throughout the body, particularly in the lymphoid tissues, antibody is produced. Rising antibody levels correspond to decreasing levels of virus in the blood, though viral replication never

completely ceases. Occasionally, a vigorous immune response appears to incite a persistent generalized lymphadenopathy in some patients.

Asymptomatic Human Immunodeficiency Virus Carriage

After the acute HIV syndrome, most patients progress to a latent stage, in which they asymptomatically harbor virus, which slowly depletes the peripheral blood CD4+ T-cell population, implying a slow deterioration of cellular immunity. This latent stage may last for years.[20] According to the most recent categorization by the Centers for Disease Control and Prevention (CDC), those placed in category A of HIV disease are defined as being patients 13 years of age or older who have documented HIV-1 infection and are either asymptomatic, have persistent generalized lymphadenopathy, or who have or have had previously acute primary HIV infection.[21]

Clinical Acquired Immunodeficiency Syndrome

The ultimate outcome of a deterioration of cell-mediated immunity may be persistent and severe constitutional symptoms, an opportunistic infection, or a malignancy. The CDC category B, which includes patients who are HIV-positive but who do not have a formally defined case of AIDS, consists of seropositive patients with one of those entities listed in Table 7-2. The CDC AIDS surveillance case definition is based on the discovery of any of several other diseases (Table 7-3) found in an HIV-positive patient.[21] In addition, as of January of 1993, all patients with CD4+ T-cell counts of fewer than 200 cells/μL (or less than 14% of total lymphocyte count) are considered to have clinical AIDS.[22]

The CDC originally subdivided these clinical categories by the CD4+ T-lymphocyte counts. Category 1 included patients with CD4+ T-cell counts of 500 or more cells/μL (or alternatively, 29% or more of total lymphocytes); category 2 patients had between 200 and 499 cells/μL (or 14% to 28%); and category 3 patients were defined by CD4+ counts below 200 cells/μL (or 14% or less). This gives some indication of how the cut-off values of 200 cells/μL and 500 cells/μL were formalized.

EPIDEMIOLOGY

The initial reports of AIDS emanated primarily from populations of male homosexuals, persons from Haiti, and hemophiliacs. It was considered then that male homosexual behavior and transfusion of infected blood products were the prime sources of viral infection. Heterosexual activity and more importantly, illicit drug use, are epidemiologic factors of rapidly rising importance. In 1991, slightly more than half of AIDS cases were in homosexual men, 5% were in homosexual men who used drugs, and almost 25% were in users of parenteral drugs (Fig. 7-2).[23] The implication of this shift for the obstetrician–gynecologist is that women are becoming a larger percentage of HIV and AIDS patients, particularly those women at risk for sexually transmitted disease (STD) and those who use illegal drugs. The fraction of AIDS cases that were

Table 7–2
Category B HIV Infection in Adults or Adolescents*

Examples of Conditions Fitting This Category Include:

- Bacillary angiomatosis
- Oropharyngeal candidiasis
- Vulvovaginal candidiasis that is persistent, frequent, or poorly responsive to therapy
- Moderate or severe cervical dysplasia or carcinoma in situ
- Constitutional symptoms (eg, fever or diarrhea) lasting longer than 1 month
- Oral hairy leukoplakia
- Herpes zoster occurring on at least two occasions or over more than one dermatome
- Idiopathic thrombocytopenic purpura
- Listeriosis
- Pelvic inflammatory disease, especially if complicated by tubo-ovarian abscess
- Peripheral neuropathy

*Category B consists of HIV-positive patients ≥ 13 years of age who do not have clinical AIDS (see Table 3) but who have a condition indicative of defective cell-mediated immunity or have a condition considered to have a clinical course or to require management that is complicated by their HIV infection.

Centers for Disease Control and Prevention: 1993 revised classification system for HIV infection and expanded surveillance case definition for AIDS among adolescents and adults. MMWR 41(RR-17):1–19, 1992.

Table 7–3
Category C HIV Infection in Adults or Adolescents

Clinical Conditions Included in the 1993 AIDS Surveillance Case Definition:

- CD4+ T-cell count <200 cells/μL (or <14% of total)
- Esophageal, bronchial, tracheal, or pulmonary candidiasis
- Invasive cervical cancer
- Disseminated or extrapulmonary coccidioidomycosis
- Extrapulmonary cryptococcosis
- Chronic (> 1 month) intestinal cryptosporidiosis
- Cytomegalovirus disease beyond liver, spleen, or nodes
- Cytomegalovirus retinitis (with vision loss)
- HIV-related encephalopathy
- Chronic (> 1 month) herpes simplex ulcers or herpetic bronchitis, pneumonitis, or esophagitis
- Disseminated or extrapulmonary histoplasmosis
- Chronic (> 1 month) intestinal isosporiasis
- Kaposi's sarcoma
- Burkitt's lymphoma
- Immunoblastic lymphoma
- Primary lymphoma of the brain
- Disseminated or extrapulmonary *Mycobacterium avium* complex or *Mycobacterium kansasii*
- *Mycobacterium tuberculosis* (any site)
- Disseminated or extrapulmonary other *Mycobacteria* species
- *Pneumocystis carinii* pneumonia
- Recurrent pneumonia
- Progressive multifocal leukoencephalopathy
- Recurrent *Salmonella* septicemia
- Toxoplasmosis of the brain
- Wasting syndrome due to HIV infection

Centers for Disease Control and Prevention: 1993 revised classification system for HIV infection and expanded surveillance case definition for AIDS among adolescents and adults. MMWR 41(RR-17):1–19, 1992; and Centers for Disease Control and Prevention: Recommendations for prophylaxis against *Pneumocystis carinii* pneumonia for adults and adolescents with human immunodeficiency virus. MMWR 4(RR-14):1–11, 1992.

reported in women in the United States in 1991 was 12% overall, higher in some states.[24] In the decade of the 1990s, HIV infection has become one of the major causes of mortality among women of reproductive age in the United States.[25]

The rate of HIV-seropositivity among women varies with the population studied and the risk factors the population presents. Women attending STD clinics have an HIV-positivity rate of 3%, significantly associated with (1) the use of intravenous

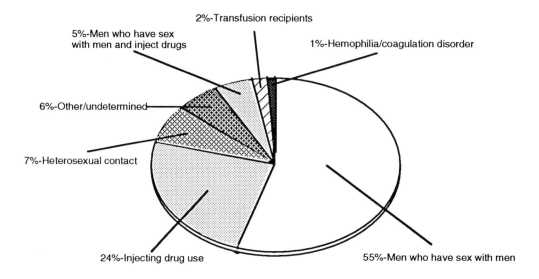

N = 43,014

Figure 7–2.   Reported adult and adolescent AIDS cases, by exposure category, United States, 1991. (Centers for Disease Control: Recommendations for prophylaxis against *Pneumocystis carinii* pneumonia for adults and adolescents with human immunodeficiency virus. MMWR 44[RR-14]:1–11. 1992)

drugs, (2) having sex with a user of intravenous drugs, or (3) having genital warts.[26] One report of women admitted to the hospital with pelvic inflammatory disease described an HIV-positivity rate of 16.7% of 30 patients whose exposure was primarily associated with multiple sexual partners and cocaine use.[27] Women from an inner-city population presenting for first trimester abortion were reported to have a seropositivity rate of 0.87%.[28]

Surveys of pregnant women in various populations have been conducted in the last few years because of the growing rates of HIV infection in children, specifically neonates. Physicians treating some low-risk populations report no confirmed HIV infections in their pregnant patients.[29] Other groups, specifically those in large cities and patients with significant use of "crack" cocaine and exposure to other STDs, report rates ranging from 0.6% to as high as 5.1%.[30,31] In some areas, the prevalence of HIV-positivity has been observed to significantly rise over time.[32] Of perhaps greatest significance is the finding from many of these studies that half or more of HIV-positive gravidas have no self-reported risk factors for the infection, implying that universal screening is necessary to adequately characterize and treat this epidemic.[33]

Risk Factors

Specific risk factors for HIV infection in women include illicit drug use and sexual exposure to drug users; prostitution; multiple sexual partners; blood or blood-product transfusion before 1985 (when adequate screening for HIV was implemented); living in areas of high HIV-1 prevalence; being born in an HIV-1 endemic area; and having or having had STDs.[18,34] Also, in most reports, black and Hispanic women have significantly higher rates of HIV than Caucasian women. It should be underscored that "crack" cocaine use, multiple STDs, and multiple sexual partners are perhaps the most significant risk factors. But the clinician must always remember that most HIV-positive women have *no* self-reported risk factors.

DIAGNOSIS

Early in the AIDS epidemic, diagnosis of the disease was based on the demonstration of the clinical syndrome of immunodeficiency in addition to opportunistic infections and malignancies. Since 1985, however, serologic testing is the major mode of diagnosis of HIV infection. Serologic testing is essentially the only method of detection of asymptomatic or latent HIV carriage.

Serologic Testing

Clinical laboratory testing for HIV is based on the detection of antibodies to various protein and glycoprotein antigens that are contained in the virus. The most commonly used screening tests to detect HIV antibody are the numerous enzyme-linked immunosorbent assay (ELISA) kits commercially available. Specific antibodies detected by this method include antibody to the p24 viral core antigen and antibodies to the surface glycoproteins gp120 and gp41. Enzyme-linked immunosorbent assay testing is highly sensitive, in the range of 99.4% to 99.8%. The specificity of some ELISAs is not as good, however; false-positive rates as high as 70% are reported in some low-risk populations.[35] Depending on the degree of purity of the HIV antigens used for the assay, false-positive results may occur in the presence of many other disease states, including chronic liver disease, autoimmune disease, and myeloma.[36] One report even implicated influenza vaccine as the cause of false-positive ELISA tests for HIV antibody.[37] For this reason, one positive ELISA test should always be repeated; two consecutive positive ELISAs have a sensitivity of 99.7% and a specificity of 98.5%.[38]

Patient serum specimens that are positive to two or more ELISA tests are confirmed as positive by being subjected to the Western blot or an equivalent test. The Western blot test uses HIV-1 antigens, which are electrophoresed to produce discrete bands. These bands are then "blotted" onto nitrocellulose paper and exposed to the suspect serum sample. If the sample contains antibodies to any of the antigen fractions, these antibodies adhere to the specific band and are subsequently detected. The Western blot test is more specific than the ELISA technology; it thus constitutes the confirmatory test for HIV-seropositivity after two separate positive ELISAs.[35]

Unfortunately, if a patient with early HIV infection is tested for antibody before a significant antibody response is measurable, the result is negative. This is theoretically clinically important, although it is rarely encountered unless one is testing patients with suspected acute HIV syndrome. Especially for research purposes, tests have been developed to detect viral antigen, most commonly p24

core antigen. In addition, viral culture methods are available that are purportedly able to detect virus in 97% of HIV-infected individuals. These methodologies are not widely available and therefore are not clinically useful at the present time.[35]

Screening for Human Immunodeficiency Virus

Because fairly sensitive and specific methods exist for detecting HIV in serum, the question arises of when and whom to screen for HIV. Although initially it was felt that the identification of the HIV-positive individual might be a damaging and discriminatory act, it is clear that the knowledge of HIV-positivity is medically positive and allows some beneficial strategies to be initiated for the patient. For the obstetrician–gynecologist, three patient groups are clearly defined: the pregnant patient, the office gynecology patient, and the surgical patient.

Voluntary HIV testing is recommended for pregnant women because of the potential intervention that may be undertaken for the patient and for her infant.[34] Initially, whether the patient is seropositive or not, any associated risky behavior (eg, drug abuse, prostitution) may be addressed. In addition, seropositive gravidas may be reassured that HIV carriage seems to have little effect on pregnancy or pregnancy outcome, nor does the pregnancy alter the course of disease due to HIV.[39] There is, however, about a 20% to 30% chance of vertical transmission of the virus to the fetus–neonate.[18] Investigation is still ongoing but it appears that such things as p24 antigenemia, prolonged maternal fever during pregnancy, and chorioamniotic membrane inflammation are markers for higher vertical transmission rates.[40] The European collaborative study also implicated preterm delivery (before 34 weeks gestation) as a risk factor for transmission of HIV to the infant.[41] All of this enables the physician to inform the mother of the specifics of the disease with relation to pregnancy. Identification of the seropositive gravida also allows the screening and counseling of family members and sexual partners, appropriate pediatric care after the delivery of the infant, and avoidance of breastfeeding because this has been implicated in postnatal HIV transmission.[42]

The prospect of an otherwise potentially normal infant contracting HIV infection from an HIV-positive mother is disturbing and has led to the initiation of a multicenter study by the National Institutes of Health. Patients who were HIV-positive but otherwise not candidates for zidovudine (AZT) therapy (ie, their CD^+ T-cell counts were not depressed and they were asymptomatic) were treated in a randomized, prospective fashion with either placebo or AZT from between 14 and 34 weeks gestation (oral medication) to delivery, with AZT being given intravenously during labor. The infants were subsequently treated with oral medication for the first six weeks of life. A recent communication from the institutes provided the interim result that this type of prophylaxis reduced the vertical transmission rate of HIV from 25.5% to 8.3% in the study population.[42a] This type of positive action further supports the concept of HIV screening in pregnancy.

A major impetus for both the gravida and the gynecologic patient to undergo HIV testing is the availability of early therapeutic measures to enhance and prolong life (Table 7-4). Emotional support and counseling and the use of antiretroviral therapy and prophylaxis for opportunistic infections are positive activities that may be of immense benefit to the seropositive individual.[43] The gynecologic patient benefits from knowing her HIV-positivity because that knowledge may influence the clinical decisions that must be made with respect to conditions such as cervical dysplasia, which may be more aggressive and demands closer follow-up in the HIV-positive women, and salpingitis, which may be less responsive to antibiotics and require earlier surgical intervention in HIV-infected women.[44–46]

The question of routine preoperative screening for HIV is a thorny one. On the practical side, it is estimated that in hospitals that have more than one case of newly diagnosed AIDS per 1000 discharges per year, routine admission testing would identify another 110,000 cases of HIV infection per year in the United States.[47]

For the general patient, the arguments regarding counseling, prophylaxis, and other issues still hold. For the patient being admitted to the hospital for a surgical procedure, however, the knowledge that she is HIV-positive may prompt an evaluation of her immunologic status (eg, CD4+ T-cell count) and a discussion of whether the intended operative procedure is essential (ie, has the risk–benefit ratio for that operation changed significantly). At the least, a more aggressive approach to any postoperative infection may be necessary.

Of course, the entire discussion of early intervention in the course of HIV infection makes it log-

Table 7–4
Intervention Strategies in HIV-Positive Patients

All Patients

Counseling, psychosocial support

Contact testing and counseling

Health maintenance (eg, nutrition)

Immunologic monitoring

Prophylaxis (eg, *Pneumocystis carinii* pneumonia)

Immunizations

Antiretroviral therapy

Tuberculosis testing

Pregnant Patients

As above

Vertical transmission counseling

Avoidance of invasive monitoring if possible

Proscription of breastfeeding

Informed pediatric follow-up

Gynecologic Patients

As above

More liberal use of colposcopy

More frequent follow-up of CIN

More aggressive therapy of PID

Preoperative Patient

As above

Immunologic evaluation preoperatively

Postponement of purely elective procedures

More aggressive postoperative care

CIN, cervical intraepithelial neoplasia; PID, pelvic inflammatory disease.

ical that *any* individual benefits from knowing his or her HIV status. With the proven benefits of AZT therapy in early disease, it is foolish for anyone to take an ostrich's view of things and refuse to know their HIV serostatus.[48] This comment does not spare the physician either, who should be more aware of this logic than anyone.

Conversely, another question often raised is screening of the physician rather than the patient for HIV. With the publicity surrounding the case of the HIV-positive Florida dentist, some patient groups are serious in their attempts to encourage HIV screening of surgeons and others who perform invasive procedures.[49] The physician, who is at risk for HIV exposure simply because of his profession, should be knowledgeable of his or her own HIV serostatus. The odds of transmission of HIV from an infected surgeon or dentist to the patient are apparently small, however, with no documented cases beyond the five reported in Florida; this lends little additional support to the overall recommendations for the screening of physicians.[50–52]

TREATMENT

Human immunodeficiency virus is a virus. As with all viral diseases, modern medicine has yet to find a cure. This is troublesome in the case of most viral entities (eg, herpes, human papillomavirus). Because HIV-1 infection is universally lethal, the lack of a cure is all the more frightening. Strategies to fight HIV infection and AIDS are prevention (which is the ideal) and treatment (which is, at most, temporization).

Prevention

Human immunodeficiency virus is typically spread by sexual contact or exposure to blood products, often through the parenteral use of illicit drugs. It is therefore reasonable that avoidance of infected sexual partners, contaminated blood, and illegal drugs is a straightforward and comprehensive recommendation. This is true to some extent but the translation of this simple statement to actual patient behavior is problematic.

It should be clear from earlier comments that more than half of HIV-seropositive individuals give no self-reported risk factors for HIV exposure. In contrast, many of these persons are actually attending clinics for STD treatment or pregnancy termination or management. This indicates that these patients are definitely sexually active. It is simple to deduce that their next sexual partner will not be warned about the possibility of contracting HIV; the urgency of impending sexual activity is not conducive to honest interpersonal communication. Furthermore, the drive to obtain the next injection of illegal drug will not be restrained to ensure that the needles being used are clean. Therefore, the task of the healthcare worker—to identify behavior that puts the patient at risk for HIV infection and attempt to modify that behavior—is difficult at best.

Despite these observations, modifications of behavior are attempted with those patients exhibiting high-risk behavior. Injecting drug users are counseled to (1) stop using drugs, (2) use clean needles and syringes if drugs are to be injected, and (3) appropriately disinfect needles and syringes that are to be reused. Bleach is commonly used as a disinfectant in these circumstances, although it is not as safe as using new needles and syringes and it is not as effective as boiling for 15 minutes.[53]

Patients who are sexually active should be informed that abstinence or monogamy with a seronegative individual is the safest form of sexual activity for avoiding HIV and other STDs. If these recommendations are refused, then noninsertive sexual activity or barrier methods (eg, condoms) are better than unprotected insertive sexual activity. Condoms should be examined for holes and should not be used with oil-soluble lubricants because these destroy the latex and cause possible leakage. Overall, however, condoms seem to decrease the risk of acquiring HIV infection from a seropositive partner by only 69%, a point worth repeating to recalcitrant patients.[54]

Finally, the original percentage of patients with AIDS who were infected by HIV-positive blood and blood products administration has decreased markedly since 1985. At that time, the CDC recommended screening of all blood and blood products for HIV-1 antibodies and the development of a method of voluntary, anonymous risk assessment of donors.[55] Therefore, since 1985, the risk of HIV-1 transmission of the virus in this manner has become extremely low. In addition, since 1992, donated blood has also been screened for HIV-2.[56]

Therapy of Human Immunodeficiency Virus Infection

The first step in providing therapy for HIV-positive individuals is identifying them. For the obstetrician–gynecologist, it has already been mentioned that the pregnant woman and the gynecologic patient with STD, pelvic inflammatory disease, cervical dysplasia (especially due to human papillomavirus), and women with apparent risk factors (eg, drug use, multiple sexual partners) should all be offered voluntary HIV screening and counseling. The question then arises regarding who should not be offered HIV screening in a routine obstetric and gynecologic clinic or office. The American College of Obstetricians and Gynecologists, through its committee on ethics, recommends that the obstetrics–gynecology physician offer screening to all women.[57] Additionally, the CDC recommends that all hospitals with an HIV-seroprevalence rate of 1.0% or more routinely offer screening to all patients between the ages of 15 and 54.[58] It may therefore be generalized that the obstetrics–gynecology practitioner should be active in the pursuit of HIV serologic testing in any patient coming under his or her care.

The patient found to be HIV-positive may be managed in several different ways (see Table 7-4), with many different goals. Besides the psychosocial and counseling aspect of the patient's circumstances, specific medical treatments are in order, depending on the stage of the illness. For all patients, certain baseline laboratory tests should be performed (Table 7-5).[59] As soon as possible after diagnosis, because immunologic responsiveness deteriorates with advancing HIV disease, patients should receive primary or booster vaccinations for influenza A and B, hepatitis B, pneumococcus, *Haemophilus influenzae*, and the usual childhood diseases (eg, measles–mumps–rubella, polio, diphtheria, tetanus).[60]

Ongoing medical care of the HIV-positive patient should include nutritional evaluation because there may be a tendency for infected individuals to experiment with "alternative therapies" in the form of special diets and supplements. Generally, nutritional factors do not seem to play a major role except in advanced stages of the disease. Reasoned selection and appropriate storage and preparation

---

Table 7–5

Baseline Diagnostic Testing in HIV-Positive Patients

- Complete blood count, with WBC differential and platelet count*
- Baseline liver and renal function test, electrolytes
- Tuberculin skin test (IPPD), with accompanying intradermal anergy battery (*Candida,* mumps, tetanus)*
- VDRL or RPR (with confirmatory FTA-ABS)
- Genital STD testing (*Neisseria gonorrhoeae* and *Chlamydia trachomatis,* as a minimum)
- CD4 + T-cell count and percentage*
- Hepatitis B screen (including antigen and antibodies)
- Glucose 6-phosphate dehydrogenase
- Papanicolaou smear

---

*Considered to be essential.

American Medical Association Advisory Group on HIV Early Intervention: HIV early intervention. Physician guidelines, 2nd ed, p 8. Chicago, American Medical Association, 1994.

of food is important to prevent some of the opportunistic infections that target HIV-positive individuals (eg, *Salmonella,* toxoplasmosis, *Listeria*).[61] Dental considerations, including general dental hygiene and the oral manifestations of HIV infection and some opportunistic infections and malignancies, dictate cooperation from a dentist familiar in the care of HIV-positive patients. Liberal consultation with mental health professionals and neurologists is recommended for situational depression or other coping problems that almost certainly arise, as well as for evaluation of possible neurologic manifestations of HIV or the associated opportunistic infections or malignancies.

Laboratory monitoring should include CD4 + T-cell counts every 6 months if the initial count was more than 500 cells/μL. Counts between 200 and 500 cells/μL should be followed every 3 months. Counts of 200 or fewer cells/μL dictate retroviral therapy and prophylaxis against *Pneumocystis carinii* pneumonia (PCP). In addition, this alone fits the surveillance definition of overt AIDS, even in the absence of other indicator conditions. Finally, at CD4 + T-cell counts of fewer than 100 cells/μL, prophylaxis for *Mycobacterium avium-intracellulare* should be initiated as well as toxoplasmosis prophylaxis if the patient is seropositive for *Toxoplasma gondii.*[59]

The only approved drug for retroviral therapy in HIV infections is zidovudine (previously and commonly known as AZT). The drug is a thymidine analogue that inhibits HIV reverse transcriptase, thus slowing the replication of the virus. Zidovudine has been used to increase survival length in HIV-positive individuals and decrease the rate and severity of opportunistic infections. Most exciting is the finding that asymptomatic patients with CD4 + T-cell counts below 500 cells/μL treated with AZT have a delayed deterioration of their immune system and a delay in developing clinical AIDS.[48] Unfortunately, survival is not beneficially affected by use of AZT in asymptomatic patients. One nucleoside analogue is didanosine, which is used in AZT-intolerant patients, patients not responding to AZT, and patients who have been on AZT for more than 4 months. Zalcitabine is used in combination with AZT in patients with CD4 counts of fewer than 300 cells/μL. Trials of other medications, including stavudine and a non-nucleoside reverse transcriptase inhibitor, are in progress. The reader is referred to a conference on HIV-therapy guidelines for specific protocols for use of AZT and other antiretrovirals.[62]

It should be mentioned that AZT use is not contraindicated for use in pregnancy. A pregnant patient is treated under the same protocols as the non-pregnant HIV-positive individual. Zidovudine may cause a degree of neonatal anemia and growth retardation in some patients but it has been found to be relatively safe and well-tolerated when given to pregnant women.[63] In addition, the pharmacokinetics of AZT in the gravida are similar to those in the nonpregnant woman.[64]

Because the ubiquitous protozoan organism *P carinii* causes pneumonia in 80% of patients with AIDS, prophylaxis against PCP has become standard when patients' CD4 counts fall below 200 cells/µL.[22,65,66] The most common regimen is a double-strength tablet of trimethoprim–sufamethoxazole given orally, either once a day or three times a week. If the patient has previously suffered a bout of PCP, the daily regimen is preferable. The daily regimen is also effective to some degree against recurrent flares of toxoplasmosis in patients who are seropositive for that organism. Other drugs used as prophylaxis for PCP include aerosolized pentamidine, 300 mg monthly by jet nebulizer, and assorted other medications (eg, dapsone, atovoquone, clindamycin).[22] Another unusual infection that requires prophylaxis when CD4 counts dip below 100 cells/µL is the *M avium* complex or organism, which is treated with oral rifabutin, 300 mg/day, continued indefinitely unless limited by toxicity.[67]

The rapidity with which tuberculosis (TB) can run through a population of HIV-infected individuals has been blamed for much of the increase in outbreaks of TB—outbreaks which are often multidrug-resistant tuberculosis. It is especially important that HIV-positive patients be initially screened for TB by skin testing, including tests for anergy (skin tests with *Candida*, mumps, and tetanus antigen), which is not uncommon in HIV-positive persons. Any signs or symptoms of TB should prompt immediate evaluation and treatment, usually with a multiple-drug regimen that includes isoniazid, rifampin, pyrazinamide, and either streptomycin or ethambutol. Exposure of an HIV-positive individual to TB should be followed aggressively, with preventive therapy and repeated skin testing to document whether seroconversion has occurred. It should also be noted that a positive skin test in an HIV-seropositive patient is one of 5 mm induration rather than the usual 10 mm used for the definition of a positive result. (Also, induration of 2 mm or more to any of the test antigens indicates that the patient is not anergic.) Chest roentgenography should be used freely in HIV-infected patients who have abnormal skin tests, anergy, recent exposure, or history of past TB infection.[68] This has been summarized by the CDC, including recommendations in cases of multidrug-resistant tuberculosis.[69]

The above information on the treatment of HIV-positive individuals has been published for the practitioner by the American Medical Association in *HIV Early Intervention. Physician Guidelines* (2nd ed), which is available from the AMA's Division of Health Science, 515 North State Street, Chicago, Illinois 60610. With the American College of Obstetricians and Gynecologists' push to have the specialty of obstetrics and gynecology declared a primary-care specialty, it becomes increasingly important for the obstetrics–gynecology practitioner to be intimately aware of the different strategies for treating HIV-positive patients on a routine basis.

FINAL MISCELLANY

In any discussion of HIV infection and AIDS, two topics invariably surface: HIV-2 and the so-called "stealth virus," HIV-negative AIDS.

Human Immunodeficiency Virus Type 2

As previously mentioned, HIV-2 is endemic to Africa and causes AIDS, although HIV-2 is somewhat less virulent than HIV-1. Human immunodeficiency virus type 2 appears to have spread throughout West Africa, primarily by heterosexual activity, although homosexual men and parenteral drug users appear to be the source for some European cases. France and Portugal have the highest rates of HIV-2 incidence in Europe, presumably predicated on former colonial associations with West Africa. In Portugal, more than 12% of AIDS cases are due to infection with HIV-2. In the United States, 32 patients with HIV-2 infection have been reported since 1987, primarily in the northeastern region of the country. West African origin or travel is the primary etiologic factor. The CDC recommends that HIV-2 testing be considered in (1) persons from an endemic area, (2) sex partners or needle-sharing partners of persons from an endemic area or of persons known to be HIV-2–positive, (3) persons receiving blood components or nonsterile injections in a country where HIV-2 is endemic, and (4) children born to women with any of these risk factors. Specific serologic tests for HIV-2 are available, just as for HIV-1; it is important to perform both tests because there is only a 60% or so cross-reactivity between the two viruses. Many laboratories use a combination HIV-1–HIV-2 screening test that is followed-up by either HIV-1 Western blot or by HIV-2 enzyme immunoassay followed by HIV-2 Western blot as the confirmatory tests. Counseling of HIV-2–positive patients is similar to that of HIV-1–positive patients, except that the period between infection and disease may be longer in the case of HIV-2 infection.[17,70]

Human Immunodeficiency Virus–Negative Acquired Immunodeficiency Syndrome

Finally, there are many reports of clinical immunosuppression and opportunistic infections (basically AIDS-like disease) in patients who are HIV-seronegative. It is theorized that there may be an unidentified virus similar to HIV active in the population of several countries. There was much media coverage of these cases, generating intense public interest and anxiety. One colorful appellation of this malady is "stealth virus," for obvious reasons. Close immunologic, virologic, and epidemiologic study, however, revealed that these patients had a variety of immunologic defects, were epidemiologically unrelated, and probably represented our technical ability to identify subtle immunologic disturbances that were previously unknown. It appears that immunologic monitoring expertise has become so developed in the decade of intense research on AIDS that patients are being found with diseases that are amenable to laboratory investigation for the first time. The syndrome is now called idiopathic CD4 + T lymphocytopenia and is considered a hodgepodge of previously undiscovered immunologic abnormalities worth further study but not worth further hysteria.[71]

REFERENCES

1. Centers for Disease Control. Kaposi's sarcoma and *Pneumocystis* pneumonia among homosexual men—New York City and California. MMWR 30: 305, 1981
2. Gottlieb MS, Schroff R, Schanker HM, et al: *Pneumocystis carinii* pneumonia and mucosal candidiasis in previously healthy homosexual men: evidence of a new acquired cellular immunodeficiency. N Engl J Med 305:1425, 1981
3. Masur H, Michelis MA, Greene JB, et al: An outbreak of community-acquired *Pneumocystis carinii* pneumonia: initial manifestation of cellular immune dysfunction. N Engl J Med 305:1431, 1981

4. Landesman SH, Vieira J: Acquired immune deficiency syndrome (AIDS). A review. 143:2307, 1983
5. Miller B, Stansfield SK, Zack MM, et al: The syndrome of unexplained generalized lymphadenopathy in young men in New York City. Is it related to the acquired immune deficiency syndrome? JAMA 251:242, 1984
6. Harris C, Small CB, Klein RS, et al: Immunodeficiency in female sexual partners of men with the acquired immunodeficiency syndrome. N Engl J Med 308:1181, 1983
7. Sonnabend J, Witkin SS, Purtilo DT: Acquired immunodeficiency syndrome, opportunistic infections, and malignancies in male homosexuals. A hypothesis of etiologic factors in pathogenesis. JAMA 249:2370, 1983
8. Popovic M, Sargadharan MG, Read E, et al: Detection, isolation, and continuous production of cytopathic retroviruses (HTLV-III) from patients with AIDS and pre-AIDS. Science 224:497, 1984
9. Gallo RC, Salahuddin SZ, Popovic M, et al: Frequent detection and isolation of cytopathic retroviruses (HTLV-III) from patients with AIDS and at risk for AIDS. Science 224:500, 1984
10. Schupbach J, Popovic M, Gilden RW, et al: Serological analysis of a subgroup of human T-lymphotropic retroviruses (HTLV-III) associated with AIDS. Science 224:503, 1984
11. Centers for Disease Control: Summary of notifiable diseases, United States, 1991. MMWR 40(53): 15, 1991
12. Bryan CS: Is there divine justice in AIDS? Why now, and not before? South Med J 83:199, 1990
13. Poiesz BJ, Ruscetti FW, Gazdar AF, Bunn PA, Minna ID, Gallo RC: Detection and isolation of type-C retrovirus particles from fresh and cultured lymphocytes of patients with cutaneous T-cell lymphoma. Proc Natl Acad Sci USA 77:7415, 1980
14. Yoshida M, Miyoshi I, Hinuma Y: Isolation and characterization of retrovirus from cell lines of human adult T-cell leukemia and its implication in the disease. Proc Natl Acad Sci USA 79:2031, 1982
15. Kalyanaraman VS, Sarngadharan MG, Robert-Guroff M, et al: A new subtype of human T-cell leukemia virus (HTLV-II) associated with a T-cell variant of hairy cell leukemia. Science 218:571, 1982
16. Rosenblatt JD, Gasson JC, Glaspy J, et al: Relationship between human T-cell leukemia virus-II and atypical hairy cell leukemia: a serologic study of hairy cell leukemia patients. Leukemia 1:397, 1987
17. O'Brien TR, George JR, Holmberg SD: Human immunodeficiency virus type 2 infection in the United States. Epidemiology, diagnosis and public health implications. JAMA 267:27759, 1992
18. Viscarello RR: Human immunodeficiency virus infection in obstetrics and gynecology. In Pastorek JG (ed): Obstetric and gynecologic infectious disease, pp 579. New York, Raven Press, 1994
19. Reitz MS, Gallo RC: Human immunodeficiency virus. In Mandell GL, Douglas RG, Bennett JE

(eds): Principles and practice of infectious diseases, 3rd ed, pp 1344. New York, Churchill Livingstone, 1990

20. Pantaleo G, Graziosi C, Fauci AS: The immunopathogenesis of human immunodeficiency virus infection. N Engl J Med 328:327, 1993

21. Centers for Disease Control and Prevention: 1993 revised classification system for HIV infection and expanded surveillance case definition for AIDS among adolescents and adults. MMWR 41(No. RR-17):1, 1992

22. Centers for Disease Control: Recommendations for prophylaxis against *Pneumocystis carinii* pneumonia for adults and adolescents with human immunodeficiency virus. MMWR 44(RR-14):1, 1992

23. Centers for Disease Control: Summary of notifiable diseases, United States, 1991. MMWR 40(53):16, 1991

24. Centers for Disease Control: The second 100,000 cases of acquired immunodeficiency syndrome, June 1981—December 1991. MMWR 41:28, 1992

25. Chu SY, Buehler JW, Berkelman RL: Impact of the human immunodeficiency virus epidemic on mortality in women of reproductive age, United States. JAMA 264:225, 1990

26. Quinn TC, Glasser D, Cannon RO, et al: Human immunodeficiency virus infection among patients attending clinics for sexually transmitted diseases. N Engl J Med 318:197, 1988

27. Sperling RS, Friedman F, Joyner M, Brodman M, Dottino P: Seroprevalence of human immunodeficiency virus in women admitted to the hospital with pelvic inflammatory disease. J Reprod Med 36:122, 1991

28. Lindsay MK, Peterson HB, Taylor EB, Blunt M, Willis S, Klein L: Routine human immunodeficiency virus infection screening of women requesting induced first-trimester abortion in an inner-city population. Obstet Gynecol 76:347, 1990

29. Horowitz GM, Scott RT, Hankins GDV: Results of a prenatal screening program for the human immunodeficiency virus in a cross-sectional population. J Reprod Med 36:773, 1991

30. Wenstrom KD, Zuidema LJ: Determination of the seroprevalence of human immunodeficiency virus infection in gravidas by non-anonymous versus anonymous testing. Obstet Gynecol 74:558, 1989

31. Ellerbrock TV, Lieb S, Harrington PE, et al: Heterosexually transmitted human immunodeficiency virus infection among pregnant women in a rural Florida community. N Engl J Med 327:1704, 1992

32. Lindsay MK, Peterson HB, Willis S, et al: Incidence and prevalence of human immunodeficiency virus infection in a prenatal population undergoing routine voluntary human immunodeficiency virus screening, July 1987 to June 1990. Am J Obstet Gynecol 165:961, 1991

33. Minkoff HL, Landesman SH: The case for routinely offering prenatal testing for human immunodeficiency virus. Am J Obstet Gynecol 159:793, 1988

34. American College of Obstetricians and Gynecologists: Human immunodeficiency virus infections. ACOG Tech Bull 169, June 1992

35. Sloand EM, Pitt E, Chiarello RJ, Nemo GJ: HIV testing. State of the art. JAMA 266:2861, 1991

36. Steckelberg JM, Cockerill FR: Serologic testing for human immunodeficiency virus antibodies. Mayo Clin Proc 63:373, 1988

37. Mac Kenzie WR, Davis JP, Peterson DE, Hibbard AJ, Becker G, Zarvan BS: Multiple false-positive serologic tests for HIV, HTLV-I, and hepatitis C following influenza vaccination, 1991. JAMA 268:1015, 1992

38. Centers for Disease Control: Update—serologic testing for HIV antibody, United States, 1988 and 1989. MMWR 39:380, 1990

39. Alger LS, Farley JJ, Robinson BA, Hines SE, Berchin JM, Johnson JP: Interactions of human immunodeficiency virus infection and pregnancy. Obstet Gynecol 82:787, 1993

40. St. Louis ME, Kamenga M, Brown C, et al: Risk for perinatal HIV-1 transmission according to maternal immunologic, virologic, and placental factors. JAMA 269:2853, 1993

41. European Collaborative Study: Risk factors for mother-to-child transmission of HIV-1. Lancet 339:1007, 1992

42. Van de Perre P, Simonon A, Msellati P, et al: Postnatal transmission of human immunodeficiency virus type 1 from mother to infant. A prospective cohort study in Kigali, Rwanda. N Engl J Med 325:593, 1991

42a. NIAID, Clinical Alert, February 22, 1994

43. Centers for Disease Control and Prevention: 1993 Sexually transmitted diseases treatment guidelines. MMWR 42(RR-14):10, 1993

44. Centers for Disease Control: Risk for cervical disease in HIV-infected women—New York City. MMWR 39:846, 1990

45. Maiman M, Fruchter GR, Serur E, Remy JC, Feuer G, Boyce J: Human immunodeficiency virus infection and cervical neoplasia. Gynecol Oncol 38:377, 1990

46. Korn AP, Landers DV, Green JR, Sweet RL: Pelvic inflammatory disease in human immunodeficiency virus-infected women. Obstet Gynecol 82:765, 1993

47. Janssen RS, St. Louis ME, Satten GA, et al: HIV infection among patients in U.S. acute care hospitals. Strategies for the counseling and testing of hospital patients. N Engl J Med 327:445, 1992

48. Volberding PA, Lagakos SW, Koch MA, et al: Zidovudine in asymptomatic human immunodeficiency virus infection. A controlled trial in persons with fewer than 500 CD4-positive cells per cubic millimeter. N Engl J Med 322:941, 1990

49. Centers for Disease Control: Transmission of HIV infection during an invasive dental procedure—Florida. MMWR 40:21, 1991

50. Rogers AS, Froggatt JW, Townsend T, et al: Investigation of potential HIV transmission to the patients of an HIV-infected surgeon. JAMA 269:1795, 1993

51. Dickinson GM, Morhart RE, Klimas NG, Bandea CI, Laracuente JM, Bisno AL: Absence of HIV transmission from an infected dentist to his patients. JAMA 269:1802, 1993

52. von Reyn CF, Gilbert TT, Shaw FE, Parsonnet

KC, Abramson JE, Smith MG: Absence of HIV transmission from an infected orthopedic surgeon. A 13-year look-back study. JAMA 269:1807, 1993

53. Centers for Disease Control: Use of bleach for disinfection of drug injection equipment. MMWR 42:418, 1993
54. Weller SC: A meta-analysis of condom effectiveness in reducing sexually transmitted HIV. Soc Sci Med 36:1635, 1993
55. Centers for Disease Control: Provisional public health service inter-agency recommendations for screening donated blood and plasma for antibody to the virus causing acquired immunodeficiency syndrome. MMWR 34:1, 1985
56. Centers for Disease Control: Testing for antibodies to human immunodeficiency virus type 2 in the United States. MMWR 41(No. RR-12):1, 1992
57. American College of Obstetricians and Gynecologists Committee on Ethics: Human immunodeficiency virus infection: physicians' responsibilities. ACOG Committee Opinion No. 130, American College of Obstetricians and Gynecologists, Washington, DC, November 1993
58. Centers for Disease Control and Prevention: Recommendations for HIV testing services for inpatients and outpatients in acute-care hospital settings. MMWR 42(No. RR-2):1, 1993
59. American Medical Association Advisory Group on HIV Early Intervention: HIV early intervention. Physician guidelines, 2nd ed, p 8. Chicago, American Medical Association, 1994
60. Centers for Disease Control and Prevention: Recommendations of the advisory committee on immunization practices (ACIP): use of vaccines and immune globulins in persons with altered immunocompetence. MMWR 42(No. RR-5):1, 1993
61. Raiten DJ: Nutrition and HIV infection: a review and evaluation of the extant knowledge of the relationship between nutrition and HIV infection. Bethesda, MD, Life Science Research Office of the Federation of American Societies for Experimental Biology, 1990
62. National Institute of Allergy and Infectious Diseases: Preliminary guidelines take more patient-tailored approach to HIV therapy. NIAID AIDS Agenda Summer 1:11, 1993
63. Sperling RS, Stratton P, O'Sullivan MJ, et al: A survey of zidovudine use in pregnant women with human immunodeficiency virus infection. N Engl J Med 326:857, 1992
64. O'Sullivan MJ, Boyer PJJ, Scott GB, et al: The pharmacokinetics and safety of zidovudine in the third trimester of pregnancy for women infected with human immunodeficiency virus and their infants: phase I acquired immunodeficiency syndrome clinical trials group study (protocol 082). Am J Obstet Gynecol 168:1510, 1993
65. Miller-Catchpole R, Rapoza NP: Prophylactic treatment for opportunistic infections in HIV-positive patients: aerosolized pentamidine. JAMA 263:2510, 1990
66. Phair J, Munozo A, Detels R, et al: The risk of *Pneumocystis carinii* pneumonia among men infected with human immunodeficiency virus type 1. N Engl J Med 322:161, 1990
67. Public Health Service Task Force on Prophylaxis and Therapy for *Mycobacterium avium* Complex: Recommendations on prophylaxis and therapy for disseminated *Mycobacterium avium* complex disease in patients infected with the human immunodeficiency virus. N Engl J Med 329:898, 1993
68. American Medical Association Advisory Group on HIV Early Intervention: HIV early intervention. Physician guidelines, 2nd ed, p 15. Chicago, American Medical Association, 1994
69. Centers for Disease Control: Guidelines for preventing the transmission of tuberculosis in health-care settings, with special focus on HIV-related issues. MMWR 39(No. RR-17):1, 1990
70. Centers for Disease Control: Testing for antibodies to human immunodeficiency virus type 2 in the United States. MMWR 41(No. RR-12):1, 1992
71. Smith KD, Neal JJ, Holmberg SC: Unexplained opportunistic infections and CD4+ T-lymphocytopenia without HIV infection. An investigation of cases in the United States. N Engl J Med 328:373, 1993

Ambulatory Gynecology, Second Edition,
edited by David H. Nichols and Patrick J. Sweeney.
J. B. Lippincott Company, Philadelphia, © 1995.

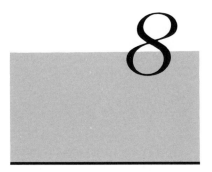

8

Contraception

Patrick J. Sweeney

After the introduction of the birth control pill in 1960, interest in the field of contraception increased exponentially. During the ensuing decades, researchers succeeded in improving the oral contraceptive by decreasing the dose of synthetic hormones required to achieve the same level of contraceptive efficacy. The newer dosages and combinations simultaneously decreased the incidence of side effects, resulting in greater acceptance by women. Although much of the attention and research was focused on the pill, the overall demand for contraceptive services also increased because of many factors, including (1) public concern about over-population, (2) personal and economic reasons to limit family size, (3) conscious decision of couples to delay childbearing in an effort to achieve certain career or material goals, (4) increased percentage of teens and young adults engaging in sexual intercourse, and (5) enactment of Title X of the Social Security Act, a nationwide program aimed at providing low-income and uninsured populations access to contraceptive services and supplies.

The field of contraception, however, has been and likely will continue to be a battlefield on which politicians, social scientists, healthcare professionals, religious leaders, and others struggle to determine the future of reproductive rights in the United States. Controversy and contraception seem inseparable. For example, litigation, both real and anticipated, resulted in the practical elimination of the intrauterine device (IUD) as an available method of contraception for couples in the United States between the years 1985–1988. Moreover, each year, legislation is introduced that would require parental consent before dispensing contraceptives to minors, even though 44% of girls and 64% of boys have had sexual intercourse by their 18th birthday and there is no compelling evidence to indicate that parental consent requirements would decrease adolescent sexual activity.[1] School-based clinics, even those located in schools with high adolescent pregnancy rates, are often prohibited from *discussing* (much less dispensing) contraceptives. Furthermore, the "gag rule"—overturned in early 1993— would have restricted access to contraceptive services by withdrawing family planning funds from small agencies that would have been unwilling or unable to comply with the prohibition of abortion counseling in federally funded clinics.

Contraceptive research in the United States has often been criticized for its lack of vision and its focus on the female reproductive system. After a relatively quiet decade (1975–1985), researchers introduced several new contraceptive methods, including an improved IUD (1988), a long-acting subdermal implant (1990), a female condom (1993), and a vaginal ring (clinical trials are underway).

The purpose of this chapter is to provide the practitioner with up-to-date information on the advantages and disadvantages of the available methods of contraception excluding natural family planning, fertility-awareness techniques, and surgical sterilization.

SELECTION OF METHOD

Some women have already decided on a specific method of birth control before their office visit; others have not. For the former group, the practitioner's role is to determine that the woman has no medical contraindications to her chosen method and that she is thoroughly informed about its mechanism of action, advantages and disadvantages, effectiveness, and cost. In addition, it is helpful to inquire about the reasons for her choice, making sure that she is aware of alternate methods that might be equally or more acceptable.

For the woman who is uninformed or undecided about a specific method, the practitioner or a designee should provide an objective and comprehensive comparison of all contraceptive options, covering the following:

- Effectiveness and failure rates
- Mechanisms of action
- Advantages, disadvantages
- Side effects, risks
- Noncontraceptive benefits
- Cost

Printed materials appropriate to the patient's reading level may be useful during these discussions. Ultimately, barring contraindications, the woman should be provided with the contraceptive of her choice. This may be particularly true for adolescents because not receiving a desired method may provide additional justification for not using contraception.[2] When discussing effectiveness, the provider should be cognizant of the potential effects that patient age, income, and pregnancy inten-

tion might have on compliance. Younger women (aged 15 to 24 years) are more likely to have higher failure rates than women older than the age of 25 years.[3-5] Studies correlate low income with higher failure rates, although low income may be a marker for low educational level or other variables that might adversely effect compliance.[4,5] Although one might assume that patients who want to prevent a pregnancy would be more motivated to use a given method than those who merely intend to delay a pregnancy, this "pregnancy intention" variable may also vary with age and socioeconomic status.

INITIAL EVALUATION

Patients requesting a method of contraception should be evaluated with a routine medical history and general physical examination. Although recommended as part of any routine gynecologic visit, the sexual history assumes increased importance for such patients. The frequency of sexual intercourse, number of partners, stability of a relationship, and pattern of sexual activity all have implications for the selection of the most appropriate contraceptive.

BARRIER METHODS

Condoms

Aside from abstinence, the condom is probably the oldest method of fertility control, dating back to at least the 18th century. Although evidence suggests that female-dependent barrier contraceptives should receive more attention in sexually transmitted disease (STD) risk-reduction programs, condoms continue to be perceived as providing the highest level of protection from STDs.[6] For this reason, condom use has gained increased acceptance and respectability. Sexually active young adults who were once willing to risk contracting an STD rather than use a condom have been forced to reconsider. The lethality of the acquired immunodeficiency syndrome (AIDS) has had a dramatic impact on sex education programs, media campaigns, television programming, and condom use rates. Several manufacturers target their product advertising toward women but some researchers suggest that condom-promotion programs targeted to women must alter existing attitudes and be culturally sensitive if they are to be successful.[7,8] One survey reports that college women were more than four times as likely to use condoms for contraception in 1989 than in 1975.[9] Although this increased use is encouraging, patients need to be reminded that condom use does not guarantee protection from AIDS. "Individuals likely to become infected or known to be infected with human immunodeficiency virus (HIV) should be aware that condom use cannot completely eliminate the risk of transmission to themselves or to others."[10] Nevertheless, it should be emphasized to patients at risk that condoms can provide a high degree of protection against HIV infection if they are used correctly and consistently. The European Study Group on Heterosexual Transmission of HIV followed 563 couples in which one partner was infected with HIV. Among the 24 couples who consistently used condoms, none of the noninfected partners became infected; of the 44 couples who inconsistently used condoms, six of the female partners became HIV-positive.[11] A study reported that women in drug treatment programs who had been surgically sterilized were *less* likely to use condoms than were nonsterilized women.[12] Health care providers must be aware of this fact and ensure that women who choose to be surgically sterilized are adequately counseled regarding their continued need for STD protection if they or their partners engage in risk-taking behaviors.

Effectiveness

All barrier methods of contraception are subject to considerable variability in effectiveness rates. Perfect use (ie, correctly using a condom for every act of sexual intercourse) should result in contraceptive effectiveness rates of 98% to 99%.[13] Allowing for human error, forgetfulness, and lack of motivation, more typical rates are in the range of 88%.[14] Nevertheless, condom use should be encouraged, particularly among patients at high risk for HIV infection. Table 8-1 summarizes the failure rates for various contraceptive methods.

Mechanism of Action

The condom is a physical barrier, collecting the ejaculate in a rubber sheath that covers the penis during intercourse. After withdrawal, the condom is carefully removed to avoid spillage of its contents and is discarded. About 20% of the 72 brands of condoms available in the United States also have a spermicidal coating. Spermicide on the *inner* surface of the condom appears to be effective in immobilizing sperm; however, if the condom should break, leak, or come off, the effectiveness of a spermicidal coating on the *outer* surface has not been

Table 8–1

Percentage of Women Experiencing a Contraceptive Failure During the First Year of Typical Use and the First Year of Perfect Use, United States

Method (1)	% of Women Experiencing an Accidental Pregnancy within the First Year of Use	
	Typical Use (2)	Perfect Use (3)
Spermicides	21	6
Cap		
Parous Women	36	26
Nulliparous Women	18	9
Sponge		
Parous Women	36	20
Nulliparous Women	18	9
Diaphragm	18	6
Condom		
Female (Reality)	21	5
Male	12	3
Pill	3	
Progestin Only		0.5
Combined		0.1
IUD		
Progesterone T	2.0	1.5
Copper TCu380A	0.8	0.6
Depo-Provera	0.3	0.3
Norplant (6 Capsules)	0.09	0.09
Female Sterilization	0.4	0.4
Male Sterilization	0.15	0.10

(Adapted from Hatcher RA, Trussell J, Stewart F, et al. Contraceptive technology, 16th ed: New York, Irvington, 1994.)

established.[13] Although the possibility of condom breakage depends on many variables, a study by Hatcher and Hughes reported 443 breaks in 46,657 uses (about 1%).[15] Other researchers report breakage rates of 2%.[16]

Contraindications

The only medical contraindication to use of a condom is an allergic sensitivity of either partner to latex or other products used in its manufacture. If the sensitivity is to the latex (and not the lubricant or spermicide), natural skin condoms made from lamb intestine may be used. In addition to being more expensive than the latex varieties, natural skin condoms are more porous and therefore are not protective against STDs. Patients should be advised to purchase reputable brands of condoms, keep them away from excessive heat, and avoid petroleum-based products as lubricants.

Advantages

The condom has many advantages that make it an ideal method of contraception for many individuals, including those with minimal resources and limited access to family planning services. They are:

1. Inexpensive, often available free or at significant savings from clinics
2. Available without a prescription
3. Significant protection from STDs
4. Convenient, easy to carry on person
5. Disposable

Noncontraceptive Benefits

Patients who complain of dyspareunia secondary to vaginal dryness may find a lubricated condom beneficial, although a small amount of water-soluble vaginal lubricant may be equally effective. Also, the slightly thickened rim at the base of the condom may act as a mild tourniquet, helping to sustain an erection.

Nonlatex Condoms

Researchers are developing condoms made from latex substitutes that will be more resistant to temperature, humidity, and ozone effects, making them more marketable worldwide. They would also provide an alternative for those with allergic reactions to latex. The proposed polyurethane condom could be used with petroleum-based lubricants; however, the poor elasticity of polyurethane may require the development of various sizes. The female condom, approved by the United States Food and Drug Administration (FDA) in May 1993, is a polyurethane product.

Female Condom

The newest barrier contraceptive on the United States market is the Reality female condom, having received FDA approval in May 1993 (Fig. 8-1). Designed to line the interior of the vagina, the polyurethane pouch also covers some of the external genital area. It is the first female-controlled barrier method officially recognized as a means for preventing STDs.[17] Public-health professionals and family planning agencies are hoping that the female

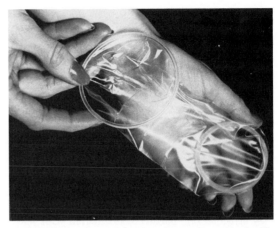

Figure 8–1.   The Reality female condom, the *first female condom approved by the FDA*, is a barrier method of contraception that also provides protection from sexually transmsitted diseases. (Courtesy of the Female Health Company.)

condom will be an acceptable alternative to women who want the STD protection provided by condoms but feel uncomfortable demanding that their male partners wear them.

Effectiveness

Because of the perceived need for a female-controlled barrier contraceptive that provides protection from STDs, the FDA modified the development program for the Reality condom to accelerate its availability to American women. Consequently, pregnancy rates were based on perfect use and typical use patterns over a 6-month period. One-year estimates of typical (or "user") failure rates for the Reality condom range from 21% to 26%. As with other barrier contraceptives, if the female condom is used correctly with every act of intercourse the "method" failure rate is significantly lower—in the range of 3%.[18] The Reality condom was only tested in humans for the ability to prevent pregnancy.

Contraindications

Similar to the male condom, the only absolute contraindication to using the female condom is sensitivity to compounds used in the manufacture of the product or the lubricant.

Advantages

The female condom is a barrier contraceptive that is available without a prescription, controlled by the woman, protective against STDs, and disposable. It is made of polyurethane, which is strong, soft, and transmits heat easily. Although it can be inserted up to 8 hours before intercourse, most women insert it between 2 to 20 minutes before engaging in sex. The Reality condom is unaffected by atmospheric conditions that are likely to be experienced during normal storage such as heat, cold, and humidity.

Disadvantages

Some problems reported by users include vaginal or penile irritation and infections of the vagina, cervix, and urinary tract. Although resistant to normal storage conditions, the Reality condom is packaged with an expiration date 18 months from manufacture. The female condom is intended for one-time use; consequently, a new device must be used with each act of sexual intercourse, including repeated intercourse in the same evening. It must be removed before standing and as with the diaphragm and the male condom, care must be taken to avoid tearing the sheath with fingernails or jewelry. Partly because polyurethane is more expensive than latex, the Reality condom costs more than male condoms.

Other Considerations

The female condom is new and although simple to use, it is recommended that patients practice inserting it without having sex to gain some familiarity with the device and how it looks. For the first two to three acts of intercourse, it is advisable for the woman to use her hand to guide her partner's penis into the vagina to prevent the penis from entering underneath or beside the sheath. The Reality condom is prelubricated; however, couples may want to add more lubricant, depending on individual comfort and preference. The man should *not* wear a condom if the woman is using the Reality condom; friction between the male partner's latex condom and the female partner's polyurethane condom may result in displacement and improper functioning.

Diaphragm

Effectiveness

It is difficult to quote effectiveness–failure rates for diaphragm use. There are many confounding variables, including patient age, education, motivation, marital status, socioeconomic status, understanding of the method, and frequency of intercourse. Consequently, reported failure rates range from 1.9 per 100 woman-years to 18%.[13,19]

Mechanism of Action

Although classified as a "barrier" method of contraception, patients must not be misled into thinking that the diaphragm acts in the same way as a condom—by *physically* keeping the sperm from entering the cervical canal. A diaphragm *must* be used with a spermicide, and it is through the spermicide that it exerts its maximal effect.

Advantages

One of the more attractive advantages of the diaphragm over barrier methods such as condoms and foams is the ability to insert the device up to 6 hours before intercourse. Many couples complain about or fail to comply with the "interruption" of sexual foreplay necessitated by other methods. In addition, diaphragm use is under the control of the woman and may provide some protection against STDs. Studies report that women using female-dependent contraceptives (diaphragm and sponge) had significantly lower rates of gonorrhea and trichomoniasis when compared with women using condoms.[20] Although STD-prevention programs have concentrated their promotional campaigns on condom use, it is possible that female-dependent barrier methods deserve increased attention.

Disadvantages

Diaphragms must be fitted and therefore require a visit to a health care provider to obtain a prescription. This indirectly increases the start-up cost of the method by adding the expense of an initial visit, evaluation, Pap smear, and other routine tests. Because they are reusable, diaphragms must be cleaned and cared for after removal to prevent deterioration.

Contraindications

The only medical contraindications to the use of a diaphragm are (1) allergy to either the materials from which the device is made or the spermicide, or (2) cervicovaginal anatomic abnormalities that preclude an adequate fit.

Important Considerations

Patients should receive explicit instructions on the insertion and use of the diaphragm. It is preferable to allow the patient to practice inserting and removing the device while in the office or clinic setting. While the patient practices the technique in the privacy of the examining room, the provider can see another one to two patients and return later to check for fit and proper insertion and to answer any questions. Patients must be told that the diaphragm *must remain in place for 6 to 8 hours after intercourse* and that a second act of intercourse within that time should be protected by inserting additional foam or other spermicidal agent into the vagina. The use of spermicides usually eliminates the need for lubrication; however, if a lubricant is desired, a water-based product should be selected. The effects of petroleum-based agents on latex are just as damaging to diaphragms as they are to condoms; although the diaphragm is made of thicker rubber, it is not disposable and repeated exposure may result in deterioration.

All vaginal barrier methods of contraception—diaphragm, sponge, cervical cap—could potentially increase the risk of toxic shock syndrome (TSS). If used correctly and removed within the recommended time frame, however, the chances of TSS are probably minimal. The risk of death from TSS is estimated to be only 0.3 per 100,000 users, considerably less than the risk of death from pregnancy-related complications.[13] Nevertheless, patients should be informed of the signs of TSS and should wash their hands thoroughly before insertion or removal of vaginal barriers.

Vaginal Sponge

The first contraceptive sponge was approved by the FDA in 1983. It is a small, polyurethane, circular sponge, about 4 cm in diameter. It is imbedded with spermicide, which is activated by wetting the sponge before vaginal insertion. Similar in action to the diaphragm, the sponge has the additional advantages of being available without a prescription, providing protection for up to 24 hours, and being disposable. Because the spermicide is contained within the sponge, it is more convenient and portable, and there is no need to insert additional spermicide for subsequent acts of intercourse within the 24-hour period.

Effectiveness rates are probably similar to those for the diaphragm. There is, however, some suggestion that failure rates may be twice as high for parous women as they are for nulliparas.[21]

Patients should be told to be sure to moisten the sponge adequately before insertion, otherwise it may absorb vaginal secretions, making intercourse uncomfortable and removal of the sponge more difficult. After removal, the sponge may be discarded but should be checked to verify that it did not tear during removal, leaving pieces in the vagina. The sponge should not be used during menstruation, after a recent miscarriage or elective abortion, or for 6 weeks postpartum.

Cervical Cap

Cervical caps are cup-shaped plastic or rubber devices that resemble small diaphragms with deeper domes. Although available in Europe for many years, cervical caps have not been successfully marketed in the United States. Only one, the Prentif Cavity Rim (Lamberts [Dalston] Ltd., England), is available in the United States, having received FDA approval in 1988. The Prentif Rim is a soft rubber cap designed to fit snugly over the cervix and is available in four sizes. Spermicide is placed inside the cap before insertion, and the cap may be left in place for up to 48 hours—one advantage over the diaphragm. If left in place for longer than 48 hours, the risk of infection or ulceration increases.

Failure rates are similar to those quoted for the diaphragm. Reported pregnancy rates range from 8% to 17% in one study and from 17% to 20% in another.[22,23] Nearly perfect users (defined as women who wore the cap for a maximum of 72 hours, used spermicide 100% of the time, and did not report unprotected sexual intercourse) are reported to have a first-year pregnancy risk of 6.1%.[24]

Contraindications

The same contraindications to diaphragm use are applicable to the cervical cap—allergy to cap material or spermicide or anatomic abnormality that interferes with a good fit. In addition, the cap is contraindicated for women who have cervical/vaginal infections, cervical/uterine malignancies, or an abnormal Pap smear. Although the potential for cervical caps to cause or accelerate Pap smear abnormalities is a concern, studies are not conclusive.[13,24,25] Patients should be informed of this concern and the FDA guidelines, which *mandate* a Pap smear before cap use and *recommend* a repeat Pap smear 3 months later.

Spermicides

As the name implies, a spermicide is a chemical agent that kills sperm. Supplied as foams, creams, gels, suppositories, and a paper-like film, spermicides may be used alone or as an adjunct or backup to other methods of contraception. The active ingredient in spermicides available in the United States is either nonoxynol-9 or octoxynol; both disrupt the sperm cell membrane. Spermicides are lethal to many bacterial and viral organisms as well and have been shown to reduce the risk of transmitting STDs. Maximal protection against STDs can be achieved by using a spermicide in conjunction with a condom.

Effectiveness

Hatcher and coworkers summarized more than 20 studies of spermicide failure rates and concluded that the initial-year failure rate among perfect users would be about 3%, whereas more typical users could expect failure rates of about 21%.[13] Patient understanding and compliance are major factors in determining the maximum level of effectiveness that can be achieved.

Contraindications

The only method-dependent contraindication is an allergy to either the spermicidal chemical or one of the components of the base ingredients.

Advantages

The advantages of the spermicides are fairly straightforward—safe, effective, partially protective against STDs, and available without a prescription. Some preparations (film, suppositories) are convenient to carry (eg, in a purse) but could be difficult to use if exposed to warm temperatures.

Disadvantages

Some couples may find the messiness unpleasant; others may find that it inhibits their enjoyment of oral–genital stimulation. The limited time frame for effectiveness (1 hour) precludes advance preparation and may add to a couple's anxiety and embarrassment.

Important Considerations

A standard dose of spermicide is effective for about 1 hour; consequently, a second dose should be applied if more than 1 hour has elapsed. Some preparations are maximally effective immediately (foam, cream, gel); others require 5 to 15 minutes to melt or dissolve (film, suppository). Couples must be told that a complete, new application of spermicide must precede each act of intercourse. For those who find this troublesome or messy, a condom is an excellent alternative for additional intercourse. The spermicide must be left undisturbed

for 6 to 8 hours after intercourse, and douching within this time period is prohibited. Therefore, this method is not recommended for women who are uncomfortable with the residual foam or gel.

ORAL CONTRACEPTIVES

Combination Oral Contraceptives

Oral contraceptives (birth control pills) were introduced in the United States in 1960. Entire textbooks have been devoted to the research, development, and clinical applications of oral contraceptives. Clearly, one section of one chapter cannot do justice to what Hatcher and colleagues have called one of the most extensively studied medications ever taken by human beings.[13] This section focuses on the major characteristics of the pill and discusses some of the issues surrounding its use—cardiovascular effects, recommendations for menopausal patients, and the additional risks for smokers.

Since their introduction more than 30 years ago, oral contraceptives have been the subject of continuous research, aimed at improving the pill by decreasing the amount or strength of hormones while maintaining effectiveness. Available in monophasic, biphasic, and triphasic preparations, the low-dose combined oral contraceptives are the results of these labors. Combined oral contraceptives that are available in the United States contain one of two estrogens and one of seven progestins, each in varying doses, making the number of possible combinations difficult to imagine. Progesterone-only pills, also called mini-pills, contain no estrogen and are discussed briefly at the end of this section.

Mechanism of Action

Through a variety of submechanisms, oral contraceptives exert their effect by suppressing ovulation, interfering with implantation, altering ovum transport, and decreasing sperm capacitation.

Effectiveness

Failure rates for oral contraceptives must be interpreted with caution. Theoretically, the lowest expected first-year failure rate is 0.1%.[14] Despite the ease of the method, however, many pill takers have difficulty using the pill correctly. Among typical users, average failure rates range from 3.8% to 8.7% in the first year. In both high- and low-failure–

rate groups, older women have lower failure rates than women younger than age 25 years.[3]

Advantages

The oral contraceptive is an extremely popular method of birth control, particularly among women under age 30 years. The American College of Obstetricians and Gynecologists estimates that more than 50 million women in the United States have used the oral contraceptive pill.[26] Its popularity may be explained by its many advantages, which include:

- Safety; oral contraceptives are extremely safe, particularly for young women and nonsmokers
- Effectiveness
- Convenience; one small pill per day
- Continuous protection
- No embarrassment or interruption of sexual foreplay
- Reversibility
- Woman having complete control

Disadvantages

Although a popular choice of contraception, the contraceptive pill suffers from a high attrition rate; 25% to 50% of women who start taking the pill discontinue it within 1 year.[13] Some of the disadvantages include:

- Prescription required
- Expense; the woman must budget not only for the pills but also for annual visits to her provider
- A pill must be taken every day, even though sexual intercourse might be limited or sporadic
- Potential side effects—most commonly, missed periods, irregular spotting, nausea, breast tenderness, and headaches; many of these can be alleviated by altering the estrogen–progestin ratio

Noncontraceptive Benefits

Oral contraceptives are well known for their ability to decrease menstrual flow and its associated cramping. This benefit alone would make the contraceptive pill an ideal choice for a sexually active young woman with moderate to severe dysmenorrhea. Additional noncontraceptive benefits include (1) reduced incidence of functional ovarian cysts,[27,28] (2) decreased incidence of benign breast disease, (3) protection against some organisms known to cause pelvic inflammatory disease (PID),[29,30] (4) improvement of iron deficiency ane-

mia, and (5) protection against ovarian and endometrial cancers.[31–34] Although there are conflicting reports, there is considerable evidence to suggest a possible reduction in the incidence of rheumatoid arthritis among women who took oral contraceptives—particularly among those for whom there is a family history of the disease.[35]

Contraindications

The absolute and relative contraindications to the use of oral contraceptives are listed in Table 8-2.

Other Important Considerations

Several issues surrounding oral contraceptive use have received increased attention in recent years—among them, the effects of oral contraceptives on lipid levels and cardiovascular disease, the detrimental effect of smoking, the controversy concerning the risk of breast cancer, and the advisability of prescribing oral contraceptives to "older" women.

CARDIOVASCULAR DISEASE, LIPID LEVELS, AND ORAL CONTRACEPTIVES. Much has been written about oral contraceptives and their association with three types of cardiovascular disease—myocardial infarction, cerebrovascular accident, and thromboembolism. Early studies were based on higher dose formulations, which are no longer prescribed. In addition, many of the studies failed to control for smoking, now recognized to be the major culprit. An update of the Royal College of General Practitioner's study revealed that for current oral contraceptive users, the risk of myocardial infarction was increased only if they smoked.[36] The large prospective Nurses' Health Study reported that past use of oral contraceptives had little or no impact on the risks of subsequent cardiovascular diseases.[37] Although the link between cardiovascular disease and lipids has been well known, the fractionation and subfractionation of lipids and the degree to which each is harmful have at times been confusing. Beginning with triglycerides and cholesterol, the latter was initially broken down into high-density lipoproteins (HDL), intermediate-density lipoproteins, and low-density lipoproteins (LDL). Shortly after the fractionation of lipids into HDL and LDL, manufacturers of oral contraceptives began studying the effects of the various hormone combinations found in oral contraceptives on these two fractions. It is desirable to have a high HDL to LDL ratio because HDL is believed to have a protective effect on cardiovascular disease. Generally, estrogens increase HDL and decrease LDL; pro-

Table 8–2
Possible Contraindications to Use of Combined Oral Contraceptive Pills

Absolute Contraindications

1. Thrombophlebitis or thromboembolic disorder (or history thereof)
2. Cerebrovascular accident (or history thereof)
3. Coronary artery or ischemic heart disease (or history thereof)
4. Known or suspected breast carcinoma (or history thereof)
5. Known or suspected estrogen-dependent neoplasia (or history thereof)
6. Pregnancy
7. Benign or malignant liver tumor (or history thereof)
8. Known impaired liver function at present time
9. Previous cholestasis during pregnancy

Strong Relative Contraindications

10. Severe headaches, particularly vascular or migraine headaches that start after initiation of oral contraceptives
11. Hypertension with resting diastolic BP of 90 mmHg or greater, or a resting systolic BP of 140 mmHg or greater on three or more separate visits, or an accurate measurement of 110 mmHg diastolic or more on a single visit
12. Mononucleosis, acute phase
13. Elective major surgery or major surgery requiring immobilization planned in next four weeks
14. Long-leg cast or major injury to lower leg
15. Over 40 years old, accompanied by a second risk factor for the development of cardiovascular disease (such as diabetes or hypertension)
16. Over 35 years old and currently a heavy smoker (15 or more cigarettes a day)
17. Abnormal bleeding

Other Considerations That May Suggest That Pills are not the Ideal Contraception

- Diabetes, prediabetes or a strong family history of diabetes
- Sickle cell disease or sickle C disease
- Active gallbladder disease
- Congenital hyperbilirubinemia (Gilbert's disease)
- Undiagnosed, abnormal genital bleeding
- Over 50 years old
- Completion of term pregnancy within past 10–14 days
- Weight gain of 10 pounds or more while on the pill
- Cardiac or renal disease (or history thereof)
- Conditions likely to make patient unreliable at following pill instructions (mental retardation, major psychiatric illness, alcoholism or other chemical abuse, history of repeatedly taking oral contraceptives or other medication incorrectly)
- Lactation
- Family history of death of a parent or sibling due to myocardial infarction before age 50. *Myocardial infarction in a mother or sister is especially significant and indicates a need for lipid evaluation.*
- Family history of hyperlipidemia

(Adapted with permission from Hatcher RA, Stewart F, Trussell J, et al: Contraceptive technology, 1990–1992, 15th ed, p 247. New York, Irvington, 1990.)

gestins have the opposite effect. These effects vary, however, from one preparation to the next because they depend on the relative proportions of the estrogen and progestin and on the androgenic potency of the progestin component. High-density lipoprotein has been subfractionated; HDL2 appears to be responsible for the protective effect, whereas HDL3 has no effect.[38,39] Thus, it is possible for an oral contraceptive (or any other medication) to increase total HDL without having any appreciable effect on cardiovascular risk. Although ethinyl estradiol—the estrogen component of all the low-dose combination oral contraceptives—is known to increase serum triglyceride levels, the association of serum triglyceride levels with coronary heart dis-

ease is uncertain, and raised levels are not thought to be a risk factor if HDL levels are also high. Because oral contraceptives may affect a patient's lipid profile, women at risk for cardiovascular disease based on other predisposing medical conditions or family history should probably be screened for hyperlipidemia before taking oral contraceptives.

Two new synthetic progestins—desogestrel and norgestimate—have received FDA approval after having been available in Europe for several years. A third, gestodene, is expected to receive approval in the near future. Oral contraceptive formulations containing these new progestins claim to offer several advantages over their predecessors. A review summarized the data from about 100 published reports on the safety, efficacy, and metabolic effects of these new progestins. Although the authors caution that the clinical relevance of the results could not be determined because of sample size and methodology differences, they found that compared with previously available combinations, the new formulations appeared to have (1) comparable efficacy, (2) less androgenicity, (3) less impact on carbohydrate and lipid metabolism, (4) better continuation rates, (5) comparable cycle control, and (6) minor effects on the coagulation system. Perhaps the most attractive noncontraceptive benefit of these new pills is the potential to offer protection against cardiovascular disease. The authors state, "With the new formulations, there is the real prospect that we can move from an effort to avoid a negative effect on the lipid profile to the promotion of a positive effect."[40]

SMOKING AND ORAL CONTRACEPTIVES.
Health care providers should encourage all their patients to stop smoking. Cigarette smoking and oral contraceptive use act synergistically, however, and markedly increase a woman's risk of cardiovascular complications.[41-45]

ORAL CONTRACEPTIVE USE AND BREAST CANCER.
Whether there is an increased risk of breast cancer associated with oral contraceptive use is a question that has been studied and debated for many years. Although a consensus has not yet been reached, research reports from large statistically powerful studies appear to show no *overall* increased risk of breast cancer in women using oral contraceptives. Various studies raise the possibility of an increased risk of breast cancer among certain subgroups (eg, women on high-progestin pills, women who took the pills before their first pregnancy, women who were long-term users, and women whose cancers were diagnosed premenopausally). For each subgroup, however, there are other studies that fail to demonstrate the increased risk.[13,46,47] British researchers performed a meta-analysis of 27 epidemiologic studies of breast cancer risk and oral contraceptive use (published between 1980–1989) and suggested that the risk of breast cancer may be raised about 20% in younger, nulliparous, and long-user subgroups.[48] Clearly the question of subgroup susceptibility remains to be answered; nevertheless, the lack of a consistent association makes it difficult to support a cause and effect relation. The Cancer and Steroid Hormone study, a large population-based study, found no association between oral contraceptive use and the aggregate risk of breast cancer in women up to the age of 45 years.[49] In 1988, after reviewing the available literature, the FDA concluded that the reports did not warrant any changes in oral contraceptive labeling, which states that overall evidence suggests that the use of oral contraceptives is not associated with an increased risk of developing breast cancer.[13]

PATIENT AGE AND ORAL CONTRACEPTIVE USE.
As recently as a decade ago, physicians were reluctant to prescribe oral contraceptives for their patients older than the age of 35, based on epidemiologic studies from the late 1960s and early 1970s that associated oral contraceptive use with an increased risk of cardiovascular disease. As discussed, newer low-dose combinations have not been shown to increase the risk of myocardial infarction or stroke in healthy nonsmoking women. Women in the perimenopausal age group are likely to have different lifestyles and contraceptive needs than younger single women. Their partners have generally grown older with them, the frequency of intercourse often decreases, and if they are not in a stable, monogamous relationship, they tend to have fewer partners, decreasing their risk of STDs.[50] Although surgical sterilization remains the most popular method of fertility control in women older than the age of 30 years, 5% of women aged 35 to 39 years continue to use oral contraceptives.[3] The noncontraceptive benefits of the pill—particularly regulation of menses, inhibition of hot flushes, and enhancement of bone density—may be attractive to women in this age group. As healthcare providers become more comfortable with prescribing oral contraceptives for women older than 35 years, the percentage of older women opting for the pill may well increase.[51] Low-dose contraceptives appear to be safe for nonsmoking women between 35 to 50 years of age who have no other familial or medical risk factors, particularly hypertension, diabetes, and cardiovascular disease.[52] Although patients with specific risk factors may benefit from diabetes or lipid screening, information does not support the *routine* use of lipid and diabetes screening before initiation or during the use of low-dose oral contraceptives in women older than 35 years.[53] Selected patients, therefore, may safely continue to take the low-dose oral contraceptives up to menopause; for such women, the determination of menopause can be made by obtaining a serum FSH level immediately before she starts a new cycle of oral contraceptives. Asymptomatic fibroids, which may be relatively common in this age group, should not be considered contraindications to oral contraceptives.[54]

Progestin-Only Oral Contraceptive

Commonly referred to as mini-pills, these oral contraceptives contain no estrogens and consequently appear to be the obvious alternative for women who desire oral contraceptives but for whom estrogen is contraindicated. Unfortunately, many assume that the undesirable side effects of oral contraceptives are solely due to estrogen and mistakenly believe the absolute contraindications to oral contraceptives apply only to estrogen-containing combinations. This is not true; despite the argument that theoretically the progestin-only pill should be safer than the combined preparations, the absolute contraindications listed in Table 8-2 apply to *all* oral contraceptives, including the mini-pill. Relative contraindications include a history of ectopic pregnancy or functional ovarian cysts. Because of the inconsistent inhibition of ovulation, the progestin-only pill is not recommended for women who have difficulty remembering to take their pills.

The progestin-only oral contraceptives are not nearly as popular as the combined products. Although the progestin-only pills are slightly less effective than the combination varieties, the major deterrent to their use is the irregular bleeding experienced by many women. Among women who stop taking the progestin-only pill, 48% cite menstrual disturbances as their reason for discontinuation.[55] In addition, they have fewer noncontraceptive benefits. Aside from those who have experienced estrogen-related side effects while on combination pills, the most likely candidates for the progestin-only pills are lactating women who desire hormonal contraception. Women over 35 years were once thought to be good candidates as well; however, with the liberalization of prescribing low-dose combined oral contraceptives through the perimenopausal period, the preferential use of progestin-only preparations in this age group is declining.

Over-the-Counter Availability Versus Prescription Requirement

Several reproductive rights advocates suggest that oral contraceptives should be available without a prescription, arguing that the additional time and costs associated with the office or clinic visit are barriers to maximal use. The advantages and disadvantages of over-the-counter access are summarized in Table 8-3. Unfortunately, the arguments supporting both sides of the controversy are largely anecdotal and speculative. Clearly, some relaxation of long-standing requirements is foreseeable. The federally funded Title X Family Planning Program is reevaluating its protocols and guidelines and may eliminate the previously required pelvic examination or Pap smear for women using a hormonal contraceptive. Alternative suggestions include (1) eliminating the pelvic examination as a requirement for a prescription, (2) requiring an initial pelvic examination but no subsequent examinations if the first one was normal, or (3) requiring counseling only for first-time users.[56]

INTRAUTERINE DEVICES

The story of the IUD is testimony to what we can and cannot accomplish through massive public health education and media campaigns. A popular method of contraception in the 1970s, the IUD rapidly fell from favor in the years after the publicized reports of the Dalkon Shield's association with pelvic infection, septic abortions, and infertility. For many reasons, including real and potential litigation, the IUD acquired a decidedly negative reputation, from which it has yet to recover; by 1986, all but one device (Progestasert) had been removed from the United States market. In 1988, a copper-containing T-shaped IUD (ParaGard TCu380A, GynoPharma Inc., Somerville, NJ) was reintroduced; it is the only IUD available in the United States that is effective for more than 1 year. It is unfortunate that healthcare providers and their patients have been so slow to reaccept the IUD. It is an excellent contraceptive choice for parous women who are in a stable, mutually monogamous relationship and who have no history of PID. The IUD is used extensively throughout China, a fact that contributes to its being "the most commonly used reversible method of birth control in the world."[57] A 1992 survey of women's attitudes toward contraceptives found that, among current users, the hormonal implant and the IUD had the highest satisfaction ratings—98% and 96% respectively. [58]

Effectiveness

Although the size and shape of an IUD and the presence of medication (copper, progesterone) may influence its effectiveness, failures are more likely to occur from incorrect insertion or undetected expulsion. Generally, if inserted correctly, the IUD should have low failure rates—in the range of 1% to 2%.[14] Some literature quotes failure rates from 1.7% to 6.3%, however, noting that failure rates

Table 8-3
Pros and Cons of Over-the-Counter Oral Contraceptive Availability

Issue	For	Against
Safety	OCs* among the most thoroughly studied drugs in the world Aspirin and cigarettes are more lethal than OCs OCs have many non contraceptive health benefits	OCs affect several systems, including lipid and CHO metabolism Patients with migraine headaches, epilepsy, diabetes, should be evaluated first
Knowledge of Contraindications	Screening for contraindications is based on medical history provided by the patient; patients could "self-screen" Smokers already ignore a well-known risk of chronic pulmonary disease and lung cancer	Patients not aware of medical contraindications may not understand implications Smokers may not heed warning against concominant OC use
General Health Screening	A woman's desire to use OCs should not be held "hostage" by requiring a physical examination	OC users would no longer receive annual Pap smears and screening for breast disease, STDs, and hypertension
No Protection from STDs	Irrevalent; applies to all forms of contraception except condom	OCs do not protect against STDs; patients need to be aware
Cost	Eliminate physician or clinic cost, including lab tests	Medicaid will not pay for over-the-counter medications, making the OCs *more* expensive to the poorest women
Efficacy	No evidence that prescriptive status improves compliance Current degree and effectiveness of clinical counseling highly variable Would encourage greater use, particularly among teenagers	Incorrect use and "missed pills" will increase without clinician instruction
Choice of OC	Most low-dose combinations very similar	Patients will not be able to make subtle distinctions in preparations that may affect acne, breakthrough bleeding, etc Patient may switch formulation for nonmedical reasons

*OCs, oral contraceptives.

tend to be highest among women aged 15 to 24 years.[3] A World Health Organization multicenter study of the TCu380A, covering 14 countries, reported cumulative pregnancy rates of 1.0%, 1.4%, and 1.6% at 3, 5, and 7 years of use, respectively.[59]

Mechanism of Action

The precise manner in which IUDs work is not known. They appear to establish a local inflammatory response in the endometrium, which interferes with implantation. Studies also suggest that the IUD interferes directly with the fertilization process.[60,61]

Contraindications

Although some argue that the only absolute contraindications to IUD insertion are known or suspected pregnancy and pelvic infection (active, recent, or chronic), clinicians should be aware that the manufacturer's recommendations are considerably more conservative. The package prescribing information for the ParaGard TCu380A states that the device "should not be inserted when one or more of the following conditions exist:[62]"

1. Pregnancy or suspicion of pregnancy
2. Abnormalities of the uterus resulting in distortion of the uterine cavity
3. Acute PID or a history of PID
4. Postpartum endometritis or infected abortion in the past 3 months
5. Known or suspected uterine or cervical malignancy, including unresolved, abnormal Pap smear
6. Genital bleeding of unknown etiology
7. Untreated acute cervicitis or vaginitis, including bacterial vaginosis, until infection is controlled
8. Copper-containing IUDs should not be inserted in the presence of diagnosed Wilson's disease
9. Known allergy to copper
10. History of ectopic pregnancy
11. Patient or her partner has multiple sexual partners
12. Conditions associated with increased susceptibility to infections with microorganisms; such conditions include, but are not limited to, leukemia, diabetes, acquired immunodeficiency syndrome (AIDS), intravenous drug abuse, and those requiring chronic corticosteroid therapy
13. Genital actinomycosis
14. A previously inserted IUD that has not been removed

Patients who are anemic or who suffer from dysmenorrhea or menorrhagia should be told that the IUD may aggravate their condition or symptom. Women with borderline low hemoglobin values should be given iron supplementation and have their hemoglobin rechecked in 3 months. A patient with valvular heart disease may be at increased risk for subacute bacterial endocarditis; if there is no acceptable contraceptive alternative, she may wish to discuss the advisability of the IUD with her cardiologist.

Opinions vary considerably as to whether nulliparous women are acceptable candidates for IUD insertion. The 15th edition of *Contraceptive Technology* recommends exercising caution when inserting IUDs for nulliparous women because they are more likely to experience vasovagal symptoms and postinsertion pain that would necessitate its immediate removal.[13] In addition, nulliparous women have higher expulsion rates and are more likely to experience bleeding.[63]

Advantages

The IUD is a highly effective reversible method of contraception. It is independent of sexual intercourse (unlike the barrier methods) and it does not have to be reinforced daily (unlike the pill). It provides continuous long-lasting protection; the progesterone-containing device must be changed annually but the ParaGard device is effective for 10 years.

Disadvantages

Intrauterine devices may increase menstrual cramping, flow, or both. More serious, however, are complications such as uterine perforation and pelvic infection. Women who contract a pelvic infection while an IUD is in place are at increased risk of PID, sterility, and possible hysterectomy.

Other Considerations

Opinions vary as to whether IUD insertions should be restricted to the first few days after the onset of menses. Traditionally, it was considered advisable to insert an IUD during menses to avoid interruption of pregnancy and to take advantage of the dilated cervix. Sensitive pregnancy tests have eliminated the former concern and there is some evidence that the cervix is equally dilated at midcycle.[64] Although the optimal time for insertion is the latter part of the menstrual period, or 1 to 2 days thereafter, the ParaGard TCu380A may be inserted at any time during the cycle once the possibility of pregnancy has been ruled out.

Some clinicians find it helpful to give their patients 400 mg of Ibuprofen (or similar prostaglandin synthetase inhibitor) 30 to 60 minutes before the insertion to decrease immediate postinsertion cramping. Selected patients (eg, those with a small uterus or a history of vasovagal reactions) may be candidates for a paracervical block.

The routine use of prophylactic antibiotics at the time of IUD insertion cannot be justified. A large placebo-controlled study conducted in Kenya found that a single 200 mg dose of doxycycline given 1 hour before insertion reduced the incidence of PID only slightly and insignificantly in a group of women considered to be at high risk for the disease.[65] In contrast, women in the United States who are considered candidates for an IUD who are appropriately counseled and selected should be at low risk for PID. Nevertheless, if STDs are prevalent in the community or if patient follow-up is suboptimal, one might wish to consider the use of prophylactic antibiotics at the time of insertion. One regimen is to administer 200 mg of doxycycline about 1 hour before insertion, followed by 100 mg 12 hours later. Erythromycin, 500 mg, 1 hour before and 6 hours after insertion is an alternate method that may be offered to breast-feeding women or women who cannot take tetracyclines.

INJECTIONS AND IMPLANTS

Two long-acting progestins have been approved for use in the United States—Norplant and Depo-Provera.

Norplant

The Norplant system contains six implantable, nonbiodegradable capsules containing levonorgestrel. Each capsule is 2.4 mm in diameter and 34 mm in length. A set of six capsules is inserted in a superficial plane beneath the skin of the upper arm, and the diffusion of levonorgestrel through the capsule wall provides a continuous low dose of progestin for 5 years.

Mechanism of Action

The two major mechanisms of action are ovulation inhibition and cervical mucous thickening; other mechanisms may add to these contraceptive effects.

Effectiveness

Similar to surgical sterilization, efficacy is independent of patient compliance. Failure rates during the first year of use are reported to be 0.1% to 0.2%.[66] Early concerns that the system might not be as effective in women weighing more than 70 kg appear to have been resolved with improvements in tubing design.[67] Massive obesity should still be considered a relative contraindication, however.

Advantages

The Norplant system provides 5 years of continuous, highly effective, reversible contraception. It contains no estrogen and fertility returns to levels comparable to those of the general population within 1 month of removal.

Disadvantages

The cost of the system is all "up front"; therefore, the cost–benefit to any given patient depends on duration of use. It is a relatively inexpensive contraceptive for those patients who are satisfied with it and continue to use it for the full 5 years. Insertion and removals must be performed by trained clinicians and removals may be difficult. The implants may be visible. Bleeding irregularities, including prolonged bleeding, intermenstrual spotting, and amenorrhea, are responsible for the largest percentage of removals.

Contraindications

The manufacturer lists the following contraindications:

1. Active thrombophlebitis or thromboembolic disorders
2. Undiagnosed abnormal genital bleeding
3. Known or suspected pregnancy
4. Acute liver disease; benign or malignant liver tumors
5. Known or suspected carcinoma of the breast

Clinicians should be cognizant of the potential effects progestins may have on metabolism (eg, lipids and carbohydrates) and should counsel patients to stop smoking (even though the risk associated with progestin-only methods is unknown) and to use barrier contraceptives *in addition* to Norplant if their sexual activities place them at risk of STDs.

Other Considerations

A 10% to 20% early removal rate has been reported.[68] Careful preinsertion counseling can be effective toward decreasing the number of requests for early removal. The advisability of inserting Norplant immediately postpartum in breast-feeding women needs further study. Although the manufacturer states that no data are available on use in breast-feeding mothers earlier than 6 weeks after parturition, some early reports appear to indicate that early postpartum insertion of the system appears to have no significant effect on lactation.[69] The progestin appears in the breast milk; consequently, if this is a concern to the mother, she should delay insertion until she decides to decrease or stop breast feeding.

Medroxyprogesterone Acetate

Depo medroxyprogesterone acetate (DMPA; Depo-Provera) is a long-acting injectable progestin, administered at 3-month intervals. Although DMPA has only recently received FDA approval as a contraceptive, it has been widely used in the United States to treat various causes of endometrial bleeding and has been available as a contraceptive in other countries for more than 30 years.

Mechanism of Action

Depo medroxyprogesterone acetate acts by inhibiting follicular maturation and ovulation and by producing changes in the endometrium and the cervical mucous that are unfavorable for implantation and sperm transport, respectively.

Effectiveness

First-year failure rates are similar to those of implantable progestins and surgical sterilization—about 0.3%. Long-term effectiveness clearly depends on the patient's willingness or ability to return every 3 months for subsequent injections.

Advantages

Depo medroxyprogesterone acetate is highly effective, provides continuous protection for several weeks, and is independent of sexual intercourse. It also offers privacy to the woman who does not wish to keep contraceptive supplies at home. Most users develop amenorrhea after 6 to 9 months, decreasing menstrual cramps and blood loss.

Disadvantages

Some women find the need for repeated injections a nuisance. Although, as noted earlier, most women become amenorrheic after 6 to 9 months, they may experience irregular and occasionally heavy bleeding during the first 6 months of use. Adequate counseling and preparation for these menstrual irregularities improves continuation rates. For some women, the amenorrhea is unacceptable. There is a tendency for women to gain weight while using DMPA, and the weight gain appears to increase with duration of therapy. Average reported weight gains are shown in Table 8-4.

Because DMPA is a long-acting contraceptive, there may be a slight delay to return of fertility after cessation. For women who stop using DMPA to become pregnant, about half conceive within 10 months after their last injection; 93% become pregnant within 18 months after the last injection. Although return of fertility is unrelated to duration of use, it is affected by body weight. Women with lower body weights conceive sooner than women with higher body weights after discontinuing the injections.[70]

Table 8–4
Average Weight Gain With Duration of Use of Depo Medroxyprogesterone Acetate

Years of Use	Weight Gain (pounds)
1	5.4
2	8.1
4	13.8
6	16.5

Contraindications

As might be expected, the absolute contraindications to DMPA are the same as those listed for Norplant.

Other Considerations

Although DMPA may be given to women who are contemplating Norplant, these women must understand that the two progestins are different compounds; although many of the side effects may be the same, many are different—particularly the bleeding pattern. Consequently, DMPA is an excellent long-term alternative for the woman who is not sure she wants 5 years of protection; it is *not* acceptable as a "trial" to determine how well a woman tolerates the side effects of an implantable system. Depo medroxyprogesterone acetate is safe for breast-feeding mothers and does not appear to adversely affect the composition, quality, or quantity of milk produced. Nevertheless, the manufacturer recommends initiation of DMPA 6 weeks postpartum for mothers who wish to breast-feed to minimize the amount of DMPA that is passed to the infant in the first weeks after birth. Depo medroxyprogesterone acetate may increase the rate of bone mineral loss, increasing the risk of osteoporosis. The rate of loss is greatest in the early years of use and subsequently approaches the normal rate of age-related fall.

SUMMARY

For many of our patients who desire contraception, the choice of a method is easy. Others seek varying degrees of guidance as they try to weigh the advantages and disadvantages, the risks and benefits, and the convenience, cost, and effectiveness of the various options available to them. There are medical contraindications to the use of some methods; in addition, the pattern of sexual activity, frequency of intercourse, number of partners, motivation, and other personal variables are significant factors in the selection of the most appropriate contraceptive for a given individual. Our goal should be to help our patients through this maze of options, simultaneously enabling them to develop healthy reproductive lifestyles and safe sexual practices.

REFERENCES

1. Hayes CD (ed): Risking the future—adolescent sexuality, pregnancy, and childbearing, p 41. Washington DC, National Academy Press, 1987
2. Smith PB, Weinman M, Malinak LR: Adolescent mothers and fetal loss, what is learned from experience? Psychol Rep 55:775, 1984
3. Harlap S, Kost K, Forrest JD: Preventing pregnancy, protecting health: a new look at birth control choices in the United States. New York, Alan Guttmacher Institute, 1991
4. Schirm AL, Trussell J, Menken J, Grady WR: Contraceptive failure in the United States: the impact of social, economic, and demographic factors. Fam Plann Perspect 14:68, 1982
5. Jones EF, Forrest JD: Contraceptive failure in the United States: revised estimates from the 1982 national survey of family growth. Fam Plann Perspect 21:103, 1989
6. Rosenberg MJ, Davidson AJ, Chen J, Judson FN, Douglas JM: Barrier contraceptives and sexually transmitted diseases in women: a comparison of female-dependent methods and condoms. Am J Public Health 82:669, 1992
7. Valdiserri RO, Arena VC, Proctor D, Bonati FA: The relationship between women's attitudes about condoms and their use: implications for condom promotion programs. Am J Public Health 79:499, 1989
8. Marin BV, Marin G: Predictors of condom accessibility among Hispanics in San Francisco. Am J Public Health 82:592, 1992
9. DeBuono BA, Zinner SH, Daamen M, et al: Sexual behavior of college women in 1975, 1986, and 1989. N Engl J Med 322:821, 1990
10. Leads from the MMWR: Condoms for prevention of sexually transmitted diseases. JAMA 259:1925, 1988
11. European Study Group on Heterosexual Transmission of HIV: Comparison of female to male and male to female transmission of HIV in 563 stable couples. Br Med J 304:809, 1992
12. Centers for Disease Control: HIV-risk behaviors of sterilized and non-sterilized women in drug treatment programs—Philadelphia, 1989–1991. MMWR 41:149, 1992
13. Hatcher RA, Stewart F, Trussell J, et al: Contraceptive technology, 1990–1992, 15th ed. New York, Irvington, 1990
14. Trussell J, Hatcher RA, Cates W, Stewart FH, Kost K: Contraceptive failure in the United States: an update. Stud Fam Plann 21(1):Table 1, 1990
15. Hatcher RA, Hughes MS: The truth about condoms. SIECUS Rep 17:1, 1988
16. Cates W, Stone KM: Family planning, sexually transmitted diseases, and contraceptive choice: a literature update, part I. Fam Plann Persp 24:75, 1992
17. Gollub EL, Stein ZA: Commentary: the new female condom—item 1 on a women's AIDS prevention agenda. Am J Public Health 83:498, 1993
18. Wisconsin Pharmacal Company: N 168 W22223, P.O. Box 198, Jackson, WI 53037
19. Vessey M, Lawless M, Yeates D: Efficacy of different contraceptive methods. Lancet 1:841, 1982
20. Rosenberg MJ, Davidson AJ, Chen J, Judson FN, Douglas JM: Barrier contraceptives and sexually transmitted diseases in women: a comparison of female-dependent methods and condoms. Am J Public Health 82:669, 1992
21. McIntyre SL, Higgins JE: Parity and use effectiveness with the contraceptive sponge. Am J Obstet Gynecol 155:796, 1986
22. Cagen R: The cervical cap as a barrier contraceptive. Contraception 33:487, 1986
23. Powell MG, Mears BJ, Deber RB, Ferguson D: Contraception with the cervical cap: effectiveness, safety, continuity of use, and user satisfaction. Contraception 33:215, 1986
24. Richwald GA, Greenland S, Gerber MM, Potik R, Kersey L, Comas MA: Effectiveness of the cavity-rim cervical cap: results of a large clinical study. Obstet Gynecol 74:143, 1989
25. Gollub EL, Sivin I: The Prentif cervical cap and Pap smear results: a critical appraisal. Contraception 40:343, 1989
26. American College of Obstetricians and Gynecologists: Oral contraceptives. Obstet Gynecol 106:, 1987
27. Vessey M, Metcalfe A, Wells C, et al: Ovarian neoplasms, functional ovarian cysts, and oral contraceptives. Br Med J 294:1518, 1987
28. Lanes SF, Birmann B, Walker AM, Singer S: Oral contraceptive type and functional ovarian cysts. Am J Obstet Gynecol 166:956, 1992
29. Senanayake P, Kramer DG: Contraception and the etiology of pelvic inflammatory disease: new perspectives. Am J Obstet Gynecol 138:852, 1980
30. Wolner-Hanssen P, Eschenbach DA, Paavonen J, et al: Decreased risk of symptomatic chlamydial pelvic inflammatory disease associated with oral contraceptive use. JAMA 263:54, 1990
31. Schlesselman JJ: Cancer of the breast and reproductive tract in relation to use of oral contraceptives. Contraception 40:1, 1989
32. Centers for Disease Control: Cancer and steroid hormone study of the Centers for Disease Control and the National Institute of Child Health and Human Development. The reduction in risk of ovarian cancer associated with oral contraceptive use. N Engl J Med 316:650, 1987
33. Centers for Disease Control: Cancer and steroid hormone study of the Centers for Disease Control and the National Institute of Child Health and Human Development. Oral contraceptive use and the risk of endometrial cancer. JAMA 249:1600, 1983
34. Jick SS, Walker AM, Jick H: Oral contraceptives and endometrial cancer. Obstet Gynecol 82:931, 1993
35. Hazes JMW, Dijkmans BAC, Vandenbroucke JP, de Vries RRP, Cats A: Reduction of the risk of

rheumatoid arthritis among women who take oral contraceptives. Arthritis Rheum 33:173, 1990

36. Croft P, Hannaford PC: Risk factors for acute myocardial infarction in women: evidence from the Royal College of General Practitioner's oral contraception study. Br Med J 298:165, 1989

37. Stampfer MJ, Willett WC, Colditz GA, Speizer FE, Hennekens CH: Past use of oral contraceptives and cardiovascular disease: a meta-analysis in the context of the nurses' health study. Am J Obstet Gynecol 163:285, 1990

38. Miller NE, Hammett F, Saltissi S, et al: Relation of angiographically defined coronary artery disease to plasma lipoprotein subfractions and apo-lipoproteins. Br Med J 282:1741, 1982

39. Krauss RM, Burkman RT: The metabolic impact of oral contraceptives. Am J Obstet Gynecol 167:1177, 1992

40. Speroff L, DeCherney A: The Advisory Board for the New Progestins: Evaluation of a new generation of oral contraceptives. Obstet Gynecol 81:1034, 1993

41. Petitti DB, Wingerd J, Pellegrin F, Ramcharan S: Risk of vascular disease in women: smoking, oral contraceptives, noncontraceptive estrogens, and other factors. JAMA 242:1150, 1979

42. Rosenberg L, Kaufman DW, Helmrich SP, et al: Myocardial infarction and cigarette smoking in women younger than 50 years of age. JAMA 253:2965, 1985

43. Rosenberg L, Palmer JR, Lesko SM, Shapiro S: Oral contraceptive use and the risk of myocardial infarction. Am J Epidemiol 131:1009, 1990

44. Fotherby K: Oral contraceptives, lipids, and cardiovascular disease. Contraception 31:367, 1985

45. Goldbaum GM, Kendrick JS, Hogelin GC, Gentry EM: The relative impact of smoking and oral contraceptive use on women in the United States. JAMA 258:1339, 1987

46. Murray PP, Stadel BV, Schlesselman JJ: Oral contraceptive use in women with a family history of breast cancer. Obstet Gynecol 73:977, 1989

47. Schildkraut JM, Hulka BS, Wilkinson WE: Oral contraceptives and breast cancer: a case-control study with hospital and community controls. Obstet Gynecol 76:395, 1990

48. Rushton L, Jones DR: Oral contraceptive use and breast cancer risk: a meta-analysis of variations with age at diagnosis, parity, and total duration of oral contraceptive use. Br J Obstet Gynaecol 99:239, 1992

49. Centers for Disease Control: The cancer and steroid hormone (CASH) study of the Centers for Disease Control and the National Institute of Child Health and Human Development: oral contraceptive use and the risk of breast cancer. N Engl J Med 315:405, 1986

50. Connell EB: Contraception for the perimenopausal woman. Female Patient 14:14,16,19, 1989

51. Archer DF: Oral contraceptives: the method of choice for perimenopausal women? Menopause Management Nov/Dec 10, 1992

52. Mishell D: Use of oral contraceptives in women of older reproductive age. Am J Obstet Gynecol 158:1652, 1988

53. Kjos SL, Gregory K, Henry OA, Collins C: Evaluation of routine diabetes and lipid screening after age 35 in candidates for or current users of oral contraceptives. Obstet Gynecol 82:925, 1993

54. Parazzini F, Negri E, La Vecchia C, Fedele L, Rabaiotti M, Luchini L: Oral contraceptive use and risk of uterine fibroids. Obstet Gynecol 79:430, 1992

55. Broome M, Fotherby K: Clinical experience with the progestogen-only pill. Contraception 42:489, 1990

56. Trussell J, Stewart F, Potts M, Guest F, Ellertson C: Should oral contraceptives be available without a prescription? Am J Public Health 83:1094, 1993

57. DaVanzo J, Parnell AM, Foege WH: Health consequences of contraceptive use and reproductive patterns. JAMA 265:2692, 1991

58. Forrest JD, Fordyce RR: Women's contraceptive attitudes and use in 1992. Family Planning Perspectives 25:175, 1993

59. World Health Organization: The TCu380A, Multiload 250 and Nova T IUDs at 3, 5, and 7 years of use—results from three randomized multicenter trials. Contraception 42:141, 1990

60. Alvarez F, Branche V, Fernandez E, et al: New insights on the mode of action of intrauterine devices in women. Fertil Steril 49:768, 1988

61. Ortiz ME, Croxatto HB: The mode of action of IUDs. Contraception 36(1)37, 1987

62. ParaGard T380A Prescribing Information. Sommerville, NJ, GynoPharma Inc, September 1990

63. Tyrer LB, Rothbart B, Anderson KL: Helping adolescents make the right contraceptive choice. Contemporary OB/GYN March: 37, 1990

64. White MK, Ory HW, Rooks JB, Rochat RW: Intrauterine device termination rates and the menstrual cycle day of insertion. Obstet Gynecol 55:220, 1980

65. Sinei SKA, Schulz KF, Lamptey PR, et al: Preventing IUCD- related pelvic infection: the efficacy of prophylactic doxycycline at insertion. Br J Obstet Gynaecol 97:412, 1990

66. Wyeth-Ayerst Laboratories: Prescribing information. Revised July 13, 1993

67. Shoupe D, Mishell DR: Norplant: subdermal implant system for long-term contraception. Am J Obstet Gynecol 160:1286, 1989

68. Silva PD, Glasser KE: Update on subdermal contraceptive implants. Female Patient 17:62, 1992

69. Shaaban MM, Salem HT, Abdullah KA: Influence of levonorgestrel contraceptive implants, Norplant, initiated early postpartum upon lactation and infant growth. Contraception 32:(6):623, 1985

70. Upjohn Company: Prescribing information. October, 1992

Ambulatory Gynecology, Second Edition, edited by David H. Nichols and Patrick J. Sweeney. J. B. Lippincott Company, Philadelphia, © 1995.

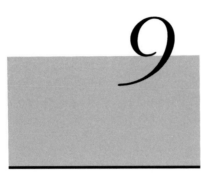

The Infertile Couple

Khalid M. Sultan, James A. Grifo, and Zev Rosenwaks

Infertility is defined as the inability of a couple to achieve a pregnancy despite unprotected intercourse for a period longer than 12 months. Primary infertility indicates that the patient has never achieved a pregnancy, whereas secondary infertility denotes that a previous pregnancy was achieved, regardless of outcome. About 30% of infertile women have primary infertility and the remaining 70% percent suffer from secondary infertility; this, however, varies by patient population. Notwithstanding, 8.4% of women ages 15 to 44 in the United States have impaired fecundity.[1,2]

The goal of the physician treating the infertile couple is not only to diagnose and treat the causes of infertility but also to provide an accurate prognosis for future fertility. Moreover, counseling of the infertile couple about realistic expectations regarding specific treatment modalities is essential. It is important to note that with passage of time, some infertile couples may achieve pregnancy spontaneously; thus, the physician's role may often be to decrease the interval required to achieve a conception.[3] This applies especially to the older female patient. It is well known that fecundity decreases more rapidly after age 35 years.[4] Thus, the manner and rapidity of the infertility work-up must not only consider the underlying etiology but also the age of the female partner.

There are six major areas to evaluate in the infertility work-up. These include tubal integrity and function, ovulatory status, the uterus and endometrium, cervical mucous, and male and peritoneal factors.

CAUSES OF INFERTILITY

Tubal Factor

The fallopian tubes serve as conduits for both the male and female gametes—not only to pick up the oocyte but also to actively transport it to the site of fertilization. Normal tubal function is necessary to provide the appropriate milieu for fertilization and early embryonic development and to maximize synchronous embryo transport to the uterine cavity.

Tubal infertility represents a major etiologic category and may result from either congenital or acquired tubal pathology. *Chlamydia trachomatis* and *Neisseria gonorrhoeae* are the major sexually transmitted organisms responsible for tubal infertility that is secondary to pelvic inflammatory disease (PID). The incidence of significant tubal damage and infertility is correlated with the severity and number of pelvic infections. Thus, most women with a history of three or more pelvic infections suffer from infertility.[5] Pelvic inflammatory disease–associated infertility is also associated with an increased incidence of subsequent ectopic gestation.[5,6] Pelvic inflammatory disease may be categorized as primary and secondary salpingitis.[5] Primary salpingitis is an ascending infection from the lower genital tract, whereas secondary salpingitis results from the direct spread of infection from other pelvic organs, most commonly the appendix.[5] It is estimated that one of every seven American women ages 15 to 44 years has been treated for PID.[7] These factors underscore the importance of early PID diagnosis and aggressive treatment.

Tubal infertility is directly related to the severity of tubal damage and the extent of adhesions. Indeed, in an effort to correlate severity of disease with future prognosis, the American Fertility Society has developed a classification system for adnexal adhesions.[8]

It should be noted that although PID represents a major cause of tubal infertility, iatrogenic tubal disruption (previous tubal sterilization procedures) also is a contributor to tubal infertility. About 13.7 million American couples aged 15 to 44 have undergone some type of sterilization procedure.[7] A significant proportion of these patients may ultimately desire children and present with infertility.

Ovulatory Factor

The cyclic maturation and monthly extrusion of a mature, fertilizable oocyte is the pivotal event of the female reproductive process. Preceding this critical ovulatory phenomenon are the central nervous system (CNS) and ovarian hormonal changes necessary to promote follicular development and endometrial proliferation. After ovulation, the follicle converts from a primarily estrogen-producing gland to a predominantly progesterone-manufacturing apparatus, a change that is necessary for converting the lush proliferative endometrium to a secretory one. The events of the menstrual cycle—namely follicle and oocyte maturation, ovulation, and conversion to a secretory endometrium—are exquisitely synchronized; the fertilized egg (early embryo) arrives at the endometrial cavity at precisely the time when the endometrium is most receptive to implantation. Any dyssynchrony between hormonal events in the CNS, the ovary, or endometrial development may result in infertility.

Although a normal ovarian follicular apparatus must be in place, normal follicular development requires an exquisitely balanced hormonal milieu consisting of appropriate follicle-stimulating hormone (FSH) or luteinizing hormone (LH) stimulation in addition to an intact positive-feedback apparatus, which ensures the elicitation of a midcycle LH surge and ovulation. The ovulatory factor requires intact hypothalamic–pituitary–ovarian axes. Any disruption in the sequence of events accompanying normal folliculogenesis and ovulation may also result in infertility.

Anovulation is often associated with amenorrhea or menstrual dysfunction. In assessing the cause of anovulatory infertility, one must consider four major potential etiologic areas: CNS disorders, ovarian abnormalities, disorders of intermediate metabolism, and nutritional factors.

Central Nervous System Disorders

Any condition—whether neoplastic, infectious, or infiltrative in nature—that interferes with hypothalamic integrity or transport of gonadotropin-releasing hormone (GnRH) from the hypothalamus to the pituitary results in a hypogonadotropic state and anovulation. Thus, tumors of the hypothalamus, pituitary stalk, or pituitary may also result in ovulatory dysfunction. Pituitary tumors associated with elevated prolactin concentrations (known as prolactinomas) may be the most common of CNS neoplasms. Often, CNS disorders include psychogenic conditions such as hypothalamic amenorrhea (ie, occurring from nutritional conditions, anorexia, or that which is stress- or exercise-induced).

Although polycystic ovary disease is often associated with multiple etiologies, one cannot exclude a central etiology for this disorder. Whereas CNS tumors are usually associated with a low gonadotropin milieu, polycystic ovary disease is characterized by an abnormal LH to FSH ratio (usually more than 3:1).

Ovary Disorders

Any disorder that results in an abnormal or absent ovarian apparatus may become an irreversible cause of infertility. These abnormalities include congenital or chromosomal defects, such as gonadal dysgenesis, or may be a result of destructive tumors and premature ovarian failure. Ovarian failure may either be a result of ovarian ablation and removal or may be due to irradiation, drugs, or chemotherapeutic agents. Although the entity of the insensitive ovarian syndrome exists, it is often difficult to separate this entity from autoimmune ovarian insensitivity and indeed, even from ovarian failure.

Disorders of Intermediate Metabolism

Proper ovarian function requires normal thyroid, adrenal, and pancreatic function. Aberrations in any of these endocrine organs may lead to anovulation and infertility. Thus, hypo- or hyperthyroidism, diabetes mellitus, adrenal enzyme deficiency disorders, adrenal hyperplasia (classic or adult-onset), Addison's disease, endocrine tumors, and Cushing's Syndrome have all been implicated in anovulatory infertility.

Nutritional Factors

Ovulatory function mandates proper nutritional status and adequate caloric intake. Thus, excessive exercise, poor nutrition, inadequate caloric intake, cachexia, and anorexia nervosa have all been associated with amenorrhea and anovulation.

Cervical Factor

Normal transport of spermatozoa from the vagina to the uterus and fallopian tubes requires their ascent through cervical mucous. Mucous in the cervical crypts may also serve as a reservoir for spermatozoa for future seeding to the upper female genital tract. Estrogen stimulation increases the daily production of cervical mucous (reaching a peak at mid-cycle) and the number of cervical crypts in the lower cervix, thus enlarging the spermatozoal storage space.[9]

Cervical mucous is a complex hydrogel composed of sugars, proteins, lipids, and various inorganic salts. The main function of these components is to provide the appropriate medium for nourishment, preservation, and migration of sperm to the fallopian tubes. It has been suggested that the intermicellar cross-linkage structure may function as a ladder, facilitating the ascent of sperm into the uterine cavity. It appears that abnormal sperm do not migrate through the cervical mucous as efficiently as normal sperm. Conditions that render cervical mucous inadequate may result in disturbed sperm penetration and infertility. Poor cervical mucous production may be due to low estrogen concentrations or may be due to infectious or anatomic disruption. It must also be emphasized that postovulatory progesterone concentrations change the quantity or quality of cervical mucous, making it impenetrable to spermatozoa.

Male Factor

The male factor is implicated in about 40% to 50% of all infertility. The male reproductive organ (the testes) is responsible for two major functions: steroidogenesis, which occurs in Leydig's cells; and spermatogenesis, which occurs in the seminiferous tubules.

Spermatogenesis encompasses proliferation of spermatogonia, meiosis (reduction–division), and spermiogenesis (the change of spermatids into spermatozoa). During the passage through the epididymis, sperm become functionally mature, although epididymal sperm have fertilized human eggs in vitro. The regulation and control of testicular function is exquisitely controlled by an interplay between the hypothalamus, pituitary, and testes. The pituitary hormones FSH and LH are required for spermatogenesis and steroidogenesis. Thus, any disruption of pituitary hormone production or testicular function leads to infertility.

Reproductive competence in the male requires adequate sexual function. Impotence or ejaculatory failure may be obvious causes of infertility. The adequacy of sexual performance must be ascertained on careful historical query. The differential diagnosis of male infertility should include hypogonadotropic hypogonadism; the presence of varicocele, cryptorchidism, chromosomal abnormality; vas deferens obstruction; and exposure to environmental toxins or drugs.

Uterine Factor

Uterine abnormalities are rarely associated with primary infertility. Recurrent pregnancy loss or premature delivery may implicate the uterus as a positive factor. Whereas the luteal phase defect is rarely associated with primary infertility, other uterine abnormalities such as Asherman's syndrome, uterine leiomyomas, and uterine anomalies are usually associated with pregnancy loss.

Asherman's Syndrome

Uterine synechiae, as described in Asherman's first published report in 1948, are usually caused by trauma and infection of the gravid uterus.[10,11] Genital tuberculosis may be a primary infectious cause of uterine synechiae. The diagnosis is established by either hysterosalpingography (HSG) or hysteroscopy. Operative hysteroscopy is generally used to lyse the synechiae; this is followed with estrogen replacement therapy (usually 1.25 to 2.5 mg of conjugated estrogens daily) for one month to promote re-epithelization of the endometrium. Success of treatment is often related to the extent and degree of scarring. These patients must be counseled relative to their increased risk of obstetric complications, including abnormal placentation.[12]

Leiomyomas

Uterine leiomyomas are the most common pelvic tumors in women.[13] Leiomyomas may cause infertility by distorting the uterine cavity, either by occluding the tubal ostia or possibly interfering with implantation.[14,15] On exclusion of all other etiologic possibilities, myomectomy is the treatment of choice, with resultant delivery rates in the 30% to 60% range. Of note, a recurrence rate of 15% to 45% has also been reported.[14]

Uterine Anomalies

Various uterine anomalies, including bicornuate, unicornuate, septate, and T-shaped uteri after diethylstilbestrol (DES) exposure in utero are associated with infertility. Careful assessment by HSG, hysteroscopy, or laparoscopy may be necessary to differentiate the septate from the bicornuate uterus. The bicornuate uterus causes minimal reproductive problems, whereas the septate uterus is often associated with reproductive failure. The distinction cannot be determined on HSG because the uterine configuration in both anomalies is the same. A laparoscopic examination or careful ultrasonographic assessment of the external contour of the uterus differentiates the two entities: the septate uterus has a smooth external configuration, whereas in the bicornuate uterus, two distinct horns can be discerned. The first description of unification of a bicornuate uterus was described by Strassmann in 1952, although this operation need rarely be performed.[16] The septate uterus can be easily corrected using transcervical hysteroscopic septum resection, with either scissors or resectoscope. The

clinical significance of uterine anomalies associated with in utero DES exposure is unclear. It should be noted that women who are DES-exposed exhibit poor reproductive performance after in vitro fertilization (IVF) when compared with women who have normal uteri.

Luteal Phase Defects

A deficiency in corpus luteum progesterone production may manifest clinically as a luteal phase defect. By definition, luteal phase insufficiency may be described as suboptimal production of progesterone, evidenced by a lag in endometrial development on histologic examination of a luteal phase endometrial biopsy. Retarded histologic development of more than 48 hours by the criteria of Hertig, Noyes, and Rock is required. The incidence of this abnormality is estimated to be 3% to 5% of primary infertility and up to 35% in cases of repeated miscarriages. The prevalence of this disorder, however, may depend on the referral pattern of a particular clinic because most investigators have found this condition infrequently. Progesterone vaginal suppositories to supplement the progesterone insufficiency and clomiphene citrate to enhance early follicular FSH secretion and follicular development have been lauded as treatment modalities. Although several investigators have debated the significance of luteal phase defects in infertility, few would withhold treatment when true progesterone insufficiency or a true lag in histologic development exists.

Peritoneal Factor

Any pathologic condition that involves the peritoneal surfaces of the pelvis and reproductive organs is considered a potential peritoneal cause of infertility. A careful laparoscopic examination of the peritoneal surface is mandatory to exclude adhesions or endometriosis.

Endometriosis

Endometriosis is described as the presence of ectopic endometrial stroma or glands outside the uterine cavity. Endometriosis is a common condition, occurring most often among women aged 30 to 40 years. Although the pathophysiology of endometriosis is controversial, several theories have been suggested to explain its etiology. These include retrograde menstruation, as described by Sampson in

1927; lymphatic or hematologic spread; and celomic metaplasia.[17] It is estimated that 10% to 25% of women with infertility may harbor endometriosis. Whereas the underlying mechanism leading to infertility in patients with severe endometriosis can be clearly explained by either tubal obstruction, pelvic adhesions, or endometriomata, it is less clear how minimal and mild endometriosis interfere with conception. In an effort to better correlate the extent of disease and future fecundity, the American Fertility Society developed a classification system for staging endometriosis (Fig. 9-1). It is hoped that refinements in our understanding of endometriosis-associated infertility will be aided by a more precise assessment of the disease in correlation with future pregnancy prognosis. It is self-evident that patients who harbor endometriomas or have significant adhesions must undergo surgical extirpation. Medical management of minimal endometriosis has not been proved to be beneficial; it may even adversely affect or delay subsequent conception.[18] Expectant management should be considered before medical or surgical treatment of infertile patients who have mild endometriosis, especially when cost, risks, and side effects are considered.[19] In vitro fertilization is a most successful treatment modality for all endometriosis stages.[20] In older patients (older than 37 years of age), IVF may be the first-line treatment of choice.

WORK-UP OF THE INFERTILE COUPLE

History

A complete history is an essential component of the infertility work-up and should include a detailed review of sexual function or dysfunction, obstetric history, and surgical history—especially previous pelvic surgery. A thorough review of possible pelvic infection, general systemic disease, or endocrinopathy should be elicited. A detailed history should be obtained from the male partner also.

Physical

A complete physical examination is necessary before initiating an infertility work-up. Body habitus is examined, fat and hair distribution are noted. The thyroid gland is palpated, and a thorough breast examination should be performed to check for discharge or secretion. A complete pelvic examination is performed, with attention to careful palpation of the uterosacral ligaments for nodularity, noting the mobility of the pelvic organs. Any fixation or thickening may denote pelvic pathology. Cervical mucous should be evaluated, with special attention given to estrogen effects: spinnbarkheit, ferning, and clarity.

Hysterosalpingogram

Hysterosalpingography is an important component of the infertility work-up because it helps to identify uterine defects such as polyps, submucous fibroids, and uterine anomalies. It also demonstrates tubal patency and lumenal integrity. The major complications of HSG include exacerbation of PID, granuloma formation, and embolization.[21] The incidence of serious infection after HSG ranges from 0.3% to 1.3%.[22] Some of these complications can be reduced by properly selecting patients and using antibiotic prophylaxis in patients with a possible history of PID. It is useful to obtain cervical cultures for *Chlamydia trachomatis* and *Mycoplasma* species as a screening method for potential undiagnosed PID. There are two forms of contrast material available—water-soluble and oil-soluble—each with distinct advantages and disadvantages. Oil-soluble contrast media enhances the image on HSG but requires a 24-hour delayed film to demonstrate tubal patency and is more likely to cause granuloma formation due to persistence of the material in the pelvis for many months.[21] Granuloma formation can be virtually eliminated by the exclusive use of water-soluble contrast media. Water-soluble contrast media provides adequate visualization of the uterine cavity and the lumenal integrity of the fallopian tubes. Moreover, it is rapidly absorbed, resulting in fewer long-term complications. Figure 9-2 shows examples of a normal and an abnormal HSG.

Postcoital Test

The postcoital test serves a dual role in assessing cervical mucous production and adequacy and the ability of sperm to penetrate cervical mucous. It provides an in vivo estimation of sperm–mucous interaction during the preovulatory phase of the menstrual cycle. It should be emphasized that cervical mucous deficiency may be the result of poor estrogen production, often associated with anovulation. A normal postcoital test, which is usually per-

THE AMERICAN FERTILITY SOCIETY
REVISED CLASSIFICATION OF ENDOMETRIOSIS

Patient's Name _____ Date _____

Stage I (Minimal) - 1-5
Stage II (Mild) - 6-15
Stage III (Moderate) - 16-40
Stage IV (Severe) - >40
Total _____

Laparoscopy _____ Laparotomy _____ Photography _____
Recommended Treatment _____
_____
Prognosis _____

	ENDOMETRIOSIS	<1cm	1-3cm	>3cm
PERITONEUM	Superficial	1	2	4
	Deep	2	4	6
OVARY	R Superficial	1	2	4
	Deep	4	16	20
	L Superficial	1	2	4
	Deep	4	16	20

POSTERIOR CULDESAC OBLITERATION	Partial	Complete
	4	40

	ADHESIONS	<1/3 Enclosure	1/3-2/3 Enclosure	>2/3 Enclosure
OVARY	R Filmy	1	2	4
	Dense	4	8	16
	L Filmy	1	2	4
	Dense	4	8	16
TUBE	R Filmy	1	2	4
	Dense	4*	8*	16
	L Filmy	1	2	4
	Dense	4*	8*	16

*If the fimbriated end of the fallopian tube is completely enclosed, change the point assignment to 16.

Additional Endometriosis: _____

Associated Pathology: _____

_____

To Be Used with Normal Tubes and Ovaries

L   R

To Be Used with Abnormal Tubes and/or Ovaries

L   R

Figure 9–1. American Fertility Society classification of endometriosis staging.

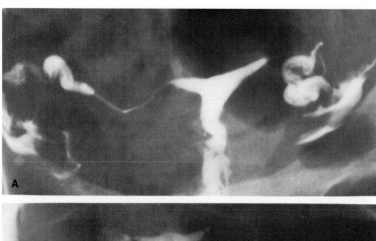

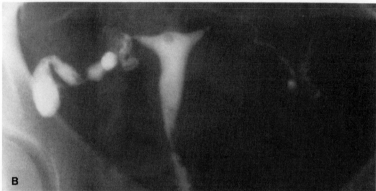

Figure 9–2. Hysterosalpingogram (**A**) Normal HSG, (**B**) Hydrosalpinx.

formed 10 to 14 hours after intercourse, provides an assessment of appropriate estrogen production; an intact, disease-free cervix; and adequate spermatozoa of normal shape and motility. Although the precise number of motile sperm per high-power field that constitutes a normal postcoital test is somewhat controversial, it is generally agreed that more than 10 motile sperm per high-power field represents an adequate test.

The cervical mucous must be evaluated for stretchability (spinnbarkheit), cellularity, and the progressive motility of the sperm present. Although the postcoital test has been used for many years, a metaanalysis by Griffith and Grimes questions its use.[23] Notwithstanding the above analysis, we consider the postcoital test a simple and useful test that rapidly indexes sperm function and cervical mucous.

Detection of Ovulation

Ovulation usually occurs about 14 to 16 days before the onset of the next menstrual period. Ovulatory menstrual cycles are characterized by their regularity, premenstrual symptoms, and often, dysmenor-

rhea. Although numerous laboratory methods have been described to assess ovulation, it should be emphasized that all known parameters for ovulation are indirect and are only presumptive signs of ovulation. It is well known that immediately preceding ovulation, the follicle undergoes rapid growth, which can be visualized on daily ultrasonographic examination. This growth is accompanied by a rising tide of estradiol, which elicits an LH surge that in turns triggers ovulation. Clinically, one can assess follicular growth by ultrasound, measuring the LH concentration in the blood or urine and if timed appropriately, one can even observe the postovulatory collapse of a follicle on vaginal ultrasonography.

A simple and inexpensive method of ovulation detection is the basal body temperature chart.[24] As described, there is a thermogenic rise associated with progesterone elevation in the luteal phase, which may range from 0.3° to 0.8°F when compared with preovulatory temperature. The temperature chart cannot precisely pinpoint the day of ovulation and is therefore only useful on retrospective examination.

One may make use of the cervical mucous examination as well as vaginal cytology because both change in characteristics in the postovulatory phase.

The mucous converts from a clear, elastic, watery fluid to one of thick and tenacious consistency.

The following laboratory methods are useful in detecting ovulation:

1. Serum progesterone more than 3 ng/mL[25]
2. Blood LH 60 mIU/mL (although this level may vary, depending on the assay used)[26]
3. Endometrial biopsy—progesterone-induced secretory histologic changes are the hallmark of ovulation; the histologic criteria of Hertig, Noyes, and Rock (1950) are often used to date secretory endometrium, primarily for assessing the adequacy of luteal function; the endometrial changes serve as an integrative biologic assay for corpus luteum function

Semen Analysis

The hallmark of the male infertility work-up is the semen analysis. It is recommended that the specimen be collected after 3 to 4 days of abstinence, although some authorities recommend a period of abstinence equal to the usual coital interval of the presenting couple.

Semen Parameters

Semen is evaluated for numerous characteristics: pH, volume, viscosity, liquefaction, concentration, sperm motility, and morphology. Table 9-1 presents normal semen parameters. Any deviation from normal parameters should be investigated by a reproductive urologist. It should be emphasized that semen profile abnormalities may be associated with many underlying pathophysiologic conditions, some of which have been described above. The details of the evaluation and treatment of the infertile male are complex and beyond the scope of this chapter.

Table 9–1
Normal Semen Parameters

Normal Semen Parameters	
Concentration	$>20 \times 10^6$/mL
Motility	>60%
Morphology (WHO)	>50% (normal oval)
Volume	2–5 mL
pH	7.0
Liquefaction	1–20 min at room temperature

TREATMENT

Ovulation Induction

Ovulation induction has been traditionally used for women with anovulation and oligo-ovulation. Its use, followed by intrauterine insemination (IUI), has been extended to also include the treatment of unexplained infertility, mild male factor, and minimal endometriosis.[27] Ovulation induction protocols should be tailored to the underlying etiology and hormone status of the patient (Table 9-2).

Clomiphene Citrate

Clomiphene citrate is an orally administered triphenylethylene derivative with antiestrogenic and weak estrogenic effects. Its efficacy relies on augmentation of endogenous FSH levels, which results in enhanced follicular development and ovulation. Clomiphene citrate treatment is reserved for patients with intact hypothalamic–pituitary axis and for women with euestrogenic chronic anovulation. It may also be useful to decrease the ovulatory interval in women who ovulate infrequently.[28] Treatment should be initiated with the lowest effective dosage—usually 50 mg/day for 5 days. It is customary to begin clomiphene citrate on the fifth day of menstrual bleeding or after progesterone withdrawal.

Gonadotropins

Human menopausal gonadotropin (hMG; a combination of FSH and LH) or purified FSH (urofollitropin; a preparation devoid of LH bioactivity) are available preparations. These agents stimulate the ovary directly, serving to supplement the absent hypothalamic and pituitary hormones in women with CNS amenorrhea. Patients with idiopathic infertility who are empirically treated with hMG and IUI have a significantly higher conception rate than women who are treated with either modality alone.[27] Careful monitoring of follicle numbers with ultrasound and serum estradiol levels minimizes the risk of ovarian hyperstimulation syndrome (OHSS).

Pulsatile Gonadotropin-Releasing Hormone

A reasonable approach to ovulation induction in women with hypothalamic amenorrhea is the use of pulsatile infusion of the native 10–amino acid GnRH.[29] This hypothalamic hormone can be delivered by miniaturized pump in a 1 to 1.5 hourly

Table 9–2
Ovulation Induction Protocols

Protocol	Dosage	Procedure	Criteria for hCG*
Clomiphene citrate (CC)	50–250 mg	Administer for 5 days, commencing day 3 or day 5 of cycle	Monitor for spontaneous LH surge or administer 10,000 units when lead follicular diameter is 18–20 mm
Human menopausal gonadotropin (hMG)	150–300 IU	Commence day 3; monitor with estradiol (E_2) and ultrasound, starting day 6; decrease hMG to 150 IU when E_2 exceeds 200 pg/mL	Administer 10,000 units when lead follicular diameter is 16–17 mm
Purified follicle-stimulating hormone (FSH)	150–300 IU	Commence day 3; monitor with estradiol (E_2) and ultrasound, starting day 6; decrease hMG to 150 IU when E_2 exceeds 200 pg/mL	Administer 10,000 units when lead follicular diameter is 16–17 mm
Gonadotropin-releasing–hormone Agonist (GnRH-a) Leuprolide acetate/hMG	Leuprolide, 1 mg SQ daily	Administer leuprolide day 21 of cycle before ovulation induction; decrease leuprolide to 0.5 mg daily on day 3; proceed with hMG stimulation, as above	Administer 10,000 units when lead follicular diameter is 16–17 mm
CC/hMG	CC, 100 mg; hMG, 150 IU	Administer CC days 2–6; commence hMG day 5 and continue until day of hCG administration while monitoring as above	Administer 10,000 units when lead follicular diameter is 18–20 mm

*Artificial insemination or intercourse 36 hours after administration of hCG.

pulse. It appears to be a safe and effective method of ovulation induction and generally decreases the incidence of OHSS and multiple gestation, although multiple follicular development and the occurrence of multiple gestation are not totally eliminated.[29,30]

Complications of Ovulation Induction

Multiple Gestation

Whereas the rate of spontaneous occurrence of twins is 1% and of triplets is 0.01%, the incidence of multiple gestations after ovulation induction with hMG is 18% to 54%; with clomiphene citrate, it is 6% to 8%.[31,32] Therefore, pregnancies after ovulation induction should be monitored ultrasonographically to screen for high-order multiple gestations. Patients must be counseled about the obstetric risks of multifetal pregnancies and when appropriate, offered selective reduction.[33]

Ovarian Hyperstimulation Syndrome

Ovarian hyperstimulation syndrome is a serious complication of ovulation induction therapy. This syndrome is characterized by ovary enlargement, with increased capillary permeability, resulting in loss of fluid from the intravascular compartment.[34] This may lead to hypovolemia, oliguria, ascites, pleural effusions, electrolyte imbalance, and hemoconcentration.[34] In the most severe cases, hypovolemic shock, thromboembolic incidents, and adult respiratory distress syndrome may ensue.[35] Human chorionic gonadotropin (hCG) administration or an endogenous LH surge and luteinization are essential prerequisites to the development of OHSS.[34] Thus, hCG must be withheld in instances in which excessive follicle numbers are observed. In mild and moderate forms, the disease process is self-limiting, requiring no active intervention other than observation and electrolyte replacement. In the severe forms, volume expanders may be required.[36] Rarely, abdominal paracentesis or thoracocentesis may be indicated when there is respiratory compromise.[36] The combination of careful ultrasonographic monitoring and evaluation of daily serum estradiol levels during ovulation induction reduces the incidence of OHSS.[37]

Artificial Insemination

For many years, artificial insemination with donor sperm was the only available method for treating male factor infertility. With the advent of contemporary sperm-separation techniques (ie, swim up, Percoll), the possibility of separating and concentrating motile spermatozoa in relatively small volumes has enabled the clinician to deliver appropriate number of spermatozoa into the uterine cavity or fallopian tubes, even for males who would otherwise be considered subfertile. Moreover, combining controlled ovarian hyperstimulation with IUI has increased the chance of achieving a pregnancy when compared with IUI alone. Intrauterine insemination is indicated for male factor infertility, idiopathic infertility, and to bypass cervical abnormalities.[38] Intrauterine insemination is superior to intracervical insemination with unwashed semen samples.

Tubal Microsurgery

The major indication for tubal microsurgery is the reversal of previous tubal ligations. Microsurgical tubal reanastomosis is reserved for instances where the fimbriae are undamaged and there is residual tubal length of at least 4 to 5 cm. Whereas tubal microsurgery was used for many years to repair damaged fallopian tubes, it is clear that with the exception of lysis of adhesions, IVF affords a more efficient method through bypassing tubal disease.

Hysteroscopy

Hysteroscopy is not only an excellent diagnostic method but may be used to correct intrauterine abnormalities. Whereas in the past, removal of submucous myomas and septa required laparotomy and hysterotomy, with modern hysteroscopic instrumentation and the resectoscope, both submucous myoma resection and septum removal can be performed as a hysteroscopically guided outpatient procedure.[39] At times, the surgeon may require laparoscopic guidance to differentiate a septate from a bicornuate uterus and at the same time minimize the occurrence of uterine perforation.[40]

Operative hysteroscopy has been highly successful in treating intrauterine synechiae, although reproductive outcomes correlate with the severity of the disease.[41,42]

Laparoscopy

Laparoscopy is a critical step in the evaluation of the infertile female. Not only is it mandatory for the diagnosis of pelvic adhesions and endometriosis, operative laparoscopy should be used to correct anatomic distortion and tubal obstruction and to ablate endometriosis. Laparoscopy is often performed in the outpatient surgical suite as a day procedure, and its usefulness in general gynecologic surgery is expanding rapidly.

Assisted Reproductive Technology

The advent of IVF in 1978 marked the beginning of a new era in the treatment of infertility. Whereas Steptoe and Edwards developed IVF to treat women with absent or irreparable fallopian tubes, it soon became apparent that IVF was an excellent method of treatment for any infertility etiology not suitably treated with conventional methods.[43] Moreover, other technologies such as gamete intrafallopian transfer, zygote intrafallopian transfer, and others have been proposed for the treatment of infertility associated with normal fallopian tubes.

In vitro fertilization has revolutionized the treatment of male factor infertility with the development of microsurgical-assisted fertilization techniques.[44] Indeed, IVF has become a simple outpatient procedure that uses ovulation induction, ultrasound-guided retrieval techniques, and simple transcervical embryo-transfer methodologies. The procedure can be performed under sedation without the need for general anesthesia, which is required for tubal transfer procedures. Success of any assisted reproductive technology depends on the age of the female partner; whereas success rates of up to 40% to 50% per transfer have been described for women younger than 30 years, such rates diminish to 5% per transfer at age 43 years. In vitro fertilization technology has been successfully used for treatment of recalcitrant endometriosis, idiopathic infertility, and severe male factor.[45]

CONCLUSION

In the past 2 decades, we have witnessed an explosive growth in our understanding of the reproductive processes. This has led to the development of novel diagnostic and treatment modalities that, accompanied with the more traditional or conventional therapies, have allowed successful treatment of most couples presenting with infertility. It is important to emphasize that our duty is not only to achieve pregnancies or accelerate the interval in which they occur but also to provide prognosis for future fertility.

Acknowledgment

We gratefully acknowledge the excellent editorial assistance of Donna Espenberg in the preparation of this manuscript.

REFERENCES

1. Hirsch MB, Mosher WD: Characteristics of infertile women in the United States and their use of infertility services. Fertil Steril 47:618, 1987
2. Mosher WD, Pratt WF: Fecundity and infertility in the United States: incidence and trends. Fertil Steril 56:192, 1991
3. Collins JA, Wrixon W, Janes LB, Wilson EH: Treatment independent pregnancy among infertile couples. N Engl J Med 309:1201, 1983
4. Stovall DW, Toma SK, Hammond MG, Talbert LM: The effect of age on female fecundity. Obstet Gynecol 77:33, 1991
5. Westrom L: Incidence, prevalence, and trends of acute pelvic inflammatory disease and its consequences in the industrialized countries. Am J Obstet Gynecol 138:880, 1980
6. Rubin GL, Peterson HB, Dorfman SF, et al: Ectopic pregnancy in the United States: 1970-78. JAMA 249:1725, 1983
7. Mosher WD: New from NCHS: fecundity and infertility in the United States. Am J Public Health 78:181, 1988
8. American Fertility Society: The American Fertility Society classification of adnexal adhesions, distal tubal occlusion, tubal occlusion secondary to tubal ligation, tubal pregnancies, Müllerian anomalies and intrauterine adhesions. Fertil Steril 49:944, 1988
9. Moghissi KS: Prediction and detection of ovulation. Fertil Steril 34:89, 1980
10. Asherman JG: Amenorrhea traumatica (Atretica). J Obstet Gynaecol Br Emp 55:23, 1948
11. Asherman JG: Traumatic intrauterine adhesions. J Obstet Gynecol Br Empire 57:892, 1950
12. Friedman A, Defazio J, DeCherney A: Severe obstetric complications after aggressive treatment of Asherman syndrome. Obstet Gynecol 67:864, 1986
13. Buttram VC Jr, Reiter RC: Uterine leiomyomata: etiology, symptomatology and management. Fertil Steril 36:433, 1981
14. Babaknia A, Rock JA, Jones HW: Pregnancy success following abdominal myomectomy for infertility. Fertil Steril 30:644, 1978
15. Hunt JE, Wallach EE: Uterine factors in infertility-an overview. Clin Obstet Gynecol 17:44, 1974
16. Strassman EO: Plastic unification of double uterus: study of 123 collected and five personal cases. Am J Obstet Gynecol 64:25, 1952
17. Sampson JA: Peritoneal endometriosis due to the menstrual dissemination of endometrial tissue into the peritoneal cavity. Am J Obstet Gynecol 14:422, 1927
18. Seibel M, Berger MJ, Weinstein FG, Taymor ML: The effectiveness of danazol on subsequent fertility in minimal endometriosis. Fertil Steril 38:534, 1982
19. Hull ME, Moghissi KS, Magyar DF, Haves MF: Comparison of different treatment modalities of endometriosis in infertile women. Fertil Steril 47:40, 1987
20. Grifo JA, DeCherney AH: Endometriosis: outcome with in vitro fertilization/embryo transfer. Assist Reprod Rev 1:110, 1991
21. Soules MR, Spadoni LR: Oil versus aqueous media for hysterosalpingography, a continuing debate based on many opinions and few facts. Fertil Steril 38:1, 1982
22. Stumpf PG, March CM: Febrile morbidity following hysterosalpingography: identification of risk factors and recommendations for prophylaxis. Fertil Steril 33:487, 1980
23. Griffith CS, Grimes DA: The validity of the postcoital test. Am J Obstet Gynecol 162(3):615, 1990
24. Luciano AA, Peluso J, Koch EI, et al: Temporal relationship and reliability of the clinical, hormonal, and ultrasonographic indices of ovulation in infertile women. Obstet Gynecol 75:412, 1990
25. Ross GT, Cargille CM, Lipsett MB, et al: Pituitary and gonadal hormones in women during spontaneous and induced ovulatory cycles. Recent Prog Horm Res 26:1, 1970
26. Frydman R, Testart J, Feinstein MC, et al: Interrelationship of plasma and urinary luteinizing hormone preovulatory surge. J Steroid Biochem 20:617, 1984
27. Serhal PF, Katz M, Little V, Woronowski H: Unexplained infertility: the value of Pergonal superovu-

lation combined with intrauterine insemination. Fertil Steril 49:602, 1988

28. Gysler M, March CM, Mishell DR Jr, Bailey EJ: A decade's experience with an individual clomiphene treatment regimen including its effect on the postcoital test. Fertil Steril 37:161, 1982

29. Saffan D, Seibel MM: Ovulation induction with subcutaneous pulsatile gonadotropin-releasing hormone in various ovulatory disorders. Fertil Steril 45:475, 1986

30. Heineman MJ, Bouckaret PXJM, Schellekens LA: A quadruplet pregnancy following ovulation induction with pulsatile luteinizing hormone-releasing hormone. Fertil Steril 42:300, 1984

31. Guttmacher AF: The incidence of multiple births in man and some other uniparae. Obstet Gynecol 2:22, 1953

32. Schenker JG, Yarkoni S, Granat M: Multiple pregnancies following induction of ovulation. Fertil Steril 35:105, 1981

33. Berkowitz RL, Lynch L, Chitkara U, et al: Selective reduction of multifetal pregnancies in the first trimester. N Engl J Med 318:1043, 1988

34. Forman RG, Ross C, Frydman R, et al: Severe ovarian hyperstimulation syndrome using agonists of gonadotropin releasing hormone for in vitro fertilization: a European series and a proposal for prevention. Fertil Steril 53:502, 1990

35. Zosmer A, Katz Z, Lancet M, Konichezky S, Schwartz-Shoham Z: Adult respiratory distress syndrome complicating ovarian hyperstimulation syndrome. Fertil Steril 47:524, 1987

36. Borenstein R, Elhalah U, Lunenfeld B, et al: Severe ovarian hyperstimulation syndrome: a reevaluated therapeutic approach. Fertil Steril 51:791, 1981

37. Schenker JG, Weinstein D: Ovarian hyperstimulation syndrome: a current survey. Fertil Steril 30:255, 1978

38. Dodson WC, Whitesides DB, Hughes CL Jr, Easley HA III, Haney AF: Superovulation with intrauterine insemination in the treatment of infertility: a possible alternative to gamete intrafallopian transfer and in vitro fertilization. Fertil Steril 48:441, 1987

39. Fayez JA: Comparison between abdominal and hysteroscopic metroplasty. Obstet Gynecol 68:399, 1986

40. March CM, Israel R: Hysteroscopic management of recurrent abortion secondary to septate uterus. Am J Obstet Gynecol 156:834, 1987

41. March CM, Israel R: Gestational outcome following hysteroscopic lysis of adhesions. Fertil Steril 36:455, 1981

42. Valle RF, Sciarra JJ: Intrauterine adhesions: hysteroscopic diagnosis, classification, treatment, and reproductive outcome. Am J Obstet Gynecol 158:1459, 1988

43. Steptoe PC, Edwards RG: Birth after reimplantation of human embryo. Lancet 2:366, 1978

44. Cohen J, Alikani M, Malter HE, Adler A, Talansky BE, Rosenwaks Z: Partial zona dissection or subzonal sperm insertion: microsurgical fertilization alternatives based on evaluation of sperm and embryo morphology. Fertil Steril 56:696, 1991

45. Jones HW Jr, Acosta AA, Andrews MC, et al: Three years of in vitro fertilization at Norfolk. Fertil Steril 42:826, 1984

Ambulatory Gynecology, Second Edition,
edited by David H. Nichols and Patrick J. Sweeney.
J. B. Lippincott Company, Philadelphia, © 1995.

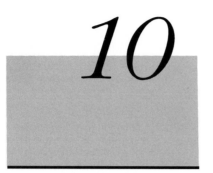

10

Applications of Gonadotropin-Releasing–Hormone Analogues in Gynecology

Robert L. Barbieri

During the past 2 decades, the centerpiece of research in gynecologic endocrinology has been the elucidation of the factors that control the menstrual cycle. A key accomplishment of this research has been the discovery of the hypothalamic decapeptide, gonadotropin-releasing hormone (GnRH; Fig. 10-1), and the realization that hypothalamic secretion of GnRH is the critical factor controlling menstrual function.[1] In humans, GnRH is secreted by neurons in the infundibular region of the hypothalamus, including the arcuate nucleus, whose neuronal processes terminate in the median eminence on the hypophysioportal capillaries.[2] The GnRH neurons are neuroendocrine transducers, which integrate multiple neural-signaling pathways (catecholamines, opioids, excitatory amino acids) and secrete the hormone GnRH in a pulsatile manner. The primary effect of GnRH is to stimulate the secretion of luteinizing hormone (LH) and follicle-stimulating hormone (FSH) from the pituitary gonadotrope. In turn, LH and FSH stimulate ovarian follicular development, including secretion of estradiol and progesterone, and the maturation of the oocyte in preparation for fertilization.

Gonadotropin-releasing hormone is secreted in a pulsatile manner, and GnRH pulse frequency and amplitude are critical variables, determining the pattern and quantity of LH and FSH secreted by the pituitary gonadotrope.

In women with ovulatory menstrual cycles, GnRH is secreted at a frequency of about 18 to 24 pulses per 24 hours in the follicular phase and with a frequency in the range of 6 to 10 pulses per 24 hours in the mid-luteal phase.[3]

In a classic series of endocrine ablation–replacement experiments, Knobil demonstrated the importance of pulsatile release of GnRH in the control of pituitary gonadotropin secretion.[4] Radiofrequency

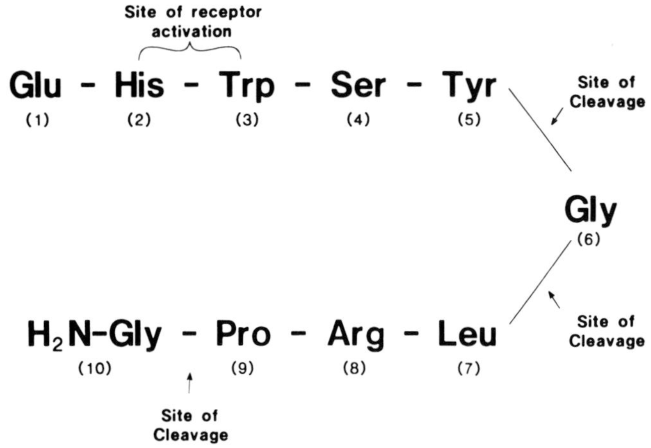

Figure 10–1. Chemical structure of hypothalamic decapeptide gonadotropin-releasing hormone (GnRH). Amino acids 2 and 3 are important for receptor activation. Degradation of GnRH occurs by cleavage of the decapeptide between amino acids 5 and 6, 6 and 7, and 9 and 10.

lesions of the arcuate nucleus were made in rhesus monkeys, thereby ablating most GnRH-secreting neurons. The ablation of the arcuate nucleus resulted in a decrease of circulating LH and FSH to undetectable concentrations. Replacement of GnRH by intravenous pulses of GnRH (1 μg/minute for 6 minutes, given every 60 minutes) restored normal patterns of LH and FSH secretion. Replacement of GnRH by chronic continuous infusion resulted in abnormally low LH and FSH secretion (Fig. 10-2). These experiments demonstrate that secretion of gonadotropins in primates depends on the intermittent secretion of GnRH.

Given that the pituitary gonadotrope responds to the pattern of GnRH secretion (pulses), it is not surprising that the plasma half-life of GnRH is short—2 to 4 minutes.[5] This short half-life and the relatively longer interpulse interval (90 minutes) ensures that a clear, clean, crisp pulse of GnRH can be detected by the pituitary. The rapid degradation of the native GnRH decapeptide is due to cleavage of the peptide bonds between amino acids 5 and 6 and 6 and 7 by endopeptidases present in the blood and pituitary tissue. In addition, a carboxamide peptidase cleaves the peptide bond between amino acids 9 and 10.[6,7] By substituting amino acids at positions 6 and 10 of the native GnRH decapeptide, analogues can be synthesized with high affinity for the pituitary GnRH receptor and a long half-life (more than 2 hours). This long half-life is partly because of resistance of these analogues to the endopeptidases. A common chemical strategy for synthesizing GnRH-agonist analogues is to substitute an "unnatural" D-amino acid (no human proteins contain D-amino acids; all human proteins are composed of L-amino acids) for the L-glycine at position 6 (Table 10-1). This change makes the GnRH ana-

logue resistant to the endopeptidases and decreases the metabolic clearance rate of the analogue. Substitutions at the tenth amino acid position further decreases the clearance rate of the analogue.

Acute administration of the GnRH analogues listed in Table 10-1 to humans results in an increase in LH and FSH secretion and an increase in ovarian steroidogenesis. Therefore, these compounds are called GnRH-agonist analogues. Chronic administration of the GnRH-agonist analogues produces an increase in LH and FSH secretion that only lasts for about the first 5 to 14 days of therapy and is followed by a paradoxical and profound decrease in the secretion of bioactive and immunoreactive LH and FSH.[8,9] The decrease in LH and FSH secretion is paralleled by a marked decrease in ovarian secretion of estradiol, progesterone, and androgens.

The cellular mechanisms by which chronic treatment with a GnRH-agonist analogue results in a paradoxical decrease in pituitary secretion of LH and FSH are not known but may involve down-regulation and desensitization of the pituitary GnRH receptor.[10] Down-regulation is a decrease in the number of available GnRH receptors. Desensitization is an uncoupling of the activated GnRH-receptor complex from intracellular signaling events, which mediate hormone action.

The clinical use of the GnRH-agonist analogues in gynecology is in the ability of these agents to reversibly decrease ovarian steroid production. Chronic administration of the GnRH-agonist analogues produces a hypoestrogenic, hypoprogestational, and hypoandrogenic state. Gonadotropin-releasing hormone–agonist analogues may be efficacious for the treatment of endometriosis, uterine myomas, abnormal uterine bleeding, the premenstrual syndrome, and ovarian hyperandrogenism.

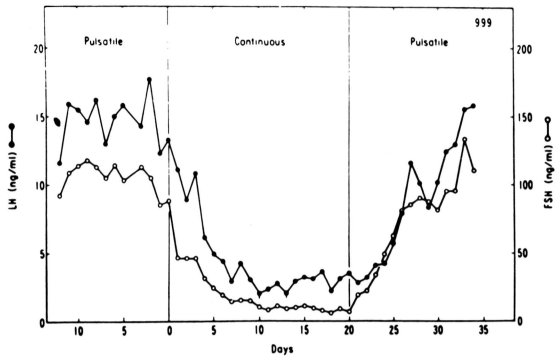

Figure 10–2. Administration of gonadotropin-releasing hormone (GnRH) at one pulse per hour produces a normal pattern of luteinizing-hormone (LH) and follicle-stimulating–hormone (FSH) secretion. Administration of GnRH as a continuous infusion results in a decrease in LH and FSH secretion. (Belchetz PE, Plant TM, Nakai Y, et al: Hypophyseal responses to continuous and intermittent delivery of hypothalamic gonadotropin-releasing hormone. Science 202:631, 1978. Reproduced with permission.)

The Unites States Food and Drug Administration (FDA) has approved two agents, nafarelin acetate (Synarel, Syntex, Palo Alto, CA) and leuprolide acetate (Lupron Tap, E. Chicago, Ill), for the treatment of pelvic pain caused by endometriosis. Additional GnRH-agonist analogues may soon be approved by the FDA but the following discussion is limited to a review of the properties of nafarelin and leuprolide.

CLINICAL PHARMACOLOGY OF GONADOTROPIN-RELEASING– HORMONE AGONISTS

As noted, replacement of the L-glycine at position 6 of the native decapeptide GnRH with various D-amino acids results in GnRH-agonist analogues with long half-lives. For nafarelin, the L-glycine is replaced by a D-naphthylalamine. For leuprolide,

the L-glycine is replaced by D-leucine, and the proline at position 9 is blocked by a N-ethyl-prolinamide group. Nafarelin and leuprolide are 45 and 15 times more potent than native GnRH on a molar basis. The half-life of nafarelin and leuprolide is in the range of 2 to 4 hours. When used at appropriate doses, both nafarelin and leuprolide are efficacious in suppressing LH and FSH secretion and ovarian steroidogenesis. Leuprolide and nafarelin differ in the route of administration and drug formulation.

Nafarelin is available as a formulation for nasal insufflation. Each nasal spray contains 200 μg of nafarelin. After a single intranasal dose of 200 μg of nafarelin, the mean peak plasma concentration is about 0.3 μg/L.[11] The ability of nafarelin to suppress gonadotropin secretion and ovarian steroidogenesis clearly depends on the dose administered. At a dose of 200 μg twice daily, the mean serum estradiol concentration is 28 pg/mL.[12,13] At a dose of 200 μg four times a day, the mean serum concentration of estradiol is 12 pg/mL.[12,13]

Table 10–1
Amino Acid Substitutions in GnRH* Analogues and Potency Compared to Native GnRH

GnRH Agonist		Potency
Nafarelin	D-Naphthylalanine[6]	100
Leuprolide	D-Leucine[6], N-ethyl-prolinamide[9]	15
Buserelin	D-Serine (tBu)[6]	50
Goserelin	D-Serine (tBu)[6], Aza-Gly-NH$_2$[10]	75
Histrelin	D-His,[6] Pro[9]	100

GnRH, gonadotropin-releasing hormone.

Leuprolide is available as two formulations: a depot preparation that is administered as an intramuscular injection every 4 weeks, and a preparation formulated for daily subcutaneous administration. The depot preparation of leuprolide is formulated by impregnating the drug in biodegradable microspheres averaging 20 microns in diameter. Immediately after intramuscular administration, there is a surge of leuprolide released into the circulation from the surface of the microspheres. After 3 days, leuprolide release becomes a zero-order process and a steady-state plasma concentration of about 0.5 µg/mL of the drug is achieved. At a dose of depot-leuprolide, 3.75 mg intramuscularly every 4 weeks, the mean circulating serum estradiol is about 13 pg/mL.[14]

INITIATION OF GONADOTROPIN-RELEASING HORMONE–AGONIST THERAPY AND MAJOR ADVERSE EFFECTS

Before initiating GnRH-agonist therapy, the clinician should confirm the diagnosis. Occasionally, case reports appear of myomas treated with GnRH agonists that eventually prove to be gastrointestinal tumors or leiomyosarcomas.

Gonadotropin-releasing–hormone agonists may be initiated in the luteal or early follicular phase of the menstrual cycle. The advantage of initiating GnRH-agonist therapy during the luteal phase of the menstrual cycle is that the progesterone and estradiol secreted by the corpus luteum partially suppresses the initial GnRH-agonist–induced increase in LH, FSH, and estradiol that occurs when a GnRH agonist is initiated in the early follicular phase.[15] Initiation of a GnRH agonist during the luteal phase of the cycle minimizes the agonist phase and results in more rapid suppression of ovarian estrogen production (Fig. 10-3).[16] A serious disadvantage to luteal-phase initiation of GnRH-agonist therapy is that the patient may be pregnant. Standard pregnancy tests may fail to detect pregnancy during the mid-luteal phase. Consequently, the recommendation is to begin treatment during the early follicular phase (cycle day 3 to 5). As noted above, initiation of GnRH-agonist therapy during the early follicular phase produces an increase in estradiol secretion and often is associated with a failure to ovulate, resulting in significant uterine bleeding during the first month of treatment. Most women become hypoestrogenic and amenorrheic within 6 weeks of starting treatment. Gonadotropin-releasing hormone–agonist treatment is associated with small but significant increases in circulating concentrations of alkaline phosphatase, aspartate transaminase, calcium, phosphate, and albumin.[13,17] Elevations in alkaline phosphatase, calcium, and phosphate may be related to increased bone resorption associated with acute hypoestrogenism. Gonadotropin-releasing hormone–agonist therapy may also be associated with increases in hemoglobin, serum iron, and total iron-binding capacity. These changes are probably due to the amenorrhea caused by these agents.

The effects of GnRH-agonist analogues on bone density remain controversial. The studies performed using the most sensitive and reliable bone-density–measurement techniques (dual x-ray absorptiometry or quantitative digital radiography)

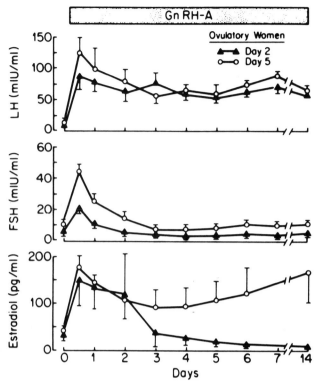

Figure 10–3. Effect of timing of initiation of gonadotropin-releasing hormone (GnRH)–agonist therapy in the early follicular phase. Normal ovulatory patients starting daily SC treatment with 100 μg of GnRH agonist ([D-Trp⁶, Pro⁹-NEt] GnRH) on cycle 2 achieve a more rapid hypogonadotropic hypogonadal response than patients commencing treatment on cycle day 5. (DeFazio J, Meldrum DR, Lu JKH, et al: Acute ovarian responses to a long-acting agonist of gonadotropin-releasing hormone in ovulatory women and women with polycystic ovarian disease. Fertil Steril 44:453–459, 1985. Reproduced with permission of the publisher, The American Fertility Society.)

suggest that 6 months of GnRH-agonist treatment results in a 2% to 10% loss of lumbar bone density.[18–20] Much of this loss in bone density is recovered after the agonist treatment is discontinued.[18–20] The clinical importance of these effects remains uncertain but warrants additional intense investigation.

GONADOTROPIN-RELEASING–HORMONE AGONISTS IN THE TREATMENT OF ENDOMETRIOSIS

Endometriosis is the presence of tissue resembling endometrial glands and stroma outside the uterine cavity. Endometriosis lesions are observed most often on the uterosacral ligaments, ovaries, pelvic peritoneum, bowel, and appendix. Women between the ages of 15 and 50 years are most frequently affected by endometriosis. The incidence and prevalence of endometriosis is not well quantified but estimates suggest that between 1% and 5% of women of reproductive age have endometriosis.[21]

STEROID-HORMONE–DEPENDENT ENDOMETRIOSIS LESIONS

Most endometriosis lesions contain high-affinity low-capacity estrogen, progesterone, and androgen receptors.[22,23] For example, Bergqvist and Feno, using a monoclonal antibody–immunoassay technique, demonstrated that of 31 endometriosis lesions examined, all contained both estrogen and progesterone receptors.[22] In endometriosis lesions, the concentration of estrogen and progesterone receptors was about 50% lower than in matched endometrial specimens.[22] Androgen receptors were present at comparable concentrations in both endometriosis lesions and matched endometrium.[23]

Both clinical and laboratory observations support the hypothesis that estradiol stimulates the growth of endometriosis lesions. Clinical observations that support this concept include the following:

1. Endometriosis is rarely observed in hypoestrogenic states, such as before menarche, after

menopause, or in association with premature ovarian failure[24]

2. In women with endometriosis, surgical castration is typically associated with regression of endometriosis lesions[25]
3. In women with endometriosis, suppression of estradiol production with GnRH agonists typically causes regression of lesions[13,26,27,28,29]

Laboratory models of endometriosis also support the concept that estradiol is a critically important factor in controlling the growth of endometriosis lesions. For example, Bergqvist and coworkers implanted human endometriosis lesions in the abdominal wall of nude mice.[30] In a hypoestrogenic environment, the implanted endometriosis lesions demonstrated decreased glandular activity. When estradiol was administered to the rats, the endometriosis lesion did not atrophy. Sharpe and coworkers autotransplanted rat endometrium to the intestinal mesentery.[31] The autotransplanted endometrium grew into cystic structures lined with endometrium. In a hypoestrogenic state (castrated animals), the endometriosis lesions atrophied. When estradiol was administered to the animals, the lesions did not atrophy. Interestingly, the administration of estradiol plus progesterone produced greater growth in the endometriosis lesions than either agent administered alone.[30,31] The efficacy of GnRH agonists in the treatment of endometriosis is probably largely due to the decrease in ovarian estradiol production produced by these agents.

ESTRADIOL CONCENTRATION REQUIRED TO SUPPRESS ENDOMETRIOSIS ACTIVITY

Multiple clinical trials suggest that GnRH agonists (1) suppress circulating estradiol concentrations; (2) reduce endometriosis disease activity, as objectively measured by pre- and post-treatment laparoscopy (Fig. 10-4); and (3) decrease pelvic pain.[13,26,27,28] An important question that remains to be answered is that of the precise estradiol concentration required to suppress the activity of endometriosis lesions. A review of multiple studies suggests that estradiol concentration of 15 pg/mL and 30 pg/mL are both efficacious in the treatment of endometriosis.[13,26,27,28]

For example, regimens used by Henzl and coworkers (nafarelin, 200 μg nasally twice daily) and

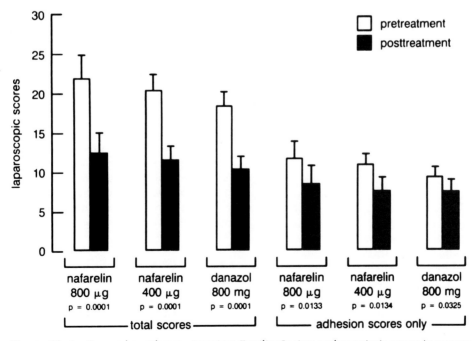

Figure 10–4. Pre- and posttherapy American Fertility Society endometriosis scores in women receiving 6 months of nasal nafarelin or oral danazol therapy. (Henzl M: N Engl J Med 361–485, 1988. Reprinted by permission of the New England Journal of Medicine.)

Cirkel and coworkers (buserelin, 300 μg nasally three times a day) both reduced circulating estradiol to 30 pg/mL and reduced the revised American Fertility Society (RAFS) endometriosis score by 43% and 51%, respectively.[13,26] In addition, the regimen studied by Henzl and coworkers reduced pelvic pain in 73% of patients.[13] In contrast, Shaw (goserelin, 3.6 mg implant every 4 weeks for 6 months), Dlugi and coworkers (leuprolide acetate, 3.75 mg intramuscularly every 4 weeks), and LeMay and coworkers (buserelin) studied regimens that reduced circulating estradiol concentrations to the range of 8 pg/mL to 15 pg/mL.[27,28,29] These regimens produced a 50% decrease in RAFS endometriosis score and decreased pelvic pain in 70% to 89% of subjects.[27,28,29] A direct comparison of these studies suggests that on average, GnRH-agonist regimens that produce circulating estradiol concentrations of 15 pg/mL or 30 pg/mL are both efficacious in the treatment of endometriosis (Table 10-2).

An important issue is whether a clinician treating a woman with endometriosis should aim for an estradiol concentration target of 15 pg/mL or 30 pg/mL.

BALANCING THE EFFECTS OF HYPOESTROGENISM IN THE TREATMENT OF ENDOMETRIOSIS: THE ESTRADIOL TARGET

Estradiol concentrations in the range of 15 pg/mL are extremely effective in causing atrophy of endometriosis lesions. Women with pelvic pain and endometriosis who are treated with doses of GnRH agonist sufficient to reduce circulating estradiol to 15 pg/mL typically experience significant relief of pelvic pain because the endometriosis lesions become atrophic. There are, however, important adverse effects associated with a circulating estradiol concentration of 15 pg/mL, including hot flashes, headaches, dry vagina, and loss of bone mineral. At an estradiol concentration of 30 pg/mL, many women experience significant relief of pelvic pain. It is likely that at an estradiol concentration of 30 pg/mL, severity of hypoestrogenic side effects is less than at estradiol levels of 15 pg/mL. When treating endometriosis with hypoestrogenism, it may be best to use a regimen that produces the *minimal* degree of hypoestrogenism necessary to cause improvement in the pelvic pain.

For women with minimal or mild endometriosis and moderate pain symptoms, an estradiol target of 30 pg/mL is often sufficient to produce significant

improvement in the pain symptoms. One strategy for achieving an estradiol concentration in the range of 30 pg/mL is to administer nafarelin at a dose of 400 μg/day. After 2 months of nafarelin treatment, if the circulating estradiol concentration is more than 30 pg/mL, the daily dose of nafarelin may be increased. If the circulating estradiol concentration is less than 30 pg/mL, the daily dose of nafarelin may be decreased. Nasal nafarelin, at a dose of 400 μg/day, produces a mean circulating estradiol concentration of about 30 pg/mL.[13] Consequently, many women require no adjustment of their nafarelin dose to achieve an estradiol target of about 30 pg/mL.

For women with severe endometriosis or endometriosis lesions that are especially sensitive to estradiol, clinicians may want to aim for an estradiol concentration target of 15 pg/mL. Strategies for achieving an estradiol concentration target of 15 pg/mL include two potential regimens: (1) leuprolide acetate, 3.75 mg intramuscularly every 4 weeks; or (2) nafarelin, 400 μg twice daily. After the disease process and the clinical symptoms are well controlled, the physician may want to consider retargeting therapy to an estradiol concentration of 30 pg/mL.

For most women with endometriosis, a circulating estradiol concentration of 15 pg/mL is associated with complete relief of pelvic pain. When the circulating estradiol concentration of these women is increased to 30 pg/mL, many continue to experience pain relief and note a decrease in the frequency and severity of their vasomotor symptoms. Some women, however, have a recurrence of pelvic pain when the estradiol concentration is increased to 30 pg/mL. This suggests that the sensitivity of endometriosis lesions to estradiol may vary from woman to woman. For women with endometriosis who only experience pelvic pain relief when the circulating estradiol concentration is less than 15 pg/mL, regimens to protect against the adverse effects of severe hypoestrogenism need to be developed. Potential novel regimens are reviewed below.

REGIMENS TO MINIMIZE THE EFFECTS OF GONADOTROPIN-RELEASING–HORMONE AGONIST–INDUCED HYPOESTROGENISM

A major deleterious effect of hypoestrogenism is a decrease in bone mineral content, especially marked at regions rich in trabecular bone. For women with estradiol concentrations of 15 pg/mL,

Table 10–2

Effects of GnRH-a on Estradiol Concentration, Reduction of Revised AFS Score, and Pain Relief in Women With Endometriosis

Subject					
Investigator	Number	Drug/Dosage	Estradiol Concentration*	Reduction in AFS Score	Pain Relief of Subjects
Henzl et al[13]	77	Nafarelin, 400 µg intranasal for 6 months	28	43	73
	79	Nafarelin, 800 µg intranasal for 6 months	15†	42	77
Cirkel et al[26]	40	Buserelin acetate, 300 µg 3 times a day intranasal for 6 months	28	51	—
LeMay et al[28]	10	Buserelin acetate, 200 µg 2 times a day SC for 5 days, then 400 µg intranasal spray 3 times a day for 25–31 weeks	8	50	72
Dlugi et al[27]	52	Leuprolide acetate, 3.75 mg IM every 4 weeks for 20 weeks	15‡	—	89
Shaw[29]	40	Goserelin, 3.6 mg implant for 6 months	12.7	50§	69.6

*At end of treatment

†Based on result from Andreyko et al.

‡Based on result from Friedman et al.

§Excluding adhesion scores

From Barbieri RL, Gordon A-MC: Hormonal therapy of endometriosis: the estradiol target. Fertil Steril 56:820–822, 1991. Reproduced with permission of the publisher, The American Fertility Society.

loss of bone mineral density may range from 3% to 15% in the lumbar vertebrae in the first 6 months of hypoestrogenism.[18–20] Regimens that may be effective in minimizing bone mineral loss due to hypoestrogenism include progestin, estradiol plus progestin, etidronate, and calcitonin.

Progestins as single agents can be effective in the treatment of endometriosis.[31] Therefore, it is not surprising that progestin plus GnRH agonists may also be efficacious in the treatment of endometriosis. Surrey and colleagues evaluated the effects of a combined regimen of the GnRH agonist histrelin (100 µg, subcutaneous daily) with norethindrone (average daily dose, 1.4 mg) in the treatment of 10 women with endometriosis.[33] This therapy significantly suppressed pelvic pain in all 10 women. In addition, this regimen reduced the AFS endometriosis dose from 14.6 before treatment to 6.4 after treatment ($p < 0.005$). The combined GnRH plus norethindrone regimen resulted in a low rate of severe vasomotor symptoms compared with that observed for GnRH agonist alone. There was a 6% decrease in lumbar spine bone density, as measured by quantitative computed tomography at the end of 24 weeks of therapy. These findings demonstrate that histrelin plus norethindrone is effective in the treatment of endometriosis. Unfortunately, at the dosages used, norethindrone was unable to block the bone loss caused by a hypoestrogenic state.

Judd and colleagues evaluated the efficacy of combined GnRH agonist plus high-dose progestin (norethindrone, 10 mg daily) in the treatment of endometriosis.[33] This dose of norethindrone has been reported to block the bone loss associated with a hypoestrogenic state.[34] Judd observed that combined GnRH agonist plus progestin therapy was associated with few vasomotor symptoms and low urinary calcium excretion. Combined therapy was efficacious in reducing pain associated with endometriosis and in rendering the surgical AFS endometriosis score.[33] Combined GnRH agonist plus high-dose progestin treatment warrants additional investigation.

Two new nonsteroidal agents that appear to be effective in blocking bone loss caused by a hypoestrogenic state are calcitonin and etidronate. Calcitonin is a hypocalcemic factor that directly inhibits bone resorption and bone-resorbing cells. Calcitonin reduces the mobilization of calcium, phosphorous, and hydroxyproline from bone. The primary stimulus for calcitonin synthesis and secretion is an increase in the concentration of circulating ionized calcium. Studies suggest that the administration of salmon or human calcitonin by parenteral or nasal routes reduces the bone resorption caused by a hypoestrogenic state. For example, Reginster and coworkers randomized 79 menopausal women (onset of menopause within 36 months of entry to trial) to a 12-month regimen of calcium (500 mg/day) or calcium plus intranasal salmon calcitonin (50 IU/day) for 5 days a week.[35] Bone mineral density in the lumbar vertebrae was measured using a dual-photon absorptiometry method. After 12 months of treatment, bone mineral density had decreased by a mean of $3.6 \pm 0.6\%$ in the calcium-only group (mean $\pm$ standard error mean) and by $1.38 \pm 0.8\%$ in the calcium plus calcitonin group ($p < 0.01$; see Fig. 10-1). The endogenous serum calcitonin concentration increased in the calcium-treated group but not in the calcitonin-treated group. Parathyroid concentration was not altered by either therapy.

This study suggests that the combination of a GnRH agonist with calcitonin may decrease the bone loss associated with GnRH-agonist therapy. The only calcitonin preparation available for use is Calcimar (Rhône-Poulenc Rorer Pharmaceuticals, Collegeville, PA), a synthetic salmon calcitonin that is approved by the FDA for the treatment of postmenopausal osteoporosis, hypercalcemia, and Paget's disease. The potency of salmon calcitonin per mole is greater than that of mammalian calcitonins. In rare individuals, salmon calcitonin may cause an allergic reaction, including bronchospasm and angioedema of the upper respiratory tract. Skin testing with 1 IU of salmon calcitonin is suggested before instituting full-dose (100 IU/day) therapy.

Etidronate disodium is an oral diphosphonate compound known to reduce bone resorption through the inhibition of osteoclastic activity.[36] Etidronate inhibits the formation, growth, and dissolution of hydroxyapatite crystals and their amorphous precursors by chemisorption to the calcium phosphate surface. Storm and coworkers reported on the effects of etidronate in blocking bone resorption in hypoestrogenic women.[38] In this study, 66 menopausal women were randomized to receive oral etidronate (400 mg/day) or placebo for 2 weeks, followed by a 13-week period in which no drugs were given.[25] This sequence was repeated 10 times for a total of 150 weeks. Oral calcium (500 mg/day) and vitamin D supplements (400 IU/day) were given to all subjects. Vertebral bone mineral content was measured using dual-photon absorptiometry. Vertebral bone mineral content increased by 5.3% in the etidronate group and decreased by 2.7% in the placebo group ($p < 0.01$). The group treated with etidronate had fewer fractures than the group treated with placebo ($p < 0.05$). Unfortunately, many women dropped out of this study before its completion. The high drop-out rate makes the results difficult to interpret.

Etidronate disodium (Didronel, Norwich Eaton Pharmaceuticals) is approved by the FDA for the treatment of symptomatic Paget's disease and heterotopic ossification. It is not approved for the treatment of postmenopausal osteoporosis. Oral etidronate is poorly absorbed (1% of dose). At a dose in the range of 5 mg/kg/day, side effects are minimal. At higher doses, gastrointestinal complaints of diarrhea and nausea may occur. The potential combination of GnRH agonists plus etidronate to prevent bone loss is attractive because of the efficacy of etidronate when used in cyclic regimens (eg, 2 weeks of etidronate, 13 weeks off drug, 2 weeks of etidronate. . .). Randomized clinical trials to evaluate combined regimens of GnRH agonist plus etidronate in the treatment of pelvic pain caused by endometriosis are eagerly awaited.

GONADOTROPIN-RELEASING–HORMONE AGONISTS IN THE TREATMENT OF ENDOMETRIOSIS: GENERAL PRINCIPLES

Duration of Therapy

The FDA has approved GnRH-agonist therapy for endometriosis for a 6-month course. This is arbitrary and based on the design of the original clinical trials of GnRH agonists. For some women, a 3-month course of therapy is effective. In other instances, therapy for 9 or 12 months may be warranted if side effects, including bone density loss, are carefully monitored.

Contraindications

There are few contraindications to GnRH-agonist therapy. These include known hypersensitivity, pregnancy, and undiagnosed vaginal bleeding.

Use Without Surgery for the Treatment of Infertility Caused by Endometriosis

There is no scientific evidence that hormone therapy improves fecundity in infertile women with endometriosis. In women with advanced endometriosis and infertility, surgery may improve fecundity.[38,39]

Use With Surgery for the Treatment of Endometriosis

In patients with advanced endometriosis scheduled for a conservative laparotomy or hysterectomy, active inflammation in the cul-de-sac and ovarian fossae may make the surgery difficult. Preoperative treatment with a GnRH agonist for 3 months may reduce the inflammatory process and simplify the surgery.

Use Before In Vitro Fertilization– Embryo Transfer

Several women with endometriosis and infertility fail to conceive after empiric hormone therapy or conservative surgery. These women often proceed to in vitro fertilization (IVF). An important clinical issue is the potential efficacy of pre-IVF GnRH-agonist therapy to improve pregnancy outcomes. Dicker and colleagues randomized 67 women with severe endometriosis and infertility (who planned to undergo a cycle of IVF) to receive a GnRH agonist for 6 months, followed by FSH and human menopausal gonadotropin (hMG) for ovulation induction ($n = 35$) or to receive FSH–hMG alone, without GnRH-agonist treatment ($n = 32$).[41] The women who received GnRH agonist before IVF had more eggs aspirated (5.2 versus 3.1; $p < 0.001$) and more embryos transferred (2.4 versus 1.7; $p < 0.04$) than the women who did not receive GnRH-agonist pretreatment. In addition, the clinical pregnancy rate per cycle was higher in the women who received GnRH-agonist pretreatment compared with controls (25% versus 4%; $p < 0.0001$). This study suggests that women with severe endometriosis and infertility should receive a course of GnRH-agonist therapy just before a cycle of IVF.

Recurrence Rates After Therapy

Gonadotropin-releasing hormone–agonist therapy produces a decrease in dysmenorrhea, dyspareunia, and pelvic pain caused by endometriosis. After discontinuing therapy, the dysmenorrhea returns quickly (within 6 months) but the dyspareunia and pelvic pain may not recur for up to 12 months.[27]

GONADOTROPIN-RELEASING– HORMONE AGONISTS IN THE TREATMENT OF UTERINE LEIOMYOMATA

Uterine leiomyomata, or myomas, are benign smooth muscle tumors that may occur in as many as 30% of women. Evidence indicates that about 50% of myomas are cytogenetically abnormal and at least 90% are clonal.[41,42] These observations suggest that many myomas arise from a somatic mutation in a myometrial cell. If myomas arise because of changes in nuclear DNA, it is unrealistic to expect that a hormonal treatment such as a GnRH agonist could cure the disease process. The activity of myomas are modulated, however, by estradiol. In premenopausal women with myomas, the induction of a hypoestrogenic state often results in a 50% decrease in the volume of the myomatous uterus, and induces amenorrhea.[43] These two effects—induction of amenorrhea and reduction of uterine volume—may offer substantial clinical benefit to women with myomas. The FDA has not yet approved any GnRH agonist for the treatment of myomas, however. The effects of GnRH agonists on uterine myomas are dose- and time-dependent.

To produce near maximal decrease in volume of a myomatous uterus, circulating estradiol concentration must be reduced to about 15 pg/mL. Reduction of circulating estradiol concentration to a range of 30 pg/mL does not produce a maximal decrease in uterine volume.[44] These findings suggest that uterine myomas are extremely sensitive to estradiol and that profound hypoestrogenism must be achieved to fully suppress myoma volume. Two effective methods for achieving a circulating estradiol concentration of 15 pg/mL is to use depot leuprolide (3.75 mg, intramuscularly every 4 weeks) or nafarelin (400 μg, twice daily).

In women with uterine myomas, nearly maximal regression in uterine volume requires about 12 weeks of GnRH-agonist treatment.[43,44] Minimal decrease in uterine volume occurs by 8 weeks of treatment. These observations may be of importance to surgeons who are planning to use a GnRH agonist before hysterectomy or myomectomy.

GONADOTROPIN-RELEASING– HORMONE AGONISTS IN THE TREATMENT OF MYOMAS: GENERAL PRINCIPLES

Primary Treatment for Symptomatic Myomas In Young Women

Uterine myomas are monoclonal, cystogenically abnormal tumors. Although GnRH agonists may decrease uterine volume and produce amenorrhea, cessation of treatment usually results in regrowth of the myoma to pretreatment size within 6 months.[43]

Consequently, clinicians should not expect treatment with GnRH agonists to produce a permanent decrease in myoma volume. Surgical therapy should be the primary treatment for women with uterine myomas.

Anemia in Women With Myomas

Numerous women with uterine myomas have menorrhagia and an iron-deficiency anemia.

For women with myomas and anemia who need a myomectomy or hysterectomy, normalization of circulating red blood cell volume is an important goal. Gonadotropin-releasing–hormone agonists, by producing hypoestrogenism and amenorrhea, are helpful when combined with iron replacement in returning red blood cell volume to normal.[43,44]

Vaginal Hysterectomy

Every gynecologic surgeon has an upper limit to the size of uterus he or she is comfortable removing by a vaginal approach. Gonadotropin-releasing–hormone agonists produce a 50% decrease in uterine volume. Logically, for a women whose myomatous uterus is too large to be removed by a vaginal approach, pretreatment with a GnRH agonist may reduce the size of the uterus so that it is possible to perform a vaginal hysterectomy.

Stovall and colleagues randomized 50 premenopausal women with uterine myomas of 14- to 18-week size (who were planning to have a hysterec-

tomy) to receive no preoperative hormone therapy (group A, $n = 25$) or 8 weeks of GnRH-agonist treatment preoperatively (group B, $n = 25$).[45] Patients in the GnRH-agonist group had an increase in hemoglobin levels (11 to 12 g/dL; $p < 0.05$) and a decrease in uterine size (1090 to 723 cm³; $p < 0.05$) during the hormone preoperative treatment. Women who received preoperative GnRH-agonist treatment were more likely to have a vaginal hysterectomy than women with no hormone treatment (76% versus 16%). The cost of the GnRH-agonist therapy was offset by the reduced hospitalization of women who received preoperative hormone therapy, compared with untreated controls (3.8 days versus 5.2 days; $p < 0.05$).

Reduced Blood Loss at the Time of Myomectomy

Friedman and colleagues randomized 18 women with uterine myomas to receive placebo (vehicle injection every 4 weeks for three doses) or GnRH-agonist treatment (depot leuprolide acetate, 3.75 mg intramuscularly every 4 weeks for three doses) before myomectomy (Fig. 10-5).[46] At surgery, the group that received preoperative GnRH agonist had about 200 mL less blood loss than the group that received placebo ($p < .05$). This difference in blood loss was primarily because of a reduction in blood lost during the uterine portion of the operation and not from the skin or abdominal wall portion of the surgery (Fig. 10-6). The reduction in blood loss was most marked for the women with the largest myomas.

Although the magnitude of the reduction in blood loss is modest (200 mL), surgeons may want to pretreat women with large myomas before myomectomy.

Reduced Blood Loss at the Time of Hysterectomy

Lumsden and colleagues randomized 27 premenopausal women with myomas who were planning to have a hysterectomy to receive either no preoperative treatment ($n = 14$) or 3 months of preoperative GnRH-agonist treatment ($n = 13$).[47] Because of the randomization process, patients in both groups were well matched for age, parity, and uterine volume. The women who received GnRH-agonist treatment before hysterectomy had a 45% decrease

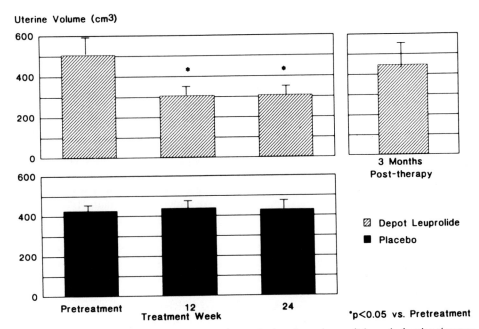

Figure 10–5. Changes in mean uterine volume during depot leuprolide and placebo therapy. Within 3 months of cessation of therapy, there is a significant increase in uterine volume. (Friedman AJ, Harrison-Atlas D, Barbieri RL, Benacerraf B, Gleason R, Schiff I: A randomized, placebo-controlled, double-blind study evaluating the efficacy of leuprolide acetate depot in the treatment of uterine leiomyomata. Fertil Steril 51:251–256, 1989. Reproduced with permission of the publisher, The American Fertility Society.)

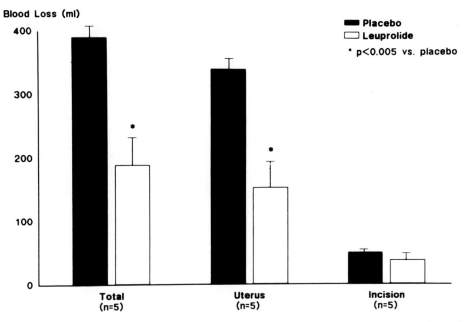

Figure 10–6. Blood loss at myomectomy for uteri having pretreatment volumes of ≥600 cm³. (Friedman AJ, Rein MS, Harrison-Atlas D, Garfield JM, Doubilet PM: A randomized, placebo-controlled, double-blind study evaluating leuprolide acetate depot treatment before myomectomy. Fertil Steril 52:728–733, 1989. Reproduced with permission of the publisher, The American Fertility Society.)

in uterine volume and reduced blood loss at the time of surgery (235 mL versus 350 mL; $p < 0.01$). The reduction in blood loss was statistically significant but of a modest amount (115 mL) from a clinical perspective. It is possible, however, that women with the largest uterine volumes may have proportionally greater reduction in blood loss when treated with a GnRH analogue before surgery.

Long-Term Treatment With Steroid Add-Back

Treatment regimens with steroid "add-back" that minimize the impact of the hypoestrogenic effects of GnRH-agonist therapy while still achieving one or more clinically important goals (reduction in uterine volume, amenorrhea) have been devised. The goal of add-back therapy is to increase the safety of prolonged GnRH-agonist treatment. Premenopausal women with clinically symptomatic myomas who refuse surgical therapy may benefit most from combined GnRH-agonist and add-back treatment.

Most studies have used a simultaneous or sequential treatment strategy. In the simultaneous strategy, GnRH agonist plus steroid add-back are started at the same time. In sequential-treatment regimens, the GnRH agonist is administered as a single agent for 3 to 6 months and then the steroid add-back treatment is initiated.

Friedman and colleagues reported the results of a simultaneous add-back regimen of GnRH agonist (leuprolide acetate, 0.5 mg subcutaneous injection daily) plus medroxyprogesterone acetate (MPA; 20 mg daily).[48] Fourteen women were randomized to receive GnRH agonist plus MPA ($n = 7$) or GnRH agonist plus placebo ($n = 7$). In this study, MPA significantly reduced the vasomotor symptoms reported by the subjects. The combination of GnRH plus MPA, however, only resulted in a 15% decrease in uterine volume, compared with a 50% decrease in uterine volume in the women who received GnRH agonist plus a placebo.

In a pilot study, Friedman evaluated a sequential add-back regimen consisting of GnRH agonist alone (leuprolide acetate, 0.5 mg subcutaneous injection daily) for 3 months, followed by the add-back of conjugated equine estrogens (CEE; 0.625 mg daily) plus MPA (10 mg daily for 10 days each month) in addition to the GnRH agonist for an additional 24 months.[49] During the first 3 months of

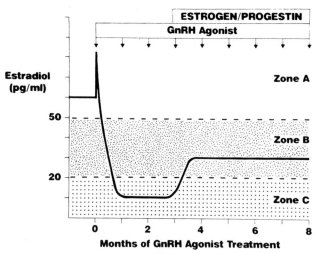

Figure 10–7. Estrogen threshold hpyothesis. (**Zone A**) Typical circulating estradiol concentrations in premenopausal women are able to support myometrial–fibroid growth and prevent rapid bone resorption. (**Zone B**) Therapeutic window; myometrial and fibroid volume may decrease at these estradiol levels but bone resorption is not accelerated. (**Zone C**) Hypoestrogenism, often attained during gonadotropin-releasing–hormone–agonist therapy may lead to myometrial-fibroid shrinkage and rapid bone resorption. Note: Estradiol values for each zone may differ among patients. (Friedman AJ, Lobel SM, Rein MS, Barbieri RL: Efficacy and safety considerations in women with uterine leiomyomas treated with gonadotropin-releasing hormone agonists: the estrogen threshold hypothesis. Am J Obstet Gynecol 163:1114–1119, 1990. Reproduced with permission of the publisher, Mosby-Year Book, Inc.)

treatment (GnRH agonist only), a 49% reduction in uterine volume was observed. After the add-back of CEE plus MPA, there was a decrease in the vasomotor symptoms reported by the subjects but no increase in uterine volume. This preliminary study suggests that some women with myomas who decline primary surgical treatment may be responsive to long-term GnRH-agonist plus steroid add-back treatment.

The early success of add-back treatment has stimulated the development of the estrogen threshold hypothesis. This hypothesis suggests that myomas are less sensitive to the effects of low doses of steroid hormones if they have been exposed to a prolonged hypoestrogenic state (Fig. 10-7).

Gonadotropin-releasing–hormone agonists are vulnerable agents for the practicing gynecologist because of the broad range of diseases which can be influenced by ovarian suppression. It is likely that every gynecologist will become an expert in the use of these agents.

REFERENCES

1. Matsuo H, Baba Y, Nair RMG, Arimura A, Schally AV: Structure of porcine LH and FSH releasing factor I. The proposed amino acid sequence. Biochem Biophys Res Commun 43:1334, 1971
2. King JL, Anthony ELP, Fitzgerald DM, Stopa EG: Luteinizing hormone neurons in human preoptic/hypothalamus: differential intraneuronal localization of immunoreactive forms. J Clin Endocrinol Metab 60:88, 1985
3. Crowley WF, Filicori M, Spratt DI, Santoro NF: The physiology of gonadotropin-releasing hormone secretion in men and women. Recent Prog Horm Res 41:473, 1985
4. Knobil E: The neuroendocrine control of the menstrual cycle. Recent Prog Horm Res 36:53, 1980
5. Handelsman DJ, Swerdloff RS: Pharmacokinetics of gonadotropin releasing hormone and its analogues. Endocr Rev 7:95, 1986
6. Griffiths EC, McDermott JR: Enzymatic inactivation of hypothalamic regulatory hormones. Mol Cell Endocrinol 33:1, 1983
7. Marks N, Stern F: Enzymatic mechanisms for the inactivation of luteinizing hormone-releasing hormone. Biochem Biophys Res Commun 61:1458, 1974
8. Meldrum DR, Chang RJ, Lu J, Vale W, Rivier J, Judd HL: Medical oophorectomy using a long-acting GnRH agonist: a possible new approach to the treatment of endometriosis. J Clin Endocrinol Metab 54:1081, 1982
9. Defazio J, Meldrum DR, Lu JKH: Acute ovarian responses to a long acting agonist of gonadotropin releasing hormone in ovulatory women and women with polycystic ovarian disease. Fertil Steril 44:453, 1985
10. Conn PM, Crowley WF Jr: Gonadotropin releasing hormone and its analogues. N Engl J Med 324:93, 1991
11. Barbieri RL: Critical drug appraisal: nafarelin. Drug Therapy 21:23, 1991
12. Barbieri RL: Hormonal therapy of endometriosis: the estradiol target. Fertil Steril 56:820, 1991
13. Henzl MR, Corson SL, Moghissi K, Buttram VC, Bergqvist C, Jacobson H: Administration of nasal nafarelin as compared to oral danazol for endometriosis. N Engl J Med 318:485, 1988
14. Friedman AJ, Hoffman DI, Cornite F, Browneller RW, Miller JD: Treatment of leiomyomata uteri with leuprolide acetate depot: a double-blind, placebo-controlled multicenter study. Obstet Gynecol 77:720, 1991
15. Sheehan KL, Casper RF, Yen SSE: Effects of a superactive luteinizing hormone releasing factor agonist on gonadotropin and ovarian function during the menstrual cycle. Am J Obstet Gynecol 135:759, 1979
16. DeFazio J, Meldrum DR, Lu JKH: Acute ovarian responses to a long acting agonist of gonadotropin releasing hormone in ovulatory women and women with polycystic ovarian disease. Fertil Steril 44:453, 1985
17. Friedman AJ, Harrison-Atlas D, Barbieri RL, Benacerraf B, Gleason R, Schiff I: A randomized placebo controlled double blind study evaluating the efficacy of leuprolide acetate depot in the treatment of uterine leiomyomata. Fertil Steril 51:751, 1989
18. Johansen JS, Riis BJ, Hassager R: The effect of a gonadotropin releasing hormone agonist analogue (nafarelin) on bone metabolism. J Clin Endocrinol Metab 1988; 67:701
19. Matta WHM, Shaw RW, Hesp R, Evans R: Reversible trabecular bone density loss following induced hypoestrogenism with the GnRH analogue buserelin in premenopausal women. Clin Endocrinol 29:45, 1988
20. Dawood MY, Lewis V, Ramos J: Cortical and trabecular bone mineral content in women with endometriosis: effect of gonadotropin releasing hormone agonist and danazol. Fertil Steril 52:21, 1989
21. Barbieri RL: Etiology and epidemiology of endometriosis. Am J Obstet Gynecol 162:565, 1990
22. Bergqvist A, Feno M: Steroid receptors in endometriotic tissue endometrium, assay with monoclonal antibodies. In Genazzi AR (ed): Recent research in gynecologic endocrinology, vol 1, p 394. Carnforth, United Kingdom, Pantheon, 1989
23. Tamaya T, Motoyama T, Ohone Y: Steroid receptor levels and histology of endometriosis and adenomyosis. Fertil Steril 31:396, 1979
24. Barbieri RL, Hornstein MD: Endometriosis. In Ryan KJ, Berkowitz R, Barbieri RL (eds): Kistner's gynecology, p 320. Chicago, Year Book Medical Publishers, 1990
25. Barbieri RL: Infertility aspects of endometriosis. In Droegemueller W, Sciarra JJ (eds): Gynecology and obstetrics, p 1. Philadelphia, JB Lippincott, 1991
26. Cirkel U, Schweppe KW, Ochs H, et al: Effects of LHRH agonist therapy in the treatment of endometriosis. In Chadha DR, Willemsen WNP (eds): Gonadotropin down-regulation in gynecological practice, vol 225, p 189. New York, Alan R. Liss, 1986
27. Dlugi AM, Miller JD, Knittle J, et al: Lupron depot

in the treatment of endometriosis: a randomized placebo controlled double blind study. Fertil Steril 54:419, 1990

28. Le May A, Maheuz R, Faure N, et al: Reversible hypogonadism induced by a luteinizing hormone releasing hormone agonist (buserelin) as a new therapeutic approach for endometriosis. Fertil Steril 41:863, 1984

29. Shaw RW: Goserelin-depot preparation of LH-RH analogue used in the treatment of endometriosis. In Chadha DR, Buttram VC (eds): Current concepts in endometriosis, vol 323, p 383. New York, Alan R. Liss, 1990

30. Bergqvist A, Jeppsson S, Kullander S, et al: Human uterine and endometriotic tissue transplanted into nude mice. Am J Pathol 121:337, 1985

31. Sharpe K, Bertero MC, Muse KN, et al: Spontaneous and steroid induced recurrence of endometriosis after suppression by a gonadotropin-releasing hormone antagonist in the rat. Am J Obstet Gynecol 164:187, 1991

32. Luciano AA, Turksoy RN, Carleo J: Evaluation of oral medroxyprogesterone acetate in the treatment of endometriosis. Obstet Gynecol 72:323, 1988

33. Surrey ES, Gambone JC, Lu JKH, Judd HL: The effects of combining norethindrone with a gonadotropin releasing hormone agonist in the treatment of symptomatic endometriosis. Fertil Steril 53:620, 1990

34. Judd HL: Gonadotropin releasing hormone agonists: strategies for managing the hypoestrogenic effects of therapy. Am J Obstet Gynecol 166:752, 1992

35. Abdalla HI, Hart DM, Lindsay R, Leggate I, Hooke A: Prevention of bone mineral loss in postmenopausal women by noresthisterone. Obstet Gynecol 66:789, 1985

36. Reginster JY, Albert A, Lecart MP, et al: One year controlled randomized trial of prevention of early postmenopausal bone loss by intranasal calcitonin. Lancet 2:1481, 1982

37. Guncaga J, Lauftenburger T, Lentner C, et al: Disphosphonate treatment of Paget's disease of bone: a correlated metabolic, calcium kinetic and morphometric study. Horm Metab Res 6:62, 1974

38. Storm T, Thamsborg G, Steiniche T, Genant HK, Sorensen OH: Effect of intermittent cyclic etidronate therapy on bone mass and fracture rate in women with postmenopausal osteoporosis. N Engl J Med 322:1265, 1990

39. Olive DL, Lee KL: Analysis of sequential treatment protocols for endometriosis-associated infertility. Am J Obstet Gynecol 154:613, 1986

40. Telimaa S: Danazol and medroxyprogesterone acetate inefficacious in the treatment of infertility in endometriosis. Fertil Steril 50:872, 1988

41. Dicker D, Goldman JA, Levy T, Feldberg D, Ashkenazi J: The impact of long-term gonadotropin releasing hormone analogue treatment on preclinical abortions in the patients with severe endometriosis undergoing IVF. Fertil Steril 57:597, 1992

42. Townsend DE, Sparkes RS, Baluda MC, McClelland G: Unicellular histogenesis of uterine leiomyomas as determined by electrophoresis of glucose-6-phosphate dehydrogenase. Am J Obstet Gynecol 107:1168, 1976

43. Friedman AJ, Lobel SM, Rein MS, Barbieri RL: Efficacy and safety considerations in women with uterine leiomyomas treated with GnRH agonists. Am J Obstet Gynecol 163:1144, 1990

44. Candiani GB, Vercellini P, Fedelel, Arcaini L, Bianchi S: Use of goserelin depot for the treatment of menorrhagia and severe anemia in women with leiomyomata uteri. Acta Obstet Gynecol Scand 69:413, 1990

45. Stovall TG, Ling FW, Henry LC, Woodruff MR: A randomized trial evaluating leuprolide acetate before hysterectomy as treatment for leiomyomas. Am J Obstet Gynecol 164:1420, 1991

46. Friedman AJ, Rein MS, Harrison-Atlas D: A randomized, placebo controlled, double blind study evaluating leuprolide acetate depot treatment before myomectomy. Fertil Steril 52:728, 1989

47. Lumsden MA, West CP, Baird DT: Goserelin therapy before surgery for uterine fibroids. Lancet 1:36, 1987

48. Friedman AJ, Barbieri RL, Doubilet PM: A randomized, double blind trial of a gonadotropin releasing hormone agonist (leuprolide) with or without medroxyprogesterone acetate in the treatment of leiomyomata uteri. Fertil Steril 49:404, 1988

49. Friedman AJ: Treatment of leiomyomata uteri with short-term leuprolide followed by leuprolide plus estrogen-progestin hormone replacement therapy for two years. A pilot study. Fertil Steril 51:526, 1989

Ambulatory Gynecology, Second Edition,
edited by David H. Nichols and Patrick J. Sweeney.
J. B. Lippincott Company, Philadelphia, © 1995.

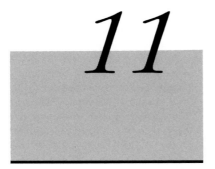

Hirsutism

Jacquelyn S. Loughlin and Susan A. Wolf

Hirsutism is the excessive growth of androgen-dependent terminal hair in women. This common clinical problem is found to have a benign etiology (polycystic ovary syndrome [PCOS], idiopathic hirsutism, nonclassic congenital adrenal hyperplasia [NC-CAH]) in most women. Nevertheless, the diagnostic evaluation must be directed to exclude the rare serious underlying disorders (androgen-secreting neoplasms, Cushing's disease) that require specific therapy.[1,2]

HISTORY AND PHYSICAL EXAMINATION

The goals of the hirsutism evaluation are to (1) exclude serious underlying disease, (2) establish a diagnosis, and (3) serve as a basis for treatment. A thorough medical history and physical examination are the initial steps and often distinguish those women with benign etiologies from those with potentially life-threatening conditions. The essential elements of the evaluation are listed in Table 11-1.

History

A proper history must include the characterization of the onset and progression of symptoms, a menstrual history, a family history, and a complete drug history. Typically, symptoms arise peri- or postpubertally and progress gradually with idiopathic hirsutism, polycystic ovary syndrome (PCOS), and NC-CAH. The abrupt onset or rapid progression of hirsutism or virilization at any age is suspicious for an androgen-secreting tumor.

The presence of regular menses is reassuring and characteristic of women with idiopathic hirsutism. Oligomenorrhea is a common feature of PCOS and NC-CAH. Premenopausal women with androgen-secreting tumors may also experience oligomenorrhea or amenorrhea. Postmenopausal bleeding may occur in older women with neoplasms. For more information about menstrual abnormalities accompanying hirsutism, see Chapter 4.

A complete drug history is essential. A generalized increase in vellus body hair (hypertrichosis) is a side effect of many commonly prescribed drugs

Table 11–1
Hirsutism Evaluation

History	Examination
Age of onset	Height, weight, blood pressure
Duration/progression of symptoms	Distribution and grade of hirsutism
Menstrual pattern	Acanthosis nigricans
Drug history	Virilization
Family history	Stigmata of Cushing's syndrome; abdominal/pelvic mass

including phenytoin, diazoxide, minoxidil, cyclosporine, glucocorticoids, penicillamine, and psoralens. Hirsutism has been reported with administration of danazol, metyrapone, some 19-nortestosterone derivatives used in oral contraceptives, and androgens. Combined estrogen–androgen replacement therapy for menopausal symptoms and topical testosterone therapy for lichen sclerosis have been associated with hirsutism and virilization.[3–5] Surreptitious use of anabolic steroids by female athletes must also be considered in the differential diagnosis.

The medical history may reveal the cause of the abnormal hair growth. Anorexia nervosa, hypothyroidism, porphyria, and some neurologic conditions are associated with hypertrichosis. Some hyperprolactinemic women have mild adrenal androgen elevations and clinical hirsutism.

Because the endowment and distribution of hair follicles varies among ethnic groups, the diagnosis of hirsutism must be considered within this context. Women of Mediterranean descent generally have more hair than Nordic or Oriental women. A benign etiology is more likely when a family history of hirsutism is elicited.

Finally, the woman should be questioned about the method and frequency of hair removal. This is one way of assessing the extent of hair growth as well as the efficacy of medical treatment.

Physical Examination

On physical examination, the first task is to differentiate androgen-independent (hypertrichosis) from androgen-dependent (hirsutism) hair growth. Recognition of the normal hair patterns in women is critical. In McKnight's study of normal Caucasian women, the prevalence of hirsutism was 9%.[6] Seventeen percent of the women had hair on the breast (periareolar) or chest, 26% had facial hair, and 35% had lower abdominal hair. Hair patterns that are distinctly abnormal in women include terminal hair on the upper back and upper abdomen.[6,7] The distribution and density of the excess terminal hair should be recorded and graded as to severity. The Ferriman and Gallwey score (Fig. 11-1) is a semiquantitative method in which hair growth in 11 body areas is graded (scale, 0 to 4) and summed.[7] Only nine of these areas are androgen sensitive and a "hormonal" score of eight or more is rarely seen in normal women. An alternative to the Ferriman and Gallwey score is based on assessment of facial hair.[15] With this method, terminal hair in a full-beard distribution constitutes severe hirsutism. Photographs, with the patient's consent, are another method of documenting the hirsutism and monitoring the response to therapy.

Virilization develops when significant and sustained hyperandrogenemia exists, as with androgen-secreting tumors. Clitoromegaly, temporal balding, increased muscle mass, deepening of the voice, loss of female body contour, and breast atrophy are signs of virilization. Normally, the clitoral index (length × width mm²) is less than 35 mm². A clitoral index of more than 100 mm² or transverse diameter of more than 1.2 cm are abnormal. The severity of the virilization is directly correlated with the testosterone production rate. Benign conditions associated with virilization are ovarian hyperthecosis and cases of severe insulin resistance. Virilization coexisting with manifestations of Cushing's syndrome is suspicious for adrenal carcinoma. The presence of virilization always mandates a thorough evaluation to exclude an androgen-secreting tumor.

Abdominal–pelvic examination may reveal a mass. Adrenal carcinomas are often large at the time of diagnosis. Many of the virilizing ovarian neoplasms (eg, Sertoli–Leydig cell tumors) are palpable. In the obese woman, the abdominal–pelvic examination may be limited. Ultrasound evaluation of the ovaries is useful in this situation.

The skin should be examined for the presence of acanthosis nigricans. Acanthosis nigricans describes the verrucous, velvety, hyperpigmented skin changes on the nape of the neck, axillae, and groin that are markers of insulin resistance.

Careful surveillance for the clinical manifestations of Cushing's syndrome are an important part of the physical examination. These manifestations include "moon" face, malar flush, acne, increased cervicodorsal or supraclavicular fat, wide purple striae, centripetal obesity, proximal muscle weakness, hypertension, and easy bruising. Women with Cushing's syndrome frequently have irregular menses, carbohydrate intolerance, osteoporosis, and emotional disturbances.

LABORATORY EVALUATION

The laboratory investigation need not be extensive. As a minimum, all patients should have serum total testosterone and dehydroepiandrosterone sulfate (DHEAS) determinations. Gonadotropin levels are not necessary unless ovarian failure is suspected. An elevated luteinizing hormone (LH) to follicle-stimulating hormone (FSH) ratio is frequently found in PCOS but is not critical in making the diagnosis. A basal (8 AM) follicular phase 17-hydroxyprogesterone (17-OHP) level is useful to screen for NC-CAH. A serum level greater than 200 ng/dL requires adrenocorticotropic hormone (ACTH)–stimulation testing to confirm a diagnosis of NC-CAH. Mild elevations of basal 17-OHP have been described in the normal luteal phase and in PCOS. Serum prolactin and thyroid-stimulating–hormone (TSH) measurements should be obtained in women with menstrual abnormalities or galactorrhea.

If the history and examination are suggestive of Cushing's syndrome, an overnight dexamethasone suppression test should be performed. This is a good screening test for Cushing's syndrome but is insufficient to establish the diagnosis. An alternative to the overnight dexamethasone suppression test is a 24-hour urine collection for free cortisol determination. If abnormal results are obtained with either of these tests, further evaluation for Cushing's syndrome is indicated.

In a virilized patient, if an adrenal tumor is suspected but the DHEAS level is normal or minimally elevated, an adrenal computed tomography (CT) or magnetic resonance imaging (MRI) scan should be obtained. Some adrenal tumors are deficient in one or more of the enzymes needed for normal steroidogenesis. Steroid precursors, proximal to the enzymatic block, accumulate. Measurement of the 24-hour urinary excretion of 17-ketosteroids, 17-hydroxycorticosteroids (17-OHCS), and creatinine may be helpful. The urinary 17-ketosteroid levels are significantly elevated in most virilizing adrenal carcinomas. Testosterone-secreting adrenal tumors have also been reported and must be considered in the differential diagnosis when the serum total testosterone levels exceed 200 ng/dL. Testosterone metabolites are not reflected in the urinary 17-ketosteroid determinations.

Selective bilateral ovarian and adrenal vein catheterization and sampling may be necessary in the virilized patient suspected of having a tumor that cannot be localized by noninvasive techniques (adrenal CT or MRI, pelvic ultrasound). If selective vein catheterization techniques are unavailable, surgical exploration is indicated. Fortunately, these cases are rare. Suppression and stimulation tests are notoriously unreliable in localizing tumors and therefore are not recommended. The important elements of a laboratory evaluation of hirsutism are given in Table 11-2.

ETIOLOGY AND DIFFERENTIAL DIAGNOSIS OF HIRSUTISM

Hirsutism may be caused by one or more of several possible etiologies. These are outlined in Table 11-3 and discussed in the following sections.

Ovarian Causes of Hirsutism

Polycystic Ovary Syndrome

The most common ovarian cause of hirsutism is PCOS. Polycystic ovary syndrome is comprised of a heterogenous group of disorders, with many possible initiating factors, all leading to the syndrome of chronic anovulation and hyperandrogenism.[8] Despite intensive investigation, the etiology of PCOS remains unclear. Abnormalities in pituitary gonadotropin secretion have been demonstrated in PCOS.[8–14] Also, the production rates of testosterone and androstenedione are increased, leading to hyperandrogenemia.[15] In most women with PCOS, the androgen excess is of ovarian origin and is gonadotropin-dependent.[16–19] Ovarian androgen production is also stimulated by chronic hyperinsulinemia, which may occur in PCOS.[28–32] Several investigators have reported dysregulation of the cytochrome P-450 17-α-hydroxylase/17,20-lyase activities in women with PCOS.[18,20,27] Adrenal androgen excess may also be present.[21–23] Sex hormone–binding globulin (SHBG) concentrations are usually low, especially in the obese women with PCOS. Many of these women have insulin resistance and hyperinsulinemia. The high insulin levels suppress SHBG, and it appears that insulin is a more potent regulator of SHBG than is hyperandrogenism.[24] With low levels of SHBG, the bioavailable testos-

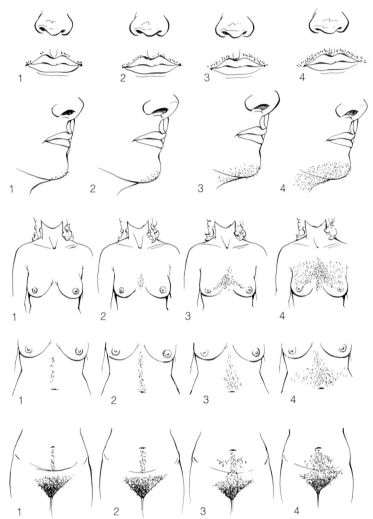

Figure 11–1. Hirsutism scoring standards, showing the spectrum from minimal hirsutism (grade 1) to frank virilization (grade 4) in several body regions. The scores in each of these areas are summed: a total score of 8 or more indicates hirsutism. (Redrawn from Hatch R, Rosenfield RL, Kim MH, Tredway D: Hirsutism: Implications, etiology, and management. Am J Obstet Gynecol 140:815, 1981. Used by permission. Adapted from Ferriman D, Gallwey JD: Clinical assessment of body hair growth in women. J Clin Endocrinol Metab 21:1440, 1961 and Lorenzo EM: Familial study of hirsutism. J Clin Endocrinol Metab 31:556, 1970.)

terone (free, unbound) is increased. In clinical practice, measurement of free testosterone is unnecessary because the development of hirsutism constitutes a bioassay.

Most women with PCOS give a history of irregular menses and a gradual onset of hirsutism, either beginning at puberty or in the early 20s.[25,26] This history distinguishes them from women with androgen-secreting tumors, who often report a sudden onset and rapid progression of hirsutism or virili-

zation. In addition to hirsutism, the physical examination may reveal acanthosis nigricans and symmetrically enlarged ovaries. Unilateral ovary enlargement has been reported but is uncommon. An ultrasound examination may show multiple small (less than 10 mm diameter) cysts, often clustering along the periphery of the ovary. The ultrasound findings are not pathognomonic of PCOS and may occur with other hyperandrogenic conditions, including tumors.

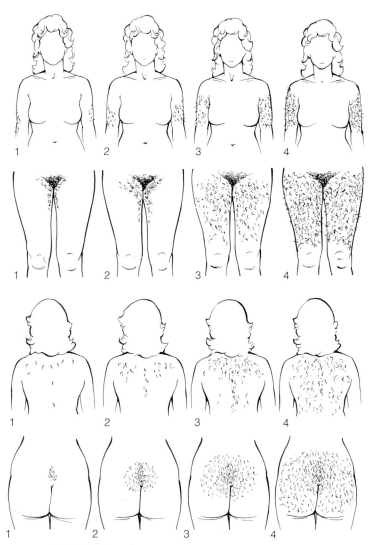

Figure 11–1. (*Continued*)

As mentioned, most women with PCOS have a normal or mildly elevated testosterone level, although the free testosterone is increased. A persistently elevated testosterone level of more than 200 ng/dL should make one suspect an androgen-secreting tumor. The finding of a coexisting pelvic mass requires laparotomy. In the absence of a pelvic mass, an ultrasound scan of the pelvis and CT or MRI scan of the adrenals are indicated. If noninvasive imaging fails to detect a tumor, selective ovarian and adrenal vein catheterization, with sampling for androgen determinations, may be helpful.

Up to 50% of women with PCOS have mild elevations of DHEAS.[21,22] The level in PCOS is less than 700 μg/dL (or less than 2.5 times the upper limit of normal for the reference laboratory). If the DHEAS level is more than 700 μg/dL, one must suspect an adrenal etiology for the hirsutism. Women with PCOS may have mildly increased 17-OHP concentrations. If the basal follicular-phase 17-OHP is more than 200 ng/dL, an ACTH-stimulation test should be performed to rule out NC-CAH. In PCOS, 17-OHP increases after ACTH stimulation but not to the high levels observed in NC-CAH.

The treatment of hirsutism secondary to PCOS depends on whether the woman desires pregnancy. If hirsutism and irregular menses are the only con-

Table 11–2
Hirsutism—Laboratory Assessment

Tests for All Patients
Total testosterone
DHEAS
8 AM follicular phase 17-hydroxyprogesterone (17-OHP)

Additional Tests to be Considered

PROBLEM:	APPROPRIATE TEST:
Oligomenorrhea	Prolactin, TSH
NC-CAH suspected	ACTH-stimulation test
Cushing's syndrome suspected	Overnight dexamethasone suppression test or 24-hour urinary free cortisol excretion
Ovarian tumor suspected or limited pelvic exam	Pelvic ultrasound
Adrenal tumor suspected	CT or MRI
Failure to localize tumor	Selective ovarian and adrenal vein catheterization and sampling

cerns, a form of ovarian suppression should be initiated. This may be accomplished with combination oral contraceptive pills or a gonadotropin-releasing–hormone (GnRH) agonist analog. The addition of an antiandrogen, such as spironolactone, improves the clinical response. If the hirsutism is refractory to treatment with a combination of ovary suppression and an antiandrogen, low doses of dexamethasone may be added.

Any therapy for hirsutism must be administered

Table 11–3
Hirsutism—Differential Diagnosis

Ovarian causes
    Polycystic ovary syndrome (+/− adrenal hyperfunction)
    Hyperthecosis
    Insulin resistance
    Tumor
Adrenal causes
    Nonclassic congenital adrenal hyperplasia
    Cushing's syndrome
    Adrenocortical tumor (adenoma or carcinoma)
Idiopathic
Obesity
Drug-induced

for at least 6 months before evaluating its efficacy because successful treatment can prevent only new terminal hair growth. Electrolysis destroys the existing terminal hair follicles and should be used in addition to medical treatments to optimize results.

Hyperthecosis

Stromal hyperthecosis and stromal hyperplasia are two disorders associated with increased ovarian synthesis of androgens. These are both pathologic diagnoses and may be suspected clinically but require ovarian biopsy to secure the diagnosis. Stromal hyperplasia is the nonneoplastic proliferation of ovarian stromal cells. It is most commonly encountered in women aged 60 to 80 years. These women have bilateral ovarian enlargement, up to 7 cm diameter. Stromal hyperplasia is associated with androgen hypersecretion in addition to obesity, hypertension, and glucose intolerance.[33,34]

Hyperthecosis is characterized by focal luteinization of islets of stromal cells. There may also be small stromal nodules of smooth muscle, Leydig cell hyperplasia, Leydig cell tumors, stromal luteomas, and thecomas.[33–35] Again, hyperthecosis is a pathologic diagnosis. Clinically, patients with this disorder give a history similar to women with PCOS but are more severely androgenized.[35–39] Testosterone production rates are significantly greater than those seen in PCOS and correlate with the degree of virilization.[40,41] Because of high circulating testosterone levels, the clinical presentation may be similar to that of patients with androgen-secreting tumors. Obesity, hypertension, and insulin resistance are common in women with hyperthecosis.

These women generally respond poorly to medical treatment with oral contraceptive therapy.[42] Administration of a GnRH-agonist analog to achieve ovarian suppression combined with subsequent hormonal replacement therapy may be more effective in hyperthecosis. Antiandrogens can also be added to the therapeutic regimen. Bilateral oophorectomy should be considered in cases of severe virilization if the woman has completed her family.

Androgen-Secreting Ovarian Tumors

An ovarian tumor should be suspected when a woman gives a history of abrupt onset or rapid progression of hirsutism. These women most often present with manifestations of severe androgen excess, such as clitoromegaly, deepening of the voice, temporal balding, increased muscle mass, and breast atrophy, in addition to hirsutism. Tumors should also be suspected if the onset of hirsutism occurs after age 30 years. Plasma testosterone levels typically exceed 200 ng/dL and may be in the normal male range.[43] Because plasma testosterone levels fluctuate, several determinations should be elevated before proceeding to invasive tests or surgical exploration.[44] Suppression of high plasma testosterone levels by oral contraceptives or a GnRH-agonist analog has been observed in women with tumors.[45,46] Therefore, endocrine suppressibility cannot be used to exclude the presence of a tumor.

An adnexal mass may be palpable on pelvic examination. If the woman has a "suspicious" history and a testosterone measurement of more than 200 ng/dL, an ultrasound of the pelvis and adrenal CT or MRI scan is recommended. If one of these imaging techniques localizes an occult tumor, surgical exploration is indicated. If a mass is not detected by noninvasive imaging, selective catheterization and sampling of the ovarian and adrenal veins for hormone determinations may be required. Catheterization studies are technically difficult and occasionally, the results are misleading. This test is indicated only when other attempts at localization have failed.[47,48,50,51] If catheterization studies are not available, surgical exploration should be considered.

The most common androgen-secreting tumor is the Sertoli–Leydig cell tumor.[49] These tumors comprise 0.5% of all ovarian neoplasms. Only a third of

women with this tumor develop endocrinologic manifestations of androgen excess. The average age of women with Sertoli–Leydig cell tumors is 25 years, and 90% of women with this tumor are younger than age 50 years.[33,34,49,50] Almost all Sertoli–Leydig cell tumors (98.5%) are unilateral. These tumors vary greatly in size but most are between 5 to 15 cm in diameter and are palpable on examination. The treatment in young women with stage 1A tumors is unilateral oophorectomy. Tumors of more advanced stage, poor differentiation, or rupture may require more extensive surgery and adjuvant therapy.[33,34]

Hilus cell tumors originate from hilar Leydig cells. These tumors occur most frequently in postmenopausal women, with the average age being 50 years. Seventy-five percent of patients with hilus cell tumors exhibit signs of hirsutism or virilization, and plasma testosterone levels are elevated. These tumors are usually small and may be difficult to detect, even at laparotomy. Almost all of the tumors reported in the literature have been benign. Because these patients are usually menopausal, a total abdominal hysterectomy with bilateral salpingo-oophorectomy is performed.[33,34,50]

Gonadoblastomas are uncommon germ cell tumors, usually seen in patients with gonadal dysgenesis and a Y-chromosome cell line. Eighty percent of the patients are phenotypic females. Amenorrhea and virilization are common clinical presentations. Leydig-like cells in the tumor may be capable of androgen secretion and are likely to be responsible for the virilization. These tumors may be associated with a dysgerminoma or a seminoma. In 10% of patients, gonadoblastomas may coexist with a more malignant form of germ cell tumor such as an endodermal sinus tumor, embryonal carcinoma, choriocarcinoma, or immature teratoma. These germ cell tumors carry the same prognosis as when they occur without a gonadoblastoma. Pure gonadoblastomas are not malignant. The tumors are bilateral in a third of cases and may vary in size from microscopic to large masses, which may be calcified. The treatment is bilateral gonadectomy.[33,34]

Gynandroblastoma is an extremely rare sex cord–stromal tumor, found to produce androgens.

The luteoma of pregnancy is a nonneoplastic androgen-producing ovarian tumor, which forms as a result of solid proliferation of luteinized cells. These tumors may be up to 20 cm in diameter, with an average size of 6 cm. Multiple tumors occur in half of all cases. Most patients with these tumors are multiparous women in the 20- to 40-year-old age group. Luteomas are more common in black women. Patients are often asymptomatic and the tumor is discovered at the time of cesarean section or postpartum tubal ligation. During the second half of pregnancy, virilization is noted by 25% of patients. Two thirds of female children born to virilized mothers are also virilized. The natural course of the luteoma of pregnancy is regression of the tumors during the postpartum period. The elevated androgen levels usually normalize by 2 weeks postpartum. Tumors may recur in subsequent pregnancies.[33,34]

Hyperreactio luteinalis, as in luteoma of pregnancy, depends on human chorionic gonadotropin (hCG) stimulation. In this condition, there are multiple cystic structures, often bilateral. It is more frequent in women with trophoblastic disease but may be seen in normal twin or singleton pregnancies. Virilization of the mother but not of the female offspring has been reported. In most cases, the cysts involute spontaneously and no intervention is necessary.[33,34]

The common epithelial tumors of the ovary with functional stroma are another important category of tumors associated with increased androgen production. Although in this case the tumor does not secrete androgens, the tumor stimulates androgen production by the surrounding stroma. These tumors may be benign, malignant, or metastatic. The treatment is surgical.[33,34]

Adrenal Causes of Hirsutism

Nonclassic Congenital Adrenal Hyperplasia

Among the adrenal causes of hirsutism are the nonclassic forms of congenital adrenal hyperplasia (late-onset, adult-onset, attenuated, or acquired congenital adrenal hyperplasia). Attenuated forms have been described for the 21-hydroxylase, 11-β-hydroxylase, and 3-β-hydroxysteroid dehydrogenase enzymes necessary for cortisol synthesis. This discussion focuses on the 21-hydroxylase deficiency, which is the most common and best characterized. With a partial 21-hydroxylase deficiency, high concentrations of substrate, 17-OHP, are needed to maintain normal cortisol production. Cortisol precursors accumulate and are shifted into androgen synthetic pathways (17-OHP → androstenedione → testosterone). Biochemical and clinical hyperandrogenism may result.

Nonclassic congenital adrenal hyperplasia is inherited as an autosomal recessive disorder, similar to classic congenital adrenal hyperplasia. The gene encoding 21-hydroxylase is closely linked to the major histocompatibility complex (HLA) on the short arm of chromosome 6.[52] This genetic linkage has permitted identification of specific haplotypes associated with NC-CAH. These include HLA-B14, HLA-DR1, and HLA-Aw33.[52–57,71,72] Only homozygotes develop clinical symptomatology, although a cryptic form of the disorder exists. The latter patients have a biochemical profile similar to symptomatic homozygotes but have a normal phenotype.[53,58,59] Heterozygote carriers are asymptomatic.

The true incidence of NC-CAH among hirsute women is not known. It has been estimated from a low of 1.2% to as high as 20%, with most reports citing an incidence in the range of 1% to 6%.[54,60–63] This disorder is more common in certain ethnic populations, with disease frequencies of 3.7% for Ashkenazi Jews, 1.9% for Hispanics, and 0.1% for a mixed Caucasian population.[64]

Women with NC-CAH are clinically indistinguishable from those with PCOS or idiopathic hirsutism. Symptoms generally emerge around the time of puberty or postpubertally. The clinical presentation varies and may wax and wane over time. Hirsutism, acne, and menstrual irregularities are frequently reported but frank virilization is uncommon. The ultrasound appearance of the ovaries may resemble that seen in PCOS.[58,64] Short adult stature is not a consistent feature. The family history may be unrevealing. Clearly, there are no unique historical or clinical features that discriminate between NC-CAH and the other common causes of hirsutism, PCOS and idiopathic hirsutism.[54,58,61–63,65,66]

A distinctive pattern of peripheral androgen concentration is not found in NC-CAH. Androstenedione and total testosterone are frequently elevated, whereas DHEAS is usually normal.[54,58,62] A basal (7 to 9 AM) 17-OHP level is a useful screen for NC-CAH, provided certain guidelines are followed. The blood sample must be obtained between 7 and 9 AM because 17-OHP follows a circadian variation, as does cortisol, with levels declining later in the day.[63] Also, the blood sample must be drawn in the follicular phase of the menstrual cycle in ovulatory women. Mild elevations of 17-OHP occur in the normal luteal phase and in women with PCOS.[62,67] A follicular-phase basal 17-OHP of more than 200 ng/dL warrants further evaluation with an ACTH-stimulation test.[58,60] In Azziz's study of 164 hirsute women, only five had basal 17-OHP levels of more than 200 ng/dL.[60] In four of the five women, the ACTH-stimulated 17-OHP level was more than

1200 ng/dL, consistent with a diagnosis of NC-CAH. The positive predictive value of a basal 17-OHP of more than 200 ng/dL for an abnormal ACTH-stimulation test was 80% (95% confidence interval, 28.4% to 99.5%) and the negative predictive value of a basal 17-OHP less than 200 ng/dL was 100% (95% confidence interval, 97.3% to 100%). Although the basal 17-OHP level appears to be a useful screen for selecting women for ACTH stimulation tests, it may be argued that it is just as cost-effective to obtain a single ACTH-stimulated 17-OHP level, which definitively excludes or confirms the diagnosis of NC-CAH.

21-Hydroxylase deficiency is the only NC-CAH for which reliable diagnostic criteria for the ACTH-stimulation test exists. The test is performed in the morning at 8 AM. A baseline blood sample (time 0) is obtained for 17-OHP determination. Cosyntropin (Cortrosyn, ACTH 1-24), 0.25 mg, is administered by intravenous bolus and an additional blood sample for 17-OHP is obtained at 30 or 60 minutes. A stimulated 17-OHP level of more than 1500 ng/dL establishes the diagnosis of NC-CAH.[54,55,58–60,62,68,71] Heterozygote carriers and some hyperandrogenic women with PCOS have stimulated 17-OHP levels that are above the normal range but they never attain the high levels observed in NC-CAH. This test may be performed in conjunction with an overnight dexamethasone (1 mg) suppression test. If this is done, the basal 17-OHP levels are suppressed but the stimulated values are not significantly affected, so the same diagnostic criteria apply.[69]

The clinical manifestations of NC-CAH traditionally have been managed with glucocorticoid administration. Although glucocorticoids frequently correct the associated menstrual abnormalities and acne, they appear to be less effective in controlling the hirsutism.[60] Greater clinical improvement has been reported with antiandrogen treatment.[70]

Cushing's Syndrome

Cushing's syndrome is characterized by excess cortisol production and abnormal cortisol dynamics. This serious endocrinopathy is a rare but potentially life-threatening cause of hirsutism and must be considered in the differential diagnosis. Cushing's syndrome is subdivided into ACTH-dependent (85%) and ACTH-independent (15%) causes. Hypercortisolism secondary to a pituitary ACTH-secreting tumor or corticotrope hyperplasia is called Cushing's disease and comprise most (80%) ACTH-dependent causes. Cushing's disease primarily affects women of reproductive age (20 to 40 years). Hirsutism is reported by 64% to 81% of women

with Cushing's syndrome, and oligomenorrhea or amenorrhea occurs in 55% to 80%.[73]

Ectopic ACTH-secreting tumors show a prediliction for males. Tumors of the lung, thymus, pancreas, and thyroid have all been associated with the ectopic ACTH syndrome. The typical Cushing's phenotype often is absent in these patients. Anorexia and weight loss occur secondary to the underlying malignancy, and metabolic aberrations are common. Other distinguishing features include hypertension, hyperpigmentation, weakness, and edema.[73–75] Ectopic corticotropin-releasing factor (CRF) secretion stimulates pituitary ACTH secretion and is an extremely rare cause of Cushing's syndrome.[73,76]

Adrenocorticotropic hormone–independent Cushing's syndrome may be iatrogenic (common) or due to an adrenal adenoma, carcinoma, or micronodular adrenal disease. Pure cortisol-secreting adrenal adenomas are not usually associated with hirsutism. Clinical evidence of hyperandrogenism, in addition to hypercortisolism, may occur with adrenocortical carcinomas. The carcinomas often are palpable as an abdominal–flank mass and cause pain.[73,75] Iatrogenic or factitious causes of Cushing's syndrome include exogenous glucocorticoids and more rarely, ACTH administration.[73]

The signs and symptoms that are clinically most useful in differentiating true Cushing's disease from simple cushingoid obesity are the centripetal obesity, wide violaceous striae, proximal muscle weakness, easy bruising, osteopenia, and emotional disturbances. "Moon" face, malar flush, increased cervicodorsal and supraclavicular fat, hypertension, and carbohydrate intolerance are less specific.

A single-dose overnight dexamethasone suppression test is an easily performed, inexpensive screen for Cushing's syndrome. Dexamethasone, 1 mg, is administered orally at 11 PM. The following day, an 8 AM serum cortisol level is obtained. Normally, the basal cortisol is suppressed to less than 5 μg/dL.[78] False-negative tests occur about 3% of the time.[76] False-positive tests are encountered more frequently (15% to 20%).[73,76] Potential sources of error include laboratory error; failure to take the medication on time; decreased absorption (alcoholics); increased metabolism secondary to other drugs (phenytoin, phenobarbital, primidone); renal failure; and depression.[73,76] An abnormal overnight dexamethasone suppression test (8 AM cortisol more than 5 μg/dL) warrants further evaluation. It *does not* establish a diagnosis of Cushing's syndrome.

The next step is to seek biochemical evidence of hypercortisolism. Measurement of the 24-hour urinary free cortisol excretion (UFC; normal less than 100 μg/24 hours) is simple and reliable. Creatinine excretion is also determined to verify that the urine collection is complete. If the UFC excretion is elevated, a standard low-dose (0.5 mg every 6 hours for 48 hours) and high-dose (2 mg every 6 hours for 48 hours) dexamethasone suppression test is performed.[79]

The standard low- and high-dose dexamethasone suppression test is based on an intact negative-feedback system. This test is key in the differential diagnosis of Cushing's syndrome. Low-dose dexamethasone suppresses the 24-hour urinary 17-OHCS excretion in endocrinologically normal individuals. In pituitary-dependent Cushing's disease, the 24-hour urinary 17-OHCS excretion is suppressed by more than 50% from baseline after high-dose dexamethasone administration. In contrast, no suppression occurs in most patients with Cushing's syndrome secondary to ectopic ACTH secretion or adrenocortical tumors.[73,76,79–81]

About 15% of Cushing's disease cases do not meet the diagnostic criterion (17-OHCS more than 50% suppression) for the high-dose dexamethasone test. Orth and coworkers state that "*Any* degree of suppression, as long as it is *significant* (ie, greater than daily variation and assay error) and *reproducible* is indicative of Cushing's disease."[73] Periodic hormonogenesis has been well documented in a few cases of Cushing's disease and may explain the occasional paradoxical response to dexamethasone.[82,83] Some ACTH-secreting tumors—most notably the bronchial or thymic carcinoids—satisfy the suppression criterion, which may lead to an incorrect diagnosis of Cushing's disease.[168] The diagnostic accuracy of the standard high-dose dexamethasone suppression test for pituitary disease may be improved by use of more stringent criteria (17-OHCS more than 64% suppression, UFC more than 90% suppression) and consideration of both the 17-OHCS and UFC responses in the interpretation.[80] Using these criteria, no patients with ectopic ACTH secretion were incorrectly diagnosed. An overnight 8-mg dexamethasone suppression test with an 8 AM serum cortisol determination compares favorably with the standard high-dose test but requires further validation.[81] A CRF stimulation test, with measurement of ACTH and cortisol levels, is another approach to the differential diagnosis of Cushing's syndrome.[73,81]

If Cushing's disease is suspected, MRI (with or without gadolinium contrast enhancement) of the pituitary is indicated.[73,81] Magnetic resonance imaging scanning is more sensitive than CT scanning for the detection of ACTH-secreting pituitary adenomas. Selected cases may require bilateral inferior petrosal sinus catheterization, with simultaneous sampling of both petrosal sinuses and a peripheral vein for ACTH to differentiate between ectopic ACTH secretion and Cushing's disease. A central to peripheral ACTH ratio of 2:1 or higher is consistent with pituitary Cushing's disease.[73,168,169] This technique may localize the tumor to the right or left hemipituitary before surgical resection.

In patients who fail to demonstrate suppression on high-dose dexamethasone, a peripheral ACTH level, determined by radioimmunoassay, assists in discriminating between hypercortisolism due to ectopic ACTH production and an adrenocortical tumor. Adrenocorticotropic hormone levels are elevated in the ectopic ACTH syndrome and low or undetectable with cortisol-secreting adrenal tumors.[73,76,81] Whereas high resolution adrenal CT or MRI scanning may detect adrenal masses as small as 1 cm, localization of an ectopic ACTH-secreting tumor frequently proves more difficult. A CT scan of the chest is the first step because most of the ACTH-secreting tumors are located in the thorax. With these disorders, primary treatment is surgical removal of the tumor.

Adrenal Neoplasms

Adrenocortical tumors are a rare cause of hirsutism. Both adrenal adenomas and carcinomas may produce an excess of androgens, resulting in severe hirsutism and virilization. These tumors function autonomously, independent of trophic hormone control. Some tumors are deficient in one or more of the enzymes necessary for normal adrenal steroidogenesis. Therefore, no characteristic serum or urinary steroid pattern exists.[50,73,77,84] Tumors with decreased 11-β-hydroxylase or 21-hydroxylase activity do not produce hypercortisolism and Cushing's syndrome. Frequently, the adrenal carcinomas synthesize large quantities of weak androgenic precursors (dehydroepiandrosterone [DHEA], DHEAS, androstenedione). These tumors may escape detection and attain a large size before clinical manifestations of hyperandrogenism occur. Conversely, a small adrenal adenoma that secretes testosterone may cause severe hirsutism and virilization within a few months. The presence of virilization and the stigmata of Cushing's syndrome is particularly worrisome and suggests a diagnosis of adrenocortical carcinoma.

Gabrilove and associates reviewed all reported cases of virilizing adrenal adenoma in 1981.[85] The clinical features of women with virilizing adenomas and carcinomas were similar, consisting of severe hirsutism, deepening of the voice, clitoromegaly, and oligomenorrhea. The biochemical profile of these patients varied. Serum testosterone levels were significantly elevated (more than 200 ng/dL) in 13 of 16 women with adenomas. An increased serum testosterone level (560 ng/dL) was reported in one woman who had adrenocortical carcinoma but it was not measured in seven additional cases. Twenty-four-hour urinary 17-ketosteroid determinations were available for 31 of 34 adenoma cases. Increased urinary 17-ketosteroids (range, 17.5 to 450 mg/24 hours) were present in 24 of 31 cases of virilizing adrenal adenoma. In five of eight cases of virilizing carcinoma reviewed, urine 17-ketosteroids were significantly increased (range, 51 to 1227 mg/24 hours). Clearly, the urinary 17-ketosteroids may be normal or elevated with virilizing adrenocortical tumors but if extreme increases are detected, a carcinoma is more likely than an adenoma.[50,73,77,85]

In recent years, urinary 17-ketosteroid determinations have been superseded by measurement of the serum DHEAS. Dehydroepiandrosterone sulfate has a high production rate, long half-life, and no diurnal variation. Consequently, serum levels are relatively constant. A DHEAS level exceeding 700 μg/dL (2.5 times the upper limit of normal for reference laboratory) warrants further evaluation of the adrenal glands. It is essential that the clinician recognize that DHEAS may be normal despite the presence of an adrenal tumor. Dehydroepiandrosterone, androstenedione, or other intermediates in adrenal steroid synthesis may be significantly elevated in these cases. Therefore, if the clinical history and examination are suspicious for a tumor, noninvasive imaging of the adrenals is indicated. Tumors are almost always visible on high-resolution CT or MRI scans.[81] Treatment of adrenal neoplasms is surgical.[50,73,77,85,86]

Idiopathic Hirsutism

Idiopathic hirsutism is a diagnosis of exclusion. These women have simple hirsutism (no virilization) accompanied by regular menses. Serum androgen concentrations are normal. It is assumed that these women develop hirsutism because of increased sensitivity of the hair follicle to normal androgen levels. Androgen use by the hair follicle may be enhanced, with increased 5-α-reductase activity and dihydrotestosterone (DHT) formation in the skin. Several studies report elevated 3-α-androstanediol glucuronide (a metabolite of DHT) in women with idiopathic hirsutism, supporting the above hy-

pothesis. Antiandrogens (+/- oral contraceptives) and depilation are the recommended treatments.

Obesity

Obesity is frequently associated with hirsutism, even in the absence of PCOS. Obesity, independent of androgen levels, reduces SHBG. This increases the fraction of biologically active androgens. Weight loss is recommended.[87]

TREATMENT OF HIRSUTISM

There are no drugs that are FDA-approved specifically for the treatment of hirsutism. The medical therapies fall into three categories: (1) drugs that suppress ovarian androgen secretion, (2) drugs that suppress adrenal androgen secretion, and (3) drugs that block peripheral androgen activity at the hair follicle. To achieve the best cosmetic result, medical therapy should be combined with a physical method of hair removal. Unfortunately, the beneficial effects of medical therapy are confined to the treatment period, necessitating ongoing therapy. The risk to benefit ratio of any medical treatment must be carefully considered because hirsutism usually has a benign etiology.

Ovarian Suppression

Oral Contraceptives

Combination oral contraceptives have been widely used to treat hirsutism. The progestin component suppresses pituitary LH and LH-dependent ovarian androgen secretion. The estrogen component increases hepatic synthesis of SHBG—thereby reducing the biologically active free testosterone concentration—and antagonizes peripheral androgen activity. Oral contraceptive administration may also affect adrenal steroidogenesis. A modest decrease in DHEAS levels occurs in both normal and hirsute women treated with oral contraceptives.[88–91] The precise mechanism leading to the decline in adrenal androgen secretion is not known, and this effect may depend on the type of progestin in the oral contraceptive.

The original studies examined the effect of high-dose oral contraceptives on androgen levels in hirsute women. After 3 to 4 weeks of administration, plasma testosterone and androstenedione concentrations were significantly reduced.[92–95] Sex hormone–binding globulin concentrations increased in most women. Subsequent studies demonstrate that low-dose oral contraceptives are equally effective in suppressing the hyperandrogenemia, increasing SHBG levels, and improving hirsutism.[96–100]

Either monophasic or multiphasic oral contraceptives may be prescribed. When selecting an oral contraceptive, consideration should be given to the progestin component.[101,102] Preparations containing progestins with the least intrinsic androgenic activity are preferred. The new generation of progestins (desogestrel, gestodene, norgestimate) have minimal androgenic activity.[103] Whether oral contraceptives containing a gonane progestin are superior to other oral contraceptives in the treatment of hirsutism remains to be determined. The same guidelines as for prescribing oral contraceptives for contraception apply when using these drugs to control hirsutism. The lowest effective dose oral contraceptive should be used.

Oral contraceptives are most effective in hirsute women who have functional ovarian hyperandrogenism (PCOS) but may also be used in women with idiopathic hirsutism and NC-CAH. Although biochemical abnormalities are corrected within several weeks, 6 to 9 months of treatment are necessary before subjective or objective parameters of hair growth improve. Continuous oral-contraceptive administration is recommended by some to maintain gonadotropin and androgen suppression. To achieve better cosmetic results, oral-contraceptive therapy may also be combined with an antiandrogen and with depilation techniques.

An additional benefit from oral-contraceptive use is cyclic uterine bleeding and protection against the development of endometrial hyperplasia or carcinoma. This is especially important in hirsute women with anovulation or oligo-ovulation.

Gonadotropin-Releasing–Hormone Analogs

Chronic exposure to a GnRH-agonist analog causes pituitary desensitization.[104] Gonadotropin secretion decreases, leading to suppression of gonadotropin-dependent steroidogenesis. The analog-induced suppression of the pituitary–gonadal axis is both selective and reversible. Chang and coworkers first demonstrated that GnRH-agonist treatment of PCOS women significantly decreased circulating testosterone and androstenedione levels.[16] Adrenal androgen and cortisol secretion was unaffected. This study suggested a potential role for GnRH-agonists in the management of ovarian hyperandrogenism.

Andreyko and coworkers studied the effect of long-term GnRH-agonist administration on hirsutism.[105] The drug was well tolerated and clinical improvement was noted after 6 months of treatment. The mean hirsutism score decreased significantly after 6 months of Nafarelin therapy. Hot flashes secondary to the hypoestrogenism were common, and all women became amenorrheic during treatment. As one would expect, androgen levels progressively increased after the GnRH-agonist was discontinued. Other investigators found more variable clinical responses in terms of the hirsutism.[106–108]

The optimal dosages of the various GnRH-agonists available to treat hirsutism have not been determined. Clearly, the dose depends on the potency of the analog and its route of administration. Furthermore, Rittmaster demonstrated that the doses of leuprolide acetate required to maximally inhibit ovarian estrogen and androgen secretion are different.[109] A significantly higher dose of leuprolide acetate (20 μg/kg/day, subcutaneously) was necessary to achieve maximal testosterone suppression, whereas estradiol was suppressed with a dose of 5 to 10 μg/kg/day, subcutaneously, leuprolide acetate. The therapeutic response was good in this study. Suboptimal ovarian androgen suppression due to an inadequate GnRH-agonist dose may explain some treatment failures.

The side effects of GnRH-agonist therapy are primarily related to estrogen deprivation. Women experience vaginal dryness, hot flashes, and are at increased risk for development of osteoporosis with long-term therapy. In women with hirsutism, the hypoestrogenism may be controlled by hormone replacement therapy without compromising the therapeutic efficacy of the analog. This may permit long-term GnRH-agonist administration, while minimizing the risks.[110,111]

The GnRH-agonists are expensive, and their routine use in the management ovarian androgen excess is probably not justified. Their use should be limited to women with severe hyperandogenism and hirsutism refractory to other therapeutic modalities.[110,111] This includes women with severe hyperinsulinemic hyperandrogenism or hyperthecosis.

Adrenal Suppression

Glucocorticoids

Glucocorticoids were the first medical therapy for hirsutism.[112–114] Exogenous glucocorticoids suppress pituitary ACTH secretion, which results in decreased adrenal cortisol and androgen secretion.

With a reduction in the precursor pool of weak adrenal androgens (DHEA, DHEAS, androstenedione), there is less substrate available for the synthesis of more potent androgens, testosterone and DHT. Glucocorticoids suppress the testosterone production rate and plasma testosterone levels decline.[95,115] Furthermore, chronic glucocorticoid suppression of elevated testosterone levels is associated with decreased mean LH levels in hirsute women.[116]

Several glucocorticoid preparations of varying potencies have been used in the treatment of hirsutism including hydrocortisone, 10 to 20 mg/day; prednisone, 5 to 7.5 mg/day; and dexamethasone, 0.25 to 0.75 mg/day.[95,117–120,123] Although adrenal androgens are more sensitive than cortisol to glucocorticoid suppression, a dose that selectively suppresses adrenal androgens has not been found.[120–122] Because the optimal dose of each drug has never been well defined, the lowest effective dose should be prescribed to avoid adverse effects. To minimize the risk of adrenal insufficiency during stress, the 8 AM serum cortisol should be maintained at more than 2 μg/dL. An alternate-day dosage schedule does not offer any advantage.[120]

There are conflicting data regarding the clinical response of hirsute patients to glucocorticoid therapy. The hirsutism improves in only 30% to 50% of cases. Glucocorticoids appear to have a greater beneficial effect on the acne and menstrual irregularities. The most serious complication of chronic glucocorticoid administration is adrenal insufficiency during stress. For this reason, women receiving chronic glucocorticoid treatment should be advised to wear a Medic-Alert bracelet. Other side effects include iatrogenic Cushing's syndrome, ulcers, osteoporosis, aseptic necrosis of the femoral head, and drug-induced hirsutism.

Considering the variable clinical response and the potentially serious adverse effects, glucocorticoids are not recommended as a treatment for hirsutism. If these drugs are used at all, their use should be restricted to specific indications such as treatment of NC-CAH. Even in this adrenal enzyme disorder, some investigators report better results with antiandrogens.[70,142]

Ketoconazole

Ketoconazole, an imidazole derivative, is a potent antimycotic agent. It inhibits the cytochrome P-450–dependent enzymes in both the gonad and the adrenal, thereby reducing steroid biosynthesis.[124–126] The principal gonadal block occurs at the 17,20-lyase enzyme complex, resulting in decreases of testosterone, androstenedione, and DHEA, with an increase in 17-OHP. Adrenal steroidogenesis is blocked at 11-β-hydroxylase and cholesterol side-chain cleavage.[124–126] Because of its effects on gonadal and adrenal steroidogenesis, ketoconazole has been proposed as a therapy for hyperandrogenism.[127,128]

Only a few hirsute women have been treated with ketoconazole.[129] Doses of 400 to 1200 mg/day (divided) were used. With both high-dose (800 to 1200 mg) and low-dose (400 mg) treatment, significant decreases in serum testosterone, androstenedione, and DHEA were evident after 1 month. Acne resolved in all women after 2 to 4 months of treatment. Despite rapid suppression of androgens, clinical improvement of hirsutism was not apparent until 6 months. Only 44% of women enrolled in the study completed the 6 months of ketoconazole necessary for a therapeutic effect, however. A significant dropout rate during therapy was also noted by Venturoli and colleagues.[130]

Ketoconazole, even at low doses, is not well tolerated. Within 2 to 3 months of treatment, 55% of women experienced adverse effects.[130] These included headaches, nausea, scalp hair loss, dry skin and desquamation, abdominal pain, asthenia, and hepatotoxicity. Polymenorrhea and other menstrual irregularities were common. No clinical manifestations of adrenal insufficiency were reported. Ketoconazole cannot be recommended as a first-line therapy for hirsutism. Its use should be limited to severe cases of hirsutism that are refractory to other medical therapies. Liver enzymes, particularly γ-glutamyltransferase, must be monitored during treatment. Effective contraception must be used by reproductive-aged women treated with ketoconazole.

Antiandrogens

Spironolactone

Spironolactone is an aldosterone antagonist with a structural configuration similar to testosterone.[131,132] It competitively inhibits testosterone and DHT binding to the intracellular androgen receptor and in the human genital skin fibroblast culture, it is a more potent antiandrogen than cyproterone acetate (CPA), flutamide, or cimetidine.[133] The competitive inhibition of T and DHT binding to the androgen receptor is its primary mechanism of action. During treatment, the metabolic clearance rate of testosterone is increased.[134,145] Peripheral 5-α-reductase activity is also inhibited by this antiandrogen.[135] In addition, spironolactone decreases androgen biosynthesis by reducing cytochrome P-450 17-hydroxylase activity.[132] This occurs only in tissues exhibiting high levels of 17-hydroxylase activity, such as the gonad and adrenal.

Recognition of the antiandrogenic properties of spironolactone led to its use in the treatment of hirsutism.[147] Circulating levels of testosterone decrease after 3 months of treatment.[136–140] Androstenedione concentrations are also reduced with dosages of 100 to 200 mg/day.[137–139,141] Most studies do not report a change in DHEA, DHEAS, or basal cortisol levels.[137,139,141] Despite favorable alterations in the androgen profile, hormonal parameters do not always correlate with the clinical response.[130,140]

Spironolactone is effective in the treatment of idiopathic hirsutism as well as hirsutism associated with PCOS and NC-CAH.[134,136–140,142,143,145,146] The usual dose is 50 to 100 mg twice a day. Decreases in hair shaft diameter, linear growth rate, and hair density scores occur after 3 to 6 months of therapy.[136–139,143] Acne and seborrhea also improve.[136,137] Spironolactone may be combined with oral contraceptive or glucocorticoid administration to treat hirsutism refractory to single-agent therapy.[142,146]

Spironolactone is well tolerated. It is a potassium-sparing diuretic and hyperkalemia is not a problem in women with normal renal function.[146] Side effects reported include transient polyuria and polydipsia, headache, fatigue, and mastalgia.[136,140,143,144] The most problematic side effect is the irregular vaginal bleeding that frequently occurs. Amelioration of the menstrual irregularities has been reported with a dose reduction or cyclic administration (days 4 to 22 of the menstrual cycle) of spironolactone.[136,140,144] Coadministration of an oral contraceptive may reduce the frequency of irregular bleeding episodes.[146] Women with oligomenorrhea or amenorrhea may report more regular menses during spironolactone therapy.[140,143,144] All reproductive-aged women must be advised to use effective contraception during spironolactone treatment to avoid potential feminization of a male fetus.

Cimetidine

Cimetidine is a histamine H_2-receptor antagonist with antiandrogenic properties.[148] In comparison with other antiandrogens, it has a low affinity for the androgen receptor in cultured human skin fibroblasts.[133] Therefore, it is not surprising that clinical trials using cimetidine to treat hirsutism have yielded mixed results.

In an uncontrolled study, five hirsute women were treated with cimetidine, 1500 mg/day in divided doses, for 3 months.[149] The rate of hair growth and oiliness of the skin decreased in four women. Biochemical parameters were unaltered by therapy, consistent with a peripheral site of action.[149] Reported side effects include headaches, dizziness, nausea, and irregular bleeding.[149–151]

A prospective randomized controlled trial of cimetidine versus placebo in 20 moderately to severely hirsute women was conducted by Lissak and coworkers.[150] The study spanned 3 months, during which there was monthly quantitative and semi-quantitative assessment of body hair growth. No significant differences between the treatment and control groups were noted in any of the parameters used to assess hair growth. Serum DHEA declined in the treatment group but other hormone levels were unchanged. Long-term administration of cimetidine, 1200 mg/day, improved hirsutism in only two of nine women.[151] These data suggest that cimetidine is not an effective therapy for hirsutism.

Flutamide

Flutamide is a nonsteroidal antiandrogen used to treat prostatic cancer.[152] In contrast to the other antiandrogens, it is devoid of any progestogenic, androgenic, estrogenic, or glucocorticoid activity. Its mechanism of action is to inhibit androgen-binding to specific receptors in target tissues, including the pilosebaceous unit. Although in vitro competitive-binding studies in human skin fibroblasts indicate flutamide has a low affinity for the androgen receptor, the few clinical trials conducted in hirsute women have yielded encouraging results.[133,153,154]

Cusan and coworkers administered flutamide, 250 mg twice a day, to 20 women with moderate to severe hirsutism.[153] Twelve of these women had failed medical management with oral contraceptives, spironolactone, or dexamethasone. Low-dose combination oral contraceptives were coadministered to 18 of the 20 women. After 7 months of therapy, 95% of the women (including two taking flutamide alone) had a clinically significant decrease in the hirsutism score. Seborrhea, acne, and androgenic alopecia improved more rapidly (1 to 3 months). Another study examined the effect of flutamide alone on moderate to severe hirsutism.[154] Nine women were treated with flutamide, 250 mg three times a day, for 3 months. A subjective improvement in the hirsutism was reported by seven of the nine women. Side effects noted were dry skin, hot flashes, increased appetite, headache, tiredness, nausea, dizziness, breast tenderness, and decreased libido. Menstrual irregularities occurred in 44% of the women in the flutamide-only study but five of the women had preexisting oligomenorrhea. The occurrence of unscheduled bleeding episodes was not specifically addressed in the flutamide–oral contraceptive trial. Circulating androgen and gonadotropin levels were not altered by flutamide and did not predict the response to therapy. Decreased free testosterone level was reported with flutamide–oral contraceptive therapy and was attributed to the estrogen-induced increase in SHBG.[153]

These data suggest a possible role for flutamide in the medical management of hirsutism. Additional controlled studies are necessary to confirm these results and determine whether flutamide is superior to the other antiandrogens available. All reproductive-aged women must be counseled to use contraception during antiandrogen treatment because of the potential effects on the developing fetus.

Cyproterone Acetate

Cyproterone acetate is another antiandrogen that has been widely used in Europe and Canada for the treatment of hirsutism. It is not available in the United States. Cyproterone acetate is a potent progestin. This explains its antigonadotropic effect and suppression of ovarian testosterone production.[155] As do other antiandrogens, CPA competes with testosterone/dihydrotestosterone (T/DHT) for binding to the androgen receptor. Although in vitro studies indicate CPA is a weaker antiandrogen than spironolactone, clinical trials show the two drugs to be of comparable efficacy.[133,156] Other mechanisms of action include a decrease in androgen-dependent 5-α-reductase activity in the skin and an increase in the metabolic clearance rate of testosterone.[155]

Cyproterone acetate is prescribed in a "reverse sequential" regimen because of its storage in adipose tissue. Doses of 50 to 200 mg/day are given days 5 to 14 of the menstrual cycle in combination with ethinyl estradiol, 35 to 50 μg/day, days 5 to 25 of the cycle.[155,157,158,166] Alternatively, CPA may be administered with an oral contraceptive for the first 10 days of the pill cycle.[159,160] Cyproterone acetate, 300 mg intramuscularly monthly, has also been used to treat hirsute women.[161] Only two studies have examined the clinical efficacy of different dosages of CPA.[160,162]

Significant decreases in plasma total testosterone and androstenedione have been demonstrated in some studies.[155,163,164] Dehydroepiandrosterone sulfate concentrations are unaffected by CPA.[161,162]

The clinical response does not correlate with plasma androgen concentrations. This suggests that the therapeutic effect of CPA is derived primarily from its peripheral androgen antagonism.

Hirsutism regresses in 50% to 80% of women after several months of treatment. Cyproterone acetate is equally effective in the treatment of hirsutism secondary to PCOS, NC-CAH, and idiopathic hirsutism.[70] Acne and seborrhea also improve. Reported side effects of CPA treatment include fatigue, mastalgia, depression, decreased libido, headaches, and menstrual irregularities.[158,161–164] Although high doses of CPA have been reported to inhibit adrenal steroidogenesis, doses of 50 to 100 mg/day have not been associated with adrenal insufficiency.[70,165] All reproductive-aged women must be counseled to use effective contraception during CPA treatment.

Physical Hair Removal

Physical methods of hair removal are an important adjunct to any therapy for hirsutism. Medical or surgical treatment of the underlying condition does not eliminate existing terminal hair. The conversion of vellus to terminal hair is largely irreversible. Therefore, early intervention is critical to halt this process and prevent new hair growth. Ongoing medical therapy coupled with physical hair removal yields the best cosmetic results.

Temporary hair removal is accomplished by shaving, plucking, waxing, or chemical depilatories. Shaving is a safe, effective, inexpensive method of eliminating unwanted hair. Women must be reassured that it does not increase the rate of hair growth, diameter of the hair shaft, or hair density. Despite its efficacy, many women object to shaving facial hair because they perceive it as unfeminine. Skin irritation is the only drawback of shaving.

Plucking may control sparse terminal hair growth. Possible complications include folliculitis, ingrown hairs, postinflammatory pigmentation, and scarring. It is impractical for hair removal from large areas. Waxing is useful in this circumstance. Hot wax is applied to the affected area; after the wax hardens, it is stripped off, removing the hair with it. The results last for several weeks. Professional waxing is expensive. Disadvantages of waxing are similar to those listed for plucking.

Chemical depilatories dissolve the hair shaft. Regrowth occurs in 24 to 48 hours. Unfortunately, skin irritation and dermatitis are significant problems, especially with facial application. Before depilatories are used, a skin test on the inner wrist is recommended to test for sensitivity. Bleaching makes the hair less noticeable but also causes skin irritation.

Electrolysis and thermolysis are the only permanent methods of hair removal.[167] The germinative cells of the hair follicle are destroyed by coagulation. Hair regrowth rates of 15% to 50% have been reported. Electrolysis or thermolysis is expensive and time-consuming. Complications of electrolysis or thermolysis include pain, edema, erythema, pitting, scarring, hyperpigmentation, hypopigmentation, and infection. A tattoo may occur with improperly performed electrolysis. Women should be referred only to practitioners with expertise in these techniques.

REFERENCES

1. Rittmaster RS, Loriaux DL: Hirsutism. Ann Intern Med 106:95, 1987
2. Hatch R, Rosenfield RC, Kim MH, Tredway D: Hirsutism: implications, etiology, and management. Am J Obstet Gynecol 140:815, 1981
3. Bardin CW, Swerdloff RS, Santen RJ: Androgens: risks and benefits. J Clin Endocrinol Metab 73:4, 1991
4. Urman B, Pride SM, Yuen BH: Elevated serum testosterone, hirsutism, and virilism associated with combined androgen-estrogen hormone replacement therapy. Obstet Gynecol 77:595, 1991
5. Punch MR, Ansbacher R: Autogenic masculinization. Am J Obstet Gynecol 163:114, 1990
6. McKnight E: The prevalence of "hirsutism" in young women. Lancet 1:410, 1964
7. Ferriman D, Gallwey JD: Clinical assessment of body hair growth in women. J Clin Endocrinol Metab 21:1440, 1961
8. Yen SSC: Chronic anovulation caused by peripheral androgen disorders. In Yen SSC, Jaffee RB (eds): Reproductive endocrinology, 3rd ed, p 576. Philadelphia, WB Saunders, 1991
9. Rebar R, Judd HL, Yen SSC, Rakoff J, Vandenberg G, Naftolin F: Characterization of the inappropriate gonadotropin secretion in polycystic ovary syndrome. J Clin Invest 57:1320, 1976
10. Yen SSC, Vela P, Rankin J: Inappropriate secretion of follicle-stimulating hormone and luteinizing hormone in polycystic ovarian disease. J Clin Endocrinol Metab 30:435, 1970
11. Baird DT, Corker CS, Davidson DW, Hunter WM, Michie EA, Van Look PFA: Pituitary-ovarian relationships in polycystic ovary syndrome. J Clin Endocrinol Metab 45:798, 1977
12. Lobo RA, Granger L, Goebelsmann U, Mishell DR: Elevations in unbound serum estradiol as a possible mechanism for inappropriate gonadotropin secretion in women with PCO. J Clin Endocrinol Metab 52:156, 1981
13. DeVane GW, Czekala NM, Judd HL, Yen SSC: Circulating gonadotropins, estrogens, and androgens in polycystic ovarian disease. Am J Obstet Gynecol 121:496, 1975
14. Waldstreicher J, Santoro NF, Hall JE, Filicori M, Crowley WF: Hyperfunction of the hypothalamic-pituitary axis in women with polycystic ovarian diseae: indirect evidence for partial gonadotroph desensitization. J Clin Endocrinol Metab 66:165, 1988
15. Bardin CW, Lipsett MB: Testosterone and androstenedione blood production rates in normal women and women with idiopathic hirsutism or polycystic ovaries. J Clin Invest 46:891, 1967
16. Chang RJ, Laufer LR, Meldrum DR, et al: Steroid secretion in polycystic ovarian disease after ovarian suppression by a long-acting gonadotropin-releasing hormone agonist. J Clin Endocrinol Metab 56:897, 1983
17. Wajchenberg BL, Achando SS, Okada H, et al: Determination of the source(s) of androgen overproduction in hirsutism associated with polycystic ovary syndrome by simultaneous adrenal and ovarian venous catheterization. Comparison with the dexamethasone suppression test. J Clin Endocrinol Metab 63:1204, 1986
18. Ehrmann DA, Rosenfield RL, Barnes RB, Brigell DF, Sheikh Z: Detection of functional ovarian hyperandrogenism in women with androgen excess. N Engl J Med 327:157, 1992
19. Kirschner MA, Jacobs JB: Combined ovarian and adrenal vein catheterization to determine the site(s) of androgen overproduction in hirsute women. J Clin Endocrinol Metab 33:199, 1971
20. Rosenfield RL, Barnes RB, Cara JF, Lucky AW: Dysregulation of cytochrome p450c17α as the cause of polycystic ovarian syndrome. Fertil Steril 53:78, 1990
21. Hoffman DI, Klove K, Lobo RA: The prevalence and significance of elevated dehydroepiandrosterone sulfate levels in anovulatory women. Fertil Steril 42:76, 1984
22. Lobo RA: The role of the adrenal in polycystic ovary syndrome. Semin Reprod Endocrinol 2:251, 1984
23. Lachelin GCL, Barnett M, Hopper BR, Brink G, Yen SSC: Adrenal function in normal women and women with polycystic ovary syndrome. J Clin Endocrinol Metab 49:892, 1979
24. Nestler JE, Barlascini CO, Matt DW, et al: Suppression of serum insulin by diazoxide reduces serum testosterone levels in obese women with polycystic ovary syndrome. J Clin Endocrinol Metab 68:1027, 1989
25. Raj SG, Thompson IE, Berger MJ, Taymor ML: Clinical aspects of the polycystic ovary syndrome. Obstet Gynecol 49:552, 1977
26. Goldzieher JW, Green JA: The polycystic ovary. I. Clinical and histologic features. J Clin Endocrinol Metab 22:325, 1962
27. Barnes RB, Rosenfield RL, Burstein S, Ehrmann DA: Pituitary-ovarian responses to nafarelin testing in the polycystic ovary syndrome. N Engl J Med 320:559, 1989
28. Barbieri RL, Smith S, Ryan KJ: The role of hyperinsulinemia in the pathogenesis of ovarian hyperandrogenism. Fertil Steril 50:197, 1988
29. Dunaif A, Graf M, Mandeli J, Laumas V, Dobrjan-

sky A: Characterization of groups of hyperandrogenic women with acanthosis nigricans, impaired glucose tolerance, and/or hyperinsulinemia. J Clin Endocrinol Metab 65:499, 1987

30. Jialal I, Naiker P, Reddi K, Moodley J, Joubert SM: Evidence for insulin resistance in nonobese patients with polycystic ovarian disease. J Clin Endocrinol Metab 64:1066, 1987
31. Dunaif A, Segal KR, Futterweit W, Dobrjansky A: Profound peripheral insulin resistance independent of obesity, in polycystic ovary syndrome. Diabetes 38:1165, 1989
32. Rittmaster RS, Deshwal N, Lehman L: The role of adrenal hyperandrogenism, insulin resistance, and obesity in the pathogenesis of polycystic ovarian syndrome. J Clin Endocrinol Metab 76:1295, 1993
33. Young RH, Scully RE: Sex cord-stromal, steroid cell, and other ovarian tumors with endocrine, paraendocrine, and paraneoplastic manifestations. In Kurman RJ (ed): Blaustein's pathology of the female genital tract, 3rd ed, p 607. New York, Springer-Verlag, 1987
34. Scully RE: Ovarian tumors with endocrine manifestations. In DeGroot LJ (ed): Endocrinology, 2nd ed, p 1994. Philadelphia, WB Saunders, 1989
35. Farber M, Daoust PR, Rogers J: Hyperthecosis syndrome. Obstet Gynecol 44:35, 1974
36. Judd HL, Scully RE, Herbst AL, Yen SSC, Ingersol FM, Kliman B: Familial hyperthecosis: comparison of endocrinologic and histologic findings with polycystic ovarian disease. Am J Obstet Gynecol 117:976, 1973
37. Abraham GE, Buster JE: Peripheral and ovarian steroids in ovarian hyperthecosis. Obstet Gynecol 47:581, 1976
38. Katz M, Hamilton SM, Albertyn L, Pimstone BL, Cohen BL, Tiltman AJ: Virilization with diffuse involvement of ovarian androgen secreting cells. Obstet Gynecol 50:623, 1977
39. Scully RE, Galdabini JJ, McNeely BU: Case records of the Massachusetts General Hospital. N Engl J Med 294:326, 1976
40. Bardin CW, Lipsett MB, Edgcomb JH, Marshall JR: Studies of testosterone metabolism in a patient with masculinization due to stromal hyperthecosis. N Engl J Med 277:399, 1967
41. Aiman J, Edman CD, Worley RJ, Vellios F, MacDonald PC: Androgen and estrogen formation in women with ovarian hyperthecosis. Obstet Gynecol 51:1, 1978
42. Nagamani M, Lingold JC, Gomez LG, Garza JR: Clinical and hormonal studies in hyperthecosis of the ovaries. Fertil Steril 36:326, 1981
43. Meldrum DR, Abraham GE: Peripheral and ovarian venous concentrations of various steroid hormones in virilizing ovarian tumors. Obstet Gynecol 53:36, 1979
44. Friedman CI, Schmidt GE, Kim MH, Powell J: Serum testosterone concentrations in the evaluation of androgen-producing tumors. Am J Obstet Gynecol 153:44, 1985
45. Haning RV Jr, Loughlin JS, Shapiro SS: Diagnosis and resection of an oral contraceptive-suppressible Sertoli-Leydig cell tumor with preservation of fertility and a 7-year follow-up. Obstet Gynecol 73:901, 1989

46. Kennedy L, Traub AI, Atkinson AB, Sheridan B: Short term administration of gonadotropin-releasing hormone analog to a patient with a testosterone-secreting ovarian tumor. J Clin Endocrinol Metab 64:1320, 1987
47. Moltz L, Pickartz H, Sorensen R, Schwartz U, Hammerstein J: Ovarian and adrenal vein steroids in seven patients with androgen-secreting ovarian neoplasms: selective catheterization findings. Fertil Steril 42:585, 1984
48. Surrey ES, de Ziegler D, Gambone JC, Judd HL: Preoperative localization of androgen-secreting tumors: clinical, endocrinologic, and radiologic evaluation of ten patients. Am J Obstet Gynecol 158:1313, 1988
49. Young RH, Scully RE: Ovarian Sertoli-Leydig cell tumors. A clinicopathologic analysis of 207 cases. Am J Surg Pathol 9:534, 1985
50. Freeman DA: Steroid hormone-producing tumors in man. Endocr Rev 7:204, 1986
51. Wentz AC, White RI, Migeon CJ, Hsu TH, Barnes HV, Jones GS: Differential ovarian and adrenal vein catheterization. Am J Obstet Gynecol 125:1000, 1976
52. Laron Z, Pollack MS, Zamir R, et al: Late onset 21-hydroxylase deficiency and HLA in the Ashkenazi population: a new allele at the 21-hydroxylase locus. Hum Immunol 1:55, 1980
53. Lee PA, Rosenwaks Z, Urban MD, Migeon CJ, Bias WB: Attenuated forms of congenital adrenal hyperplasia due to 21-hydroxylase deficiency. J Clin Endocrinol Metab 55:866, 1982
54. Kuttenn F, Couillin P, Girard F, et al: Late-onset adrenal hyperplasia in hirsutism. N Engl J Med 313:224, 1985
55. White PC, New MI, Dupont B: Congenital adrenal hyperplasia (first of two parts). N Engl J Med 316:1519, 1987
56. Speiser PW, Dupont B, Rubinstein P, et al: High frequency of nonclassical steroid 21-hydroxylase deficiency. Am J Hum Genet 37:650, 1985
57. Blankstein J, Faiman C, Reyes FI, Schroeder ML, Winter JSD: Adult-onset familial adrenal 21-hydroxylase deficiency. Am J Med 68:441, 1980
58. Dewailly D, Vantyghem-Haudiquet MC, Sainsard C, et al: Clinical and biological phenotypes in late onset 21-hydroxylase deficiency. J Clin Endocrinol Metab 63:418, 1986
59. New MI, Lorenzen F, Lerner AJ, et al: Genotyping steroid 21-hydoxylase deficiency: hormonal reference data. J Clin Endocrinol Metab 57:320, 1983
60. Azziz R, Zacur HA: 21-hydroxylase deficiency in female hyperandrogenism: screening and diagnosis. J Clin Endocrinol Metab 69:577, 1989
61. Chetkowski RJ, DeFazio J, Shamonki I, Judd HC, Chang RJ: The incidence of late-onset congenital adrenal hyperplasia due to 21-hydroxylase deficiency among hirsute women. J Clin Endocrinol Metab 58:595, 1984
62. Lobo RA, Goebelsmann U: Adult manifestation of congenital adrenal hyperplasia due to incomplete 21-hydroxylase deficiency mimicking polycystic ovarian disease. Am J Obstet Gynecol 138:720, 1980
63. Chrousos GP, Loriaux DL, Mann DL, Cutler GB: Late-onset 21-hydroxylase deficiency mimicking

idiopathic hirsutism or polycystic ovarian disease. Ann Intern Med 96:143, 1982

64. Hague WM, Adams J, Rodda C, et al: The prevalence of polycystic ovaries in patients with congenital adrenal hyperplasia and their close relatives. Clin Endocrinol 33:501, 1990

65. Brodie BL, Wentz AC: Late onset congenital adrenal hyperplasia: a gynecologist's perspective. Fertil Steril 48:175, 1987

66. Rosenwaks Z, Lee PA, Jones GS, Migeon CJ, Wentz AC: An attenuated form of congenital virilizing adrenal hyperplasia. J Clin Endocrinol Metab 49:335, 1979

67. Azziz R, Rafi A, Smith BR, Bradley EL, Zacur HA: On the origin of the elevated 17-hydroxyprogesterone levels after adrenal stimulation in hyperandrogenism. J Clin Endocrinol Metab 70:431, 1990

68. Gourmelen M, Pham-Huu-Trung MT, Bredon MG, Girard F: 17-Hydroxyprogesterone in the cosyntropin test: results in normal and hirsute women and in mild congenital adrenal hyperplasia. Acta Endocrinol 90:481, 1979

69. Rosenfield RL, Helke J, Lucky AW: Dexamethasone preparation does not alter corticoid and androgen responses to adrenocorticotropin. J Clin Endocrinol Metab 60:585, 1985

70. Spritzer P, Billaud L, Thalabard JC, et al: Cyproterone acetate versus hydrocortisone treatment in late-onset adrenal hyperplasia. J Clin Endocrinol Metab 70:642, 1990

71. White PC, New MI, Dupont B: Congenital adrenal hyperplasia (second of two parts). N Engl J Med 316:1580, 1987

72. Chrousos GP, Loriaux DL, Mann D, Cutler GB Jr: Late-onset 21-hydroxylase deficiency is an allelic variant of congenital adrenal hyperplasia characterized by attenuated clinical expression and different HLA haplotype associations. Horm Res 16:193, 1982

73. Orth DN, Kovacs WJ, Debold CR: The adrenal cortex. In Wilson JD, Foster DW (eds): Williams textbook of endocrinology, 8th ed, p 489. Philadelphia, WB Saunders, 1992

74. Liddle GW, Givens JR, Nicholson WE, Island DP: The ectopic ACTH syndrome. Cancer Res 25:1057, 1965

75. Imura H, Matsukura S, Yamamoto H, et al: Studies on ectopic ACTH-producing tumors. II. Clinical and biochemical features of 30 Cases. Cancer 35:1430, 1975

76. Kamilaris TC, Chrousos GP: Adrenal diseases. In Moore WT, Eastman RC (eds): Diagnostic endocrinology, p 79. Philadelphia, BC Decker, 1990

77. Bertagna C, Orth DN: Clinical and laboratory findings and results of therapy in 58 patients with adrenocortical tumors admitted to a single medical center (1951 to 1978). Am J Med 71:855, 1981

78. Melby JC: Assessment of adrenocortical function. N Engl J Med 285:735, 1971

79. Liddle GW: Tests of pituitary adrenal suppressibility in the diagnosis of Cushing's syndrome. J Clin Endocrinol Metab 20:1539, 1960

80. Flack MR, Oldfield EH, Cutler GB Jr, et al: Urine free cortisol in the high-dose dexamethasone suppression test for the differential diagnosis of the Cushing syndrome. Ann Intern Med 116:211, 1992

81. Kaye TB, Crapo L: The Cushing syndrome: an update on diagnostic tests. Ann Intern Med 112:434, 1990

82. Brown RD, Van Loon GR, Orth DN, Liddle GW: Cushing's disease with periodic hormonogenesis: one explanation for paradoxical response to dexamethasone. J Clin Endocrinol Metab 36:445, 1973

83. Liberman B, Wajchenberg BL, Tambascia MA, Mesquita CH: Periodic remisssion in Cushing's disease with paradoxical dexamethasone response: an expression of periodic hormonogenesis. J Clin Endocrinol Metab 43:913, 1976

84. Lipsett MB, Wilson H: Adrenocortical cancer: steroid biosynthesis and metabolism evaluated by urinary metabolites. J Clin Endocrinol Metab 22:906, 1962

85. Gabrilove JL, Seman AT, Sabet R, Mitty HA, Nicolis GL: Virilizing adrenal adenoma with studies on the steroid content of the adrenal venous effluent and a review of the literature. Endocr Rev 2:462, 1981

86. Richie JP, Gittes RF: Carcinoma of the adrenal cortex. Cancer 45:1957, 1980

87. Garner PR: The impact of obesity on reproductive function. Semin Reprod Endocrinol 8:32, 1990

88. Madden JD, Milewich L, Parker CR, Carr BR, Boyar RM, MacDonald PC: The effect of oral contraceptive treatment on the serum concentration of dehydroisoandrosterone sulfate. Am J Obstet Gynecol 132:380, 1978

89. Carr BR, Parker CR, Madden JD, MacDonald PC, Porter JC: Plasma levels of adrenocorticotropin and cortisol in women receiving oral contraceptive steroid treatment. J Clin Endocrinol Metab 49:346, 1979

90. Wild RA, Umstot ES, Andersen RN, Givens JR: Adrenal function in hirsutism. II. Effect of an oral contraceptive. J Clin Endocrinol Metab 54:676, 1982

91. Wiebe RH, Morris CV: Effect of an oral contraceptive on adrenal and ovarian androgenic steroids. Obstet Gynecol 63:12, 1984

92. Givens JR, Andersen RN, Wiser WL, Fish SA: Dynamics of suppression and recovery of plasma FSH, LH, androstenedione and testosterone in polycystic ovarian disease using an oral contraceptive. J Clin Endocrinol Metab 38:727, 1974

93. Givens JR: Hirsutism and hyperandrogenism. Adv Intern Med 21:221, 1976

94. Givens JR, Andersen RN, Wiser WL, Umstot ES, Fish SA: The effectiveness of two oral contraceptives in suppressing plasma androstenedione, testosterone, LH, and FSH, and in stimulating plasma testosterone-binding capacity in hirsute women. Am J Obstet Gynecol 124:333, 1976

95. Ettinger B, Goldfield EB, Burrill KC, Von Werder K, Forsham PH: Plasma testosterone stimulation-suppression dynamics in hirsute women: correlation with long-term therapy. Am J Med 54:195, 1973

96. Talbert LM, Sloan C: The effect of a low-dose oral contraceptive on serum testosterone levels in polycystic ovarian disease. Obstet Gynecol 53:694, 1979

97. Raj SG, Raj MHG, Talbert LM, Sloan CS, Hicks B: Normalization of testosterone levels using a low estrogen-containing oral contraceptive in women with polycystic ovary syndrome. Obstet Gynecol 60:15, 1982

98. Dewis P, Petsos P, Newman M, Anderson DC: The treatment of hirsutism with a combination of desogestrel and ethinyl estradiol. Clin Endocrinol 22:29, 1985

99. Cullberg G, Hamberger L, Mattsson L-A, Mobacken H, Samsioe G: Effects of a low-dose desogestrel-ethinylestradiol combination on hirsutism, androgens and sex hormone binding globulin in women with a polycystic ovary syndrome. Acta Obstet Gynecol Scand 64:195, 1985

100. Azziz R, Gay F: The treatment of hyperandrogenism with oral contraceptives. Semin Reprod Endocrinol 7:246, 1989

101. Upton GV, Corbin A: The relevance of the pharmacologic properties of a progestational agent to its clinical effects as a combination oral contraceptive. Yale J Biol Med 62:445, 1989

102. Pang S: Editorial: relevance of biological properties of progestogen of oral contraceptives in treatment of androgen excess symptoms. J Clin Endocrinol Metab 71:5, 1990

103. Fotherby K: Desogestrel and gestodene in oral contraception: a review of the European experience. J Drug Dev 4:101, 1991

104. Conn PM, Crowley WF Jr: Gonadotropin-releasing hormone and its analogues. N Engl J Med 324:93, 1991

105. Andreyko JL, Monroe SE, Jaffe RB: Treatment of hirsutism with a gonadotropin-releasing hormone agonist. J Clin Endocrinol Metab 63:854, 1986

106. Steingold K, DeZiegler D, Cedars M, et al: Clinical and hormonal effects of chronic gonadotropin-releasing hormone agonist treatment in polycystic ovarian disease. J Clin Endocrinol Metab 65:773, 1987

107. Faure N, Lemay A: Ovarian suppression in polycystic ovarian disease during 6 month administration of a luteinizing hormone-releasing hormone (LH-RH) agonist. Clin Endocrinol 27:703, 1987

108. Rittmaster RS, Thompson DL: Effect of leuprolide and dexamethasone on hair growth and hormone levels in hirsute women: the relative importance of the ovary and the adrenal in the pathogenesis of hirsutism. J Clin Endocrinol Metab 70:1096, 1990

109. Rittmaster RS: Differential suppression of testosterone and estradiol in hirsute women with the superactive gonadotropin-releasing hormone agonist leuprolide. J Clin Endocrinol Metab 67:651, 1988

110. Adashi EY: Potential utility of gonadotropin-releasing hormone agonists in the management of ovarian hyperandrogenism. Fertil Steril 53:765, 1990

111. Gagliardi C: GnRH agonists: hirsutism and hyperandrogenism. Semin Reprod Endocrinol 11:162, 1993

112. Wilkins L, Crigler JF, Silverman SH, Gardner LI, Migeon CJ: Further studies on the treatment of congenital adrenal hyperplasia with cortisone. J Clin Endocrinol Metab 12:277, 1952

113. Greenblatt RB: Cortisone in the treatment of the hirsute women. Am J Obstet Gynecol 66:700, 1953

114. Perloff WH, Channick BJ, Hadd H, Nodine JH: The Stein-Leventhal ovary: a manifestation of hyperadrenocorticism. Fertil Steril 9:247, 1958

115. Bardin CW, Hembree WC, Lipsett MB: Suppression of testosterone and androstenedione production rates with dexamethasone in women with idiopathic hirsutism and polycystic ovaries. J Clin Endocrinol Metab 28:1300, 1968

116. Karpas AE, Rodriguez-Rigau LJ, Smith KD, Steinberger E: The effect of acute and chronic androgen suppression by glucocorticoids on gonadotropin levels in hirsute women. J Clin Endocrinol Metab 59:780, 1984

117. Abraham GE, Maroulis GB, Buster JE, Chang RJ, Marshall JR: Effect of dexamethasone on serum cortisol and androgen levels in hirsute patients. Obstet Gynecol 47:395, 1976

118. Casey JH: Chronic treatment regimens for hirsutism in women: effect on blood production rates of testosterone and on hair growth. Clin Endocrinol 4:313, 1975

119. Yuen BH, Mincey EK: Role of androgens in menstrual disorders of nonhirsute and hirsute women, and the effect of glucocorticoid therapy on androgen levels in hyperandrogenic women. Am J Obstet Gynecol 145:152, 1983

120. Rittmaster RS, Givner ML: Effect of daily and alternate day low dose prednisone on serum cortisol and adrenal androgens in hirsute women. J Clin Endocrinol Metab 67:400, 1988

121. Cutler GB Jr, Davis SE, Johnsonbaugh RE, Loriaux DL: Dissociation of cortisol and adrenal androgen secretion in patients with secondary adrenal insufficiency. J Clin Endocrinol Metab 49:604, 1979

122. Rittmaster RS, Loriaux DL, Cutler GB Jr: Sensitivity of cortisol and adrenal androgens to dexamethasone suppression in hirsute women. J Clin Endocrinol Metab 61:462, 1985

123. Abraham GE, Maroulis GB, Boyers SP, Buster JE, Magyar DM, Elsner CW: Dexamethasone suppression test in the management of hyperandrogenized patients. Obstet Gynecol 57:158, 1981

124. Loose DS, Kan PB, Hirst MA, Marcus RA, Feldman D: Ketoconazole blocks adrenal steroidogenesis by inhibiting cytochrome P450-dependent enzymes. J Clin Invest 71:1495, 1983

125. Feldman D: Ketoconazole and other imidazole derivatives as inhibitors of steroidogenesis. Endocr Rev 7:409, 1986

126. Engelhardt D, Weber MM, Miksch T, Abedinpour F, Jaspers C: The influence of ketoconazole and human adrenal steroidogenesis: incubation studies with tissue slices. Clin Endocrinol 35:163, 1991

127. Carvalho D, Pignatelli D, Resende C: Ketoconazole for hirsutism. Lancet 2:560, 1985

128. Pepper GM, Poretsky L, Gabrilove JL, Ariton MM: Ketoconazole reverses hyperandrogenism in a patient with insulin resistance and acanthosis nigricans. J Clin Endocrinol Metab 65:1047, 1987

129. Martikainen H, Heikkinen J, Ruokonen A, Kauppila A: Hormonal and clinical effects of ketocon-

azole in hirsute women. J Clin Endocrinol Metab 66:987, 1988

130. Venturoli S, Fabbri R, Dal Prato L, et al: Ketoconazole therapy for women with acne and/or hirsutism. J Clin Endocrinol Metab 71:335, 1990

131. Corvol P, Michaud A, Menard J, Freifeld M, Mahoudeau J: Antiandrogenic effect of spirolactones: mechanism of action. Endocrinology 97:52, 1975

132. Loriaux DL, Menard R, Taylor A, Pita JC, Santen R: Spironolactone and endocrine dysfunction. Ann Intern Med 85:630, 1976

133. Eil C, Edelson SK: The use of human skin fibroblasts to obtain potency estimates of drug binding to androgen receptors. J Clin Endocrinol Metab 59:51, 1984

134. Boisselle A, Tremblay RR: New therapeutic approach to the hirsute patient. Fertil Steril 32:276, 1979

135. Serafini PC, Catalino J, Lobo RA: The effect of spirononlactone on genital skin 5α-reductase activity. J Steroid Biochem 23:191, 1985

136. Shapiro G, Evron S: A novel use of spironolactone: treatment of hirsutism. J Clin Endocrinol Metab 51:429, 1980

137. Cumming DC, Yang JC, Rebar RW, Yen SSC: Treatment of hirsutism with spironolactone. JAMA 247:1295, 1982

138. Milewicz A, Silber D, Kirschner MA: Therapeutic effects of spironolactone in polycystic ovary syndrome. Obstet Gynecol 61:429, 1983

139. Lobo RA, Shoupe D, Serafini P, Brinton D, Horton R: The effects of two doses of spironolactone on serum androgens and anagen hair in hirsute women. Fertil Steril 43:200, 1985

140. Evans DJ, Burke CW: Spironolactone in the treatment of idiopathic hirsutism and the polycystic ovary syndrome. J R Soc Med 79:451, 1986

141. Serafini P, Lobo RA: The effects of spironolactone on adrenal steroidogenesis in hirsute women. Fertil Steril 44:595, 1985

142. Pittaway DE, Maxson WS, Wentz AC: Spironolactone in combination drug therapy for unresponsive hirsutism. Fertil Steril 43:878, 1985

143. Barth JH, Cherry CA, Wojnarowska F, Dawber RPR: Spironolactone is an effective and well tolerated systemic antiandrogen therapy for hirsute women. J Clin Endocrinol Metab 68:966, 1989

144. Helfer EL, Miller JL, Rose LI: Side-effects of spironolactone therapy in the hirsute woman. J Clin Endocrinol Metab 66:208, 1988

145. Tremblay RR: Treatment of hirsutism with spironolactone. Clin Endocrinol Metab 15:363, 1986

146. Crosby PDA, Rittmaster RS: Predictors of clinical response in hirsute women treated with spironolactone. Fertil Steril 55:1076, 1991

147. Ober KP, Hennessy JF: Spironolactone therapy for hirsutism in a hyperandrogenic woman. Ann Intern Med 89:643, 1978

148. Funder JW, Mercer JE: Cimetidine, a histamine H₂ receptor antagonist, occupies androgen receptors. J Clin Endocrinol Metab 48:189, 1979

149. Vigersky RA, Mehlman I, Glass AR, Smith CE: Treatment of hirsute women with cimetidine. N Engl J Med 303:1042, 1980

150. Lissak A, Sorokin Y, Calderon I, et al: Treatment of hirsutism with cimetidine: a prospective randomized controlled trial. Fertil Steril 51:247, 1989

151. Golditch IM, Price VH: Treatment of hirsutism with cimetidine. Obstet Gynecol 75:911, 1990

152. Hellman L, Bradlow HL, Freed S, et al: The effect of flutamide on testosterone metabolism and the plasma levels of androgens and gonadotropins. J Clin Endocrinol Metab 45:1224, 1977

153. Cusan L, Dupont A, Belanger A, Tremblay RR, Manhes G, Labrie F: Treatment of hirsutism with the pure antiandrogen flutamide. J Am Acad Dermatol 23:462, 1990

154. Marcondes JAM, Minnani SL, Luthold WW, Wajchenberg BL, Samojlik E, Kirschner MA: Treatment of hirsutism with flutamide. Fertil Steril 57:543, 1992

155. Mowszowicz I, Wright F, Vincens M, et al: Androgen metabolism in hirsute patients treated with cyproterone acetate. J Steroid Biochem 20:757, 1984

156. O'Brien RC, Cooper ME, Murray RML, Seeman E, Thomas AK, Jerums G: Comparison of sequential cyproterone acetate/estrogen versus spironolactone/oral contraceptive in the treatment of hirsutism. J Clin Endocrinol Metab 72:1008, 1991

157. Hammerstein J, Meckies J, Leo-Rossberg I, Moltz L, Zielske F: Use of cyproterone acetate (CPA) in the treatment of hirsutism, acne and virilism. J Steroid Biochem 6:827, 1975

158. Dewhurst CJ, Underhill R, Goldman S, Mansfield M: The treatment of hirsutism with cyproterone acetate (an anti-androgen). Br J Obstet Gynaecol 84:119, 1977

159. Schmidt JB, Huber J, Spona J: Parenteral and oral cyproterone acetate treatment in severe hirsutism. Gynecol Obstet Invest 24:125, 1987

160. Barth JH, Cherry CA, Wojnarowska F, Dawber RPR: Cyproterone acetate for severe hirsutism: results of a double-blind dose-ranging study. Clin Endocrinol 35:5, 1991

161. Marcondes JAM, Wajchenberg BL, Abujamra AC, Luthold WW, Samojlik E, Kirschner MA: Monthly cyproterone acetate in the treatment of hirsute women: clinical and laboratory effects. Fertil Steril 53:40, 1990

162. Belisle S, Love EJ: Clinical efficacy and safety of cyproterone acetate in severe hirsutism: results of a multicentered Canadian study. Fertil Steril 46:1015, 1986

163. Garner PR, Poznanski N: Treatment of severe hirsutism resulting from hyperandrogenism with the reverse sequential cyproterone acetate regimen. Obstet Gynecol 29:232, 1984

164. Jones DB, Ibraham I, Edwards CRW: Hair growth and androgen responses in hirsute women treated with continuous cyproterone acetate and cyclical ethinyl oestradiol. Acta Endocrinol 116:497, 1987

165. Smals AGH, Kloppenborg PWC, Goverde HJM, Benraad ThJ: The effect of cyproterone acetate on the pituitary-adrenal axis in hirsute women. Acta Endocrinol 87:352, 1978

166. Miller JA, Jacobs HS: Treatment of hirsutism and acne with cyproterone acetate. J Clin Endocrinol Metab 15:373, 1986

167. Wagner RF, Tomich JM, Grande DJ: Electrolysis and thermolysis for permanent hair removal. J Am Acad Dermatol 12:441, 1985

168. Oldfield EH, Doppman JL, Nieman LK, et al: Petrosal sinus sampling with and without corticotropin-releasing hormone for the differential diagnosis of Cushing's syndrome. N Engl J Med 325:897, 1991

169. Tabarin A, Greselle JF, San-Galli F, et al: Usefulness of the corticotropin-releasing hormone test during bilateral inferior petrosal sinus sampling for the diagnosis of Cushing's disease. J Clin Endocrinol Metab 73:53, 1991

Ambulatory Gynecology, Second Edition,
edited by David H. Nichols and Patrick J. Sweeney.
J. B. Lippincott Company, Philadelphia, © 1995.

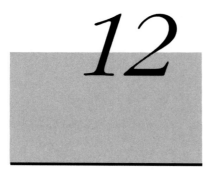

Pelvic Pain

Frank W. Ling

*If the only tool you have is a hammer, you
tend to see every problem as a nail*
Abraham Maslow

The syndrome of chronic pelvic pain continues to
frustrate both patient and physician. To some extent, perhaps this is due to the terminology itself.
"Chronic pelvic pain" may too often suggest the
cause of the pain as being an organ in the female
pelvic region. With too great an emphasis on organ-
based etiology, the patient may undergo diagnostic
and therapeutic modalities that focus too much on
the uterus, tubes, and ovaries when in reality, she
needs a more holistic approach. Using the knowledge that the body and mind are entwined inextric-
ably, physicians, in conjunction with other healthcare professionals, are increasingly aware that the
patient suffering from chronic pelvic pain must be
evaluated and treated with a different approach.
The term "gynevision" was coined to describe a
traditional, excessively narrow focus on pelvic pain
as arising from female reproductive tract organs.[1]
This tends to encourage more of a surgical approach, in which organic pathology is a top priority.

This has particularly been the case since laparoscopy has been made safer and more accessible to
more patients. The results, however, have been inadequate for both the physician and the patient and
as the result, a multidisciplinary approach to these
patients is being increasingly viewed with greater
acceptance.

The approach taken in this chapter is to briefly
touch on the traditional gynecologic conditions
treated by physicians who typically manage patients who have chronic pelvic pain. Complement-
ing this traditional approach are various aspects of
the multidisciplinary approach that are necessary to
round out a total management scheme. Regardless
of whether an individual physician chooses to incorporate any or all of the recommendations made,
ultimately, it is her or his patient who may benefit
as she is taught to better cope with and manage her
pain—both during the evaluation phase and after
any treatment that is rendered. Curing all patients
with chronic pelvic pain is an ideal and admirable.
Realistically, however, the physician should recognize that some patients are best helped by management of pain, with a goal of minimally disrupting

her life-style and enabling her to carry on her normal daily activities relating to her job, her interpersonal relationships, and her self-image.

GYNECOLOGIC CAUSES OF PELVIC PAIN— A TRADITIONAL VIEW

The traditional model for evaluating and treating chronic pelvic pain focuses primarily on gynecologic causes. The patients' histories are divided into cyclic and noncyclic categories to determine whether there is a likely menstrual cycle–related origin to the pain. For example, Table 12-1 lists the common disorders that present as cyclic pain.

In addition to the organ-based search for pathology in these patients, it should be noted that other nonmenstrual-related conditions may be exacerbated in a cyclic fashion, resulting in a differential diagnosis that must at least begin with an approach that can rule out common disorders in the female reproductive tract (ie, dysmenorrhea must be differentiated from pelvic pain that is constant throughout the month but is exacerbated at the time of the menstrual flow). Major sources of pain such as the musculoskeletal system, the urinary tract, the intestines, and psychologic factors are discussed later in this chapter. For now, they should simply be kept in mind as additional differential diagnostic considerations. Table 12-2 is a more extensive list of causes of pelvic pain that considers both gynecologic and nongynecologic etiologies.

In establishing a gynecologic basis for the chief complaint, a careful history combined with a thorough physical examination and selected laboratory tests can do a great deal to both identify the cause

Table 12–1
Causes of Cyclic Pelvic Pain

Mittelschmerz

Primary dysmenorrhea

Secondary dysmenorrhea
    Endometriosis
    Leiomyomata uteri
    Adenomyosis
    Endometrial polyps
    Intrauterine contraceptive device
    Endometritis
    Cervical stenosis

Premenstrual syndrome

Table 12–2
Etiologies of Noncyclic Pelvic Pain

Gynecologic

Uterine
    Leiomyomata uteri
    Adenomyosis
    Intrauterine contraceptive device
    Symptomatic pelvic relaxation
    Chronic endometritis
    Endometrial poyps

Extrauterine

Postoperative adhesions

Chronic pelvic infection

Endometriosis

Retained ovary syndrome

Ovarian remnant syndrome

Adnexal mass

Musculoskeletal

Low back pain

Degenerative joint disease

Fibromyositis

Muscle sprains/strains

Disk/postural causes

Urogynecologic

Chronic urinary tract infection

Urethral syndrome

Interstitial cystitis

Uninhibited bladder contractions

Gastrointestinal

Chronic constipation

Irritable bowel syndrome

Inflammatory bowel disease

Psychologic factors

Sexual victimization

Somatization disorder

Depression

of pain and minimize unnecessary intervention. Primary dysmenorrhea is most common in young women in their late teens or early 20s. Driven by prostaglandins, the pain is typically in the suprapubic area and may be described as "like labor." Associated symptoms of nausea, vomiting, or diarrhea are not uncommon. In some women, however, primary dysmenorrhea is a diagnosis of exclusion because secondary causes are ruled out by history and physical. The presence of dyspareunia should suggest a secondary cause of pain. Because primary dysmenorrhea is by definition without organic cause, the physical examination should be normal. Even when the patient is examined during her period, the abdomen will be soft and nontender, as will the uterus. It is critical that in ruling out secondary dysmenorrhea, the history and physical focus not just on the female genital tract but also other possible causes. If the history of pain is purely related to the menstrual flow itself, greater attention may be focused on the pelvic organs. Heavy menstrual flow accompanying dysmenorrhea suggests a greater possibility of uterine pathology. In older patients, symptom of pelvic heaviness may be associated with symptomatic pelvic relaxation or a pelvic mass. Deep-thrust dyspareunia strongly suggests a pelvic etiology. Conversely, urinary difficulties, chronic constipation, and pain throughout the month unrelated to the menstrual flow can help the clinician identify nongynecologic disorders.

The physical examination should identify organ-specific sites of tenderness. Specifically, the clinician should seek to identify associated pain in the posterior vaginal wall, the urethra and bladder base, the uterus, and the adnexa, all as separate structures. It is only with a greater degree of organ specificity in the pelvic examination that a more accurate clinical diagnosis can be made. Limited use of laboratory evaluation is appropriate with patients presenting with chronic pelvic pain, dysmenorrhea, or both. A complete blood count may help to identify excessive blood loss that is suggested by the history. It is unusual for a leukocyte count to be elevated in patients who do not otherwise have symptoms suggestive of infection. Similarly, sedimentation rates are nonspecific and only infrequently can help to identify the presence of a chronic inflammatory process.

Scanning techniques usually offer little additional information if specific conditions are not strongly suspected based on history and physical examination. Ultrasonography, magnetic resonance imaging, and computed tomographic scanning add little to the basic office evaluation of patients who have chronic pelvic pain. The ultimate diagnostic tool, diagnostic laparoscopy, should be used only after a thorough work-up has been undertaken and empiric therapeutic attempts have been unsuccessful. The role of surgery is discussed more fully below but it may be helpful to note that one out of three patients with chronic pelvic pain has a normal laparoscopy.[2]

With regard to therapy, specific treatment should be aimed at correcting the underlying pathology. Nonspecific treatment with agents such as birth control pills, analgesics, and nonsteroidal anti-inflammatory drugs may also have some limited value. For example, specific therapy for endometriosis or removal an intrauterine contraceptive device are specific for causes of secondary dysmenorrhea. In patients who have primary dysmenorrhea, the use of nonsteroidal anti-inflammatory drugs is extremely effective in reducing the effect of prostaglandins. If such therapy is unsuccessful,

---

Table 12–3

Nonsteroidal Anti-inflammatory Drugs for Treatment of Patients With Pelvic Pain

	Drug	Initial Dose	Subsequent Dose
FDA-approved for primary dysmenorrhea	Ibuprofen	400 mg	400–600 mg q 6 hrs
	Naproxen	500 mg	250 mg q 6–8 hrs
	Naproxen sodium	550 mg	275 mg q 6–8 hrs
	Mefenamic acid	500 mg	250 mg q 4–6 hrs
	Meclofenamate	100 mg	50–100 mg q 6 hrs
Other useful agents	Piroxicam	20 mg	20 mg q day
	Tolmetin	400 mg	400 mg q tid
	Diflunisal	1000 mg	500 mg q 12 hrs
	Oxyphenbutazone	100 mg	100 mg tid
	Phenylbutazone	100 mg	100 mg tid

the clinician should reconsider whether the patient should truly be considered to have primary dysmenorrhea. Many studies document the efficacy of various agents in the treatment of primary dysmenorrhea. No one drug appears superior to the others. Table 12-3 lists potentially useful drugs for treatment of primary dysmenorrhea.

As an alternative to nonsteroidal anti-inflammatory drugs or in conjunction with them, oral contraceptive agents have also proved to be beneficial in patients with primary dysmenorrhea. As with the nonsteroidal anti-inflammatory drugs, no single oral contraceptive agent has been proved to be more beneficial than others. All function by preventing ovulation. Even in cases of secondary dysmenorrhea, rendering a patient amenorrheic by use of oral contraceptives with no pill-free interval may be beneficial for short-term management while the chronic pain is monitored and evaluated. Gonadotropin-releasing–hormone agonists have also been used in this fashion, both as therapy and to confirm a cyclic relation of the pain. Long-acting contraceptive agents such as Norplant and Depo-Provera may also be used in this fashion, although shorter-acting (and therefore reversible) oral contraceptives may be better tolerated.

Failure to achieve a reasonable amount of pain relief after thorough evaluation and trials of therapy may result in the need for diagnostic or therapeutic surgical intervention. Under any circumstances, patients with chronic pelvic pain should be informed that the surgery that they are undergoing may not totally remove all the pain. Patients who understand the limitations of surgical intervention have more realistic expectations of how they will feel postoperatively.

MUSCULOSKELETAL CAUSES OF PELVIC PAIN

Musculoskeletal evaluation is an often overlooked component of the comprehensive evaluation of the patient with chronic pelvic pain.[3] A practitioner skilled in musculoskeletal evaluation and treatment can be crucial in identifying the actual etiology of pain. Physical therapists, when included in a multidisciplinary approach, have been extremely successful in managing such patients. Because the practicing clinician cannot practically perform a complete musculoskeletal evaluation, a screening examination can help identify those patients who would most likely benefit from referral. Table 12-4

lists clues to those patients with chronic pelvic pain who are candidates for further musculoskeletal screening. Identification of specific tender areas of the paraspinous muscles, the superficial abdominal wall, or pelvic floor with or without levator ani contraction may be a significant component of the pain picture.[4] Referral to orthopedic physical therapists is an appropriate first line of consultation. If such individuals are not available or relatively inaccessible, muscle relaxants and nonsteroidal anti-inflammatory drugs may be used effectively. Commonly used muscle relaxants is listed in Table 12-5. Medications may also be needed in conjunction with physical therapy.

As an extension to the musculoskeletal evaluation, a specific search for abdominal wall pain is appropriate. A typical bimanual examination in the course of evaluating a patient with chronic pelvic pain includes the simultaneous evaluation of multiple tissue layers, including those of the abdominal wall, the vaginal wall, and other layers in between. For example, in evaluating an anteverted uterus,

Table 12–4

Musculoskeletal Screening Examination for Patients Presenting With Chronic Pelvic Pain

History

Normal laparoscopy

History of trauma to low back or lower extremities, including motor vehicle accident or fall

Pain is altered by positional changes, particularly prolonged standing or sitting

Lack of response to previous gynecologic intervention

Exacerbation with stress

Structural Observations

Marked lumbar lordosis

Unilateral standing habits

Obesity

Scoliosis

Slouched standing or sitting habits

Dynamic Testing and Palpable Findings

Asymmetric gait (eg, limp)

Pain on standing, sitting, or laying down

Trigger-point tenderness in the abdominal wall, pelvic floor

Tenderness to palpation in the paraspinous muscles

Tenderness of abdominal wall on heel raising or leg lifting

Table 12–5
Muscle Relaxants for Patients Presenting With Chronic Pelvic Pain

Trade Names	Generic Names	Dosage
Parafon Forte	Chlorzoxazone	500 mg q tid or qid
Robaxin	Methocarbamol	500 mg 3 tabs qid
Soma compound	Carisoprodol	200 mg 1 or 2 tabs qid
	Aspirin	325 mg qid
Valium	Diazepam	2–10 mg qid

the two examining hands palpate the abdominal wall (including skin, subcutaneous tissue, fascia, and muscle); the uterus; the bladder; and the vaginal wall. Injection of a local anesthetic into the abdominal wall may prove invaluable in distinguishing visceral pain originating from deeper pelvic structures from pain originating from the abdominal wall.[5] Trigger points are hyperirritable areas that are tender when compressed and may also generate referred pain and tenderness. Trigger points typically start after some type of muscle strain that results in sensitized nerves and may commonly be found within a taut band of skeletal muscle. Common sites are shown in Figure 12-1. In his classic study, Slocumb treated 122 patients who presented with chronic pelvic pain.[6] In his series, more than half of the patients were pain-free after receiving trigger-point injections. Only 13 had surgery, and all patients who received only abdominal wall trigger-point injections were reported to have a successful response. Those with vaginal trigger points had an 84.6% response rate to their injections.

In assessing a patient for the possible use of trigger-point injections, it should be remembered that a patient's pain may be related to the abdominal wall, intra-abdominal structures, or both. Relief of pain from one source may reduce pain symptoms from the other or actually unmask a different set of symptoms. A routine physical examination of a patient who has chronic pelvic pain should include tensing of the rectus muscles, with the possible additional use of local anesthetic injections. A 22-gauge needle is recommended for superficial muscles; a length of 1 to 1.5 inches is appropriate. Twenty-five–gauge needles cause less discomfort on insertion but have the disadvantage of being less able mechanically to disrupt a trigger point and they reduce the clinician's sensitivity in passing through various tissue planes. Furthermore, a 27-gauge needle may be too flexible, thus sliding around taut fiber bands and thereby masking the

tactile clues that a clinician may use. An aseptic technique should be used and the patient should be forewarned that she may experience a muscle twitch or a flash of referred pain. The palpating fingers maintain tension on the skin, and this tension is maintained as various injection tracks are made (Fig. 12-2). The needle tip probes for the tight muscle band. If the trigger point is not identified directly, the injection may be less effective but still useful diagnostically. Successful injection results in a loss of tenderness and relaxation of the tight band, with the patient verbalizing a symptomatic difference as she palpates the affected area. Using

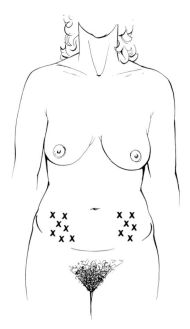

Figure 12–1. Common sites of abdominal wall trigger points amenable to injection. (Adapted from Travell JG, Simons DG: Myofascial pain and dysfunction; the trigger point manual. Baltimore, MD, Williams & Wilkins, 1983.)

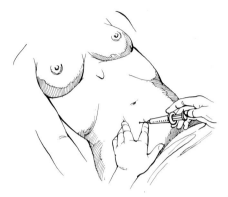

Figure 12–2. Injection of right rectus abdominis muscle trigger point. (Adapted from Travell JG, Simons DG: Myofascial pain and dysfunction; the trigger point manual. Baltimore, MD, Williams & Wilkins, 1983.)

Table 12–6
Assessment of Possible Chronic Abdominal Wall Pain

Acute process ruled out
Evaluation of chronic pelvic pain
    Any pain patient without evidence of acute process
    Examination of abdomen and low back
        Hyperesthesia of skin over pain area
        Focal trigger points with single-finger examination
        Exacerbation of trigger points with tensing of rectus muscle
        Relief from pain with local block of 0.25% bupivacaine
    Pelvic examination with abdominal wall anesthetic block
    Colposcopic examination or clinical evaluation for vulvar vestibulitis

Adapted from Slocumb JC: Neurologic factors in chronic pelvic pain: trigger points and the abdominal pain syndrome. Am J Obstet Gynecol 149:536, 1984

agents such as 0.25% bupivicaine is appropriate. Volumes of 10 mL or less are commonly adequate to provide the clinician with a clear diagnostic test.

Relief of pain after abdominal wall trigger-point injection helps the patient understand that her pain is likely not to be coming from solely intra-abdominal sources such as ovarian cysts, endometriosis, or infection. Although not necessarily therapeutic, when used in this fashion, a trigger-point injection is clearly diagnostic. As shown by Slocumb, injections can be therapeutic, either alone or in series. They should also be looked on as useful adjuncts to other forms of therapy because several sources of pain may be identified simultaneously. The assessment of possible abdominal wall pain is listed in Table 12-6.

URINARY TRACT CAUSES OF PELVIC PAIN

Because of their close developmental relation, the genital and lower urinary tracts may be difficult to differentiate as sources of pain. As long as the clinician keeps the potential of urologic origin high in the differential diagnosis, particularly when the standard gynecologic evaluation is inconclusive, patients with urogynecologic pain can be identified and treated within the context of the overall pelvic pain. Urinary complaints should be a standard part of the history for patients with chronic pelvic pain. Urgency, frequency, and dysuria may be evidence of both acute and chronic lower urinary tract problems. Recurrent urinary tract infections that yield repeated negative cultures should suggest a chronic inflammatory process of a noninfectious nature. A

history of incomplete emptying or hesitancy suggests disorders of the urethra or vesical neck. Postcoital voiding problems are also strongly associated with urethral syndrome due to chronic urethritis.[7] Dyspareunia is not an infrequent finding. A 24-hour voiding diary provides insight into the frequency of voiding, episodes of leakage, and amount of fluid intake. For example, frequency at night may relate to sensory problems of the bladder and urethra, whereas constant voiding throughout the day may suggest limited bladder capacity due to an intrinsic bladder condition.

The physical examination should include a neurologic examination of the lower extremities and perineal area. Gentle palpation of the pelvic floor musculature may be related to underlying urethral or bladder problems (eg, it has been suggested that levator ani spasm may contribute to the pain in patients who have interstitial cystitis).[8] Gentle palpation of the urethra, trigone, and bladder base may identify specific sources of pain. To fully evaluate patients with chronic pelvic pain suggestive of urologic origin, cystourethroscopy should ultimately be performed. It is usually performed in the office without anesthesia. Evaluation of the appearance of the urethra and the bladder mucosa is performed. Acute and chronic infection can be identified and anatomic abnormalities such as diverticula or tumors can also be seen. Painful conditions such as interstitial cystitis may require general anesthesia and evaluation in a hospital or outpatient surgical setting.

Urogynecologic disorders that cause pelvic pain are listed in Table 12-7. Special attention should be focused on two conditions—urethral syndrome and interstitial cystitis—because they often prove to be diagnostic and therapeutic challenges for the practicing clinician who sees patients with chronic pelvic pain.

Urethral Syndrome

Patients with urethral syndrome tend to present with urinary urgency, frequency, and dysuria. Other common symptoms include urge or stress incontinence, vulvar irritation, dyspareunia, suprapubic tenderness, and postvoiding fullness. No specific etiology has been identified, although many hypotheses have been proffered. In addition to infection, other suggested etiologies include urethral spasm, hypoestrogenism, trauma, and psychosomatic conditions. Because the symptoms are primarily similar to urinary tract infection, misdiagnosis is common and antibiotic therapy is frequently repeated, without patient response. Ultimately, the diagnosis is one of exclusion, with the diagnosis being made by cystourethroscopy.

Because the potential causes are multiple, a specific therapy may not be uniformly successful. Reeducation of voiding habits is a key element to treatment. Patients are taught to tighten and relax their pelvic floor musculature to gain control of involuntary or learned spastic behavior of the urethral sphincter. Antimicrobal agents may be used, with low-dose bedtime suppression for 3 to 6 months suggested. Urethral dilations have also been used, although the mechanism of action is unclear. Massaging the urethra when dilating has also

---

Table 12–7
Urogynecologic Causes of Chronic Pelvic Pain

Detrusor dyssynergia

Interstitial cystitis

Neoplasm

Radiation cystitis

Urethral caruncle

Urethral diverticulum

Urethral syndrome

Urolithiasis

---

been suggested. Other treatments include urethrotomy, anxiolytics, tranquilizers, psychotherapy, and periurethral steroid injections. Consultation with a urogynecologist or urologist may be extremely beneficial because these patients often present with a confusing and sometimes changing clinical picture.

Interstitial Cystitis

Interstitial cystitis may also present with findings that have been diagnosed or mistreated by previous clinicians. The diagnosis is one of exclusion, in which the patient presents with frequency, urgency, nocturia, and suprapubic pain, usually relieved by voiding. Incontinence is rare but hematuria may also occur. An elevated number of mast cells have been found in the bladder walls of patients having interstitial cystitis, suggesting an autoimmune phenomenon.[9] Others suggest a defect in the glycosaminoglycan layer of the bladder wall as a cause, which results in excessive permeability and exposure to urine.[10]

On examination, a tender bladder base may simulate the pain experienced with coitus. Urinalysis typically rules out an infectious agent, and cytology also rules out a neoplasm. Because of the discomfort, cystoscopy usually must be performed under anesthesia in an operating-room setting. The bladder is filled, emptied, and on second filling, the bladder mucosa demonstrate hemorrhage and petechiae, sometimes referred to as glomerulations. Occasionally, terminal hematuria is noted when the bladder is emptied after the first filling. Biopsy is typically nonspecific but may be useful in ruling out other conditions. Therapy for interstitial cystitis is directed at either the inflammation or the bladder wall permeability. Hydrodistention performed at the time of diagnosis may be therapeutic. Similarly, behavioral modification (using increasing voiding intervals) may help. Tricyclic antidepressants have been used providing sedative action as well as pain relief. Dimethylsulfoxide may be used as an intravesical insulation. Surgical therapies have also been used as a last resort.

GASTROENTEROLOGIC CAUSES OF PELVIC PAIN

It has been estimated that up to 60% of referrals to gynecologists for chronic pelvic pain may be attributed to gastrointestinal diagnoses, particularly irritable bowel syndrome.[11] It is often difficult to differentiate lower abdominal pain of gynecologic from that of intraperitoneal origin because of the visceral innervation. As with the other causes of pelvic pain, specific historical information can be extremely helpful. It should be noted that in some patients, symptoms of irritable bowel syndrome may be exacerbated premenstrually, thus simulating a cyclic disorder that might be misinterpreted as a gynecologic condition. Irritable bowel syndrome typically improves after bowel movements and may be worsened after eating. There may also be a sense of fullness in the rectum or of incomplete rectal evacuation. Stress-related symptoms in conjunction with irritable bowel are not uncommon. Bowel habits may also be a source of useful information. Patients who have infrequent bowel movements, with pain preceding those bowel movements, may simply have chronic constipation, whereas patients with frequent stools should be queried regarding intrinsic bowel disease that results in diarrhea. Dyspareunia, although increasing the likelihood of a gynecologic source of pain, may also be associated with patients who have irritable bowel syndrome.

With gastrointestinal symptoms, patients typically present those concerns that are bothering them. A thorough evaluation for chronic pelvic pain must include at least closer questioning regarding bowel function to not miss those subtle causes of pelvic pain that are related to the gastrointestinal tract.

The physical examination is similar to that previously described and should always include a rectal examination and an examination of the pelvic floor. Both a plain film of the abdomen and an abdominal ultrasound may identify significant findings, although the history and physical examination techniques are most effective in ruling out acute problems and most chronic conditions. In appropriate situations, flexible sigmoidoscopy, colonoscopy, or barium enema may be appropriate. Laboratory tests may include a complete blood count and stool for occult blood and white blood cell count. If white cells or blood are found, further evaluation is appropriate.

Irritable Bowel Syndrome

Irritable bowel syndrome is a common cause of lower abdominal pain, not infrequently interpreted as pelvic pain by the patient and physician. There are no identifiable structural or biochemical abnormalities. Signs and symptoms such as constipation,

diarrhea, or mucous in the stool may be present, suggesting a gastroenterologic cause of pelvic pain. The diagnosis may be suggested on pelvic examination by identification of a tender sigmoid colon or pain on rectal examination. Similarly, hard feces in the rectum may suggest this condition. Therapy for irritable bowel syndrome includes such diverse treatments as antidepressants, anxiolytics, and bulk-forming agents in addition to psychotherapy, reassurance, and stress reduction.

Because the differential diagnosis of irritable bowel syndrome includes inflammatory bowel disease and neoplasia, a thorough work-up must be used for patients suspected of having one of these other conditions. Irrespective of the ultimate diagnosis, patients who have pain related to gastroenterologic conditions may require medical therapy, surgical therapy, or psychotherapeutic support. In many instances, multidisciplinary pain management is appropriate for these patients, just as it is for any patient with chronic pelvic pain.

PSYCHIATRIC FACTORS IN PELVIC PAIN

Underlying the entire spectrum of causes for chronic pelvic pain are the psychosocial issues that complicate organic conditions and serve as the etiologies for chronic pelvic pain. The gate theory of pain takes recognizes that the individual's pain experience is directly affected by emotional factors.[12,13] Knowing that nociceptive signals are transmitted in both directions between the periphery and the central nervous system, the clinician is thereby cognizant that mood states, motivation, and other psychological factors have a role in chronic pain states. To adequately assess a patient's pain, psychological, emotional, and physical states must be evaluated. For patients with chronic pain, the exercise of trying to differentiate mental from physical pain is not useful because "mental" factors such as clinical depression, anxiety, and anger are clearly critical parts of the patient's perception of discomfort.

In this regard, patients with chronic pelvic pain are not unique from patients who have chronic pain in other areas.[14] All chronic pain complaints must be placed in the context of the patient's circumstances (ie, a patient's response to pain is affected by such diverse considerations as culture value placed on pain tolerance, the patient's perception of the risk involved with the pain, and work, social, financial and other idiosyncratic determinations).

Depression

Classically, depression may accompany chronic pain and may manifest before, after, or simultaneously with the symptoms of pain.[15] It is not uncommon for these patients to have been relegated to a dependent role, both in their personal and professional lives, because of the need to pursue diagnosis and treatment for their chronic pain. The change in life-style and self-image also contributes to the often hostile relations that these patients have with healthcare providers because they often "doctor shop," looking for cures. Although pejorative, the term "doctor shopping" should be viewed as more of a coping mechanism of the individual patient; she seeks symptomatic improvement, yet often all she seems to be told is that the pain is not real, it is "all in her head," or that she is seeking secondary gain.

In one study, 75% of patients who had depression had their first episode of major depression before the onset of chronic pelvic pain. About two thirds of patients with chronic pelvic pain had a lifetime history of depression, whereas only 17% of a control group had suffered major depression.[16] Rather than implying that the pain is not real or suggesting that the pain is "in her head," the clinician should more forthrightly address the potential coexistence of chronic pain symptoms felt in the pelvis as well as coexistent and likely related clinical depression. It is for these reasons that antidepressants may have a role in the management of some of these difficult patients.

Victimization Histories

Many patients who present with pelvic pain have or have had abusive family relationships, either as children or in adulthood.[17,18] A growing body of literature supports a potential link between chronic pelvic pain and victimization histories. Indeed, women who have suffered previous sexual trauma are more likely to have unexplained physical symptoms. This complicates both the evaluation and treatment of women with chronic pelvic pain. For example, the use of antidepressant medications appears to be less efficacious in women who have a history of sexual victimization. These patients may also be less able to develop a close relationship with their physicians, a situation that may make long-term therapeutic attempts less effective. Because they are at greater risk for other psychiatric illness such as anxiety and mood disorders, these patients

may not easily fall within the expertise of those physicians typically seeing these patients as first-line physicians. Because of the complex needs that patients with chronic pelvic pain and a history of sexual trauma may have, psychiatric consultation is appropriate relatively early in the diagnostic process. The most important factor for the clinician and the patient is that the physician be made aware of sexual trauma. The initial evaluation of patients who have chronic pelvic pain should include a gentle inquiry as to current or past sexual or physical abuse. For example, "Have you ever been touched against your will, either as a child or an adult?" is one possible entry statement. Recognition of this factor may help frame future discussions and therapeutic intervention, including supportive listening, use of community resources, referral to support groups, and treatment with antidepressants. Nortriptyline may be started, using 25 mg at bedtime and increasing by 25 mg every 3 to 4 days thereafter, as tolerated, with a maximum dosage of 100 mg/day. Fluoxetine may be given, 20 mg/day. Sertraline may be given at a dosage of 50 mg/day. The physician who prescribes such medication should be familiar with side effects and aware that other unresolved environmental stressors (eg, financial difficulties, job-related problems, interpersonal or ongoing abuse) can reduce the efficacy of the medication.

Somatization

Physicians treating patients who have chronic pelvic pain should also be cognizant of the possibility that the symptoms are one aspect of somatization disorder. Multiple physical symptoms without apparent organic causes may or may not meet diagnostic criteria for somatization disorder according to the *Diagnostic and Statistical Manual*, 4th edition. Although, with their multiple symptoms, these patients play to the sensitivity of their physicians, the diagnostic and therapeutic interventions undertaken may often be unnecessary and even potentially damaging. Also referred to as Briquet's syndrome, patients with somatization disorders present frequently with dramatic complaints and are best managed with emotional support rather than extensive intervention. These patients cannot be cured per se but they can be managed by offering them visits and support in addition to the critical factor of validating the patient's concerns. Table 12-8 is a summary of the management of somatization disorder.

Table 12–8
Management of Somatization Disorder

1. See patient regularly
2. Accept her need to be "ill"
3. Do not vary contact time in proportion to symptom severity
4. Do not make physician contact contigent upon development of somatic complaint
5. Allow patient to verbalize her concerns
6. Minimize secondary gain
7. Teach the patient to address emotions in words
8. Monitor patient for development of new pathology

ROLE OF SURGICAL MANAGEMENT FOR CHRONIC PELVIC PAIN

Surgery is a logical extension of a thorough diagnostic and therapeutic management scheme in patients who have chronic pelvic pain. The ease with which procedures can be performed, particularly through laparoscopy, should not alter the need to fully investigate more conservative modes of therapy. In some cases, however, surgical intervention, particularly in the form of diagnostic laparoscopy, may provide the patient and physician with reassurance that a suspected disease process is not present. By accurately diagnosing a particular condition or ruling out the existence of others, the patient can be more easily reassured or treated by the physician. Laparoscopy also provides easy access to therapeutic modalities such as excision of disease, lysis of adhesions, and cautery of endometriosis as well as other techniques performed by many endoscopic surgeons. Interestingly, virtually every operation described for the treatment of chronic pelvic pain can be performed using the laparoscope. Table 12-9 is a list of surgical procedures for the treatment of chronic pelvic pain.

Extensive experience with diagnostic laparoscopy for pelvic pain has not only confirmed the relatively high incidence of normal anatomy but has aided in a greater sensitivity in the diagnosis of various conditions.[2,19–21] With greater experience, subtle findings of endometriosis have been identified, so that the traditional blue or bluish-black appearances are no longer the sole types of lesions associated with this condition, known to be potentially related to pelvic pain. Vesicular, white, pink, clear, and red lesions may be proved to be endometriosis by obtaining peritoneal biopsies.

The role of patient reassurance in cases of normal pelvic findings at the time of diagnostic laparoscopy should not be underplayed. For example, pelvic pain may resolve after pathology has been excluded, simply with the passage of time.[22] It is against this background rate of resolution that many of the findings of surgical intervention must be placed. This perspective also aids in better understanding the actual benefit or lack thereof attributable to a specific surgical intervention.

Many studies document the potential relation of pain and adhesions. Lysis of adhesions has in turn been associated with improvement in many patients, although the body of evidence does not necessarily suggest that all adhesions need to be taken down to provide pain relief.[23–26] There is no evidence that cautery or laser vaporization is better if adhesiolysis is to be attempted. Similarly, there are no data to indicate that the addition of Hyskon or Dextran-70 prevents adhesion formation. INTERCEED, when used as a postoperative barrier, (Johnson & Johnson Patient Care Inc., New Brunswick, NJ) has been demonstrated to be successful in decreasing the recurrence of pelvic adhesions when used in conjunction with meticulous surgical techniques.[27] The role of INTERCEED, however, has not been well evaluated with regard to pelvic pain symptoms.

Just as adhesions cannot be diagnosed except with laparoscopy, endometriosis must be visualized and—ideally—undergo biopsy to confirm the diagnosis. The use of techniques such as excision, laser vaporization, and electrocoagulation are useful, although it is generally assumed that conservative surgical management of endometriosis is a temporary treatment, as opposed to a long-term cure. Endometriosis may be found in up to a third of all pa-

Table 12–9
Surgical Procedures for Chronic Pelvic Pain

Diagnostic laparoscopy

Lysis of adhesions

Cautery or excision of endometriosis

Uterine suspension

Uterosacral ligament resection

Presacral neurectomy

Ovarian cyst treatment

Diagnosis of pelvic congestion syndrome

Diagnosis and treatment of ovarian remnant syndrome/residual ovary syndrome

Hysterectomy

tients who have chronic pelvic pain, with the percentage depending on the particular population studied (eg, fertile versus infertile) and the diagnostic acumen of the physicians involved. Both medical and surgical therapies for endometriosis have proved beneficial in patients with pain symptoms, although no direct study comparing the two has been undertaken. Just as no uniform medical treatment has been formulated, no specific surgical therapy is optimal for every patient. To that end, it behooves the gynecologic surgeon to maximally treat whatever endometriosis is found at the time of initial endoscopic diagnosis to potentially improve pain symptoms for the short term while maximizing potential response to medical therapy for the long term. The often paradoxical relation between severe pain and minimal endometriosis or advanced endometriosis associated with minimal symptoms makes the aggressive therapy for endometriosis a clinically relevant dilemma.

Uterine suspension has been advocated as a potential surgical procedure for patients with chronic pelvic pain. Because up to a third of women have a uterus that is retroflexed–retroverted, the mere presence of this condition should not be an indication for the procedure. Insertion of a pessary is a necessary management attempt before consideration of surgical intervention. For those patients who have completed their childbearing and whose pain is recreated on palpation of the uterine fundus in the cul-de-sac, hysterectomy may be a better procedure. Laparoscopic procedures that simulate the Gilliam suspension have been described, as have other techniques for shortening the round ligaments, such as the use of falope rings.[28] Conservative measures, however, are prerequisites before surgical intervention is entertained.

The diagnosis of pelvic congestion syndrome, describing patients with extensive pelvic varicosities, has received less attention recently than when the condition was originally described by Duncan and Taylor in the 1950s.[29] Clinical studies suggest that extraperitoneal dissection at the left ovarian vein or hysterectomy with bilateral salpingo-oophorectomy may be of some benefit. Because of the vague nature of the diagnosis and the lack of convincing scientific evidence for either conservative or extirpative surgery, the clinician should make all reasonable attempts to rule out other nongynecologic diagnoses before embarking on these surgical attempts of treatment.[30,31]

Ovarian remnant syndrome may present as pelvic pain after gynecologic surgery involving the ovaries, often as a result of extensive endometriosis or adhesions due to previous surgery or infection.

Because of the active ovarian tissue, the follicle-stimulating–hormone measurement is at a premenopausal level. Because of the often close approximation with the urinary tract, careful dissection around the ureter is critical. Residual ovary syndrome or pain related to the preservation of one or both ovaries at the time of hysterectomy may be due to pelvic adhesions or displacement of the ovary from its normal anatomic position. Both oophorectomy and ovarian suspensions have been described as treatment for residual ovary syndrome.[32]

Pelvic denervation procedures such as presacral neurectomy and uterosacral ligament resection have also been described for relief of dysmenorrhea, central pelvic pain, and deep dysparuenia. Data on laparoscopic presacral neurectomy suggest that it is as effective as those results obtained with open laparotomy.[33] Other data suggest that relief of primary dysmenorrhea may be achieved in up to 80% of patients, with lower rates of success (ie, less than 50%) for secondary dysmenorrhea. The use of a uterosacral block with a local anesthetic before undertaking surgery has been suggested as a way to determine who might benefit by presacral neurotomy or uterosacral ligament resection.[34,35] Less well documented than presacral neurectomy is the use of laparoscopic uterosacral nerve ablation. Long-term follow-up of these patients reveals symptomatic relief in about 50% of patients. A review article concerning the appropriate use of either procedure suggests that their roles in the long-term management of patients with chronic pelvic pain may be limited.[36]

As with the other operations listed, few data exist regarding the efficacy of hysterectomy for patients with chronic pelvic pain. In the only study of long-term outcome of patients undergoing hysterectomy for chronic pelvic pain with presumed origins in the uterus, about one out of four patients had pain postoperatively.[37] Even in a highly selected group of cases, patients still had significant pain symptoms postoperatively. Some pain was similar to the preoperative evaluation, whereas some was even worse.

Given the unconvincing data in the literature, physicians and patients together must critically determine whether surgery can be expected to bring definitive relief. No operation has been found to be universally effective. Patients must be made aware of the potential that their pain symptoms may not be totally resolved by the surgery. The patient will not only appreciate the physician's frankness in estimating the likelihood of success, she also will be more likely to see her physician as a long-term management partner in this difficult situation. Conservative counseling on the part of the surgeon can minimize any potential deleterious effects of surgery such as hysterectomy and also maximize the possibility that the patient's expectations will be realistic.

MULTIDISCIPLINARY APPROACH TO PELVIC PAIN— A CONTEMPORARY MODEL

As an overriding philosophic approach to the patient with chronic pelvic pain, the multidisciplinary approach considers all potential sources of pain at the outset rather than only after ruling out gynecologic pathology. The benefits of such a model have been most clearly demonstrated in a study by Peters and coworkers, in which patients were randomized to either traditional or nontraditional pelvic pain therapy—the latter focusing on dietary, psychological, physiotherapeutic, and environmental as well as somatic issues.[38] Patients who underwent an evaluation process that did not necessarily include diagnostic laparoscopy but focused on a wide array of possible sources for their pelvic pain had less pain, less disturbance of their daily activities, and fewer associated symptoms. This randomized trial of two different management schemes clearly demonstrates how a clinician can collect appropriate, interested practitioners who complement his or her interests and expertise in managing such patients.

Far too often, patients are assumed to have gynecologic disorders first and having had those conditions ruled out, are told either directly or indirectly that their problem is more likely to have a psychiatric or psychosomatic etiology. Messages such as this do not fully address the needs of the patient, nor do they address potential medical conditions from which these patients suffer. Although it is not logical for a busy office practice to employ all the needed medical specialists and subspecialists in addition to nonphysician healthcare providers, a network of providers can easily be implemented over time, with the patient being managed realistically. By using an integrated, longitudinal approach, patients are less likely to embark on adventures into emergency departments, where they are evaluated by providers with no previous insight into their problems or expectation of seeing them for follow-up care. By getting to know their providers, patients are more likely to reveal their true emotional ties to their symptoms, thereby allowing more effective intervention on a psychosocial level.

In a holistic approach to these patients, counseling, surgery, behavior modification, medications, and physical therapy all potentially play a role. By having at least a working knowledge of the various diagnostic and therapeutic modalities available to the patient, the individual clinician can better aid the patient in her understanding of chronic pain, generally, and her own pelvic pain, specifically.

REFERENCES

1. Smith RP, Ling FW: "Gynevision." Obstet Gynecol 78:708, 1991
2. Cunanan RG, Courey NG, Lippes J: Laparoscopic findings in patients with pelvic pain. Am J Obstet Gynecol 146:589, 1983
3. King PM, Meyers CA, Ling FW, et al: Musculoskeletal factors in chronic pelvic pain. J Psychom Obstet Gynecol 12:87, 1991
4. Sinaki M, Merritt JL, Stillwell GW: Tension myalgia of the pelvic floor. Mayo Clin Proc 52:717, 1977
5. Adelman AA: Abdominal pain in the primary care setting. J Fam Pract 25:27, 1987
6. Slocumb JC: Neurologic factors in chronic pelvic pain: trigger points and the abdominal pelvic pain syndrome. Am J Obstet Gynecol 149:536, 1984
7. Summitt RL, Ling FW: Urethral syndrome presenting as chronic pelvic pain. J Psychom Obstet Gynecol 12(Suppl):77, 1991
8. Lilius HG, Orovisto KJ, Valtronen EJ: Origin of pain in interstitial cystitis. Scand J Urol Nephrol 7:150, 1973
9. Fall M, Johannson SL, Aldenberg F: Chronic interstitial cystitis: a heterogeneous syndrome. J Urol 137:35, 1987
10. Parsons CL, Lilly JD, Stein P: Epithelial dysfunction in nonbacterial cystitis (interstitial cystitis). J Urol 145:732, 1991
11. Reiter RC: A profile of women with chronic pelvic pain. Current Problems in Obstetric, Gynecology and Fertility 14:102, 1991
12. Wall PD: The gate control theory of pain. Brain 101:1, 1978
13. Melzack R: Neurophysiologic foundations of pain. In Steinbach RA (ed): The physiology of pain, p 1. New York, Raven Press, 1986
14. Rosenthal RH, Ling FW, Rosenthal TL, et al: Chronic pelvic pain: psychological features and laparascopic findings. Psychomatics 25:833, 1984
15. Blumer D, Heilbron M: Chronic pain as a variant of depression disease: the pain-prone disorder. J Nerve Ment Dis 170:381, 1982
16. Walker AE, Katon WJ, Harrop-Griffiths J, et al: Relationshp of chronic pelvic pain to psychiatric diagnoses and childhood sexual abuse. Am J Psych 145:75, 1988
17. Rapkin AJ, Kames LD, Darke LL, et al: History of physical and sexual abuse in women with chronic pelvic pain. Obstet Gynecol 79:92, 1990
18. Reiter RC, Shaperin LR, Gambone JC, et al: Correlation between sexual abuse and somatization in

women with somatic and nonsomatic chronic pelvic pain. Am J Obstet Gynecol 165:104, 1991

19. Vercellini P, Fedel L, Monlteni P, et al: Laparoscopy in the diagnosis of gynecologic chronic pelvic pain. Int J Gynaecol Obstet 32:261, 1990

20. Levitan Z, Eibschitz I, deVries K, et al: Value of laparoscopy in women with chronic pelvic pain and normal pelvis. Int J Gynaecol Obstet 23:71, 1985

21. Martin DC, Hubert GD, VanderZwaag R, et al: Laparoscopic appearances of perinotenal endometriosis. Fertil Steril 51:63, 1989

22. Baker PN, Symonds EM: The resolution of chronic pelvic pain after normal laparoscopy findings. Am J Obstet Gynecol 166:835, 1992

23. Steege JF, Stoot AL: Resolution of chronic pelvic pain after laparoscopic lysis of adhesions. Am J Obstet Gynecol 165:278, 1991

24. Chan CLK, Wood C: Pelvic adhesiolysis—the assessment of symptom relief by 100 patients. Aust NZ J Obstet Gynaecol 25:295, 1985

25. Daniell JF: Laparoscopic enterolysis for chronic abdominal pain. J Gynecol Surg 5:61, 1989

26. Peters AAW, Trimbos-Kemper GCM, Admirella C, et al: A randomized trial on the benefit of adhesiolysis in patients with intraperitoneal adhesions and chronic pelvic pain. Br J Obstet Gynaecol 99:59, 1992

27. Malinack LR: Interceed R (T&C) as an adjuvant for adhesion reduction: clinical studies. In de Zerega GS, Malinak LR, Diamond MP, et al (eds): Treatment of post surgical adhesions, p 193. New York, Wiley-Liss, 1990

28. Massouda D, Ling FW, Muram D, et al: Laparoscopic uterine suspension utilizing falope rings. J Reprod Med 32:859, 1987

29. Duncan CH, Taylor HC: A psychosomatic study of pelvic congestion. Am J Obstet Gynecol 64:1, 1952

30. Rundqvist E, Sandholm LE, Larsson G: Treatment of pelvic varicosities causing lower abdominal pain with extraperitoneal resection of the left ovarian vein. Ann Chir Gynaecol 73:339, 1984

31. Beard RW, Reginald PQ, Wadsworth J: Clinical features of women with chronic lower abdominal pain and pelvic congestion. Br J Obstet Gynaecol 95: 193, 1988

32. Bukovsky I, Liftshitz Y, Langer R, et al: Ovarian residual syndrome. Surg Gynecol Obstet 167:132, 1988

33. Perez JJ: Laparoscopic presacral neurectomy—results of the first 25 cases. J Reprod Med 35:625, 1990

34. Black WT: Use of presacral sympathectomy in the treatment of dysmenorrhea: a second look after twenty-five years. Am J Obstet Gynecol 89:16, 1964

35. Lee RB, Stone K, Magelessen D, et al: Presacral neurectomy for chronic pelvic pain. Obstet Gynecol 68:517, 1986

36. Vercellini P, Fedele L, Bianchi S, et al: Pelvic denervation for chronic pain associated with endometriosis: fact or fancy? Am J Obstet Gynecol 165:745, 1991

37. Stovall TG, Ling FW, Crawford DA: Hysterectomy for chronic pelvic pain of presumed uterine etiology. Obstet 75:676, 1990

38. Peters AAW, vanDorst E, Jellis B, et al: A randomized clinical trial to compare two different approaches in women with chronic pelvic pain. Obstet Gynecol 77:740, 1991

Ambulatory Gynecology, Second Edition,
edited by David H. Nichols and Patrick J. Sweeney.
J. B. Lippincott Company, Philadelphia, © 1995.

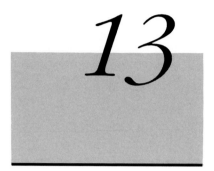

13

Sexual Assault

Dorothy J. Hicks

RAPE AND THE MANAGEMENT OF THE RAPE VICTIM

Epidemiology of Rape

Forcible rape is one of the fastest growing violent crimes in the United States; it is estimated that one forcible rape occurs every 5 minutes. The 1992 Uniform Crime Reports (UCR) show there is an 18% increase in reported rapes since 1988.[1] In 1992, 109,062 rapes were reported to law enforcement—a rate of 84/100,000 and a 2% increase from 1991. Eighty-six percent of occurrences were rape by force; the rest were attempted rape. At best, it is estimated that only one in four rapes are reported.

Forcible rape, as defined for the Uniform Crime Reports, is the carnal knowledge of a female forcibly and against her will. Assaults or attempts to commit rape by force or threat of force are also included; however, statutory rape (without force) is not included in these statistics. This definition is no longer sufficient in light of our present knowledge and many states have changed or are in the process of changing from the old rape laws to sexual battery laws. These newer statutes, which are more inclusive, are similar to homicide statutes. They describe degrees of sexual battery against any person, regardless of age.

> *Sexual battery means oral, anal or vaginal penetration by or union with the sexual organs of another or the anal or vaginal penetration of another by any other object; however, sexual battery shall not include acts done for bona fide medical purposes.*
> **Florida State Law 794.0111**

Under the newer statutes, "penetration" is no longer necessary; "union with" is sufficient; "consent" is the key word. The age of consent varies from state to state; in Florida, the age of consent is 12 years of age and there is no statutory rape law. The concept of marital rape is recognized in 12 states but such charges are usually prosecuted as assault and battery. People who work with these victims have long known that rape is violence and not a sexual act but the general public usually considers the victim of sexual battery to be as guilty as the offender.

Little was written on the subject until the late 1950s, and most of those articles were in law enforcement and sociology journals. In 1971, Amir published one of the first studies of forcible rapes in Philadelphia.[2] In 1971, Evrard was one of the first gynecologists to discuss the medical, social, and legal implications of this crime.[3] In 1979, Brownmiller's tome explored rape from the dawn of history to the present time.[4] In the 1970s, the women's movement in the United States provided the impetus to make the country aware of (1) the plight of rape victims, and (2) that rape is a violent rather than a sexual act. Progress is still being made in helping victims of sexual battery survive this trauma.

The Rapist

Anyone who comes into contact with rape victims must understand the dynamics of sexual battery and know something about the sex offender if they are to be of real help to the victims. It is recognized that rape is a crime of violence, the motive for the attack being anger, hostility, or the need to humiliate, degrade, or overpower someone. Rape is not the craving for sex that it is commonly thought to be; rape is violence. Attitudes are changing and law enforcement, the courts, and medical personnel are taking a different approach to both the rape victim and the attacker. The attack is only the beginning of problems for the victim; her difficulties intensify and compound after the assault. All victims need psychological and medical treatment. The "nuisance" offenders—the "peeping toms" who once were thought to be harmless—are no longer ignored by the authorities. These offenders often progress to rape and rape–homicide as they become older and more aggressive. Ideally, all sex offenders should be provided psychotherapy, although some must be incarcerated.

Rape is a repetitive crime; therefore, once a rapist is apprehended, he is usually charged with several assaults. Each rapist has a modus operandi; he does the same thing in the same way every time. At least half the men are married and many others have a relationship with an adult female. One man in a therapy program volunteered the information that he would "have sex with my girlfriend" and then "stop and rape a woman on my way home."

The victim was just a "thing" to him. He chose her because she was vulnerable and fit his pattern. Many men say they could not recognize the victim once the attack was over.

Groth, who has worked extensively with sex offenders, divides the crime into three categories: power rape, anger rape, and sadistic rape.[5] At one time, rapists were thought not to progress; however, it is now known that as they continue to rape, many become more violent.

Power Rape

In the power rape, the goal of the rapist is sexual conquest but not sexual gratification. Overpowering his victim is the objective; by controlling her, the rapist compensates for his feelings of worthlessness and inadequacy. These men are usually in the younger age groups, and their victims are of the same age or younger.

The power rapist may stalk his victim. He often kidnaps her, holds her for a time, and rapes her repeatedly. He uses only enough force to subdue his victim and makes her submit to his advances. Physical injury to the woman is not common. Because the attack never lives up to his fantasy, the attacker rapes again and again in an effort to find the "right" victim.

Because the offenders are usually young, these cases are often plea-bargained to a charge of assault or breaking and entering and are never reported as rape. The "date" or acquaintance rape is in this class. About 55% of all rapes reported are in this category.

Anger Rape

In the anger rape, the expression of anger and hostility is more spontaneous and episodic than the power rape. The attack may be triggered by sudden stress, such as an argument; the victim is the target of the attacker's rage. The offender wants to hurt and degrade his victim, so he forces her to do such things as perform fellatio, sodomy, and other sexual acts that may offend her. He also uses more physical force than necessary to get her to submit, and the victim may have significant physical injuries. This man strikes when his frustrations and anger build to the point of eruption.

Sadistic Rape

Sadistic rapes constitute only about 5% of the reported rapes. The sadistic offender intentionally harms and mistreats his victim, who in many cases does not survive the attack. It is common for the sexual areas of the woman's body to be the focus of violence, such as biting, burning, or insertion of foreign objects. The attack is premeditated but the victim, chosen at random, is just someone who is vulnerable and happens along at the "right" moment. Physical force is eroticized. The sadistic rapist often has a Jekyll-and-Hyde type of personality. He is the most dangerous of the rapists, his aim being to punish and destroy his victim, literally or figuratively.

Rehabilitation

The recidivism rate for rapists is high; some workers in this field believe that it may be as great as 90% if they are incarcerated without psychotherapy. Because of this, the authorities have become interested in rehabilitation programs for sex offenders. Although some sex offenders may never learn to control their emotions, intensive psychotherapy helps many realize that violence, not sex, is the motive for their crimes.

The average length of treatment is 3 years, although it may take longer, and the offenders are never considered to be "cured" but are "recovering." The State of Florida had three such programs but in 1990, funding was withdrawn after 14 years. The recidivism rate after therapy was 6% (corrected to 1% for sex crimes). Psychological therapy is less expensive than sending offenders to prison, and the end result is better for both the offender and the community.

The Victim

Examination

After I was raped, it was very hard for me to deal with people. I was afraid of almost everything. I had the kind of job that required me to be active and independent but I couldn't make decisions; I couldn't do anything. I was afraid to go out alone. My boyfriend couldn't understand what had happened to me, so he left me. My life was a disaster. It was 3 months before I could do anything by myself.

Susan is a 29-year-old rape victim. She, like many other young women, had problems gaining control of her life after being raped. She moved, changed jobs, and lost contact with her friends and family. Susan was not battered but was held at gunpoint for 5 hours. It has been 2 years but she still has nightmares about the rape and is still in therapy.

Rape victims need comprehensive, expert care if they are to survive the incident and return to a functioning state.[6] Even victims of uncompleted rape need psychological counseling and guidance. Ideally, only people who understand the nature of the crime and are empathetic should come into contact with these patients and their significant others; this includes hospital personnel as well as police. The manner in which these patients are managed from the outset sets the course for the entire postrape period, including the prosecution of the rapist, and determines how rapidly and successfully the victim recovers from the trauma.

The crisis of rape may produce a post-traumatic stress disorder. Rape victims are emergencies and must be treated as such. Because few are hysterical or injured physically, it is often difficult to realize how traumatized they are. The most common emotion experienced by the victim of a rape is fear—absolute terror that she will be killed. Because of this, victims are usually exhausted and quiet and they may even withdraw.

A private quiet area should be available to the rape victim and the significant person or persons with her, so that she is not a part of the busy emergency room atmosphere. She should be escorted to this place immediately and examined as soon as possible after her arrival. The word rape should never be used in her presence. Rape is a legal term, and the judgment can only be rendered by a jury.

The patient should never be left alone once she reaches the hospital. If no significant others or police are with her, a nurse or counselor should stay until the doctor arrives.

It is essential that the victim be given control of her life as soon as possible after the attack, and no unnecessary questions should be asked by hospital personnel. If the police are not present, she should be asked whether she wishes to report the crime. She should be encouraged to do so but no pressure should be put on her. In many cases, explaining to the patient that rape is a repetitive violent crime rather than a sexual act and that the purpose of the rapist is to hurt and humiliate her may help her to decide. Only if the victim agrees should the police be notified. In Florida, unless the patient is under the age of consent (12 years old), it is not necessary to report the crime to the police but the law varies from state to state.

The gender of the people caring for the patient is usually not important. Although a female nurse should always be present during the examination of a female patient, the gender of the doctor is seldom an issue. In fact, coming into contact with a normal, understanding male is generally psychologically therapeutic for the female rape victim. Although most older male victims are more comfortable with a male physician, it is the attitude of the examiner that is the most important factor.

The nurse should be supportive and understanding and allow the patient to talk if she wishes to do so.

The victim should never be rushed and although the nurse should allow the patient to ventilate, she or he should not ask the patient to recite the details of the crime. Nothing but the basic information that is needed to start a chart should be obtained at this time. Appropriate consent forms must be signed to allow examination, treatment, photographs, and collection of evidence. If the patient is a young child, the parent or responsible party must sign. If the patient is old enough to understand, both the child and the parent should sign the consent forms. Each signature should be witnessed and dated.

It is essential that the victim be given control of her life as soon as possible after the attack. If the physical trauma is such that it demands immediate attention, the forensic portion of the examination may be delayed until the patient is stable; it may be performed in the operating room if necessary.

TAKING THE HISTORY. The physician should obtain an accurate but not detailed history of the crime.[7] If the police are present, it is helpful for the examiner to obtain a skeleton history of the crime from the police before seeing the patient. The doctor should ask the patient only about things that are pertinent to the examination. Forcing the victim to go over the crime again and again is not good for her mental health. The physician must ask, however, about sodomy, fellatio, invasion of the vagina by fingers or foreign bodies, and any other sexual acts performed during the attack. Patients are often too embarrassed to tell anyone but the doctor about these things. Teenagers and elderly patients are particularly likely to confide only in the doctor.

The medical chart should be written as much as possible in terms that laypersons understand because it will be used primarily by the police and attorneys (Fig. 13-1). Black ink is the best color to use because the chart will be photocopied many times. The examiner should leave the investigation

of the crime to the police; this is not the function of the physician and may jeopardize the case when it goes to trial. The victim is often confused immediately after the attack, and the details she gives about the crime itself may be wrong. It is the work of trained police investigators, not the examiner, to piece together an accurate account of the crime.

If the patient is an adult, no one except the doctor and nurse should be in the examining room with the victim unless she requests otherwise. The teenager should be examined without a parent present but the young child is more cooperative if a parent is with her. Police officers should never be in the room.

The date and time of the examination should be documented and the date and time of the assault noted. The patient's parity and gravidity, the date of her last menstrual period, the date and time of her last consensual intercourse, and whether or not contraception was used are important. The reasons for these and any other questions should be explained to the victim as the examination proceeds.

An abbreviated past history should be obtained, including any allergies and significant illnesses or surgery. Whether the patient has had hepatitis or venereal disease and the treatment given are of importance to the people who will be handling the specimens. This is no longer significant in many areas, however, because the human immunodeficiency (HIV) virus is so prevalent that all specimens are handled as though the material is infectious.

Has the victim been sexually assaulted before? This is significant because a patient who has been previously assaulted sexually—whether as a child or an adult—and has never resolved the trauma will have an unusually strong reaction to this attack.

The history of the attack should contain the essentials but not the details of the crime. How many attackers were there? Did she know them? Were they relatives? What did they look like? Answers to these questions may determine how she will react.

Did the rapist have a weapon? Did she resist the attack? Patients with the most severe physical injuries are often those who fought the rapist. Was she held down or restrained? If so, with what? Answers to these questions guide the physician to look for bruises, rope burns, and other injuries.

Where was the patient when the rapist approached her? Where did he take her? Where did the attack occur? Did she have to remove all her clothes or only her underpants? Answers to these questions also help the examiner and may explain

FILE COPY

RAPE TREATMENT CENTER

JACKSON MEMORIAL HOSPITAL   UNIVERSITY OF MIAMI SCHOOL OF MEDICINE

PATIENTS
ADDRESS_____

PLACE OF EXAM_____ DATE: _____

PERSONAL HISTORY   TIME: _____

PARA ___ ___ ___ ___ GR. _____

LMP: DATE_____NORMAL ABNORMAL

LAST COITUS: DATE_____TIME:_____

CONTRACEPTION: YES NO TYPE:_____

DOUCHE BATH DEFECATE VOID SINCE ASSAULT

VENEREAL DISEASE: YES NO TYPE_____RX_____

HEPATITIS: YES NO WHEN_____RX_____

HISTORY OF ASSAULT_____

DATE:_____TIME:_____

LOCATION: _____

NO. OF ASSAILANTS_____RACE: B W L O UNK

ATTACKER: KNOWN_____UNK_____RELATIVE_____

THREATS: YES NO TYPE_____

RESTRAINTS: YES NO TYPE_____

WEAPON: YES NO TYPE_____
RESIST: YES NO
                    ORAL ANAL VAGINAL DIGITAL FOR. BODY
TYPE OF SEX: _____ _____ _____ _____ _____

PENETRATION: _____ _____ _____ _____ _____

EJACULATION: _____ _____ _____ _____ _____

COMMENTS:_____

BIRTHDATE_____RACE_____M S W D SEP

POLICE DEPT. _____CASE #_____

OFFICER_____

GENERAL EXAM: (bruises, trauma, lacerations, marks)
NO HISTORY·

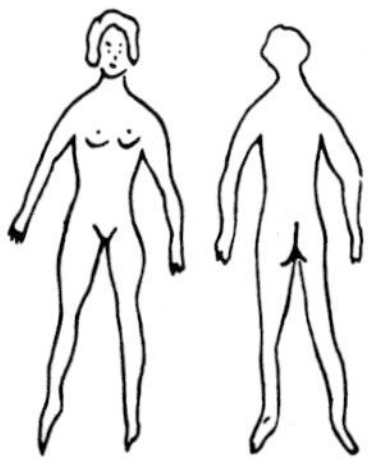

PELVIC EXAM: (include signs of trauma, bleeding, foreign bodies)
VULVA_____

HYMEN_____

VAGINA_____

CERVIX_____

FUNDUS_____

ADNEXAE_____

RECTAL_____

JMH-02-5662-6
8-1-78

PAGE 1	**SEXUAL BATTERY FORM**

Figure 13–1.   Rape-treatment–center form. (*continued*)

FILE COPY
RAPE TREATMENT CENTER
MIAMI, FLORIDA

JACKSON MEMORIAL HOSPITAL   UNIVERSITY OF MIAMI SCHOOL OF MEDICINE

PHYSICIAN_____ NURSE _____ COUNSELOR _____

TESTS   HEIGHT_____   WEIGHT_____   **TREATMENT**

GC CULTURE: ORAL ANAL CERVICAL OTHER _____   V.D. PROPHYLAXIS: YES   NO TYPE _____

VDRL: YES NO (5cc venous blood - red top)   PREGNANCY PROPHYLAXIS: YES NO TYPE _____

PAP TEST: YES NO   TETANUS: YES NO OTHER MEDS:_____

EVIDENTIAL SPECIMENS, TESTING AND RECEIPT

RESULTS OF PRELIMINARY TESTS: A.P.: NEGATIVE   WEAK   MODERATE   STRONG

SPERM: NONE 1-5   6-10   10 +   MOTILE   NON-MOTILE

SPECIMENS OBTAINED:	GIVEN TO POLICE	OTHER TREATMENT
10 cc VENOUS BLOOD (red top)_____	_____	X-RAY_____
FINGER NAIL SCRAPINGS _____	_____	SURGICAL CONSULT _____
PUBIC HAIR COMBINGS_____	_____	PSYCH. CONSULT_____
VAGINAL { SMEAR_____ SWAB_____	_____ _____	OTHER: (Explain)_____ _____
CERVICAL { SMEAR_____ SWAB_____	_____ _____	_____
VAGINAL ASPIRATE _____	_____	_____
RECTAL { SMEAR_____ SWAB_____	_____ _____	_____
ORAL { SMEAR_____ SWAB_____	_____ _____	_____
SALIVA SPECIMEN _____	_____	GIVEN TO POLICE

CLOTHING (number)_____ { TYPE _____
                              CONDITION _____

FOREIGN BODIES (number) _____ { TYPE _____
                                      LOCATION _____

OTHER SPECIMENS_____   PHOTOGRAPHS: YES NO TAKEN BY_____

TOTAL NUMBER SPECIMENS _____   **TOTAL TO POLICE** _____

RECEIPT OF EVIDENCE: THE ABOVE EVIDENCE HAS BEEN RECEIVED BY ME ON (DATE) _____ AT

(TIME)_____   (OFFICER'S SIGNATURE)_____

PHYSICIANS SIGNATURE:_____

WITNESS SIGNATURE_____

JMH-02-5662-6
8-1-78

PAGE 2 | **SEXUAL BATTERY FORM**

Figure 13–1.   (Continued)

foreign bodies found in the victim's hair or on her skin, such as lint, dirt, or leaves.

Whenever possible, the patient's own words should be used and put into quotation marks. If an interpreter is used, the name of the interpreter should be documented.

A general note on the patient's emotional state may be made but it is not necessary to elaborate. It is also not necessary to draw blood samples for alcohol or drug levels unless the police specifically request them.

PHYSICAL EXAMINATION. Figure 13-2 shows the instruments and supplies needed for an examination.[8] The patient should be completely disrobed and garbed in a hospital gown. This is particularly true for young victims; physical abuse often accompanies sexual abuse when a child is the object of an attack. The light should be good so injuries can be seen easily. Documentation of findings not related to the rape incident is not required. Old track marks, tattoos, and scars may prejudice a jury. Any abrasions, ecchymoses, contusions, lacerations, and scratches must be described accurately and their size recorded in inches so laypersons can appreciate the extent of the victim's injuries. Most laymen are not skilled in the metric system and cannot visualize the size of lesions described in centi-meters; jurors are usually laymen. Bruises from gripping by the fingers of the offender are commonly found on the victim's neck, upper arms, breasts, and medial aspects of the thighs.

Because tooth marks may identify an offender, any bite marks should be carefully documented and photographed. Whenever possible, a forensic dentist should be called in for consultation. Tooth marks may be as individual as fingerprints.

If the patient has been beaten or slapped on the face, the lips and mucosa of the oral cavity should be inspected for lacerations or bruises.

If the patient resisted and scratched the attacker, scrapings should be taken from underneath her fingernails. An orange stick may be used for this, and the scrapings and the orange stick placed in a clean white envelope and sealed. Broken nails should be clipped and preserved in a similar manner; a piece of nail found at the scene of the crime may match the broken edge. Any foreign bodies should be identified and saved.[9]

If the attacker ejaculated on the patient's skin or in the hairy areas, the semen may be identified by inspection. Under direct light, the dried seminal stain is a scaly, glistening pale yellow. Under a Wood's lamp (filtered ultraviolet light), this area fluoresces. Filter paper or cotton-tipped applicators moistened with saline may be used to lift the semen

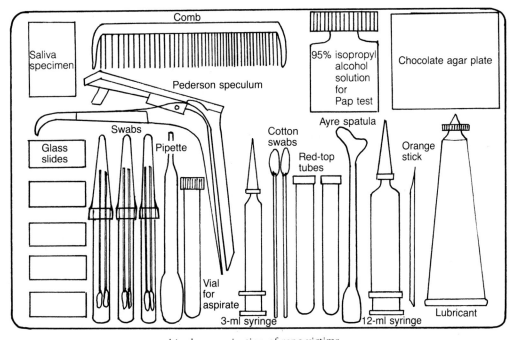

Figure 13–2.   Instruments used in the examination of rape victims.

from the skin surface. If there is evidence of semen in the hair, the hairs may be clipped and put in a white envelope, which is then sealed. Any positive findings should be carefully documented.

If the patient described fellatio, her mouth and pharynx should be swabbed with cotton-tipped applicators and an air-dried smear made. Special attention should be paid to the areas between the teeth and cheeks, behind the upper central incisors, and under the tongue. If ejaculation occurred, semen may sometimes be recovered from the nasal mucous by having the patient blow her nose into a piece of clean cloth. This should be performed even if the patient has drunk something or brushed her teeth since the attack. If she did clean her mouth, she should be asked what she used. Washings from the mouth are difficult to obtain and are usually less satisfactory than swabs and smears. A culture for gonorrhea should be taken from the nasopharynx, plated on chocolate agar, provided with a carbon dioxide atmosphere, and incubated as soon as possible. If sodomy occurred, the perirectal area should be inspected carefully. Any evidence of lubricant should be recorded and the material collected. The tone of the external sphincter should be noted and any splits in the perianal area should be described carefully. Washings from the rectum may be obtained with difficulty by placement of a saline-filled syringe into the anus and injection of the material into the lumen (5 to 10 mm saline). After about 2 minutes, the fluid may be retrieved and placed into a test tube and the tube capped. Specimens may also be obtained from the rectum with cotton-tipped swabs, from which an air-dried smear is made. The swabs should be free of feces. Both the swabs and the smear are sent to the forensic laboratory. A culture for gonorrhea should also be taken from the rectum. Digital exploration of the rectum should be performed and if indicated, a proctoscope should be used. If the adult patient denies that fellatio or sodomy has occurred, it is usually not necessary to subject her to these examinations.

Most victims have been violated vaginally, in which case, careful inspection of the external genital area is indicated. Any matted pubic hair may be cut out with scissors and placed in a clean white envelope. The hair should then be combed briskly and the comb and combings placed in a separate clean envelope. Some law enforcement agencies demand that the pubic hair be plucked because most of the information needed to identify hair is found in the root portion.[10] Identification of hair samples may be helpful in some instances but it is not absolute identification. Because plucking pubic hair is painful and traumatic and because 40 to 50 hairs are needed if the specimen is to be valid, our examiners comb briskly, with the understanding that if hairs are to be a factor in the prosecution, the patient will consent to plucking. Only 14% of the reported cases are prosecuted.

If cunnilingus occurred, moistened cotton swabs may be used to obtain specimens of the attacker's saliva from the areas involved. The forensic laboratory can examine these for secreted substances.

The inner aspect of both thighs and the vulva should be inspected for abrasions, contusions, lacerations, and foreign materials. Unless the attack was brutal, there is seldom any obvious injury in the vulvovaginal area of women who are sexually active or have delivered children vaginally. Some examiners use colposcopes in an effort to identify abrasions of the vestibular and vaginal tissues.[11] If bruises or lacerations are noted, they should be described accurately. A clock face is usually used to document the location (eg, 5 o'clock, 7 o'clock). Many examiners believe that most perihymenal and introital injuries occur between 9 and 3 o'clock, whereas the most common location for penetration tears is between 4 and 8 o'clock. If the trauma is recent, some bleeding is commonly seen. Toluidine blue may be used to stain the areas.[12]

It is important to inspect the hymenal area. On the chart, the word "marital" and "virginal" should be avoided. If the woman has been sexually active or has had previous vaginal surgery, "parous," "remnants," and "old scarring" are terms better suited to this examination. Any evidence of recent invasion should be described but it is not necessary to describe remnants (hymenal tags).

Careful inspection of the vaginal canal and cervix should be performed next. Most patients are tender and sore because there was no natural lubrication of the vagina during the assault. Because lubricant interferes with the forensic tests, only water may be used to moisten the speculum. The speculum of choice is a Pederson because it is narrow. If a tampon is present, it should be removed and sent to the forensic laboratory as evidence.

Any laceration of the vaginal walls or cervix should be described in detail. The color and viscosity of secretions in the vaginal canal should be described. Ideally, nonabsorbent cotton-tipped swabs should be used to obtain samples from the proximal portion of the vagina and an air-dried smear made on a glass slide. Similar swabs should be taken from the fornices and an air-dried smear made. The endocervical canal should be avoided in victims who have had consensual intercourse within 3 weeks because spermatozoa can remain motile for several days and morphologically intact in the endocervical mucous for up to 17 days postexposure. Consequently, sperm identified in the cervical mucous may have been present long before the sexual assault occurred.

After swabs have been taken, 2 mL of sterile saline may be injected into the vagina and retrieved by a pipette. This pipette should be a disposable one-piece unit, so that there is no chance of contamination from a previous examination. The solution should be retrieved, placed in a glass tube, capped, and labeled "vaginal aspirate." After all the forensic specimens have been taken, a Papanicolaou (Pap) test may be performed; if performed earlier, scraping the cervix with the spatula may cause bleeding, which interferes with the forensic tests. The Pap test often provides a permanent record of sperm.

Cultures for gonorrhea and *Chlamydia trachomatis* should be taken from the endocervical canal and sent to the clinical laboratory.[13]

A bimanual pelvic examination should be done. This reveals gross pathology, such as ovarian cysts and pregnancy. The vaginal epithelium should be palpated carefully; lacerations in the mucosa are often more easily palpated than visualized.

A sample of the patient's saliva should be obtained so the laboratory can check for her secretor status. A secretor is a person whose body fluids contain a water-soluble form of the antigens of the ABO blood group in the red blood cells. About 80% of the population are secretors. The other 20% are called nonsecretors. If the victim is a secretor, her blood-group antigens may be secreted in her vaginal fluids and coat the sperm in the vagina. Sperm of secretors can be typed according to the blood-group antigens. If the sperm type is the same as the victim's blood type, and if she is a secretor, there is always the possibility that the sperm may been typed falsely by having been coated by her secretor substance. The victim's secretor status must be determined to eliminate this possibility. A small square of clean white cloth or a piece of filter paper may be used. It is important that no one but the patient touch the material so that it is not contaminated. The specimen should then be put into a clean container and sealed.

Venous blood should be drawn and placed into two tubes. One is sent for serology and the second to the forensic laboratory for sophisticated testing; our forensic laboratory uses a tiger-top tube. If the police request toxicology tests, we collect a specimen of urine from the patient. Unless specifically requested, however, this is not performed routinely.

The patient may be concerned about acquired immunodeficiency syndrome.[14] If she wishes to be tested for the virus, blood should be drawn and placed in a tiger-top tube. In Florida, the patient must request a test for HIV; it cannot be performed unless the patient requests it, and there are strict guidelines that must be followed. The patient must be given pre- and post-test counseling and should have follow-up tests 3 and 6 months after the initial test if the tests are negative. Human immunodeficiency virus has added to the rape victim's problems. Most patients are well aware that they are at risk, although there are no reliable reports on the incidence of HIV infection after rape. Florida permits the victim to request HIV testing of the sex offender once they are charged with the crime.[15]

After completion of the physical examination, the examiner should make a wet mount from the vaginal aspirate and examine it under the microscope. The number of sperm per high-power field and whether they are motile should be recorded. Sperm usually remain motile in the vaginal canal for only 4 to 6 hours because of the acidity of the vagina. They may, however, be found in the vaginal canal for more than 72 hours. If no sperm are found, the aspirate may be checked for acid phosphatase (AP), an enzyme found in large quantities in the seminal fluid of man and ape.[16] There are small quantities of acid phosphatase in vaginal fluid, fecal material, red blood cells, and occasionally, saliva. A high level of AP in the vagina is generally accepted as evidence of the presence of semen. The qualitative test is considered positive only when a deep purple color develops within 10 seconds after the dye is added to the solution. We no longer test for AP because the forensic laboratory used by our police is testing all specimens for DNA. DNA is thought to be as individual as fingerprints.[17]

All specimens must be carefully labeled with the name of the patient, the location from which it was obtained, the date, and the initials of the person taking the material. All specimens should be placed in a paper bag and the bag sealed with evidence tape and properly identified. A plastic bag should never be used; it permits moisture to develop, causing an overgrowth of bacteria, which may destroy the specimen. Ideally, the bag should be handed directly to a police officer. If no one is there to receive the specimens, the bag should be placed in a refrigerator and the refrigerator locked. Signatures must be obtained each time the evidence is transferred from one person to another, so that the chain of evidence remains intact.

Clothing worn by the victim at the time of the attack is important evidence. Whenever possible, only the police should deal with the clothing; this keeps hospital personnel out of the chain of custody for the clothing. If this is not feasible, the clothing should be identified, handled as little as possible, placed in a paper bag, and the bag sealed.

All injuries should be photographed. Whenever possible, photographs should be taken by a police photographer so there is no question as to who took the pictures and their whereabouts since that time. If this is impossible, the exposed film should be given to the police so they can have it developed; the chain of evidence thereby remains intact.

The physician and hospital personnel should never become involved in the detailed history of the crime itself. "Rape" is a legal term, not a medical diagnosis, and it is impossible for the examiner to state that the patient was raped; the physician was not there and can say only that the evidence does or does not support the patient's immediate history. If the chart is legible and written in terms that laypersons can understand, the examiner often does not have to appear at the trial; the chart is sufficient.

Medical Treatment

All victims of sexual battery, even if they have not been brutalized, benefit from medical and psychological care. Such care should be available regardless of whether the patient decides to report the crime to the authorities. Although the victim must be allowed to make the decision, she should be encouraged to obtain treatment as soon as possible after the attack.

Medical treatment consists of examination to be sure that there has been no physical damage, accurate description of any trauma, and proper collection of specimens for evidence if the case is to be reported to the police. Tetanus toxoid and prophylactic medication for venereal disease and pregnancy should be offered when indicated. X-ray films and specialty consultations should be ordered whenever indicated. Severe injuries take precedence over the forensic examination and should be dealt with first.

The most common medication used for the prevention of syphilis and gonorrhea in our area is cephtriaxone sodium, 250 mg for adults and 125 mg for children, given intramuscularly. Penicillin is no longer used because the incidence of penicillin-resistant gonorrhea is almost 50%. If desired, probenecid, 1 g orally, followed by 4.8 million U aqueous penicillin, given intramuscularly, half in each buttock, may be used. Both of these medications prevent incubating syphilis and treat gonorrhea.

If the patient is allergic to either of those medications, spectinomycin, 2 g given intramuscularly, treats gonorrhea but does not prevent syphilis. Doxycycline, 300 mg perorally, followed in 1 hour by a second 300-mg peroral dose, may also be used.

If the patient appears likely to follow a medical regimen on her own, tetracycline, 500 mg perorally every 6 hours for 14 days, or doxycycline, 100 mg twice daily for 10 days, may be used instead to treat *Chlamydia trachomatis*, a disease of increasing significance.

The risk of pregnancy post-rape is thought to be about 1%. This should be explained to the patient and she should be offered prophylactic medication to prevent pregnancy. Treatment should be withheld, however, from patients who are adamant against pregnancy termination should conception occur. All patients do not take medication as prescribed and a fetus may be at risk.

If pregnancy is suspected, a pregnancy test should be performed before medication is given. We prefer a quantitative β-subunit assay for human chorionic gonadotropin because this test is capable of determining pregnancy 10 days after ovulation.

Prophylaxis for pregnancy is usually effective if given within 72 hours after exposure, before implantation of the fertilized ovum. Hormone therapy in the form of the "morning-after pill" is the most popular. Several different drugs may be prescribed. The combination tablet of ethinyl estradiol and norgestrel (Ovral) is the most commonly used: two tablets given orally, followed by two tablets in 12 hours.[18] Compliance is good because only one dose needs to be taken after leaving the hospital and usually there are no side effects.

Ethinyl estradiol (0.5 mg/day for 5 days) and diethylstilbestrol (25 mg twice a day for 5 days) are other drugs commonly used. Compliance is poor with these medications because of the length of treatment and because nausea is a problem in about 75% of patients. An antiemetic should also be given: trimethobenzamide (250 mg perorally, 45 minutes before each dose of diethylstilbestrol) or prochlorperazine and isopropamide (10 mg twice a day, perorally) are effective.

If pregnancy does occur, menstrual extraction may be performed within 2 weeks of the missed period. Legal abortion is also available.

Patients should be offered a follow-up examination 6 weeks after the initial procedure. At this time, cultures for gonorrhea, a test for chlamydia, and a serologic test for syphilis should be repeated and the psychological state of the patient assessed by the counseling staff. Many times, patients who initially felt they needed no counseling will now accept help for themselves and their significant others.

The Elderly Victim

Attempted and completed assaults on the elderly are more frequent than one would expect. In our series at the Rape Treatment Center, 5% of rape victims were older than 50 years of age; the oldest was 98 years of age. Most were assaulted in their homes; 88% were raped by someone they did not know, compared with 35% in the younger age groups. Of elderly victims, 21% were raped by several offenders; only 9% of younger victims were "gang" raped.[19] The completion ratio among the elderly, as reported by a study done by the Law Enforcement Assistance Administration, was the highest of any age group. Because completed rape attacks are more serious than attempted rapes, the victimization suffered by the older woman is usually more severe than that of younger women.

The older victim is more likely to have body trauma than the younger victim: 63% versus 19%, respectively. Only 5% of the younger women had vaginal trauma, whereas 38% of the elderly had injuries in the vaginal area.

Examination of the older woman is essentially the same as that of the younger victim. Elderly patients need more understanding than others, however, because they usually believe rape is a crime of passion and therefore have greater anxiety and guilt feelings than younger women. The dynamics of the rape experience must be explained to them.

The older victim usually has heightened reactions to the attack because of her vulnerability. She may not have the support systems available to younger victims, and she may be physically less flexible. The mores and values of her generation may also hinder her adjustment. She often cannot ventilate her feelings about the rape because of her reluctance to discuss sexual matters, even with her husband. Some of these women have minimal emotional support, and it is essential that they be linked with agencies that can help them resolve some of these problems. These victims in particular should not be forced to make changes in their life-styles unless they are absolutely necessary; this intensifies their feelings of inadequacy.

The Young Victim

From 1974, when the Rape Treatment Center at Jackson Memorial Hospital in Miami was started, until child sexual abuse became a recognized problem in 1984, only a third of our victims were younger than the age of 17 years. Since 1985, however, 50% of the victims have been younger than the age of 12 years and 70% have been younger than the age of 18 years. The youngest victim we have seen was 2 weeks old. This increase in the number of children has occurred in all areas of the United States; it is not peculiar to our center.[20] The younger the victim, the more likely it is that the offender is someone well known to her or in a position of authority.

Although the law and the age of consent vary from state to state, it is usually mandatory to report cases of sexual abuse of children to the child protection services in the area; HRS is the agency in Florida. The Florida State Health and Rehabilitative Services agency has an 800 number to which abuses can be reported, and this agency investigates and decides the question of custody of the child. The examiner is cleared of responsibility once the crime is reported. In our area, because HRS accepts only those cases involving children who are abused by "caretakers," we also call the police department in whose jurisdiction the alleged assault occurred; the police investigate every case reported to them.

Any case of vaginal bleeding or venereal disease in a young child should be considered sexual assault until proven otherwise. Although fondling is the most common form of sexual abuse of a child, finger penetration and even penile penetration are not unknown.

The child should be completely undressed if an examination is to be performed because it is necessary to inspect the entire body; physical abuse often accompanies sexual abuse. The physician should suspect repeated fondling of the genitalia if the child does not object to examination of the genital area; most youngsters allow you to look but object to anyone touching the vulva unless they know from experience that it will not be unpleasant.

No child should be held down to perform an examination of this sort. Physically restraining her is tantamount to assaulting her. If the child is uncooperative, mild sedation is usually enough for the small child. We weigh the patient and give them chloral hydrate syrup, 50 mg/kg, perorally. A "lytic cocktail" may also be used of Demerol, 2 mg/kg; Thorazine 1 mg/kg; and Phenergan, 1 mg/kg, in a single intramuscular injection. If this is not successful, the child should be examined in the operating room under anesthesia.

In the child, as in the adult, lesions should be documented.[21] A throat culture for gonorrhea should always be taken from children; they almost never admit to fellatio. The size of the hymenal opening should be documented and the edges of the hymen described; the presence or absence of irregularities or tears should be noted. If there are only hymenal lacerations and no bruises on the vulvar area or inner aspects of the thighs, the examiner should be suspicious of sexual battery rather than a "fall"; the vulvar area is so vascular that any trauma usually causes some bruising. Cultures for gonorrhea and chlamydia should be taken from the vagina; nasopharyngeal swabs should be used instead of the larger cotton-tipped swabs. A culture for gonorrhea should be taken from the anal canal.

The source of any vaginal bleeding must be determined. If it is impossible to examine the vagina carefully with a pediatric speculum or an otoscope, an examination with the patient under general anesthesia must be performed. It is not uncommon to find that a lunate laceration in the vaginal vault is the source of the bleeding. This is characteristic of finger penetration and resultant laceration from a fingernail of the offender.

Appropriate prophylactic treatment should be offered to the young patient when indicated. For prevention of syphilis and gonorrhea, the same medications may be used as in the adult but the dosage is adjusted for the patient's weight. Tetracycline should not be used in younger children.

Both the parents and the child may be candidates for psychological counseling.

Counseling the Victim

Psychological Reaction

Psychological reactions to rape may be viewed within the framework of general crisis theory. A "crisis" may be defined as a stressful life event, a hazard that poses a threat, real or imagined. Tension increases, and a period of disorganization follows. If the threat is not dealt with successfully, the threatened person may become an emotional, behavioral, or even physical invalid.

To successfully resolve a crisis, the patient must be able to deal effectively with loss. Rape is a form of loss, and the depth of the feeling associated with rape is said to be the same as that associated with the loss of a child. The rape victim may lose several things: virginity, self-esteem, status, interpersonal relationships. This in turn intensifies her feelings of worthlessness.

The elements needed to modify the effects of this stress are immediate action and authority, not force.

The victim must be allowed to regain control of her life but to do so, she may need expert guidance. Medical and psychological care should be offered as soon as possible after the attack because as time passes, the patient builds up her defenses and may use denial as a coping method.

Responses to rape vary with the victim's age, personal situation, family or peer support system, and previous coping mechanisms.[22] If these factors are strong, the patient has a good chance of dealing with the crisis effectively.

In 1972, a crisis intervention scheme for victims of rape was described by Fox and Scherl.[23] Their design divided the reactions of rape victims into three predictable sequential phases: (1) the acute reaction, (2) the outward adjustment, and (3) the integration and resolution of the experience. In 1974, Burgess and Holmstrom identified a rape trauma syndrome, which they divided into two phases: (1) the immediate or acute phase, and (2) the long-term phase, the reorganization process.[24] These concepts are essentially the same. Both agree that rape is a social crisis because it involves not only the victim but also her family and all others who come into contact with her. Contrary to public opinion, rape is not a woman's problem; it is everyone's problem.

The acute phase is a period of disorganization. It begins immediately after the rape and may last for a few days or a few weeks. It is during this period that the victim must deal with practical concerns. Whom will she tell? Will she report the crime to the police? Will she seek medical treatment? Is her home safe? Her immediate emotional reactions are shock and disbelief: why me? She experiences guilt, humiliation, anger, and fear. Some patients express a desire for revenge. Many victims are vocal, whereas others have an intensified calm. The patient who is too controlled is more worrisome than the patient who can express her concerns.

The somatic complaints persist for several weeks. Vaginal soreness secondary to the attack, gastrointestinal symptoms, tension headaches, and genitourinary problems such as discharge and burning are not unusual.

The period of outward adjustment follows. During this time, the patient seems to be doing well. Many victims cope by denying that the experience ever happened and try to suppress it. That is rationalizing rather than adjusting, however. The patient may refuse counseling. It is essential that she be supported during this stage and not be challenged.

The reorganization phase may last for months or even years. It is during this period that the patient is most receptive to counseling. The patient is often depressed, especially if she has focused her anger on herself rather than the offender. She may direct her anger toward other males, which may result in many problems. Many victims have nightmares and somatic complaints. The victim may change her residence several times because she does not feel safe in her home. Over a period of months, she may develop an aversion to all sexual activity. Fears and phobias are common. Although the patient is depressed, she is now willing to talk about her experience and will accept counseling. She needs guidance to integrate her feelings about herself and the offender. Unless this is accomplished, she will remain emotionally handicapped.[25]

Approaches

Counseling at the Rape Treatment Center in Miami follows a crisis intervention model. It assumes that the patient was a normal, functioning person before the rape and that adequate coping mechanisms can be mobilized. If an underlying mental illness is discovered, a psychiatrist is consulted.

The crisis counselor encourages the patient to verbalize her fears and discuss her nightmares. The victim is encouraged to mobilize her anger and direct it at the offender. The counselor supports her and sustains her hope. The counseling is issue-oriented and guides the victim to make her own decisions and increase her independence. The counselor must be available so the victim can communicate her fears and feelings.

The family or significant others are encouraged to become involved in the counseling. A network of family and friends gives the patient the sense of support that is essential for her recovery. This is especially true when a child is the victim.

Summary

The degree of trauma experienced by the rape victim can be understood most easily if one considers that rape, invasion of the body without permission, is the ultimate invasion of privacy. The experience generates self-criticism and guilt, which lead to depression. All victims of sexual battery need understanding and expert medical and psychological care if they are to return to satisfactory levels of functioning. Their lives and the lives of all those around them will be affected by the experience. This is especially true when a child is the victim. If not provided comprehensive care, many victims develop a post-traumatic stress syndrome.[26,27]

BATTERED WOMEN

Demographics

As defined by Lenore Walker, the battered woman is any woman who has been physically and psychologically abused by her spouse or significant other. Federal Bureau of Investigation statistics show that in the United States, 2 million cases of women being battered are reported to law enforcement agencies each year; the number of actual cases is thought to be 3 to 4 million. One woman is battered every 15 seconds and 32% of these women are victimized again within 6 months. Most of the victims are women and 95% of the offenders are men. Women are also known to batter men but most of these cases go unreported. Another 3 to 4 million who have been battered in the past remain in the abusive relationship. Battering also occurs in the gay and lesbian communities.

History

The first significant legal limitation on the use of violence against wives occurred in 1796, when English Common Law decreed that a husband could not use a stick thicker than his thumb to beat his wife. Alabama, in 1981, was the first state to make it illegal for husbands to beat their wives. Today, although it is against the law in all states for a husband to beat his wife, many people still consider spouse abuse a personal and not a legal matter. The battered woman syndrome has been recognized by the American Psychological Society and is listed under Post Traumatic Stress Disorder in the revised third edition of the *Diagnostic and Statistical Manual*.

Signs

The gender bias study found that battering is the single largest cause of injury to women in the United States but it is unusual for the woman to reveal the cause of her injuries. The battered woman may be an insecure, dependent, nonassertive, and self-deprecating individual who is often immobilized and unable to take action to change her lot. The battered woman is usually unable to share her difficulty with others and is socially isolated. She is ashamed, feels she has been in some way responsible for the abuse, and is also afraid that the offender will beat her more if she tells. For these reasons, it is important for the physician to be alert to signs of possible battered woman syndrome.

Battered women most commonly present to the emergency area but it is not unusual for them to present to the offices of the obstetrician–gynecologist or family practitioner. The abuse may be physical, sexual, psychological, or economic or it may be a combination of these. Recurring injuries of the face, neck, and breasts from "falling" and personality changes such as depression are the most common findings and should make the examiner suspect possible battery. It is often relatively simple to uncover a history of repeated abuse on questioning because most of these women are waiting to find someone who understands and is interested enough to help them; they are relieved to share their secret.

Management

Once they are identified, it is important that the underlying causes are found and dealt with appropriately. It is usually necessary for several disciplines to become involved if these patients are to be cared for properly: medical, psychiatric, social service, and law enforcement. Florida law requires the police to notify the nearest shelter of *all* police reports within 24 hours. Typically, treatment is needed for a long time, until the home situation is resolved or the woman can become independent. Practical suggestions for management of battered woman syndrome are outlined in the January 1989 American College of Obstetrics and Gynecology Technical Bulletin.

Battering is a well-known problem, and there are more than 1200 shelters in the United States that offer "safe space" to abused women and their families. The physician must be aware of such facilities in his or her locale and be prepared to inform patients about their alternatives. It is a challenge to all physicians to identify these patients and attempt to help them.

REFERENCES

1. United States Department of Justice, Federal Bureau of Investigation: Uniform crime report on crime in the United States. Washington, DC, 1992
2. Amir M: Patterns in forcible rape, p 296. Chicago, University of Chicago Press, 1971
3. Evrard JR: The Medical, social and legal implications. Am J Obstet Gynecol 111(2):197, 1971
4. Brownmiller S: Against our will. Men, women and rape. New York, Plenum Press, 1979
5. Groth N: Men who rape. New York, Plenum Press, 1979
6. Hicks DJ, Weisberg MP: Sensitive emergency management of rape victims. Emerg Med Rep 9:114, 1988
7. Hicks DJ: The patient who's been raped. Emergency Medicine 20:106, 1988
8. Bureau of Crime Victims Rights, State of Florida Department of Legal Affairs: Evidence collection protocol for sexual assault, 1991
9. Gaudette BD: Forensic aspects of textile fibers examinations. In Faferstein R (ed): Forensic science handbook, vol 2, pp 209, 1988
10. Bisbing RE: Forensic identification and associations of human hair. In Faferstein R (ed): Forensic science handbook, p 185. Prentice-Hall, 1982
11. Slaughter L, Brown CRV: Colposcopy to establish physical findings in rape victims. Am J Obstet Gynecol 166:83, 1992
12. Bays J, Lewman LV: Toluidine blue in the detection at autopsy of perineal and anal lacerations in victims of sexual abuse. Arch Pathol Lab Med 116(6): 620, 1992
13. Glaser JB, Schachter J, Beves S, et al: Sexually transmitted diseases in postpubertal female rape victims. J Infect Dis 164(4):726, 1991
14. Claydon E, Murphy S, Osborne EM, et al: Rape and HIV. Int J STD AIDS 2(3):200, 1991
15. Fla Stat 960.003; Fla Stat 775.0875
16. Gomez R, Wunsch C, Davis J, et al: Qualitative and quantitative determinations of acid phosphatase activity in vaginal washings. Am J Clin Pathol 64:423, 1975
17. Evett IW, Buffery C, Willott G, et al: A guide to interpreting single locus profiles of DNA mixtures in forensic cases. Forensic Sci Soc 31(1):47, 1991
18. Jones W, Porter J: Postcoital contraception. Med J Aust 1(2): 68, 1981
19. Hicks DJ, Moon DM: Sexual assault of the older woman. In Stuart I, Greer J (eds): Sexual aggression: men, women and children. New York, Van Nostrand, 1984
20. Law Enforcement Administration Assistance: National Criminal Justice Information and Statistics Services. Washington, DC, 1992
21. Muram D: Child sexual abuse. In Pediatric and adolescent gynecology, p 365. Philadelphia, WB Saunders, 1994
22. Bowie SI, et al: Blitz rape and confidence rape: implications for clinical intervention. Am J Psychother 44(2):180, 1990
23. Fox SS, Scherl DJ: Crisis intervention with victims of rape. Soc Work 37:37, 1972
24. Burgess AW, Holmstrom LL: Rape: victims of crisis. Robert J. Brady Publishers: Bowie MD, 1974
25. Hilberman E: The rape victim. Washington, DC, American Psychiatric Association, 1976
26. Moscarello R: Posttraumatic stress disorder after sexual assault: its psychodynamics and treatment. J Am Acad Psychoanal 19(2):235, 1991

27. Psychiatric Clinics of America: Entire issue devoted to sexual abuse, 1989

Suggested Reading

American College of Obstetrics and Gynecology. Obstet Gynecol 124, 1989

Finkelhor D, Yilo K: License to rape: sexual abuse of wives free press, 1989, New York

Hicks DJ: Review of battered women syndrome: clinical practice in sexuality, vol 9. 1993

Saltzman LE, Mercy JA, Rosenberg ML, et al: Magnitude and patterns of family intimate assault in Atlanta, Georgia, 1984. Violence Vict 5(1):3, 1990

Straus MA, Gelles RJ: Societal changes In family violence from 1975 to 1985 as revealed by two national surveys. J Marriage Fam 48:465, 1986

Walker L: The battered woman syndrome. New York, Springer, 1984

Walker L: Terrifying love. New York, Harper & Row, 1989

Ambulatory Gynecology, Second Edition, edited by David H. Nichols and Patrick J. Sweeney. J. B. Lippincott Company, Philadelphia, © 1995.

14

Psychosexual Gynecology

Gloria A. Bachmann

For generations, the psychosexual aspects of gynecology were largely ignored, with emphasis on the reduction of mortality and serious morbidity being of primary concern to both practicing gynecologists and researchers. Because progress toward increased life expectancy has been achieved since the turn of the century, greater attention is being given to preserving function and improving psychosexual outcomes and quality of life. In the care of the female patient, addressing psychosexual health is of utmost importance. Ambulatory gynecology patients, when compared with community controls, show higher levels of psychological symptoms. Patient psychosexual health and well-being are also affected by gynecologic pathology and the intervention it necessitates.[1-4] In addition, certain psychosexual characteristics may be the etiology of or a significant contributor to various gynecologic conditions, such as premenstrual syndrome (PMS), infertility, polycystic ovary disease and endometriosis.[5-9] The quality of physician education and patient counseling regarding gynecologic health, as well as the degree of empathy shown to the woman who has pelvic pathology, may either exacerbate or improve psychosexual outcome. Being available to

the patient, informing her in a caring manner about treatments she may need, and clarifying misconceptions about her diagnosis often beneficially alter the patient's psychological outlook. Written materials and videotapes about her condition and a verbal physician–patient exchange that addresses the psychosexual implications of the dysfunction positively affect gynecologic wellness and overall health.

This chapter reviews the psychosexual effects of several gynecologic disorders. Data are presented on pelvic conditions that may possibly be exacerbated by the patient's psychosexual characteristics. The management and care of the woman who presents with a sexual dysfunction will also be addressed.

ENDOMETRIOSIS AND CHRONIC PELVIC PAIN

Ten percent to 20% of ambulatory gynecologic visits are for the evaluation and treatment of chronic abdominal and pelvic pain, and 30% of laparoscopies are performed for this reason.[10,11] Because endometriosis (which often presents as chronic pelvic pain and dysmenorrhea) may adversely affect fertility and sexuality, in many women, laparoscopy is performed to exclude endometriosis before any treatment other than analgesics is offered. Endometriosis patients are usually between 30 and 40 years of age and when compared with normal controls, have either delayed childbearing or have had relatively few pregnancies.[12-14] Reports of endometriosis patients being of higher socioeconomic class have been debated because the diagnosis of endometriosis may be used more frequently in these women, whereas women of lower socioeconomic class with the same presenting history may be labeled as having pelvic inflammatory disease.[15,16] Although data are lacking that clearly define the frequency of endometriosis in the general population, it is estimated that the prevalence of endometriosis in menstruating women ranges from 7% to 50%.[17] Endometriosis is a chronic illness, characterized by pelvic pain, severe dysmenorrhea, infertility, and dyspareunia; over the course of the disease, the psychosexual implications become as significant as the physical ones. There are also data to suggest that psychosexual dysfunction may not be solely the outcome of the disease but that the psychosexual health of the patient may play a role in the etiology of both endometriosis and chronic pelvic pain by alternating gonadal physiologic function.[18,19] Mood disorders that affect estradiol, progesterone, and prolactin secretion (thereby altering the hormonal environment), and abnormalities of the immune system caused by environmental stresses have been hypothesized as etiologies of both endometriosis and chronic pelvic pain.[5-8] Many pelvic pain patients have a degree of pelvic pathology (endometriosis or adhesions) that does not significantly differ from patients who undergo laparoscopy for sterilization or infertility evaluation.[20] Higher frequencies of depressive disorders, substance abuse, sexual dysfunction, and a history of childhood sexual abuse are also more prevalent in this group. Pelvic pain patients characterize themselves as anxious and depressed, with multiple somatic symptoms, as compared with nonpain patients.[21-23]

The physician should proceed with an evaluation for the cause of the pain in an efficient and timely manner and outline interventions as soon as the diagnosis is made. A patient with chronic pain should be encouraged to follow one of the treatment plans that are suggested to her. If the patient refuses therapy, the physician should offer additional take-home educational materials and schedule a follow-up visit in 4 to 6 weeks so that the situation may be reassessed.[24] If the pain cycle is not intercepted early, exacerbated feelings of hopelessness, helplessness, despair, and depression may result.[12] The use of nonsteroidal anti-inflammatory drugs should be suggested at the onset of pain, before pain becomes severe. For women with pain throughout most of the menstrual cycle or endometriosis, the use of oral contraceptive pills to suppress ovarian function should be suggested to the patient. Oral contraceptive pills alleviate pain, inhibit the progression of endometriosis, regulate menstrual-cycle length, and decrease menstrual flow. The standard of care is laparoscopy for definitive diagnosis with the capability of performing laser ablation of endometrial implants and adhesions. Laparoscopic laser transection of the utero sacral ligaments for pain control has not been consistently shown to be beneficial. High-dose progestins, gonadotropin-releasing–hormone (GnRH) agonists, and danazol may be used for short-term management or after laser ablation to insure atrophy of small or missed endometrial lesions.

Endometriosis patients often experience dyspareunia, which—in addition to the negative psychological outcomes that accompany pelvic pain (depression, anxiety, loss of self-esteem, feelings of inadequacy, hopelessness and helplessness)—may cause interpersonal and intrapersonal conflicts. Pain with intercourse decreases the pleasure of sexual exchange for both partners, and anticipation of pain with coital episodes ultimately leads to vaginismus, diminished sexual desire, difficulty in becoming sexually aroused, and problems with inadequate vaginal lubrication. Initially, the couple may decrease the frequency of sexual activity but if the coital pain does not improve or exacerbates, refraining from all types of sexual intimacy (even those sexual activities requiring no vaginal penetration) may result.

Many patients are reluctant to spontaneously report sexual difficulties and all endometriosis patients should be questioned about dyspareunia, vaginismus, and lack of sexual desire. Coital activities that are pleasurable, with avoidance of uncomfortable positions, or noncoital sexual activities (if pain cannot be ameliorated with a change in position) should be encouraged during diagnosis and treatment. Physician approval of different types of sexual exchange (eg, oral–digital stimulation, mutual self-stimulation, massage) and the use of vaginal lubricants often helps the couple to continue a satisfactory sexual life and avoid further sexual problems. Assisting the couple so that sexual abstinence does not result has a beneficial effect on the relationship and the ability to achieve pregnancy, when desired. If endometriosis results in infertility, intense psychosexual support is necessary, with a team approach that combines physicians, nurses, social workers, and psychologists being the ideal health care delivery model.

When the combination of supportive office counseling and pharmacologic and surgical treatment for chronic pelvic pain and endometriosis is not sufficient to prevent or ameliorate adverse psychosexual consequences, the patient should be referred for psychological or psychiatric counseling. This is especially important for the patient who is having extreme difficulty coping or the patient who has a history of childhood abuse or other long-standing disturbances. Appropriate and early intervention decrease the psychological stresses that exacerbate gynecologic symptoms and pathology.

EFFECTS OF HORMONAL CONTRACEPTION

The role of endogenous and exogenous hormones on the psychosexual behavior of the female is of concern to both physicians and patients, especially when exogenous hormones are electively used for birth control.[25-28] Some reports suggest affective changes such as depression (listed as a side effect in the *Physician's Desk Reference*) with oral contraceptive pill use. Other data show no cause and effect between oral contraceptives and affective disorders.[29-33] A study by Goetsch and coworkers found no change in psychological functioning of women using oral contraceptives; if psychosexual dysfunction exists, it may be associated with the myths and beliefs of unfounded negative effects (such as cancer and infertility) associated with oral contraceptive pill use.[34] A 1994 Gallup survey reports that 86% of American women do not believe oral contraceptives are safe to buy without a doctor's prescription, a belief that has not substantially changed from a similar 1985 poll.[35] Long-acting levonorgestrel implants (Norplant) and medroxyprogesterone acetate (Depo-Provera) are also reported to be linked to depression, although the incidence is reported as being less than 5%.[36]

Women who are contemplating the use of a hormone-based contraceptive should be educated not only about the risks but also about the benefits, such as decreased risk of endometrial and uterine cancer. Clearly elaborating the benefits and the risks puts birth control options in perspective and possibly decreases noncompliance and potential adverse psychosexual effects. Women with a personal or family history of depression should receive in-depth counseling regarding affective disorders. Long-acting hormonal contraceptives such as Depo-Provera (which takes 6 to 8 months to clear after injection) should be recommended with caution.

PREMENSTRUAL SYNDROME (PMS)

Premenstrual syndrome, previously referred to as premenstrual tension or exaggerated menstrual molimina, appears to be the consequence of a complex interaction between ovarian steroid hormones, endogenous opiates, peptides, central neurotransmitters, prostaglandins, and the peripheral autonomic and endocrine systems.[37,38] Fifty percent to 90% of women who have ovulatory cycles experience some premenstrual symptoms, with only 3% to 5% reporting changes severe enough to disrupt their life-style.[39-41] Adolescent women who have other emotional problems tend to have an intense PMS response.[42] It is not clear why some women have an exaggerated response related to menstrual cycle changes, whereas others are almost asymptomatic or in some instances experience positive feelings.[43] Symptoms and severity are so variable between women that PMS is often difficult to diagnose and a question frequently asked by clinicians is whether PMS is a distinct pathologic entity.[44,45] Because psychosexual factors may affect cyclical ovarian activity (eg, amenorrhea occurring in freshman college coeds away from home for the first time) and menstruation to some women is a repetitive, unpleasant event that evokes psychosexual effects such as depression, anxiety, and sexual aversion, over time, profound changes in brain activity and behavior may result, triggering PMS.[46] Research suggests that (1) PMS is an autonomous mood disorder, linked to but not caused by events of the menstrual cycle; and (2) cyclic ovarian activity is the etiologic factor of PMS, regardless of ovarian hormone production.[47] The most convincing data that PMS is related to cyclic ovarian activity was summarized by Schagen van Leeuwen and coworkers, who reported:

1. Premenstrual syndrome is not present in prepubertal, postmenopausal, oophorectomized, or pregnant females.
2. Premenstrual syndrome does not occur in females who have hypothalamic hypogonadotropic amenorrhea.
3. Hysterectomy without oophorectomy does not affect PMS.

4. Gonadotropin-releasing–hormone agonists reduce PMS, with return of ovulatory cycles producing symptom recurrence.
5. Cyclic mood changes are observed during sequential estrogen–progestin replacement therapy.
6. In a dysmenorrhea study, PMS symptoms were evoked in women after hysterectomy by auto-transfusion of plasma collected during a pre-hysterectomy symptomatic perimenstrual period. Double-blind transfusion of autologous plasma sampled in an asymptomatic period produced significantly fewer symptoms.
7. In the 28-day–cycling Rhesus monkey, PMS-like symptoms can be observed in the luteal phase.
8. In severe PMS, bilateral oophorectomy produced a lasting beneficial effect in patients who had a positive response to suppression of ovulation with danazol.
9. Suppression of ovulation with estradiol implants and dermal patches in a double-blind placebo-controlled fashion significantly decreased the severity of PMS.
10. Intrasubject comparison of spontaneous ovulatory and anovulatory cycles among women with PMS suggests that symptoms are markedly reduced in the absence of ovulation.
11. Women on triphasic oral contraceptives demonstrate more premenstrual distress than women on monophasic contraceptives.
12. Only postmenopausal women who had previously suffered from PMS reacted adversely when prescribed oral contraceptives.[37]

Although PMS symptoms are numerous, with a wide range of severity, a Dutch study reports that the 10 most typical PMS symptoms described by patients (in ranked order) are:

1. Painful breasts
2. Feeling bloated
3. Irritability
4. Mood swings
5. Tension
6. Weight gain
7. Fatigue
8. Back pain
9. Abdominal pain
10. "Everything hurts"[48]

Although most women appear to report similar symptoms with each cycle, about a third show some variation over time.[49,50] Before treatment options are considered, a seven-step approach that was devised by Keye to evaluate the patient with complaints of PMS may be clinically useful.[51] The steps are to:

1. Take a complete patient history to document complaints and their relation to menstrual cycle
2. Perform prospective charting for 1 to 2 months to confirm the history
3. Evaluate patient calendars
4. Establish differential diagnosis for each of the symptoms
5. Rule out chronic underlying diseases as the cause
6. Perform a thorough psychosexual evaluation
7. Establish a patient profile that guides treatment[51]

There is no universally effective treatment regimen for PMS, and therapy is most beneficial when individualized. Because reports show that placebo treatment is as useful as surgical and chemical castration in reducing PMS symptoms, an approach using individualized pharmacologic and nonpharmacologic therapy is advised.[52-55] A wide range of pharmacologic agents are used for PMS, such as oral contraceptives, progestins (including natural progesterone suppositories), danazol, GnRH agonists, the anxiolytic alprazolam, diuretics (eg, spironolactone and hydrochlorothiazide), and prostoglandin inhibitors. It is important to judiciously prescribe each drug for a specific symptom rather than to employ a multipharmacy approach and hope for a "complete cure." Because the psychosexual implications are significant, stress-reduction therapies and intensive counseling are often beneficial, especially when combined with a healthy diet, regular exercise, and avoidance of smoking. More data are needed on vitamin and herbal remedies. The cause of PMS will ultimately be defined, as was the etiology for primary dysmenorrhea, which was considered a psychosomatic disorder for many generations. Until the pathophysiology of PMS is certain, a multidisciplinary approach is necessary to study the problem, with different strategies for diagnosing disease intensity and evaluating response to treatment. Therapy should consist of intensive education, counseling regarding life-style intervention, pharmocologic treatment for specific symptoms, and referral for counseling if psychosexual problems are significant. Physician intervention should not consist of minimizing the patient's symptoms or dismissing PMS as solely a psychosexual problem without anatomic or physiologic components.

GYNECOLOGIC TUMORS

Malignant and premalignant conditions of the pelvis affect psychological health in several ways: the patient must (1) face issues of mortality, possible infertility, and changes in anatomy resulting from the tumor and the surgery; and (2) endure any radiation and chemotherapy her condition may necessitate at the same time that her sense of self-esteem, femaleness, and sexual wholeness are altered.[56–58] The diagnosis and treatment of pelvic tumors has negative psychological (eg, depression, malaise, anxiety, mood lability) and sexual (eg, decreased libido, changes in sexual arousal, dyspareunia, and anorgasmia) effects, which are most prevalent in younger women, those who want to preserve fertility, women with nonavailable spouses and no support network, and those who derive their sense of worth and sexuality mainly from their pelvic organs.[57–59] Not all psychosexual changes are due to the personality and coping mechanisms of the woman and her environment; the tumor and its treatment also affect her overall health. Conization and LEEP procedures in younger women may affect cervical secretions, resulting in inadequate lubrication with sexual arousal. Pelvic radiation therapy or chemotherapy affects ovarian and vaginal function, causing an immediate postmenopausal state for many women.[56,60,61] Loss of estrogen often results, causing vasomotor symptoms and atrophy of the urogenital tissues which become thin and denuded, and obliteration of small blood vessels. Operative intervention may further exacerbate vaginal dysfunction by excision of additional tissue, causing stenosis—narrowing and decreased vaginal canal size. Postoperative recovery from surgery places an added burden on the psychosexual health of the woman, and if radiation or chemotherapy follows immediately, feelings of malaise, fatigue, and poor health are exacerbated. If her partner's reaction to the tumor and its treatment are negative, an additional psychological burden is placed on the patient.

Concerns raised by any type of treatment that is potentially debilitating or by a gynecologic diagnosis that elicits fear of cancer, cancer transmission through sexual intercourse, partner rejection, and loss of sexual attractiveness and desirability should be addressed at the onset of the evaluation. Many of the adverse psychosexual changes due to a pelvic pathology and necessary intervention may be explained not only at the time of the initial diagnosis but during the time when evaluation for extent of disease is occurring. If a serious gynecologic condition is diagnosed (either through biopsy, radiographic study, or other tests), it is preferable to have the woman (and her partner if possible) come to the office for an explanation of the condition rather than give the diagnosis over the phone. It is important to be honest and realistic in explaining the condition and prognosis and answering questions but it is critical to be hopeful, empathetic, and supportive. Briefly describing the problem and waiting to answer questions is often not desirable because many women and their partners are so anxious at the time of the diagnosis that they tend to forget or cannot verbalize fully their concerns and fears.

Points that should be addressed with counseling are similar to those reported by Doherty and coworkers regarding abnormal Pap smears:

- What has caused the abnormal cells?
- Will the treatment result in a cure?
- Will the abnormal cells recur after treatment?
- Have I got cancer?
- Is something seriously wrong with me?
- Will I need surgical treatment?
- Will I get worse waiting for appointments?
- Will it affect having children?
- Will I pass anything on to my partner?
- Will it affect my sex life?
- Have I caught something from my partner?
- Will I need a hysterectomy?[62]

When discussing cancer, reassure the woman and her partner that there is no possibility of cancer transmission through intercourse. It is important, however, that condoms be use by couples at risk for viral, bacterial, or parasitic transmission of infection. Emphasize to the couple that there are no changes routinely noted in sexual response after most types of surgical, radiation, or chemotherapeutic treatments and that the anatomic and physiologic changes that do affect sexual function can be treated effectively.[63] For women in whom there will be changes in the vaginal vault, preoperative instruction of dilator use should be reviewed and encouraged, especially when coitus is less frequent than twice per week.[61] Continued intercourse or mechanical dilation, supplemented with estrogen use when necessary, may prevent vaginal stenosis.[64,65] Educating the woman and her husband about physical changes that will occur with surgery and emphasizing that it will not predispose the couple to sexual abstinence can demystify the treatment and open up the discussion for reviewing practical suggestions and strategies for continued sexual exchange. Women and their partners should be provided with written information about the gynecologic tumor; given a follow-up visit in a short and specified period, not only for treatment or further evaluation but also for psychosexual support if it appears necessary; informed to call or come back sooner if an emergency or sudden change in the women's health arises; and encouraged to seek short-term counseling if major psychosexual difficulties are noted.

CLIMACTERIC

For generations, the climacteric has been regarded as a time of great hormonal upheavals in women that translate into a plethora of disturbing symptoms.[66–69] The types and prevalence of menopausal symptoms vary and include vasomotor changes (27%–85%), palpitations (9%–75%), vertigo (10%–74%), headache (16%–86%), insomnia (27%–67%), depression (21%–78%), rheumatic pains (17%–49%), fatigue (21%–93%), numbness and tingling (22%–69%), irritability (35%–92%) and weight gain (50%–70%).[69] In addition to vasomotor sequelae and annoying psychosexual and medical symptoms, researchers have reported that the climacteric evokes profound emotional changes, including feelings of internal frustration due to the loss of reproductive potential, decline in libido, increased sexual dysfunction, and insomnia.[70] In addition, some report that psychosomatic symptoms are more prevalent in menopausal women and are the major reason women seek physician help and family support at this time.[66] Other data negate the extreme, negative impact of menopause on women and show that health complaints during the menopause are not as prevalent as reported.[71] In a study conducted in Norway, the highest prevalence of complaints were reported for 2 to 3 years postmenopause and consisted of hot flashes (45%), excessive sweating (33%), vaginal dryness (22%), and mood swings (10%).[71] Like other gynecologic conditions, symptoms of the climacteric result from the interaction of endocrine changes with psychological and sociocultural factors.[28,72,73] The main treatment for climacteric symptoms and for prevention of long-term adverse effects such as osteoporosis, cardiovascular disease, and urogenital atrophy is hormone-replacement therapy, although data suggest that unaddressed psychological and sexual issues decrease the effectiveness of the replacement hormones.[74] The climacteric and not aging has been shown to be an independent influence on the psychosexual well-being of women; therefore, hormone replacement is often effective therapy. Other pharmacologic therapies should be prescribed as they would be in premenopausal women for the treatment of a specific symptom or problem. Positive psychosexual factors are noted to occur with menopause as well (eg, no fear of unwanted pregnancy, elimination of monthly menstruation). Overall, menopause is reported to have a small negative influence on the behavioral functioning of the woman. In one Dutch study, climacteric women were reported as being less interested in family members and friends and acting in a less friendly manner toward those persons.[66] Emotions, feelings, and sensations are often significantly depressed in menopause and women express feelings of nervousness, tenseness, and depression. The level of intellectual functioning may also be lower in the early perimenopausal period and on the average, women seem to be less able to concentrate and are more forgetful.[66] Because many of the climacteric symptoms women experience are universal, with their expression influenced by social, cultural, and psychological factors, intense education and counseling of these women is of extreme importance.[75] Because of the similarity in symptoms between women, self-help groups positively influence menopausal women in improving self-image and lowering conflicts in interpersonal relationships.[75]

SEXUALLY TRANSMITTED DISEASES

In addition to fears of unwanted or unplanned pregnancy, most women (regardless of age) express concern and fear about the contraction of a sexually transmitted disease (STD) with coital activity, especially in situations of a new partner or a partner with multiple or suspected multiple partners. Herpes genitalis was the first STD to have tremendous impact on women of middle- and upper-class socioeconomic status. Before herpes made headlines in the lay media, STDs such as syphilis and gonorrhea were perceived as occurring mainly in women with many partners or women of lower socioeconomic status. Although Herpes genitalis was of primary concern in the 1980s, other STDs have overshadowed this viral infection. *Chlamydia trachomatis*, with its ability to cause pelvic inflammatory disease and infertility; human papillomavirus (HPV), which is associated with cervical cancer; and human immunodeficiency virus (HIV), which is associated with incurable progressive debilitation, are the STDs women are most fearful of contracting. Although HIV infections are associated with the gravest medical consequences and social stigmatization, all STDs may lead to similar psychosexual sequelae. If the woman's partner has an STD or was treated for one in the past, even greater psychosexual disturbances may occur. Sexually transmitted disease also contributes to the loss of sexual desire or the equating of coitus with unpleasant activity, which further increases interpersonal difficulties and emotional suffering. In addition, the sexual pleasure of patients with an STD or the fear of contracting an STD may be further hampered by the use of condoms. In certain instances, the fear of contracting an infection becomes so exaggerated that the woman becomes anxious, depressed, and develops hypochondriacal fears, often necessitating frequent trips to the physician for culturing of vaginal secretions or giving the appropriate blood samples for testing. In one study, the fear of having or developing cancer was the major psychological effect reported by women who contracted genital HPV.[76] Of the 51 patients studied, 16% reported that HPV infection caused increased aggression, fighting, and suspicion of their partner, and overall, their partnership was worsened.[76] The most prevalent problem the group reported was sexual; 57% reported that their sexual life had worsened, with symptoms of inhibited sexual desire, dyspareunia, and for a few, sexual abstinence.[76]

As with other gynecologic conditions, it is important to properly inform the patient about STDs, clarify misconceptions about disease transmission, summarize the natural history, and review prevention of recurrence. Because STDs affect psychosexual health dramatically, it is important to provide extensive counseling regarding the impact of these infections on relationships and to give the woman appropriate and positive counseling regarding condom use. It is also advantageous to instruct patients in other forms of sexual gratification such as massage and mutual self-stimulation.

PREGNANCY

Generations of physicians have recognized that many pregnant women experience symptoms of depression; often, these feelings are exacerbated in the postpartum period.[77] Because pregnancy and childbirth result in major hormonal shifts and lifestyle changes, with several psychological and social factors also contributing to the postpartum stress, psychosexual consequences are expected. Some women express feelings of sadness and an inability to cope as early as 2 weeks after delivery, whereas others may not notice any changes until 6 months postpartum. The most consistent psychosocial predictor of postpartum depression is not obstetric risk history and complications but a poor marital relationship; other factors include insufficient emotional and social support by family and friends and high levels of depressive symptoms in the spouse.[78–81] Many women who develop postpartum depression tend to have a hypomanic period, either immediately before delivery or afterward, and should be monitored closely and counseled before postpartum depression occurs.[82,83] To avoid or ameliorate postpartum depression, it is important for the physician to assess psychosocial factors early in the patient's pregnancy and determine the woman's beliefs about her ability to handle the challenges of pregnancy and parenthood. Women who have frequent concerns about their ability to master the demands of motherhood often exhibit severe depressive symptoms in the postpartum periods. Women who repeatedly voice concerns about their parenting abilities during pregnancy should be provided with additional educational materials and given psychological intervention to address their concerns before the delivery.

Adverse psychosexual consequences after a spontaneous or medically induced pregnancy loss are also of concern to physicians.[84,85] The concept that (1) management of miscarriage may be enhanced by attention to psychosocial issues as well as to the physical aspects of the event, and (2) counseling should be given to mothers regarding the immediate and long-term implications is well recognized.[86] The degree of psychosexual effect from miscarriage is determined by the length of the pregnancy, the degree of bonding that has occurred, the number of children the woman has, her desire for the pregnancy, existence of a support system, and having an explanation for the miscarriage.[86,87] Not knowing the reason for a spontaneous pregnancy loss may be the most disquieting factor and should be addressed by the physician. Although in many instances the cause of the miscarriage may not be possible to determine, most women want the issue discussed and want the physician to offer a hypothesis of why it occurred.[86] Counseling on the behavioral changes linked to miscarriage and help in planning future pregnancies may also be helpful. Minimizing the loss or suggesting that a future pregnancy will compensate for the one terminated is not helpful to patients. Although there is controversy regarding whether the woman should see the dispelled fetus, studies suggest that a woman should be able to view (and hold) a fully formed fetus but that a conceptus that resembles a collection of tissue probably has no positive impact on overall well-being.[86] Couples who have dealt with recurrent pregnancy loss appear to have better coping mechanisms than do couples who have never experienced a miscarriage. Communication between the woman and her partner seems to be a major determinant of how well the pregnancy loss will be accepted. Studies of spontaneous miscarriage and medically induced termination of pregnancy occurring after prenatal diagnostic testing reveal that this is a traumatic event for the couple and that many women relate this event as being equal to or more stressful than any previous adverse life event.[87–90] In addition to grief and depression over their loss, many women feel angry and guilty. Women who have a spontaneous pregnancy loss after chorionic villus sampling feel particularly guilty because of the perceived extra risk to which they subjected their fetus; only a little more than a third would choose chorionic villus sampling again for prenatal testing.[88–90]

Regardless of circumstance, women who experience a pregnancy loss often become stressed and depressed. It is important for the physician to educate the woman and her partner early in the pregnancy, especially if prenatal diagnostic testing will be performed, so that they are aware of the rate of spontaneous pregnancy loss from the procedure. For some women, post-loss support groups are helpful and should be recommended.

If a woman elects to terminate a pregnancy, there are many other psychosexual issues that must be dealt with; for some women, this procedure evokes feelings of guilt, regret, anxiety, and dysphoria, whereas for others relief and diminished stress levels are reported.[91–95] Most of the data on elective pregnancy termination report that most women handle this event without major psychosexual distress.[93–95] The attention of healthcare providers should be directed to women who have a high degree of emotional problems preabortion, lack a support system, or have a history of psychological problems.[91,96,97] It is important to include a partner or support person in all counseling sessions because there is uniformly less distress in women with a support system.

INFERTILITY

Infertility has an enormous impact on the psychosexual health of the female, and going through an evaluation adds to the negative effect on overall well-being.[98,99] Data link psychological factors to the etiology of infertility.[99] Whatever the etiology, there are many issues infertile women must deal with—for example, sexual inadequacy, maternal yearning, marital duty, and self-esteem. As infertility treatments progress, there is a gradual decrease in sexually related activity other than coital episodes necessary for possible conception; spontaneity and pleasure are usually diminished or lost. In some instances, vaginismus may result.[100] Psychologically, women become more anxious, develop more physical complaints, and are less able to cope with stress.[101] Psychosexual consequences often depend on the motives for wanting children, preinfertility psychological and sexual health, and the spousal relationship. Whether psychological stress contributes to infertility or whether the stress occurs as a consequence of long-term infertility is not clearly understood.[101,102] For some couples, by the third unsuccessful attempt at pregnancy, impairment in the relationship begins.

Five factors seem to be important prognostic factors for future psychosexual well-being of the infertile woman:

1. The status of psychological functioning when beginning the infertility evaluation—If there is no impairment, the risk is smaller that she will experience a great emotional disturbance after 2 years of unsuccessful treatment.
2. Gender identity—If this is insecure, the risk is greater of experiencing psychosexual problems with unsuccessful treatment.
3. The relationship between the woman and her spouse—If the relationship is good, deterioration of overall well-being during fertility evaluation and treatment is blunted.
4. Desire to be a parent—Couples who want to be parents regardless of treatment outcome and

who are willing to adopt experience less distress.

5. Close communication—Ongoing communication between the couple and physician during each step of the evaluation and treatment is helpful.

An infertility investigation should be compressed into the smallest time period possible, and the couple should be told there may not be a biological baby even after all is done. Infertile couples should be treated in a way that they feel confirmed as persons and not numbers or statistics and provided with the information necessary for treatment with empathy and understanding. Support groups should be encouraged for all couples at the beginning of an infertility evaluation.

HYSTERECTOMY

Hysterectomy is the second most common operation in the United States, with 600,000 procedures performed annually at a cost exceeding $3 billion. It has historically been associated with significant psychosexual sequelae.[103] For generations, gynecologists have recognized that removal of the uterus (which has unique psychosexual significance for many women) may be associated with psychological and sexual manifestations and in the early 1970s coined the term "post-hysterectomy syndrome."

The existential importance of the uterus as a "female" organ is different in each woman and is influenced by her psychosexual makeup, upbringing, and social environment. Not only is it a childbearing organ but some women perceive the the uterus as also being a regulator and controller of body processes, an origin of female competence, a reservoir of strength and vitality, a proof and maintainer of youth and attractiveness, and a sexual organ. Adverse medical and psychological states have been attributed in the past to this organ as well. Although the Greek word for uterus (hystera) is derived from the word referring to the placenta, hystera is also used to denote exaggerated and extreme emotional lability (hysterical). Physicians before the turn of the century felt the uterus had a central position in diseases of women and that many medical conditions (hysteromniosis) of women could be traced to uterine pathology. Hysteria was thought to be due to the migration of the uterus to different parts of the woman's body, which caused a variety of unrelated symptoms.

Many women view hysterectomy as a threat to their integrity, health, reproductive function, and femininity and experience depression, anxiety, and sexual dysfunction after surgery. It appears, however, that the psychosexual problems that surface after uterine removal are often caused by pre-existing emotional problems that are exacerbated by a decline in ovarian hormones, either through oophorectomy or postoperative functional impairment of the ovaries. The risk factors associated with an increased probability of developing psychosexual problems after hysterectomy include:

1. Ovarian hormone decline
2. Preoperative history of psychosexual disturbances such as depression and diminished libido
3. Younger age group, especially in women with limited educational attainment and conflict about childbearing
4. The belief that the uterus has unique importance for maintaining psychological and sexual health
5. Poor preoperative understanding of the indications and expectations of the proposed surgery
6. The absence of pelvic pathology, especially when hysterectomy is performed for quality-of-life indications[104]

The reason that post-hysterectomy syndrome may occur in women in whom there is no uterine pathology is that a somatization disorder may have produced the symptoms that led to the surgery and the symptoms were not due to uterine dysfunction. For example, women who have cyclical mood disturbances may undergo hysterectomy for this reason and find the symptoms are not diminished afterward because they were not causally related to the uterus.

Because many factors affect psychosexual health, the causal relation of hysterectomy and subsequent psychosexual difficulties has not been scientifically established. Four percent to 23% of women studied over 3 months to 5 years post-hysterectomy are reported to become depressed.[104] Adverse psychological effects of uterine removal are ascribed to loss—not only to loss of the uterus as an organ for childbearing but also to symbolic or social loss, especially when the dominant societal view dictates that hysterectomy neuters or defeminizes women. Richards—the first author who used the term post-hysterectomy syndrome to describe depression and concomitant symptoms of hot flashes, urinary problems, headaches, dizziness, and insomnia that occur more frequently after hysterectomy as compared with other operations—attributes it to an endocrine imbalance.[105] This observation is supported by literature reporting improvement in most women placed on hormone-replacement therapy post-hysterectomy. One out of three hysterectomies in the United States is associated with bilateral oophorectomy, which causes an abrupt decline in estrogen, with associated menopause symptoms such as hot flashes, night sweats, depression, and insomnia. These symptoms are seen in women with bilateral oophorectomy, regardless of whether or not the uterus is removed, lending credence to the opinion that part or all of the post-hysterectomy syndrome in women is due to ovarian decline. When hormonal status and preoperative emotional state are considered, most prospective studies find no greater risk of postoperative mood disturbances after hysterectomy than cholecystectomy.

On the specific issue of sexual dysfunction after hysterectomy, there is no consensus.[105] Sexual function after hysterectomy may be affected if either the woman or her partner consider the entire uterus or the cervix necessary for optimal sexual function or attractiveness. In some women, the assumed natural relation of menopause with aging and loss of sexual appeal may lead to the false impression that hysterectomy leads to the same changes and that the woman will age abruptly and become sexually undesirable and dysfunctional. The incidence of sexual dysfunction after hysterectomy has been reported to range from 10% to 46%, depending on when the survey was taken, the inclusion of patients in whom hysterectomy was performed for quality-of-life reasons, and the instrument used for collection of data.[104] Whether hysterectomy causes disturbances in sexual function rather than the attendant hormonal changes that often accompany hysterectomy is not well known. It appears that sexual difficulties after hysterectomy may be due to (1) pre-existing depression or sexual problems that were either secondary to the problem that led to the hysterectomy, or (2) a psychosomatic basis that led to hysterectomy without uterine pathology.

Reviewing the literature in its totality, psychosexual difficulties after hysterectomy appear to be related to preoperative physical and emotional factors, which are influenced by the social and cultural environment of the woman and not to the hysterectomy per se. Problems are more likely to appear when hysterectomy is accompanied by ovarian hormonal decline. The physician should attempt to minimize adverse postoperative sequelae by (1) as-

sessing the psychological and sexual makeup of the patient before surgery, (2) educating the woman and her partner preoperatively, (3) reviewing the indications and the risks of the surgery, and (4) outlining the expected physiologic and anatomic changes. Even with good preoperative counseling and attention to hormone replacement postoperatively, the existential meaning of the uterus as an organ that defines femininity and as a maintainer of youth and health may lead to psychosexual difficulties in a certain subset of women. In the patient who exhibits extreme anxiety or depression after careful preparation or explanation of the procedure and the expectant results, referral for additional preoperative psychological or psychiatric counseling should be offered.

SEXUAL VICTIMIZATION OF WOMEN

Sexual Assault

Although the sexual victimization of adult women encompasses a wide spectrum of criminal acts that are commonly referred to as sexual assault, sexual contact, sexual molestation, rape, sodomy, incest, sexual violence, sexual battery, and lewdness, the common underlying thread in all of these acts is that of coerced sexual activity thrust on one individual (the victim) by another (the perpetrator) without informed consent.[106]

Sexual assault of the adult female, considered to be the most serious of the sex crimes from both a medical and legal standpoint, commonly refers to the nonconsensual, forcible sexual penetration of the victim's vagina, anus, or mouth by the perpetrator and has absorbed the historical definition of rape (ie, forced penile penetration of the victim's vagina). Because of the severely intrusive nature of the crime and the degree to which the victim is violated, in conjunction with modern considerations of the consequential possibility of contracting STDs such as HIV infection in certain situations, sexual assault often acutely damages and upsets a woman's physical, emotional, social, and sexual wellbeing on a short-term basis and creates long-term psychosexual problems, from which many victims never fully recover.

Criminal sexual contact, a lesser criminal offense, generally refers to the nonconsensual touching of sexual areas of the victim's body or unwanted viewing on the part of the victim of sexual activity engaged in by the perpetrator. Lewdness, the least intrusive of the sexual offenses and usually having the least psychosexual sequelae, generally refers to indecent exposure or the compelled viewing of pornography.

Over 650,000 aggravated sexual assaults of adults are reported each year—a figure that is especially staggering when considering that up to 80% of such assaults go unreported. It is estimated that two to five sexual assaults occur every minute in the United States and that 10% to 15% of women will be the victim of an attempted or actual sexual assault during their lifetime.[106,107] Furthermore, the perpetrator is known by the victim in up to 80% of all sexual assaults, whereas more than a third of all such assaults are committed by the victim's spouse. Although fighting back during a sexual assault increases the risk of injuries requiring medical attention, it also increases the victim's chances of escaping the perpetrator before completion of the assault.

Despite public concern regarding date rape and gang rape, most victims fail to report incidents of these sexual assaults because of fear of retaliation, feelings of humiliation or embarrassment, uncertainty about the reaction of her partner, inability to cope with the stress of criminal prosecution, or a lack of faith in the legal system. It is therefore important that the obstetrician–gynecologist who attends to the sexual assault victim make the attempt to minimize the initial trauma by approaching the patient with empathy and preparing her for physical and psychosexual reactions to the assault. The physician must also recognize poor adjustment in the period after the incident and make appropriate referrals.

New research suggests that, given the combination of certain factors, most men may be sexually aroused by violent or rough sex, although in non-sex offenders, such arousal does not provoke a sexual assault.[106] Of the sex-offenders, researchers categorize rapists as being either (1) opportunists, (2) vindictive, (3) fixed sexual fantasizers, (4) angry, or (5) sexual sadists. A common element among all sex offenders is their lack of concern for their victims. They believe their victims either desired or deserved to be sexually assaulted. Such a belief may partly explain why the rate of cure among sex offenders is low and the rate of recidivism is often high.

The 30% of perpetrators who can be described as opportunistic rapists (including date-rapists) generally act on impulse, do not display anger toward their victims, and employ minimal unnecessary force. Likewise, the least violent rapists are the 25% described as fixed sexual fantasizers, men with an internalized romantic fantasy of forcibly having sex with a woman, thereby causing her to fall in love with him.

In contrast to the opportunists and fixed sexual fantasizers, the 27% of perpetrators described as being vindictive or hating women are violent and harbor the intent to physically harm, degrade, and humiliate their victims. This is also true for the 10% of perpetrators labeled as angry—typically described as sociopaths who hate everyone. Having long criminal histories, these men are especially dangerous and are likely to seriously injure their victims. Finally, 8% of perpetrators may be described as sexual sadists. These men are sexually stimulated by the victim's manifestation of fear and mutilation during a sexual assault.

Psychosexual difficulties commonly follow a sexual assault. Nadelson and coworkers (1982) report that 1 to 2 ½ years after sexual assault, 40% of victims experience sexual difficulties, restricted dating, suspiciousness, fear of being alone, and depression stemming from the assault.[108] Feelings of fear, helplessness, suspicion, and humiliation—often described as "rape trauma syndrome"—may have a minimal effect on the victim or may overwhelm her.

Immediately after the sexual assault, many women experience a variety of emotional and somatic symptoms, commonly described as the disorganization phase. During this phase, complaints of extreme fatigue and lethargy are common. Those physically injured during the assault often complain of soreness, increased bruising, and musculoskeletal pain. Other symptoms that arise after a sexual assault include sleep disorders (nightmares and insomnia), digestive disorders, eating disorders, genitourinary problems, and dyspareunia.

In the weeks after the acute event, women who have been the victims of sexual assault often develop strong feelings of suspicion toward men and an overwhelming sense of vulnerability. Others may plan for revenge against their assailants. Often described as the reorganization phase, many women make an active attempt to guard against future assaults by installing new locks on doors and windows, changing phone numbers to unlisted ones, installing security systems, changing modes and routes of transportation (especially to avoid the site of the sexual assault), changing places of residence or employment, and changing or curtailing dating habits. Many victims may manifest a new or increased dependency on family members or friends and may fear being left alone.

As time passes, women who have experienced a sexual assault evaluate their response to the incident. Some realize they handled the situation in the best manner they could under the circumstances, whereas others conclude that their response was insufficient or inadequate and experience a diminution of their self-esteem. Feelings of helplessness, humiliation, embarrassment, inadequacy, or contamination accompanied by lability of mood, anger, irritability, and depression may persist and cause some victims to lose interest in their daily lives, families, friends, and careers. At this point, patients usually need psychiatric evaluation and treatment. Physical symptoms may include nausea and vomiting, eating disorders, insomnia or nightmares, headaches, muscle spasms and pain, malaise, dizziness, genitourinary problems, vaginitis, pelvic pain, PMS, and menstrual disturbances and are best treated with medical treatment combined with psychological care.

Finally, many sexual assault victims present with complaints of lack of sexual desire, inability to become sexually aroused, and avoidance of sexual touching or intimacy. Some women experience shame or an aversion to their own breasts and genitalia, thereby causing them to become celibate, which in turn characteristically invokes a negative response from their sexual partners. Victims who do not have sexual partners at the time of the sexual assault may experience inability in securing or maintaining sexual partners because of dyspareunia or vaginismus. In some women, the vaginismus response occurs when a pelvic examination is attempted because the examination triggers fears associated with the sexual assault (ie, loss of control and being harmed or victimized), thereby inducing involuntary pubococcygeal muscle spasm. Other women may seek increased sexuality activity with one or many partners to reaffirm their ability to experience sexual arousal and be sexually responsive.

In addition to sexual abuse, many women are physically and emotionally traumatized by their spouses and fail to be diagnosed as a victim of domestic violence by many physicians.[109] About 2 million women (about 4% of married women) are battered in the United States each year but only 2% to 5% of physicians include questions on domestic violence in the medical history.[110,111] With directed physician inquiry, it is estimated that about 20% of women will report victimization. Questions physi-

cians should ask patients regarding battering may be adapted from an abuse questionnaire developed by Braham and coworkers:

1. I noticed you have a number of bruises. Could you tell me how they happened? Did someone hit you?
2. You seem frightened of your partner. Has he ever hurt you?
3. Many patients tell me they have been hurt by someone close to them. Could this be happening to you?
4. You mention your spouse loses his temper with the children. Does he ever lose his temper with you? Does he become abuse when he loses his temper?
5. Have there been times during your relationship when you have had physical fights?
6. Do your verbal fights ever include physical contact?
7. Have you ever been in a relationship where you have been hit, punched, kicked, or hurt in any way? Are you in such a relationship now?
8. You mentioned your spouse uses drugs or alcohol. How does your spouse act when drinking or on drugs?
9. Does your spouse or boyfriend consistently control your actions or put you down?
10. Sometimes when others are overprotective and as jealous as you describe, they react strongly and use physical force. Is this happening in your situation?
11. Your partner seems very concerned and anxious. Was he responsible for your injuries?[111]

It is important that the examination rooms or bathrooms of the physician's office contain educational materials on battering and phone numbers for women to call for help or advice. The materials should not be left in an area where other patients or healthcare providers are present because many battering victims are embarrassed or reluctant to pick up the information in a public area.

The immediate and long-term care of sexual assault and battering victims is best served by a multidisciplinary team that involves the integrated effort of physicians, nurses, psychologists, and social workers to ensure the appropriate medical and psychological management of the patient. Every center that treats trauma should have a standardized protocol for identifying battered women among female trauma victims.[110] In addition to treatment provided for injuries, potential pregnancy, and STDs, attention must be directed toward the psychosexual health of the woman. The gynecologist can direct the team caring for the victim to ensure that all aspects of her evaluation and treatment are being addressed; the gynecologist should not be expected to handle the medical and psychosexual needs of the woman singularly.

SEXUALITY

Sexuality is a complex human response that is characterized by a wide range of variation between and among individuals and is modulated by three basic components: (1) motivation (desire or libido); (2) psychosocial attitudes and beliefs; and (3) endocrine profiles. That patterns of sexual behavior in the human are more varied than in other mammals and can be explained by the extensive learning process unique to humans and the effect that a variety of psychosexual attitudes and beliefs have on sexual function. Acting as a counterbalance are the endocrinologic processes responsible for both limiting the possibilities and dictating common patterns of sexual behavior. Because of similar endocrine profiles, societies with vastly diverse cultures, mores, and institutions have common patterns of sexual behavior that include (1) the sequence of activities involved in self-or mutual stimulation to achieve orgasm; (2) the physiologic changes that occur with sexual response; (3) pleasure as the most frequent motivation for sexual activity; (4) the tendency to pair off when engaging in sexual activity; and (5) the universal practice of coitus.[112]

Likewise, sexual desire is a neurohumoral process of the brain that must be psychologically primed for sexual arousal to occur. Sexual desire can be self-manipulated by the individual, to an extent, through the reception of visual or other sensory stimulation that initiates arousal—or conversely, by ignoring or suppressing sexually arousing thoughts or stimuli.

The changing endocrine profile of women at various times over the reproductive and postreproductive lifespan is complex, and emphasis is generally placed on estrogen levels and metabolism. For example, the menopause is conceptualized as progressive ovarian follicular failure, culminating in estrogen deficiency. Ovarian and adrenal androgens also have a pivotal function in both men and premenopausal and postmenopausal women, especially in their impact on sexual development and function. Androgens affect development of the fetus and are also substrates for reproductive and postmenopausal estrogen biosynthesis but by different metabolic pathways. In contrast to the male, in the absence of fetal testicular androgen, the female genital tubercle forms into a clitoris and the urogenital groove stays open as the vaginal introitus. As with the male, the resultant female genital morphology is both permanent and complete by the 14th fetal week. At 6 weeks gestational age, fetal androgens in the male begin acting on parts of the brain, especially in the hypothalamus and limbic system, which effect patterns of male behavior. In the absence of fetal androgens, the central nervous system develops in the female pattern and at puberty, gonadotropins are secreted in a cyclic pattern.

The relation of adult female sexual function and sex hormones has been studied, with attempts to isolate endocrine effects (estrogen, progesterone, and androgen) from those that are sociocultural.[113–115] A population often evaluated to determine the influence of hormones on sexual function is postmenopausal women.

The effect of hormone-replacement therapy (especially androgens) on sexual behavior in postmenopausal women has been studied for more than five decades.[113] Diverse hormone-replacement–therapy formulations (varying estrogens, estrogen–progestogen, and estrogen–androgen combinations); dosages; duration; and routes of administration have been employed, making data difficult to compare.[114] Also, the study populations vary (ie, perimenopausal and natural and surgical menopausal subjects, with or without various levels of sexual dysfunction). Although disparate methods for the evaluation of subjective and objective sexual responses and other psychological parameters are employed in the studies, some global conclusions regarding the role of hormone-replacement therapy of sexual and other related physiologic responses may be extracted. Estrogens alone result in decreased atrophic vaginitis and increased vaginal blood flow, reduced vaginal dryness, and dyspareunia in postmenopausal women.[114] These reduced beneficial gynecologic effects often provide the environment for more satisfactory sexual response but probably do not exert a direct effect on sexual behavior. Similarly, estrogen–progestin combinations do not appear to directly enhance sexual function in the older woman. Androgens, either alone or in combination with estrogen, appear to enhance sexual motivation.[116] Although coital frequency depends on many factors, such as partner availability, desire, and function, androgens appear to positively influence coital and orgasmic frequency. The relation of sexual response to specific androgen blood level requires further investigation; there are no dependable data correlated to an androgen blood level to the need for postmenopausal replacement of this hormone. In surgically postmenopausal women who lose all ovarian hormone production, androgens or androgens with estrogens seem to be of benefit and may enhance sexual responsiveness more than estrogens alone.[116] With the addition of androgens, body image was more positive and women reported a greater mean frequency of sexual desire, masturbation, female-initiated sexual activity, and arousal than estrogen only or untreated groups.[116–118]

When examining the effects of oral contraceptives on sexuality, it appears that women who are using oral contraceptives are more likely to have a current sexual partner and report an increased frequency of premarital sexual activity and sexual partners when compared with nonusers.[119] Oral contraceptive pill users do not report an increase in self-stimulation, however. Considering these factors, oral contraceptive pill users appear to show higher sexual motivation and orgasmic adequacy, less inhibition during intercourse, and the ability to more easily express their preferred frequency of intercourse. In addition, they are more likely to be positive toward their partner. No differences seem to exist between users and nonusers regarding sexual fantasy, arousal to erotic imagery, or gender-role behavior. Of interest, despite the lower levels of free testosterone in oral contraceptive pill users, there is a positive association with frequency of sexual intercourse and a negative association with restrictive sexual preferences.[120]

Although the impact of hormones on sexual function is of great importance, the cause of sexual dysfunction is often multifactorial; therefore hormone use alone is usually not effective for treatment. The prevalence of sexual dysfunction in gynecologic patients is high and ranges from 19% to 33% in outpatients and up to about 50% in inpatient samples.[121] The physician may not elicit discussion about sexual problems a woman is experiencing unless he or she asks direct questions. In a study at Robert Wood Johnson Medical School, of 887 consecutive patients, only 3% spontaneously cited a sexual problem; an additional 16% raised sexual concerns only with direct inquiry.[121] Although sexual history–taking is often shunned by gynecologists because of the increased time involved and the issue of how to manage the patient who reports sexual difficulties, this study found that asking two questions, "Are you sexually active?" and "Are

you having any sexual difficulties such as decreased vaginal lubrication, pain with intercourse, or diminished sexual desire?" uncovered many sexual difficulties without adding a lot of time to the office visit. Most of the difficulties reported could be taken care of in the office. It is helpful to gear the examples of difficulties cited to the age of the patient and use problems that are commonly seen in that subgroup of women. Adolescent problems include anxiety about sexual performance, guilt, fears of bodily damage, fears of intimacy, and concerns about pregnancy, STDs, and homosexuality. Women in early adulthood often report orgasmic dysfunction and the sexual problems related to pregnancy, whereas women between the ages of 30 and 40 years typically complain of sexual communication problems, especially if the marital unit is not a happy one and there are different levels of sexual desire between partners. Women in the perimenopausal and menopausal years begin to experience ovarian hormone changes and often note decreased vaginal lubrication, dyspareunia, and diminished sexual desire. In the postmenopausal years, chronic illness and partner loss or dysfunction play a greater role in defining the sexual function and activity of older women. Older couples who adhere to the sexual script that they had used for their entire sexual life usually experience more sexual problems and are more likely to become sexually abstinent than couples who are willing to experiment with different sexual activities.

Common sexual dysfunctions the gynecologist often sees in the office include anorgasmia, dyspareunia, loss of sexual desire, and vaginismus. Anorgasmia is often reported in women who (1) lack information or are misinformed regarding orgasm, (2) believe that orgasm is spontaneous and not learned, (3) adhere to rigid female role scripting, and (4) fear loss of control with orgasm. Treatment of orgasmic difficulties usually involves long-term counseling and is one of the sexual dysfunctions that often must be referred to a therapist. One approach that the gynecologist may want to employ was developed by Lobitz and LoPiccolo, a nine-step masturbation desensitization plan.[122] The plan begins with the patient examining herself while naked and practicing Kegel exercises and progresses to the patient's partner stimulating her genitals manually or with a vibrator after she has achieved orgasm through self-stimulation. This plan is most successful when the woman is simultaneously counseled regarding sexual and communication issues.

Dyspareunia, when due to an organic etiology

(eg, endometriosis, vaginal dryness), is treated by pharmacologic or surgical interventions. Dyspareunia may either be caused entirely or partially by psychological factors, however, including a history of trauma to the pelvic area and relationship difficulties. When dyspareunia is related to psychological factors, it is more difficult to treat and may require referral to a therapist. Lazarua developed seven areas that should be covered in the medical history of women with dyspareunia:

- Behavior. Are there deficits and shortcomings in sexual technique?
- Effect. Is guilt, anger, fear, or shame a primary or contributory factor? Are feelings of love and physical attraction conspicuously present or absent?
- Sensation. Because dyspareunia presents as a sensory complaint, this modality requires a detailed initial assessment.
- Imagery. Are there intrusive images (negative mental pictures) that disrupt sexual enjoyment? Is there a poor or distorted body image?
- Cognition. Do negative self-statement, irrational self-talk, and erroneous notions play a significant role in undermining the client's sexual participation?
- Interpersonal. What basic interaction and personal climate exists between the partners in sexual and nonsexual settings?
- Drugs (biological). Is the patient on any medication, especially antihypertensive drugs, tranquilizers, or sedatives? Is there evidence of proper hygiene?"[123,124]

The gynecologist should address each of these points and if no short-term resolution is apparent, referral is necessary.

Vaginismus is probably the most perplexing and frustrating problem to the patient and gynecologist. Because of the involuntary contraction of the pubococcygeus and related muscles surrounding the vaginal opening, the patient is often unable to have full or in some cases any penile penetration. Many women present for help with this condition when they desire pregnancy, although some women with vaginismus achieve pregnancy without medical assistance. There is no consensus regarding the etiology of this sexual dysfunction but it has been described as a psychosomatic disorder, a phobia, a conditioned response, and a conversion reaction. Although there are limited data on the prevalence of vaginismus, gynecologists see this condition several times annually in their practice. It presents in varying degrees of severity, ranging from extreme discomfort with speculum insertion to inability to use a speculum at all. Of interest, although there are several possible etiologies, ranging from a specific traumatic event to an underlying psychodynamic conflict, the role of the spouse is viewed as a major contributor in the continuance if not the cause of vaginismus. Prognosis is good, and regardless of the cause, the most successful treatment is with the use of vaginal dilators.[125] Women with this condition should be instructed in the gradual insertion of larger dilators into the vaginal introitus under conditions of relaxation and patient control. Systematic desensitization is often used in conjunction with vaginal dilators. It does not appear to be important for the partner to be involved in the process during the early stages of treatment; the partner should become involved only after the woman has made substantial progress.

Probably the most difficult sexual dysfunction to define is low sexual desire. Because there is no consensus on what constitutes a low frequency of sexual exchange and what is the norm for ideal sexual activity, no "normal" coital frequency can be used as a measure for each patient. Sexual desire problems most often surface when one spouse is not happy with the couple's sexual activity and requests treatment. Women at risk for loss of sexual desire, as described by LoPiccolo, include women who:

1. Have not learned to perceive or perceive accurately their own levels of physiologic sexual arousal; perception of arousal (such a genital sensations) is diminished or mislabeled
2. Have not learned how to facilitate arousal in themselves
3. Use a limited set of cues to define a situation as sexual
4. Use a limited set of cues to define their own sexual arousal
5. Have limited expectations for their own ability to be aroused
6. On the basis of the above, tend not to perceive themselves as very sexual[126]

Assessment of this problem should include a measure of the couple's and the woman's actual and desired sexual behavior in addition to several other parameters of psychological health, such as perception of body image and relationship to partner. Evaluation of hormonal status (especially androgens) is important, especially if the patient has had a surgical menopause. If there is a specific dysfunction such as anxiety or depression, treatment should be individualized. In-office education that encourages couple communication and the use of fantasy and erotic stimuli should be offered. Referral to a therapist for extensive counseling of select patients should be considered, regardless of the age of the couple.

In summary, the sexual dysfunctions and difficulties of the gynecologic patient can be successfully assessed in the office, with management consisting of education, counseling, and pharmacologic and surgical intervention. Treatment by the gynecologist is effective in more than 90% of women, with fewer than 10% needing referral.[121] In women who do not improve sexual functioning through the treatments offered, work with a therapist in the community is ideal, so that the gynecologist can have continued input into the woman's care.

REFERENCES

1. Slade P, Anderton KJ: Gynaecological symptoms and psycological distress: a longitudinal study of their relationship. J Psychosom Obstet Gynaecol 13:51, 1992
2. Slade P, Anderton KJ, Faragher EB: Psychological aspects of gynaecological outpatients. J Psychosom Obstet Gynaecol 8:77, 1988
3. Byrne P: Psychiatric morbidity in a gynaecology clinic: an epidemiological survey. Br J Psychiatry 144:28, 1984
4. Gath D, Osborn M, Bungay G, et al: Psychiatric disorders and gynaecological symptoms in middle aged women: a community survey. Br Med J 294:213, 1987
5. Koninckx PR: Pelvic endometriosis: a consequence of stress. Contrib Gynecol Obstet 16:56, 1987
6. Gleicher N, Dmowski WP, Siegel I, et al: Lymphocyte subsets in endometriosis. Obstet Gynecol 63:463, 1984
7. Brosens IA, Koninckx PR, Corveleyn PA: A study of plasma progesterone, oestradiol-17b, prolactin, and of the luteal phase appearance of the ovaries in patients with endometriosis and infertillity. Br J Obstet Gynaecol 85:246, 1987
8. Ader R, Cohen N: Behaviourally-conditioned immunosuppression. Psychosom Med 37:333, 1975
9. Bruce-Jones W, Zolese G, White P: Polycystic ovary syndrome and psychiatric morbidity. J Psychosom Obstet Gynaecol 14:111, 1993
10. Dicker RC, Greenspan JR, Strauss LT, et al: Complications of abdominal and vaginal hysterectomy among women of reproductive age in the United States. Am J Obstet Gynecol 144:841, 1982
11. Gambone JC, Lench JB, Slesinski MJ, et al: Validation of hysterectomy indications and the quality assurance process. Obstet Gynecol 73:1045, 1989
12. Low WY, Edelmann RJ: Psychosocial aspects of endometriosis: a review. J Psychosom Obstet Gynaecol 12:3, 1991
13. Houston DE, Noller KL, Melton LJ, Selwyn BJ, Hardy RJ: Incidence of pelvic endometriosis in Rochester MN 1970–1979. Am J Epidemiol 125: 959, 1987
14. Barbieri RL: Etiology and epidemiology of endometriosis. Am J Obstet Gynecol 162:565, 1990
15. Houston DE, Noller KL, Melton LJ, Selwyn BJ: The epidemiology of pelvic endometriosis. Clin Obstet Gynecol 31:787, 1988
16. Chatmann DL: Endometriosis in the black woman. Am J Obstet Gynecol 125: 987, 1976
17. Hammond CB, Hancy AF: Conservative treatment of endometriosis. Fertil Steril 30:497, 1978
18. Lewis DO, Comite F, Mallouh C, et al: Bipolar mood disorder and endometriosis: preliminary findings. Am J Psychiatry 144:1588, 1987
19. Walker E, Katon W, Jones LM, Russo J: Relationship between endometriosis and affective disorder. Am J Psychiatry 146:380, 1989
20. Walker E, Katon W, Harrop-Griffiths J, Holm L, Russo J, Hickok LR: Relationship of chronic pelvic pain to psychiatric diagnoses and childhood sexual abuse. Am J Psychiatry 145:75, 1988
21. Castelnuovo-Tedesco P, Krout BM: Psychosomatic aspects of chronic pelvic pain. Int J Psychiatry Med 1:109, 1970
22. Rosenthal RH, Ling FW, Rosenthal JL, McNeeley SG: Chronic pelvic pain: psychological features and laparoscopic findings. Psychosomatics 25:833, 1984
23. Slocumb JC, Kellner R, Rosenfield RC, Pathak D: Anxiety and depression in patients with the abdominal pelvic pain syndrome. Gen Hosp Psychiatry II:48, 1989
24. Weinstein K: The emotional aspeects of endometriosis: what the patient expects from her doctor. Clin Obstet Gynecol 31:866, 1988
25. McEwen BS: Basic research perspective: ovarian hormone influence on brain neurochemical functions. In Gis LH, Kase NG, Berkowitz RL (eds): The premenstrual syndromes. New York, Churchill Livingstone, 1988
26. Gandelman R: Gonadal hormones and sensory function. Neurosci Biobehav Rev 7:1, 1983
27. Adams DB, Gold AR, Burt AD: Rise in female-initiated sexual activity at ovulation and its suppression by oral contraceptives. N Engl J Med 299:1145, 1978
28. Adler EM, Bancroft J, Livingstone J: Estradiol implants, hormone levels and reported symptoms. J Psychosom Obstet Gynecol 13:223, 1992
29. Grounds D, Davies B, Mowbray R: The contraceptive pill, side effect and personality: report of a controlled double blind trial. Br J Psychiatry 116:169, 1970
30. Kane FJ: Evaluation of emotional reactions to oral contraceptive use. Am J Obstet Gynecol 126:965, 1976
31. Parry BL, Rush AJ: Oral contraceptives and depressive symptomatology: biologic mechanisms. Compr Psychiatry 20:347, 1979
32. Vessey MP, McPherson K, Lawless M, Yeates D: Oral contraception and serious psychiatric ill-

ness: absence of an association. Br J Psychiatry 146:45, 1985

33. Marcotte DB, Kane FJ, Obrist P, Lipton MA: Physiologic changes accompanying oral contraceptive use. Br J Psychiatry 116:165, 1970

34. Goetsch, Burnette MM, Wiener AL, Koehn KA, Vanin J, Clements J-N: An investigation of the influence of expectancy on affective and physical changes associated with oral contraceptive use. J Psychosom Obstet Gynaecol 12: 209, 1991

35. Murphy P: Poll shows women still skeptical of contraceptive safety. American College of Obstetrics and Gynecology News Release, 1994

36. Speroff L, Darney P: Long-acting steroid methods. A clinical guide for contraception, p 117. Baltimore, Williams & Wilkins, 1992

37. Schagn van Leeuwen JH, te Velde ER, Koppeschaar HPF, et al: Is premenstrual syndrome an endocrine disorder? J Psychosom Obstet Gynaecol 14:91, 1993

38. Kimmel S, Gonsalves L, Youngs D, Gidwani G: Fluctuating levels of antidepressants premenstrually. J Psychosom Obstet Gynaecol 13:277, 1992

39. Rubinow DR, Roy-Byrne P: Premenstrual syndromes: overview from a methodological perspective. Am J Psych 141:29, 1984

40. Reid RL, Yen SSC: Premenstrual syndrome. Am J Obstet Gynecol 139:85, 1981

41. Andersh B, Wendetam C, Hahn L, Ohman R: Premenstrual complaints. I. Prevalence of premenstrual symptoms in a Swedish urban population. J Psychosom Obstet Gynaecol 5:39, 1986

42. Chaturvedi SK, Chandra PS, Issac MK, et al: Premenstrual experiences: the four profiles and factorial patterns. J Psychosom Obstet Gynaecol 14:223, 1993

43. Freeman EW, Rickels K, Sondheimer SJ: Premenstrual symptoms and dysmenorrhea in relation to emotional distress factors in adolescents. J Psychosom Obstet Gynaecol 14:41, 1993

44. Steiner M, Haskett RF, Carrol BJ: Premenstrual tension syndrome: the development of research diagnostic criteria and new rating scales. Acta Psychiatr Scand 62:177, 1980

45. Endicott J, Halbreich U: Retrospective report of premenstrual depressive changes: factors affecting confirmation by daily ratings. Psychopharmacol Bull 18:109, 1982

46. Fioroni L, Facchinetti F, Gerrutti G, Nappi G, Genazzani AR: Personality traits in secondary amenorrhea. J Psychosom Obstet Gynaecol II:67, 1990

47. Dennerstein L, Brown JB, Gotts G, Morse CA, Farley TMM, Pinol A: Menstrual cycle profiles of women with and without premenstrual syndrome. J Psychosom Obstet Gynaecol 14:259, 1993

48. Schagen van Leeuwen JH, teVelde ER, Kop WJ, vander Ploeg HM, Haspels AA: A simple strategy to detect significant premenstrual changes. J Psychosom Obstet Gynaecol 14:211, 1993

49. Ekholm U-B, Hammarback S, Backstrom T: Premenstrual syndrome: changes in symptom pattern between two menstrual cycles. J Psychosom Obstet Gynaecol 13:107, 1992

50. Ekholm U-B, Hammarback S, Backstrom T: Premenstrual tension syndrome: a study comparing

symptom ratings during two consecutive menstrual cycles. J Psychosom Obstet Gynaecol 12: 291, 1991

51. Keye WR Jr: The clinical approach to evaluation and treatment. In The premenstrual syndrome. Philadelphia, WB Saunders, 1988

52. Metcalf MG, Livesey JH, Wells JE: Mood and physical symptom cyclicity in women with the premenstrual syndrome: unexpected response to placebo treatment. J Psychosom Obstet Gynaecol 12:273, 1991

53. Casson P, Hahn PM, Van Vugt DA, Reid RL: Lasting response to ovariectomy in severe intractable premenstrual syndrome. Am J Obstet Gynaecol 162:99, 1990

54. Casper RF, Hearn MT: The effect of hysterectomy and bilateral oophorectomy in women with severe premenstrual syndrome. Am J Obstet Gynecol 162:105, 1990

55. Muse KN, Cetel NS, Futterman LA, Yen SSC: The premenstrual syndrome: effects of "medical ovariectomy." N Engl J Med 311:1345, 1984

56. Krum S, Lamberti J: Changes in sexual behavior following radiation therapy for cervical cancer. J Psychosom Obstet Gynaecol 14:51, 1993

57. Andersen B, Racher N: Treatment for gynecologic cancer: a review of the effects on female sexuality. Health Psychol 2:203, 1983

58. Tamburini M, Filiberti A, De Palo G, Ventafridda V: Psychological and sexual dimension of gynecological cancer. Br J Sex Med 170, 1987

59. Campion MJ, Brown JR, McCance DJ, et al: Psychosexual trauma of an abnormal cervical smear. Br J Obstet Gynaecol 95:175, 1988

60. Hartman P, Diddle AW: Vaginal stenosis following radiation therapy for carcinoma of the cervix uteri. Cancer 30:426, 1972

61. Mickal A, Torres JE, Schlosser JV: Complications of therapy for carcinoma of the cervix. Am J Obstet Gynecol 112:556, 1972

62. Doherty IE, Richardson PH, Wolfe CD, Raju KS: The assessment of the psychological effects of an abnormal cervical smear result and subsequent medical procedures. J Psychosom Obstet Gynaecol 12:319, 1991

63. Seibel M, Freeman MG, Graves WL: Sexual function after surgical and radiation therapy for cervical carcinoma. South Med J 75:1195, 1982

64. Pitkin RM, Bradbury JT: The effects of topical estrogen on irradiated vaginal epithelium. Am J Obstet Gynecol 91:175, 1965

65. Adelusi B: Coital function after radiotherapy for carcinoma of the cervix uteri. Br J Obstet Gynaecol 87:821, 1980

66. Groeneveld FPMJ, Bareman FP, Barentsen R, et al: The climacteric and well-being. J Psychosom Obstet Gynaecol 14:127, 1993

67. Hunter MS, Battersby R, Whitehead M: Relationship between psychological symptoms, somatic complaints and menopausal status. Maturitas 8: 217, 1986

68. McKinlay JB, McKinlay SM, Brambilla DJ: Health status and utilization behaviour with menopause. Am J Epidemiol 125:110, 1987

69. Ballinger CB: Psychiatric morbidity and the menopause. Survey of a gynaecological outpatient clinic. Br J Psychiatry 131:83, 1977

70. Tropeano G, Saini S, Dell'Acqua S: Psychological and psychosomatic symptoms of the climacteric. J Psychosom Obstet Gynaecol 12:229, 1991

71. Holte A: Prevalence of climacteric complaints in a representative sample of middle-aged women in Oslo, Norway. J Psychosom Obstet Gynaecol 12:303, 1991

72. Greene JS: A factor analytic study of climacteric symptoms. J Psychosom Res 20:425, 1976

73. Chakravarti S, Collins WP, Thom MH, Studd JWW: Relation between plasma hormone properties, symptoms and response to oestrogen treatment in women approaching the menopause. Br Med J 1:983, 1979

74. Hunter D: Emotional well-being, sexual behaviour and hormone replacement therapy. Maturitas 12:159, 1990

75. Leysen B, DeMunter A, Buytaert Ph: Image of the climacteric woman: a comparison of women attending a university menopause clinic and women participating in a self-help group. J Psychosom Obstet Gynaecol 13:299, 1992

76. Filiberti A, Tamburini M, Stefanon B, et al: Psychological aspects of genital human papillomavirus infection: a preliminary report: J Psychosom Obstet Gynaecol 14:142, 1993

77. Affonso D, Lovett S, Paul S, et al: Predictors of depression symptoms during pregnancy and postpartum. J Psychosom Obstet Gynaecol 12:255, 1991

78. Paykel E, Emms E, Fletcher J, Rassaby E: Life events and social support in puerperal depression. Br J Psychiatry 136:339, 1980

79. Pitt B: "Atypical" depression following childbirth. Br J Psychiatry 114:1325, 1986

80. Kumar R, Robson J: A prospective study of emotional disorders in childbearing women. Br J Psychiatry 144:35, 1984

81. O'Hara M, Rehm L, Campbell S: Postpartum depression: a role for social network and life stress variables. J Nerv Ment Dis 171:336, 1983

82. Watson J, Elliott S, Rugg A, Brough D: Psychiatric disorder in pregnancy and the first postnatal year. Br J Psychiatry 144:453, 1984

83. Cox J, Connor Y, Kendell R: Prospective study of the psychiatric disorders of childbirth. Br J Psychiatry 140:111, 1982

84. Stirzinger R, Robinson GE: The psychological effects of spontaneous abortion. Can Med Assoc J 140:799, 1989

85. Peppers LG, Knapp RJ: Maternal reactions to involuntary fetal/infant death. Psychiatry 43:155, 1989

86. Chalmers B, Meyer D: A cross-cultural view of the psychosocial management of miscarriage. J Psychosom Obstet Gynaecol 13:163, 1992

87. Lloyd J, Lawrence KM: Sequelae and support after termination of pregnancy for fetal malformation. Br Med J 290:907, 1985

88. Robinson GE, Carr ML, Olmsted MP, Wright C: Psychological reactions to pregnancy loss after prenatal diagnostic testing: preliminary results. J Psychosom Obstet Gynaecol 12:181, 1991

89. Robinson GE, Garner DM, Olmsted MP, Shime J, Hutton EM, Crawford BM: Anxiety reduction following chorionic villi sampling and genetic amniocentesis. Am J Obstet Gyncol 159:953, 1988

90. Spencer JW, Cox DN: Emotional responses of pregnant women to chorionic villi sampling or amniocentesis. Am J Obstet Gynecol 157:1155, 1987

91. Rizzardo R, Magni G, Desideri A, Cosentino M, Salmaso P: Personality and psychological distress before and after legal abortion: a prospective study. J Psychosom Obstet Gynaecol 13:75, 1992

92. Lazarus A: Psychiatric sequelae of legalized elective first trimester abortion. J Psychosom Obstet Gynaecol 4:141, 1985

93. Barnett W, Freudenberg N, Willie R: Eine regionale Prospektivstudie psychisher Folgeerscheinungen der Notlagenabrupto. Fortschr Neurol Psychiatr 54:106, 1986

94. Burnell GM, Norfleet MA: Women's self-reported responses to abortion. J Psychol 121:71, 1987

95. Holmgren K: Time of decision to undergo a legal abortion. Gynecol Obstet Invest 26:289, 1988

96. Cohen L, Roth S: Coping with abortion. J Hum Stress 10:140, 1984

97. Franco KN, Tamburrino MB, Campbell NB, Pentz JE, Jurs SG: Psychological profile of dysphoric women post abortion. J Am Med Wom Assoc 44:113, 1989

98. Moller A, Fallstrom K: Psychological consequences of infertility: a longitudinal study. J Psychosom Obstet Gynaecol 12:27, 1991

99. deParseval GD: Clinical remarks concerning parents (potential and real) after different "treatments" for the sterility of couples. J Psychosom Obstet Gynaecol 13:65, 1992

100. Scholl GM: Vaginismus and infertility. J Psychosom Obstet Gynaecol 12:45, 1991

101. Strauss B, Appelt H, Bohnet HG, Ulrich D: Relationship between psychological characteristics and treatment outcome in female patients from an infertility clinic. 13:121, 1992

102. Wasser SK, Isenberg DY: Reproductive failure among women: pathology or adaption? J Psychosom Obstet Gynaecol 5:153, 1986

103. Bachmann GA: Hysterectomy: a critical review. J Reprod Med 35:9, 1990

104. Bachmann GA: Pyschosexual aspects of hysterectomy. Women's Health Issues 1:1, 1990

105. Richards DH: A post-hysterectomy syndrome. Lancet 2:983, 1974

106. Bachmann GA: Sexual abuse and sexual assault. In Moore TR, Reiter RC, Rebar RW, Baker VV (eds): Gynecology and obstetrics: a longitudinal approach. New York, Churchill Livingstone, 1993

107. Lurvey L, Trupin S: Emergency Department evaluation of the sexual assault victim. J Clin Pract Sex 9:1, 1993

108. Nadelson CC, Notman MT, Zackson H, Gornick J: A follow-up study of rape victims. Am J Psychiatry 139:1266, 1982

109. Bachmann GA, Ramondetta L: Treatment of battered women. J Clin Pract Sex 9:1, 1993

110. McLeer SV, Anwar R: A study of battered women presenting in an emergency department. AJPH 79:65, 1989

111. Hamberger KL, Saunders DG, Hovey M: Prevalence of domestic violence in community practice and rate of physician inquiry. Fam Med 24:283, 1992

112. Lief HI: Sexuality and sexual health. In Sexual

problems in medical practice. Chicago, American Medical Association, 1984

113. Salmon UJ, Geist SH: Effect of androgen upon libido in women. J Endocrinol 3:235, 1943

114. Walling N, Andersen BL, Johnson SP: Hormonal replacement therapy for postmenopausal women: a review of sexual outcomes and related gynecologic effects. Arch Sex Behav 19:119, 1990

115. Longcope C: Adenal and gonadal androgen secretion in normal females. Clin Endocrinol Metab 15:213, 1986

116. Sherwin BB, Gelfand MM, Brender W: Androgen enhances sexual motivation in females: a prospective, crossover study of sex steroid administration in the surgical menopause. Psychosom Med 47 (B):339, 1985

117. Bellerose SB, Benik YM: Body image and sexuality in oopherectomized women. Arch Sex Behav 22:435, 1993

118. Sherwin BB, Gelfand MM: The role of androgen in the maintenance of sexual functioning in oophorectomized women. Psychom Med 48:397, 1987

119. Bancroft J, Sherwin BB, Alexander GM, Davidson DW, Walker A: Oral contraceptives, androgens, and the sexuality of young women: I. A comparison of sexual experience, sexual attitudes, and gender role in oral contraceptive users and non-users. Arch Sex Behav 20(A):105, 1991

120. Bancroft J, Sherwin BB, Alexander GM, Davidson DW, Walker A: Oral contraceptives, androgens, and the sexuality of young women: II. The role of androgens. Arch Sex Behav 20(B):121, 1991

121. Bachmann GA, Leiblum S, Grill J: Graduate education. Brief sexual inquiry in gynecologic practice. Obstet Gynecol 73:425, 1989

122. Lobitz WC, LoPiccolo J: The role of masturbation in the treatgment of orgasmic dysfunction. Arch Sex Behav 2:163, 1972

123. Lazarus AA: Multimodal behavior therapy. New York, Springer, 1976

124. Lazarus AA: Psychological treatment of dyspareunia. In Leiblum S, Previn LA (eds): Principles and practices of sex therapy. New York, The Guilford Press, 1980

125. Leiblum S, Pervin LA, Campbell EH: The treatment of vaginismus: success and failure. In Leiblum S, Pervin LA (eds): Principles and practices of sex therapy. New York, The Guilford Press, 1980

126. LoPiccolo L: Low sexual desire. In Leiblum S, Previn LA (eds):Principles and practices of sex therapy. New York, The Guilford Press, 1980

Ambulatory Gynecology, Second Edition,
edited by David H. Nichols and Patrick J. Sweeney.
J. B. Lippincott Company, Philadelphia, © 1995.

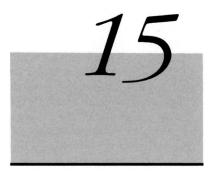

15

Medical Management of Ectopic Pregnancy

Kevin E. Bachus and Charles B. Hammond

The implantation of an embryo at a site other than the uterine endometrium has been recognized for centuries as a serious complication of conception and continues to be a major health concern for women. In 1970, the number of reported ectopic pregnancies was estimated at 17,800, with a mortality rate of 35.5 per 10,000 pregnancies in the United States alone.[1] In addition to this high mortality rate, a fivefold increase in the number of women hospitalized for ectopic pregnancy has been reported by the Centers for Disease Control and Prevention (CDC) during the last 2 decades. Whereas the incidence of ectopic pregnancy was once reported to occur at a rate of one in 200 live births, many studies report ectopic rates as high as one in every 44 live births.[2] One emergency room report listed one ectopic pregnancy for every 13 visits by pregnant patients in the first trimester.[2]

Factors responsible for this dramatic increase in the number of ectopic pregnancies include concomitant increases in disease states that alter normal tubal anatomy and physiology and consequently slow ovum transport. Such conditions as prior pelvic infection, tubal damage by prior ectopic pregnancy or failed sterilization, salpingitis isthmica nodosa, intrauterine device (IUD) use, and possibly assisted reproductive technologies contribute to this increased risk. Additionally, increased awareness of the severity of this diagnosis has led to increased surveillance on the part of healthcare workers. Improvements in the sensitivity and availability of assays for the β-subunit of human chorionic gonadotropin (hCG-β), improved resolution of abdominal and vaginal ultrasound, and aggressive use of laparoscopy have assisted physicians in the diagnosis and treatment of this clinical entity. Consequently, these improved technologies have increasingly enabled the physician to make the diagnosis well before the pregnancy ruptures from its ectopic implantation site, allowing earlier therapeutic intervention. As a result, despite the increase in the number of women hospitalized for ectopic pregnancy from 4.5 to 11.8 per 1000 pregnancies, the risk of death has declined 10-fold for the years 1970 through 1987.[1]

Despite the decline in mortality, patients with ectopic pregnancies still suffer from the morbidity of recurrent ectopic gestations and subsequent infertility. Traditional surgical procedures such as salpingectomy, with or without oophorectomy, in many cases have been replaced with salpingotomy or salpingostomy and with laparoscopic salpingostomy. These trends in surgical management parallel an increasing interest in preserving fertility options with a concurrent diminution of surgical invasiveness. In an effort to further improve subsequent fertility and decrease surgical morbidity for patients with an unruptured ectopic gestation, chemotherapy has been proposed as an alternative to surgical therapies. Certain chemotherapeutic modalities appear to be successful, especially if they are used within specific guidelines. This chapter discusses the indications, limitations, and routes of administration of different chemotherapeutic agents for patients with ectopic pregnancy and reviews the available literature, with regard to post-treatment tubal patency and intrauterine pregnancy rates. An understanding of the indications and limitations of medical management depends on a basic knowledge of the pathophysiology and the diagnostic strategies involved with ectopic pregnancies. A full discussion is beyond the scope of this chapter but a brief review of the pathophysiology and diagnostic approaches is appropriate.

PATHOPHYSIOLOGY

Damage to the fallopian tube by infection, surgery, prior ectopic or postoperative adhesion formation increases ectopic rates to as high as 27%.[3-5] Probably the most important risk factor for an ectopic pregnancy is a history of pelvic infection because evidence of prior salpingitis occurs in nearly half of all patients with ectopic pregnancies.[6-8] As a consequence of infection, the plicae of the endosalpinx may become agglutinated and entrap the embryo as it travels toward the uterus. Westrom and colleagues found that women with laparoscopically confirmed acute salpingitis who were followed prospectively for reproductive outcome had a sixfold higher ectopic rate compared with noninfected controls.[6] A history of prior ectopic pregnancy also increases the recurrence risk to 15% with one and to 20% with two prior ectopic pregnancies.[9]

Another pathologic tubal finding considered a risk for ectopic pregnancy is salpingitis isthmica nodosa. The finding of numerous tubal lumenal diverticula in this condition appears to increase the ectopic pregnancy risk by an unknown mechanism. It is suggested that mechanical entrapment within these diverticula is not the primary etiology but it appears to be more related to dysfunction of normal tubal transport mechanisms.[10,11] Contraceptive failure is also reported to increase ectopic pregnancy risk. Failure of elective tubal sterilization may result in an increased ectopic pregnancy risk of up to 60%, depending on the techniques used.[12] This is secondary to intraperitoneal fistulas, which have been reported in about 11% of women after tubal ligation.[13] Pregnancies that result despite IUDs are also at increased risk for being ectopic. By inducing a sterile inflammatory reaction in the uterine cavity, the IUDs are more effective in preventing intrauterine pregnancy (compared with ectopic pregnancies), resulting in a 5% ectopic risk should conception occur with an IUD in place.

Altered tubal motility may be an etiology for the apparent increased ectopic pregnancy rate noted in women in whom estrogen or progesterone levels are elevated over usual physiologic concentrations.[12,14] Conceptions that occur despite the attempted interruption of pregnancy by the high-estrogen "morning after pill" are 10 times more likely to result in an ectopic pregnancy.[15] Patients exposed to diethylstilbestrol in utero have a 5% to 13% risk of ectopic pregnancy.[16] Through a similar mechanism, changes in endogenous estrogen production, such as that which occurs with ovulation induction with human menopausal gonadotropins, is postulated to contribute to the surprisingly high rate (7%) of ectopic pregnancy in patients undergoing ovulation induction for in vitro fertilization, despite the intrauterine placement of embryos. Whether this is due to mechanical propulsion of the embryo into the fallopian tube or whether transtubal migration occurs is uncertain. Conception despite the use of the progestin-only "minipill" also result in a fivefold increase in the ectopic pregnancy rate.[12,17] Progestin-containing IUDs have 5% to 15% higher ectopic pregnancy rates compared with inert IUDs. In many cases, however, it is unclear whether the non-physiologic hormone profiles in these women act to increase ectopic rates by directly altering tubal motility or whether a subtle form of inherent tubal damage is already present.

The anatomic distribution of ectopic pregnancies studied by Breen from a series of 654 patients

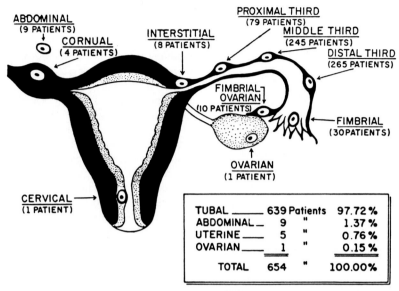

Figure 15–1.   Incidence of ectopic pregnancy by anatomic site. (Breen JL: A 21-year study of 654 ectopic pregnancies. Am J Obstet Gynecol 106:1004, 1970. With permission.)

revealed that 97.7% are tubal, 1.4% abdominal, 0.2% cervical, and 0.2% ovarian (Fig. 15-1).[18] For those pregnancies in the tube, histopathologic examination reveals that, contrary to popular belief, many ectopic pregnancies are extraluminal. This occurs as the implanting trophoblast invades the lamina propria and tubal muscularis before eventually gaining sufficient size to rupture the tubal serosa.[19] The anatomic location of the pregnancy may be important in deciding whether medical or surgical management is most appropriate. Isthmic, cornual, and even cervical locations are considered relative contraindications for conservative surgical management because of the dangers associated with hemorrhage or subsequent tubal occlusion.[20] If diagnosed early, however, these conditions have been successfully managed medically.[21–23]

SIGNS AND SYMPTOMS

The most frequent symptoms of ectopic pregnancy are abdominal pain, amenorrhea, or irregular vaginal bleeding (Table 15-1).[24] Physical examination most frequently reveals adnexal or abdominal tenderness (Table 15-2). Palpation of a pelvic adnexal mass is found only 50% of the time, of which 20% are found on the side opposite the confirmed ectopic pregnancy. Unfortunately, these signs and symptoms are not pathognomonic of an ectopic pregnancy. Other pathologic entities in the differential diagnosis include threatened or incomplete abortion, ruptured corpus luteum, dysfunctional uterine bleeding, adnexal torsion, endometriosis, degenerating uterine leiomyomata, and salpingitis. For any patient presenting with these signs and symptoms, however, an accurate diagnosis is made only 50% of the time without further evaluation.

Table 15–1
Symptoms of Ectopic Pregnancy

	Frequency of Occurrence (%)
Abdominal pain	90–100
Amenorrhea	75–95
Vaginal bleeding	50–80
Dizziness, fainting	20–35
Urge to defecate	5–15
Pregnancy symptoms	10–25
Passage of tissue	5–10

Weckstein LN: Current perspective on ectopic pregnancy. Obstet Gynecol Surv 40:259, 1985. With permission.

Table 15–2
Signs of Ectopic Pregnancy

	Frequency of Occurrence (%)
Adnexal tenderness	75–90
Abdominal tenderness	80–95
Adnexal mass*	50
Uterine enlargement	20–30
Orthostatic changes	10–15
Fever	5–10

Weckstein LN: Current perspective on ectopic pregnancy. Obstet Gynecol Surv 40:259, 1985. With permission.
*20% on the side opposite the ectopic pregnancy.

Furthermore, in the patient without these clinical signs or symptoms, ectopic pregnancy should still be considered and appropriately investigated in those patients with a suggestive history for ectopic pregnancy.

DIAGNOSTIC STRATEGIES

Human Chorionic Gonadotropin

Advances in laboratory techniques have greatly improved the ability to detect ectopic pregnancy, often in the unruptured state. Critical to the early recognition of ectopic pregnancy is the development of increasingly sensitive qualitative and quantitative assays for hCG. The development of radioimmunoassay (with an assay sensitivity of less than 5 mIU/mL) resulted in positive pregnancy tests in nearly 100% of patients with a diagnosed ectopic pregnancy.[25] Concurrent with the improved sensitivity of hCG assays, the ability to discriminate normal from ectopic pregnancy has also improved. Early studies found lower serum-hCG concentrations in patients with ectopic pregnancies, compared with normal intrauterine pregnancy at the same gestational age.[26,28] A single hCG value is limited in its use, however, because the actual gestational age is often uncertain. Furthermore, considerable overlap exists for any single hCG value between ectopic and intrauterine pregnancies. Consequently, attention has turned toward serial measurements of hCG values because studies by several groups found a slower rate of rise in ectopic pregnancy compared with normal intrauterine preg-

nancy (Figs. 15-2 and 15-3).[27–30] For a viable intrauterine pregnancy, 1.4 to 2.2 days are needed to observe a doubling of the hCG value. If such a doubling time is not observed or if hCG does not increase by 66% over a 2-day interval, the risk of *abnormal* pregnancy (nonviable intrauterine or ectopic pregnancy) is high.[31] Despite the improved discriminatory value of these serial quantitative hCGs, 15% of normal pregnancies fail to show this rate of rise and 13% of ectopic pregnancies exhibit a normal rate of increase. Another drawback of serial hCGs is the necessity to wait 24 to 48 hours between samples. This has led for a search for other parameters that give more immediate information with regard to the relative risk of ectopic pregnancy.

Progesterone

Single serum progesterone has been used in patients suspected of having an ectopic pregnancy in an effort to avoid the delay required for serial quantitative hCG determinations. As a consequence, a significantly shorter time to establish a diagnosis has been reported, with a decrease in the percentage of patients with subsequent tubal rupture.[32] The discriminatory zone for progesterone in distinguishing normal intrauterine pregnancy from ectopic pregnancy varies somewhat between studies, but when abnormally low increases the suspicion for an abnormal gestation, including ectopic pregnancy. In a small retrospective study by Yeko and coworkers, 15 ng/mL was reported to differentiate normal from abnormal pregnancies; 24 patients with viable intrauterine pregnancies had serum progesterone concentrations of more than 15 ng/mL, whereas all 28 patients with ectopic pregnancies and 17 of 18 nonviable intrauterine pregnancies had values of less than 15 ng/mL.[33] Another retrospective study by Matthews and associates produced similar findings.[34] In a larger prospective study, however, only 81% of patients with ectopic gestation and 11% of those with viable intrauterine pregnancies had a serum progesterone level of less than 15 ng/mL.[32] In this same study, only one of 67 patients with ectopic pregnancy had a serum progesterone concentration of more than 25 ng/mL and no viable intrauterine pregnancies were identified when the progesterone level was less than 5 ng/mL. This led to the following conclusions: (1) a serum progesterone concentration of more than 25 ng/mL is suggestive of normal intrauterine pregnancy; (2) a serum progesterone concentration of less than

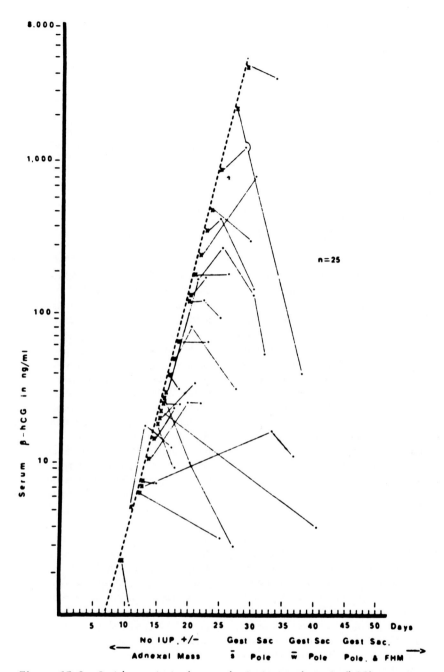

Figure 15–2.   Serial quantitative human chorionic gonadotropin (hCG) concentrations for 25 patients with ectopic pregnancies. Broken line represents average hCG progression for the first 30 days of normal pregnancy. (Cartwright PS, DiPietro DL: Ectopic pregnancy: changes in serum human chorionic gonadotropin concentrations. Obstet Gynecol 63:76, 1984. With permission.)

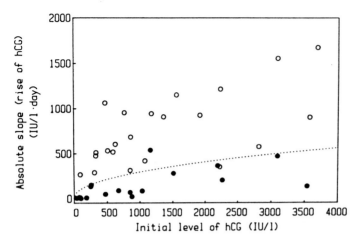

Figure 15–3. Slope of serum human chorionic gonadotropin (hCG) rise as a function of initial hCG level. (*Open circles*) Intrauterine pregnancies. (*Filled circles*) Ectopic pregnancies. (Lindblom B, Hahlin M, Sjoblom P, et al: Serial human chorionic gonadotropin determinations by fluoroimmunoassay for differentiating between uterine and ectopic gestation. Am J Obstet Gynecol 161:397, 1989. With permission.)

5 ng/mL is suggestive of abnormal pregnancy, whether intrauterine or ectopic in location; and (3) values between 5 and 25 ng/mL are indeterminate because considerable overlap exists between normal and abnormal pregnancies. As a consequence of these and other studies, the use of serum progesterone measurements has been added to many of the diagnostic algorithms for ectopic pregnancy (Fig. 15-4).[35] Nevertheless, no single serum marker has sufficient sensitivity or specificity to adequately distinguish all ectopic or abnormal gestations from normal intrauterine pregnancies. Consequently, they are used in conjunction with other investigative procedures such as ultrasound.

Ultrasound

Ultrasonography has greatly added to the ability to detect ectopic pregnancy. Using abdominal scanning, Kadar and colleagues report that the discriminatory zone in which a gestational sac may be visualized *in the uterus* is 6000 to 6500 mIU hCG/mL, using the International Reference Preparation (IRP) for hCG.[36] This information is somewhat limited, however, because of the resolution of the transabdominal ultrasound at the time this study was completed. Development of the transvaginal ultrasound transducer, with its increased resolution, has dramatically reduced this discriminatory zone, yielding information regarding the location of the gestational sac at early gestational ages (Fig. 15-5). Although Bernaschek and colleagues report a 2-mm gestational sac at 4 weeks and 2 days with an hCG of 141 mIU/mL (Second International Standard [IS]), most authors suggest that the discriminatory zone for an intrauterine gestational sac using the

transvaginal probe to be 750 to 1000 mIU/mL (2nd IS) or 1500 mIU/mL (IRP).[37,38]

Concurrent with this increased resolution for detecting an intrauterine gestational sac, transvaginal ultrasound is more accurate in identifying an adnexal gestational sac (Fig. 15-6). In a study of 22 patients with surgically proven ectopic pregnancies, Shapiro and colleagues found the vaginal-probe technique to be accurate in detecting an adnexal mass 91% of the time, in contrast to abdominal ultrasound, which identified the mass only 50% of the time.[39] Obviously, the ability to define these discriminatory zones at an earlier gestational age has greatly aided the physician in the diagnosis of ectopic pregnancy before tubal rupture and diminished the consequent mortality and morbidity. The addition of color Doppler-flow techniques has aided in locating early intrauterine as well as ectopically located pregnancies. As a consequence of improvements in ultrasound technology, earlier confirmation of intrauterine or ectopic pregnancy is possible. The size and characteristics of any adnexal mass are important, not only for diagnosis but for counseling patients regarding the probability of successful conservative surgical or medical management.

Culdocentesis

The finding of nonclotting blood in the posterior cul-de-sac has been reported to be 70% to 97% predictive of ectopic pregnancy.[40] Despite its high predictive value for a positive result, a negative culdocentesis does not rule out ectopic pregnancy because many early ectopic gestations do not result in intraperitoneal bleeding. With the increased res-

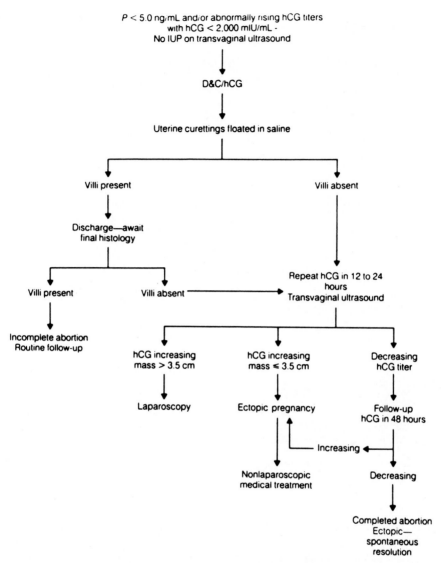

Figure 15–4. Treatment algorithm for patients with abnormally rising human chorionic gonadotropin titers or low serum progesterone concentrations. (Stovall TG, Ling FW: Some new approaches to ectopic pregnancy. Contemp Obstet Gynecol 37:37, 1992. With permission.)

olution of ultrasound, the physician may detect gestational-sac location with increasing frequency before extensive intraperitoneal bleeding and tubal rupture, obviating the need for culdocentesis in many instances. Additionally, vaginal sonography can give valuable information regarding the amount of free fluid in the pelvis, alerting the physician to the increased possibility of intraperitoneal hemorrhage. Where sensitive ultrasound or laparoscopy is not readily available, culdocentesis is still an appropriate diagnostic tool. Under such circumstances, a negative culdocentesis may be used to reassure the physician that other diagnostic modalities such as a serum progesterone or serial quantitative hCG measurements may be performed before committing a stable patient to an operative procedure. Conversely, if culdocentesis is positive, immediate operative intervention is usually prudent to determine the source of the intra-abdominal bleeding.

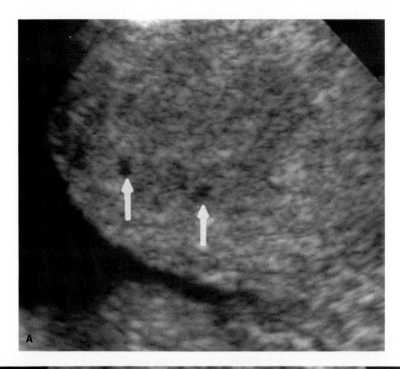

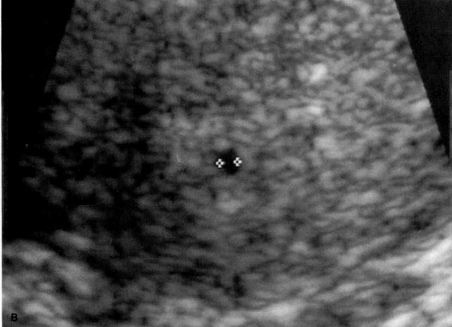

Figure 15–5. Transvaginal ultrasound showing two intrauterine gestational sacs (*arrows*) at 4 weeks and 2 days from last menstrual period. (**A**) Increased magnification of one gestational sac of 1.4 mm (calipers) surrounded by a double-ring sign. (**B**) Patient had undergone ovulation induction with gonadotropins. (Scott JS, DiSaia PJ, Hammond CB, Spellacy WN: Danforth's obstetrics and gynecology, 7th ed. Philadelphia, JB Lippincott, 1994.)

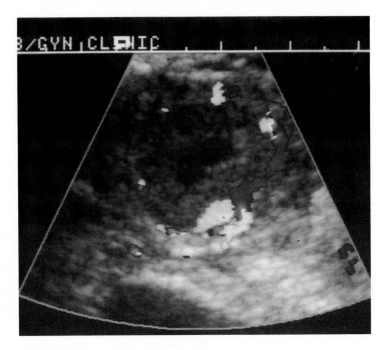

Figure 15–6. Transvaginal ultrasound showing a gestational sac in the left adnexa. Pulsed color Doppler ultrasound of the vessels in the region surrounding the gestational sac help to identify it as an ectopic pregnancy. (From Scott JS, DiSaia PJ, Hammond CB, Spellacy WN: Danforth's obstetrics and gynecology, 7th ed. Philadelphia, JB Lippincott, 1994.)

Dilation and Curettage

With quantitative hCGs that fail to rise appropriately or serum progesterone concentrations of less than 5 ng/mL, endometrial curettage may be useful in localizing the chorionic villi within the uterine cavity and therefore avoid the need for laparoscopy. This does not rule out the possibility of combined (heterotopic) pregnancy but in the general population, this risk is small, estimated to occur between one in 4000 and one in 30,000 pregnancies. In patients undergoing assisted reproductive techniques, however, this risk may be as high as 2% to 3%.[41]

Laparoscopy

Despite the increasing usefulness of serial hCG and ultrasound, coupled with rapid progesterone determination, a definitive diagnosis of ectopic pregnancy is often made by direct visualization through the laparoscope. The appropriate indications for laparoscopy require considerable experience in interpreting the above investigative steps. Patients considered to be good candidates for laparoscopy are those who are at high risk for ectopic pregnancy based on:

1. History
2. Symptoms of acute pelvic pain
3. Vaginal bleeding
4. Inappropriately rising quantitative hCG values
5. Low serum progesterone concentration
6. Absence of an intrauterine gestational sac, using transvaginal ultrasound, when concomitant hCG concentrations are more than 1500 mIU/mL (2nd IS)

All of these findings, however, are often absent in documented ectopic pregnancies; therefore, certain clinical acumen is necessary. Even direct visualization by laparoscopy is not infallible. In an effort to avoid the grave circumstances of missing the diagnosis of a ruptured ectopic pregnancy, laparoscopy may occasionally be performed too early. In this circumstance, the ectopically located pregnancy may not have reached sufficient size to be identified at the time of laparoscopy. The incidence of this false-negative finding has been found by Samuelsson and Sjovall to occur in four of 166 ectopic pregnancies.[42] Conversely, incorrectly identifying an ectopic pregnancy in patients who were later confirmed to have a viable intrauterine pregnancy was reported by the same authors to occur in six of 120 patients studied. Because the sensitivity of testing has increased with more liberalized use of laparoscopy for the diagnosis, false-negative and false-positive findings at the time of laparoscopy likely will continue to occur. This leaves the physician in the uncomfortable position of occasionally needing to reoperate should the hCG continue to rise with no evidence of a developing intrauterine pregnancy. Alternatively, patients with ectopic pregnancies that were not visible at the time of diagnostic laparoscopy may be amenable to medical treatment in an effort to avoid further surgery.

TREATMENT

Expectant Management

The oldest "treatment" for ectopic pregnancy is expectant management because this was the only means of therapy available for centuries. It was not until 1884, when Lawton Tait first published a series studying five patients, that extirpative treatment was advocated as "clearly a chief element of success in modern abdominal surgery."[43] Nevertheless, in lieu of the increasing sensitivity for the diagnosis, an occasional patient is undoubtedly appropriate for expectant management when the ectopic growth is self-limiting. With the potential life-threatening circumstances surrounding tubal rupture, some guidelines are appropriate for this expectant form of treatment. As presented in Table 15-3, the results from reported series are mixed. Generally, expectant management is more success-

ful in patients with lower hCG concentrations that plateau or fall.[44,45] It is unclear whether this treatment has any distinct advantage or disadvantage versus surgical or medical management, with regard to tubal patency or intrauterine pregnancy rates. Clearly, avoidance of surgical intervention when the ectopic pathology is self-limiting would be preferable, provided this does not compromise the tubal patency rate or the ability to achieve pregnancy in those patients desiring fertility options.

Surgical Management

Extirpation of the involved fallopian tube through a laparotomy incision was the preferred surgical intervention for many years; however, many thought that this may have contributed to the subsequent compromised fertility rates of 20% to 70%.[46,47] With irreparable tubal rupture and extensive hemorrhage, salpingectomy is still the treatment of choice; however, because of earlier diagnosis (afforded by the methodologies described previously), tubal rupture and hemorrhage are seen more infrequently. Consequently, more conservative approaches such as salpingotomy or salpingostomy were developed as alternatives to salpingectomy for

Table 15-3
Expectant Management in Ectopic Pregnancy

Author	Cases (n)	Resorption (n) (%)	Tubal Patency		Pregnancy Rate		Ectopic Rate	
			(n)	(%)	(n)	(%)	(n)	(%)
Lund, 1955[98]	119	68 (57)	—	—	32/43	(74)	11/43	(26)
Ohel, 1980[99]	1	1 (100)	1/1	(100)	—	—	—	—
Mashiach, 1982[100]	5	4 (80)	1/1	(100)	—	—	—	—
Adoni, 1986[101]	11	11 (100)	—	—	—	—	—	—
Carp, 1986[102]	14	11 (79)	5/5	(100)	3/5	(60)	1/5	(20)
Dericks-Tan, 1987[103]	12	12 (100)	7/10	(100)	—	—	—	—
Garcia, 1987[104]	13	12 (92)	7/10	(7)	3/3	(100)	0/3	(0)
Sauer, 1987[44]; 1989[105]	10	10 (100)	—	—	—	—	—	—
Fernandez, 1988[106]	14	10 (71)	6/6	(100)	3/6	(50)	—	—
Letterie, 1989[107]	1	1 (100)	—	—	—	—	—	—
Carson, 1991[108]	9	6 (67)	—	—	—	—	—	—
Total	209	146 (70)	27/33	82	41/57	(72)	12/51	(24)

Modified from Stovall TG, Ling FW: Expectant management of ectopic pregnancy. In Diamond MP, DeCherney AH (eds): Obstetrics and gynecology clinics of North America, ectopic pregnancy. Philadelphia, WB Saunders, 1991; 18:136.

patients who desire to preserve fertility.[48] When subsequent ectopic rates declined with such conservative treatment measures (with concomitant increases in subsequent intrauterine pregnancy rates), these procedures became the preferred surgical therapy.[49–51] These techniques quickly became amenable to a laparoscopic approach and are replacing laparotomy as the preferred means of intervention because of the diminished level of invasiveness, length of hospital stay, and postoperative recovery time.

These surgical approaches are effective but may still compromise future fertility. Because surgery of the fallopian tube is considered a risk factor for future tubal occlusion or ectopic pregnancy, chemotherapeutic agents that inhibit trophoblastic growth have been investigated as a medical means for treating such patients. The benefits of medical management are obvious. If surgery can be avoided, the operative morbidity and hospital costs can be reduced. Considerable interest still exists regarding the potential for improved fertility outcome with the chemotherapeutic approach, when contrasted to patients treated surgically. As mentioned, medical management offers some patients the opportunity to avoid reoperation if conservative surgical approaches fail to completely remove all of the trophoblastic tissue or if laparoscopy was performed too early to visualize the actual ectopic site. Bengtsson and colleagues reported on 15 patients treated with methotrexate as second-line therapy for persistent trophoblast after conservative surgery.[52] This low-dose treatment was successful in 14 of 15 patients, with the mean time for decline to nonpregnant values being 24 days.

Medical Treatment

Chemotherapy has long been successful in arresting trophoblastic cell growth. In 1956, Li and colleagues first reported on the use of methotrexate in treating patients with gestational trophoblastic disease.[53] Success in treating this disease state led investigators to study its use in treating normal, albeit ectopically placed, trophoblastic tissue. Consequently, a growing number of different chemotherapeutic agents and different routes of administration have been studied in an effort to treat ectopic pregnancy in the most effective and least morbid fashion. The list of chemotherapeutic agents used to treat ectopic gestation include methotrexate, actinomycin D, prostaglandins, hyperosmolar glucose, potassium chloride, Trichosanthin, RU-486

(Mifepristone), and anti-hCG antibody. The routes of administration differ from systemic (methotrexate, actinomycin D, Trichosanthin, RU-486, and anti-hCG antibody) to direct local injection of the ectopic (methotrexate, prostaglandins, potassium chloride, and hyperosmolar glucose) and are discussed individually.

Systemic Administration

Methotrexate

Methotrexate is considered the prototype drug for medical management of patients with ectopic pregnancy because of its long record in effectiveness and patient safety in treating patients with gestational trophoblastic disease.[54] In addition to its use with abnormal trophoblastic cells, it inhibits cell growth from normal trophoblastic cells grown in vitro.[55] Furthermore, a growing number of clinical studies in patients treated for ectopic pregnancy have been encouraging. Methotrexate is a potent folate antagonist, which inhibits dihydrofolate reductase, an enzyme necessary for conversion of dihydrofolic acid to tetrahydrofolic acid. As a consequence, thymidylate incorporation into DNA is inhibited, preventing cellular proliferation. Folinic acid administration does not reverse this deficiency; however, administration of citrovorum factor (folinic acid) is used to reduce toxic side effects to nontrophoblastic tissue.[56] Folinic acid's effect is to resume normal folate metabolism as it is converted to 5-methyltetrahydrofolate, which is beyond the enzymatic block of methotrexate.

REPORTED SERIES. Studies on the use of methotrexate for conditions other than gestational trophoblastic disease were slow in coming. One of the earliest reports of medical management using methotrexate in patients with ectopic pregnancies was that of Hreshchyshyn and coworkers, who successfully treated a patient with an abdominal pregnancy in 1965.[57] In 1982, Tanaka and colleagues successfully treated a patient for interstitial pregnancy, with normal tubal patency demonstrated on follow-up hysterosalpingogram.[58] Miyazaki and associates then studied a group of eight patients (with total doses ranging from 60 to 300 mg), of which seven were successfully treated.[59] In this study, however, diagnosis was based on ultrasound and not on laparoscopy. Follow-up hysterosalpingogram (HSG) revealed tubal patency in four out of five patients studied. Two patients subsequently achieved pregnancy without further therapy. Treatment of a patient with a cervical pregnancy with methotrexate was then reported by Farabow and colleagues; however, the patient ultimately needed surgical intervention.[60] Subsequently, several reports have demonstrated efficacy in treating this rare form of ectopic pregnancy.

In 1986, Ory and colleagues used methotrexate to treat six patients with ectopic pregnancy.[61] In this study of documented ampullary tubal pregnancies confirmed by laparoscopy, medical treatment was initiated if the unruptured tubal diameter was 4 cm or less and no more than 100 mL of free blood was found in the peritoneal cavity at the time of laparoscopy. The treatment regimen was intravenous methotrexate (1 mg/kg) with intramuscular leucovorin rescue (0.1 mg/kg) on alternate days, for a total of four doses of each medication. Five of six patients were successfully treated; two patients required blood transfusions and one required salpingectomy for hemorrhage. This single treatment failure occurred in a woman with an advanced gestation, as evidence by quantitative hCG of more than 25,000 mIU/mL and fetal cardiac activity on ultrasound at the time therapy was begun.

In a study by Sauer and colleagues, 20 of 21 patients with ectopic pregnancies were successfully treated; two required transfusion—one of whom also required laparotomy.[44] Both of these patients with complications also had evidence of advanced gestation, with fetal cardiac activity on sonogram. Subsequent reproductive potential, determined by

HSG, was performed in 20 patients (of whom five were expectantly managed), with 15 (75%) showing patency of the involved tube. At a year, two had achieved pregnancy and two had repeat ectopic pregnancy.

Using ultrasound, urinary hCG-β, and endometrial curettage alone but forgoing laparoscopy in establishing the diagnosis of ectopic pregnancy, Ichinoe and colleagues treated 23 patients with methotrexate, with successful resolution in 22 (96%).[62] Ten of 19 patients (53%) had tubal patency, and four patients reported subsequent pregnancies. Stovall and coworkers also reported a 94% rate of successful ectopic resolution among 36 patients.[63] In this series, two had tubal rupture after chemotherapy, one of which was delayed by 23 days. Similar to the other series, both of these complications had more advanced gestations, with hCG concentrations of more than 15,000 mIU/mL, and one had fetal cardiac activity. A follow-up report in 1991 revealed similar results among 100 patients treated as outpatients.[64] As seen in Table 15-4, successful resolution of ectopic pregnancy is achieved in 70% to 96% of patients, with subsequent tubal patency rates of about 70%. In one of the largest series, intrauterine pregnancy rates of 59% (33 of 56) were found, with ectopic rates of 7% (four of 56) of those attempting pregnancy.[65] Although a multidose protocol (as described by Ory) is probably most commonly employed, a single dose of methotrexate without citrovorum rescue has also been reported,

Table 15–4
Methotrexate Management of Ectopic Pregnancy

Author	Cases (n)	Success (n) (%)	Tubal patency (n) (%)
Miyazaki et al, 1983[59]	8	7 (88)	4/5 (80)
Goldstein, 1986[109]	13	12 (92)	4/4 (100)
Ory et al, 1986[61]	6	5 (82)	4/7 (57)
Garcia et al, 1987[45]	10	7 (70)	NR NR
Ichninoe et al, 1987[62]	23	22 (96)	10/19 (53)
Sauer et al, 1987[44]	21	20 (95)	15/20 (75)
Stovall et al, 1989[63]	36	34 (94)	NR NR
Stovall et al, 1990[65]	57	49 (85)	NR NR
Total	174	156 (90)	37/55 (67)

NR, not reported.

Modified from Ory SJ: Chemotherapy for ectopic pregnancy. In Diamond MP, DeCherney AH (eds): Obstetrics and gynecology clinics of North America, Ectopic Pregnancy. Philadelphia, WB Saunders, 18:129, 1991.

with good success. In a study reported by Stovall and associates, 29 of 30 patients were successfully treated with a single dose of methotrexate (50 mg/m^2) without citrovorum rescue, with no side effects.[66]

PATIENT SELECTION. Although the results from the above studies are encouraging, successful treatment of an ectopic pregnancy ultimately requires complete resolution of the trophoblastic tissue and accompanying tubal dilation without the need for further surgical intervention. Optimally, this resolution occurs in the absence of pelvic pain or hemorrhage and preserves tubal architecture so that tubal patency and future fertility are maximized. A review of the literature finds a failure of resolution of the ectopic pregnancy in only 5.9% of 118 treated cases.[67] In most of these cases, higher levels of hCG-β (more than 5000 mIU/mL) or a fetal heart beat was observed. Consequently, many authors recommend the following criteria as important to the success of medical management: (1) a hemodynamically stable patient, (2) involved tubal diameter of less than 3 to 4 cm, (3) unruptured fallopian tube without significant intra-abdominal hemorrhage, and (4) no fetal cardiac activity on sonogram. Additionally, some concern regarding a safe threshold of hCG concentrations has been discussed; however, exclusion criteria based on hCG concentrations alone have not been established. It is clear that values of more than 15,000 mIU/mL have higher failure rates, more protracted treatment courses, and higher complication rates. Active hepatic or renal disease; known methotrexate sensitivity; evidence of bone marrow suppression (platelet count less than 100,000; hemoglobin less than 11 mg%; or leukocyte count less than 3000); active peptic ulcer disease; or expected poor compliance for follow-up are additional limitations when methotrexate is considered.

In addition to the use of methotrexate for primary treatment of ectopic pregnancy, another indication for methotrexate has been reported when conservative surgery has not eliminated all trophoblastic tissue.[52,68,69] This complication generally follows laparoscopic surgery and is recognized postoperatively by failure of quantitative hCG concentrations to fall to zero. In one large series, this persistent hCG production required additional treatment in 4.8% of patients.[70] If conservation of the tube is desired for future fertility, a medical form of therapy may increase the likelihood of avoiding removal of the involved tube. Alternatively, if diagnostic laparoscopy fails to give a definitive diagnosis, chemotherapy may be discussed as an alternative to reoperation. Although not as much data exists regarding the use of chemotherapy in this situation, the use of these agents as primary therapy without any prior operative intervention supports its use.

SIDE EFFECTS. A major concern for the use of methotrexate has been the potential of known toxicity and side effects. This toxicity is dose-dependent and influenced also by the duration of therapy. Gastrointestinal side effects such as mucositis, stomatitis, nausea, and diarrhea are the most common; however, hepatotoxicity and bone marrow suppression, including leukopenia and thrombocytopenia, have also been reported. Other side effects include renal toxicity, alopecia, dermatitis, photosensitivity, pneumonitis, and anaphylaxis. Serious side effects have been observed more commonly at high doses and are rarely reported with the lower doses combined with folinic acid rescue that are ordinarily used to treat ectopic pregnancy. In a series reported by Sauer and coworkers, a 24% incidence of side effects was noted.[44] Other larger series have reported toxicity rates of 8% to 23%.[71,72] These side effects most commonly are mild and resolve within 2 to 4 days after completion of therapy. In an effort to reduce the rate of side effects, reduction in the daily dose of methotrexate or the concurrent administration of leucovorin rescue has been advocated.[67] Additionally, others have used direct injection into the amniotic sac at the time of diagnostic laparoscopy or transvaginal sonography in an effort to reduce the treatment dosage and time required with parenteral administration.[73,74]

Of additional concern in women treated with such chemotherapeutic agents is any potential contribution to teratogenicity in subsequent pregnancies, tumor-formation risks, higher subsequent miscarriage rates, and possible ovulatory dysfunction due to direct toxic effects on the ovary. Because of the relatively short course with low-dose therapy, these outcomes have not been verified.[75] Long-term experience using higher doses in patients treated for gestational trophoblastic disease demonstrates no evidence of these adverse outcomes and suggests that these are unlikely complications.

RU-486

The success of RU-486 as an abortifacient has led investigators to study its effect in extrauterine pregnancies. It was hypothesized that ectopic trophoblast growth would be arrested by the antagonistic effect of the drug on corpus luteum progesterone production. Kenigsberg and colleagues used 650 mg of the progesterone antagonist RU-486 to treat a patient with persistent ectopic pregnancy and without change in hCG levels for 7 days.[76] One treatment course of methotrexate resulted in successful resolution of the pregnancy, with diminution of hCG levels. Two other reports (with a total of 28 patients) used 200 mg of RU-486 daily for 4 days.[77,78] Five of 28 patients continued to show increasing hCG-β levels. Furthermore, because of the uncertainty of efficacy for this form of chemotherapy, surgical intervention (1 week after oral RU-486) was performed in 24 of 28 patients. A quantitative hCG of more than 1000 mIU/mL appeared to be a high-risk factor for documented increases in hematosalpinx volume at the time of second-look surgery. Pathologic examination of 25 samples revealed necrotic trophoblast. Unfortunately, no controls using expectant management alone were used as comparison. A patient with an ovarian heterotopic pregnancy was unsuccessfully treated, as reported by Levin and colleagues.[79] Although RU-486 may have a place in the medical management of ectopic pregnancy, not enough data are available to support its use over methotrexate or prostaglandins.

Actinomycin D

The RNA polymerase inhibitor actinomycin D has been used in one reported case for the treatment of ectopic pregnancy.[23] This chemotherapeutic agent has less liver and renal toxicity than methotrexate but has similar bone marrow and mucositis toxicity. Administration is by intravenous route and therefore limits its attractiveness as an outpatient therapy. Despite its success in this particular patient, who had bilateral patent tubes demonstrated after treatment, no extended series exist to advocate widespread use.

Trichosanthin

A drug frequently used for mid-trimester abortion in China, Trichosanthin has been used to treat ectopic pregnancy. Lu and Jin treated 71 patients with ectopic pregnancy with Trichosanthin, with a reported success rate of 86% and subsequent fertility rate of 83%.[80] A case report using this same drug administered by injection into the ectopic gestation laparoscopically was also reported.[81]

Anti-hCG Antibody

A phase I clinical trial using monoclonal anti-hCG antibody appeared to induce a resolution of the ectopic pregnancy in one of three patients.[82] Salpin-

gectomy was needed in two patients, however, for persistent hCG elevations. Larger trials are needed to evaluate the efficacy of this particular medical therapy.

Local Injection

Methotrexate

Feichtinger and Kemeter were the first to report transvaginal sonography for injection of methotrexate (10 mg) into the ectopic pregnancy.[83] A follow-up study of eight additional patients showed successful resolution of the ectopic gestation without further treatment in 89% of patients.[84] Leeton and Davidson used 50 mg of methotrexate in two patients, with complete resolution.[85] One patient had a demonstrable fetal heart beat on ultrasound, yet resolution was successful. Pansky and colleagues used 12.5 mg of local injection of methotrexate through the laparoscope in 1989.[73] In this study, 24 of 27 patients required no additional surgery, with a 90% tubal patency rate, as determined by subsequent hysterosalpingography in 21 of 24 patients.[73,86] Strict selection criteria of patients included an unruptured tube, a pregnancy diameter of less than 3 cm, no active bleeding, and no additional pelvic pathology.

Despite Pansky's success, not all authors have been so successful in their experience with needle aspiration of the involved pregnancy using injection of methotrexate. Of nine patients in Robertson and colleagues' study, five eventually needed surgery secondary to the persistence of ectopic trophoblastic tissue.[87] Tubal patency rates of 90% to 100% are reported in two studies; however, little data exists on the effect of tubal injection on human fertility rates. In rabbits, a randomized prospective trial examined the nidation index after intratubal injection of methotrexate and found no difference when compared with controls using Ringer's solution.[88] This small animal study has obvious limitations with regard to subsequent pregnancy rates in humans. Larger series of patients among different groups of investigators are needed before this form of therapy can be recommended.

Prostaglandins

Prostaglandin F (PGF) and prostaglandin E (PGE) compounds have also been reported for direct-injection treatment of ectopic pregnancy. Presumably, these drugs exert their effect by smooth-muscle contraction and constriction of blood vessels and have been injected directly into tubal pregnancies or the corpora lutea for their luteolytic effect. In one study of three patients treated by PGE_2 injection, all required subsequent surgery.[89] Gastrointestinal discomfort such as vomiting and diarrhea was noted as the most common side effect.

Prostaglandin $F_{2\alpha}$ causes increased tubal peristalsis and vasospasm of the arteries of the mesosalpinx. In two studies by Lindblom, PGF_{2a} (0.5 to 1.5 mg) was injected intratubally and within the corpus luteum.[90,91] Eight of nine patients treated in this manner were successfully treated. Somewhat higher doses of PGF_{2a}, with local injection within the tube and corpus luteum concurrent with systemic administration of PGE_2, were successful in 16 of 18 patients.[92] Severe hemodynamic and cardiac side effects were experienced in three of 18 patients. These side effects included pulmonary edema, malignant hypertension, atrioventricular block, and severe cardiac arrhythmia. Other potential side effects of PGF_{2a} also include immediate bronchospasm, hypotension or hypertension, or cardiac conduction disturbances. In an expanded series of 71 patients treated with prostaglandins, 81% successfully avoided additional surgery.[93] Tubal patency was demonstrated in 22 of 24 subsequent hysterosalpingograms, compared with five of eight patients surgically treated. In a series by Vejtorp and coworkers, a 90% success rate with no side effects was found if the original treatment protocol of Lindblom was used.[94]

Potassium Chloride

Robertson and colleagues were successful in one out of three attempts at locally injecting 20% solution of potassium chloride to induce cardiac arrest in an ectopic fetus.[95] Timor-Tritsch and colleagues reported another successful case.[96] Not enough experience is documented to recommend this as a routine form of treatment for ectopic pregnancy. In the case of heterotopic pregnancy, however, the effect of systemic, antimetabolic, or vasoactive chemotherapeutic agents is preferably avoided. Consequently, potassium chloride or hyperosmolar glucose is a potential alternative.

Hyperosmolar Glucose

Hyperosmolar glucose as an alternative to prostaglandins or methotrexate was used in a study by Lang and colleagues.[97] In this randomized study comparing hyperosmolar glucose with PGE_2, none of the nine patients treated with direct injection of glucose into the ectopic pregnancy needed further surgery. One of nine patients systemically treated with PGE_2 required additional surgery, with six patients reporting severe abdominal pain as side effects.

CONCLUSIONS

More experience with methotrexate and prostaglandins has been reported in the literature and should be considered first until more experience advocates the safety and effectiveness of the other agents. Despite chemotherapy having been used to treat ectopic pregnancy since the early 1960s, only recently have investigators studied the efficacy and morbidity in a systematic manner. Larger series support the concept that if careful patient selection criteria are used to identify qualified patients for this form of outpatient therapy, good success (94%) in resorption of the ectopic trophoblast can be anticipated. It is also clear that early identification of an ectopic gestation is important for any form of conservative treatment to be successful in preserving tubal patency and improving the chances of future intrauterine pregnancies. Some information regarding tubal patency using these more conservative selection criteria suggests that more than 60% to 70% of ectopic pregnancies medically treated result in patency of the involved tube. Unfortunately, series with large enough numbers to establish meaningful pregnancy rates, especially in comparison with conservative surgical procedures, have not been performed. Systemic methotrexate is the chemotherapeutic modality most commonly employed. Localized injection of methotrexate administration shows promising results. Nevertheless, too few studies are reported in the literature to advocate its preferential use. Local injection does make sense, however, in the rare case of heterotopic pregnancy. Based on the clinical experience with these different agents, it would appear that given the appropriate indications, medical management of ectopic pregnancy is a safe and effective means of therapy, providing an alternative to surgical management for this increasingly common complication of pregnancy.

REFERENCES

1. Nederlof KP, et al: Centers for Disease Control: Ectopic pregnancies—United States, 1979 to 1987. MMWR 39(SS-4):9, 1990
2. Stovall TG, Kellermann AL, Ling FW, et al:

Emergency department diagnosis of ectopic pregnancy. Ann Emerg Med 19:1098, 1990

3. Brenner PF, Roy S, Mishell DR Jr: Ectopic pregnancy: a study of 300 consecutive surgical treated cases. JAMA 243:673, 1980

4. Stovall TG, Ling FW: Expectant management of ectopic pregnancy. In Diamond MP, DeCherney AH (eds). Obstetrics and gynecology clinics of North America, ectopic pregnancy, p 18. Philadelphia, WB Saunders, 1991

5. Nagamani M, London S, St Amand P: Factors influencing fertility after ectopic pregnancy. Am J Obstet Gynecol 149:533, 1984

6. Westrom L, Bengtsson LPH, Mardh PA: Incidence, trends, and risk of ectopic pregnancy in a population of women. Br Med J 282:15, 1981

7. Bone NL, Greene RR: Histologic study of uterine tubes with tubal pregnancy: a search for evidence of previous infection. Am J Obstet Gynecol 82:1166, 1961

8. Miles JH, Clark JJ: Pathogenesis of tubal pregnancy. Am J Obstet Gynecol 105:1230, 1969

9. DeCherney AH, Maheaux R, Naftolin F: Salpingostomy for ectopic pregnancy in the sole patent oviduct: reproductive outcome. Fertil Steril 37:619, 1982

10. Majmudar B, Henderson PH, Simple E: Salpingitis isthmica nodosa: a high-risk factor for tubal pregnancy. Obstet Gynecol 62:73, 1983

11. Green LK, Kolt ML: Histological findings in ectopic tubal pregnancy. Int J Gynecol Pathol 8:255, 1989

12. Tatum HJ, Schmidt FH. Contraception and sterilization practices and extrauterine pregnancy: a realistic perspective. Fertil Steril 28:407, 1977

13. Shaw A, Courey NG, Cunanan RG: Pregnancy following laparoscopic tubal electrocoagulation and division. Am J Obstet Gynecol 192:459, 1977

14. McBain JC, Evans JH, Pepperell RJ, Robinson HP, Smith MA, Brown JB: An unexpectedly high rate of ectopic pregnancy following the induction of ovulation with human pituitary and chorionic gonadotrophin. Br J Obstet Gynaecol 87:5, 1980

15. Morris JM, Van Wagenen G: Interception: the use of post-ovulatory estrogen to prevent implantation. Am J Obstet Gynecol 115:101, 1973

16. Kaufman RH, Noller K, Adam E, et al: Upper genital tract abnormalities and diethylstilbesterol-exposed progeny. Am J Obstet Gynecol 148:973, 1984

17. Beral V: An epidemiologic study of recent trends in ectopic pregnancy. Br J Obstet Gynaecol 82:775, 1975

18. Breen JL: A 21 year survey of 654 ectopic pregnancies. Am J Obstet Gynecol 106:1004, 1970

19. Budowick M, Johnson TRB, Genadry R, Parmley TH, Woodruff JD: The histopathology of the developing tubal ectopic pregnancy. Fertil Steril 34:169, 1980

20. Thorton KL, Diamond MP, DeCherney AH: Linear salpingostomy for ectopic pregnancy. Obst Gynecology Clin North Am 8(1):95, 1991

21. Fernandez H, DeZiegler DD, Bourget P, Feltain P, Frydman R: The place of methotrexate in the management of interstitial pregnancy. Hum Reprod 6(2):302, 1991

22. Bateman BG: Methotrexate treatment of tubal pregnancy. Am J Obstet Gynecol 164:231, 1991

23. Alteras M, Cohen I, Cordoba M, Ben-Nun I, Ben-Aderet N: Treatment of interstitial pregnancy with actinomycin D. Br J Obstet Gynaecol 95(2):1321, 1988

24. Weckstein LN: Current perspective in ectopic pregnancy. Obstet Gynecol Surv 40:259, 1985

25. Schwartz RO, DePietro DC: Beta-hCG as a diagnostic aid for suspected ectopic pregnancy. Obstet Gynecol 56:197, 1980

26. Pittaway DE, Wentz AC, Maxon WS, et al: The efficacy of early pregnancy monitoring and serial chorionic gonadotrophin determination and real-time sonography in an infertility population. Fertil Steril 44:190, 1985

27. Batzer FB, Schlaff S, Goldfarb AF, et al: Serial beta-subunit human chorionic gonadotropin doubling time as a prognosticator of pregnancy outcome in an infertile population. Fertil Steril 35:307, 1981

28. Kadar N, Caldwell BV, Romero R: A method of screening for ectopic pregnancy. Obstet Gynecol 58:162, 1981

29. Lindblom B, Hahlin M, Sjoblom P: Serial human chorionic gonadotropin determinations by fluoroimmunoassay for differentiating between intrauterine and ectopic gestation. Am J Obstet Gynecol 161:397, 1989

30. Cartwright PS, DiPietro DL: Ectopic pregnancy: changes in serum human chorionic gonadotropin concentrations. Obstet Gynecol 63:76, 1984

31. Kadar N, Freedman M, Zachar M: Further observation on the doubling time of human chorionic gonadotropin in early asymptomatic pregnancy. Fertil Steril 545:783, 1980

32. Stovall TG, Ling FW, Cope BJ, Buster JE: Preventing ruptured pregnancy with a single serum progesterone. Am J Obstet Gynecol 160:1425, 1989

33. Yeko TR, Gorrill MJ, Hughes LH, et al: Timely diagnosis of early ectopic pregnancy using a simple blood progesterone measurement. Fertil Steril 48:1048, 1987

34. Matthews CS, Coulson PB, Wild RA: Serum progesterone levels as an aid in the diagnosis of ectopic pregnancy. Obstet Gynecol 68:390, 1986

35. Stovall TG, Ling FW: Some new approaches to ectopic pregnancy. Contemp Obstet Gynecol 37:37, 1992

36. Kadar N, DeVore G, Romero R: Discriminatory hCG zone: its use in the sonographic evaluation for ectopic pregnancy. Obstet Gynecol 58:156, 1981

37. Bernaschek G, Rudelstorfor R, Csaicsich P: Vaginal sonography versus human chorionic gonadotropin in early detection of pregnancy. Am J Obstet Gynecol 156:608, 1988

38. Nyberg DA, Filly RAA, Mahoney BS, et al: Early gestation: correlation of hCG levels and sonographic identification. Am J Radiol 144:951, 1985

39. Shapiro BS, Cullen M, Taylor KJW, DeCherney AH: Transvaginal ultrasonography for the diagnosis of ectopic pregnancy. Fertil Steril 50:425, 1988

40. Cartwright PS, Vaughn B, Tuttle D: Culdocentesis and ectopic pregnancy. J Reprod Med 29:88, 1984
41. Dimitri E, Subak Sharpe R, Mills M, et al: Nine cases of heterotopic pregnancies in four years of in vitro fertilization. Fertil Steril 153:107, 1990
42. Samuelsson S, Sjovall A: Complication and prophylaxis against complication in gynecological laparoscopy. Lakartidningen 70(28):2570, 1973
43. Tait L: Five cases of extra-uterine pregnancy operated upon at the time of rupture. Br Med J 1250, 1884
44. Sauer MV, Gorrill MJ, Rodi IA, et al: Nonsurgical management of unruptured ectopic pregnancy: an extended clinical trial. Fertil Steril 48:752, 1987
45. Garcia AJ, Aubert JM, Sama J, Dosimovich JB: Expectant management of presumed ectopic pregnancy. Fertil Steril 48:395, 1987
46. Leach RE, Ory SJ: Modern management of ectopic pregnancy. J Reprod Med 34:324, 1989
47. Shenker J, Eyal Z, Polishuk W: Fertility after tubal surgery. Surg Gynecol Obstet 135:74, 1972
48. DeCherney A, Kase N: The conservative surgical management of unruptured ectopic pregnancy. Obstet Gynecol 54:451, 1979
49. Langer R, Bukovsky I, Herman A, Sherman D, Sadovsky G, Caspi E: Conservative surgery for tubal pregnancy. Fertil Steril 38:427, 1982
50. DeCherney AH, Polan ML, Kort H, et al: Microsurgical techniques in management of ectopic pregnancy. Fertil Steril 34:324, 1980
51. Sherman D, Langer R, Sadovsky G: Improved fertility following ectopic pregnancy. Fertil Steril 37:497, 1982
52. Bengtsson G, Bryman I, Thornburn J, Lindblom B: Low dose oral methotrexate as second-line therapy for persistent trophoblast after conservative treatment of ectopic pregnancy. Obstet Gynecol 79:589, 1992
53. Li MC, Hertz R, Spencer DB: Effect of methotrexate treatment on choriocarcinoma and chorioadenoma. Proc Sci Exp Biol Med 93:361, 1956
54. Hammond CB, Weed JC, Currie JL: The role of operation in the current therapy of gestational trophoblastic disease. Am J Obstet Gynecol 136:844, 1980
55. Sand PK, Stubblefield P, Ory SJ: Methotrexate inhibition of normal trophoblast in vitro. Am J Obstet Gynecol 155:324, 1986
56. Goldstein DP, Goldstein PR, Bottomly P, et al: Methotrexate with citrovorum rescue for nonmetastatic gestational trophoblastic neoplasms. Obstet Gynecol 48:321, 1976
57. Hreshchyshyn MM, Naples JD, Randall CL: Amethopterin in abdominal pregnancy. Am J Obstet Gynecol 93:286, 1965
58. Tanaka T, Hayashi H, Kutsuzawa T, et al: Treatment of interstitial ectopic pregnancy with methotrexate: report of a successful case. Fertil Steril 37:851, 1982
59. Miyazaki Y, Shiina Y, Wake N, et al: Studies on nonsurgical therapy of tubal pregnancy. Nippon Sanka Fujinka Gakkai Zasshi 35:489, 1983
60. Farabow W, Fullton J, Fletcher V, Velat CA, White JT: Cervical pregnancy treated with methotrexate. NC Med J 44:91, 1988
61. Ory SJ, Villanueva AL, Sand PK, Tamura RK: Conservative treatment of ectopic pregnancy with methotrexate. Am J Obstet Gynecol 154:1299, 1986
62. Ichinoe K, Wake N, Shinkai N, Shiina Y, Miyasaki Y, Tanaka T: Nonsurgical therapy to preserve oviduct function in patients with tubal pregnancies. Am J Obstet Gynecol 156:484, 1987
63. Stovall T, Ling F, Buster JE: Outpatient chemotherapy of unruptured ectopic pregnancy. Fertil Steril 51:435, 1989
64. Stovall TG, Ling FW, Gray LA: Methotrexate treatment of unruptured ectopic pregnancy: a report of 100 cases. Obstet Gynecol 77:749, 1991
65. Stovall TG, Ling FW, Buster JE: Reproductive performance with methotrexate treatment of ectopic pregnancy. Am J Obstet Gynecol 162:1620, 1990
66. Stovall TG, Ling FW, Gray LA: Single dose methotrexate of ectopic pregnancy. Obstet Gynecol 77:754, 1991
67. Pansky P, Golan A, Bukovsky I, Caspi E: Nonsurgical management of tubal pregnancy. Necessity in view of changing clinical practice. Am J Obstet Gynecol 164:888, 1991
68. Higgins KA, Schwartz MB: Treatment of persistent trophoblastic tissue after salpingostomy with methotrexate. Fertil Steril 45:427, 1986
69. Rose PG, Cohen SM: Methotrexate therapy for persistent ectopic pregnancy after conservative laparoscopic management. Obstet Gynecol 76: 947, 1990
70. Pouly JL, Mahnes H, Mage G, Canis M, Bruhat MA: Conservative laparoscopic treatment of 321 ectopic pregnancies. Fertil Steril 46:1093, 1986
71. Stovall TG, Ling FW, Buster JE: Outpatient chemotherapy of unruptured ectopic pregnancy. Fertil Steril 51:435, 1989
72. Ichinoe K, Wake N, Shinkai N, Shiina Y, Miyzaki Y, Tanaka T: Nonsurgical therapy to preserve oviduct function in patients with tubal pregnancies. Am J Obstet Gynecol 56:484, 1987
73. Pansky M, Bukovsky I, Golan A, et al: Local methotrexate injection: a nonsurgical treatment for ectopic pregnancy. Am J Obstet Gynecol 161:393, 1989
74. Tulandi T, Bret DM, Atri M, Senterman M: Treatment of ectopic pregnancy by transvaginal intratubal methotrexate administration. Obstet Gynecol 77:627, 1991
75. Walden M, Bagshawe K: Reproductive performance of women successfully treated for gestational trophoblastic tumor. Am J Obstet Gynecol 15:1108, 1976
76. Kenigsberg D, Porte J, Hull M, Spitz IM: Medical treatment of residual ectopic pregnancy: RU-486 and methotrexate. Fertil Steril 47:702, 1987
77. Paris FX, Henry-Suchet J, Tesquier L, et al: The value of an antiprogesterone steroid in the treatment of extrauterine pregnancy. Rev Fr Gynecol Obstet 81:607, 1986
78. Paris FX, Henry-Suchet J, Tesquir L, et al: Interet d un steroide action antiprogesterone dans le traitement de la grossesse ectrauterine. Rev Fr Gynecol Obstet 81:33, 1986
79. Levin JH, Lacarra M, d'Ablaing G, Grimes DA,

Vermesh M: Mifepristone (RU 486) failure in an ovarian heterotopic pregnancy. Am J Obstet Gynecol 163:543, 1990

80. Lu PX, Jin YC: Ectopic pregnancies treated with trichosanthin. Clinical analysis of 71 patients. Chin Med J (Engl) 102:365, 1989

81. Egarter C, Hussllein P, Yeung HW: Trichosanthin injection in tubal pregnancy. Gynecol Obstet Invest 31(2):119, 1991

82. Frydman R, Fernandez H, Troalen F, et al: Phase I clinical trial of monoclonal anti-human chorionic gonadotropin antibody in women with an ectopic pregnancy. Fertil Steril 52:734, 1989

83. Feichtinger W, Kemeter P: Conservative treatment of ectopic pregnancy by transvaginal aspiration under sonographic control and injection of methotrexate. Lancet 1:381, 1987

84. Feichtinger W, Kemeter P: Treatment of unruptured ectopic pregnancy by needling of sac and injection methotrexate or PGE$_2$ under transvaginal sonography control. Arch Gynecol Obstet 246:85, 1989

85. Leeton J, Davidson G: Nonsurgical management of unruptured tubal pregnancy with intra-amniotic methotrexate: preliminary report of two cases. Fertil Steril 501:67, 1988

86. Pansky M, Bukovsky I, Golan A, et al: Tubal patency after local methotrexate injection for tubal pregnancy. Lancet 2:967, 1989

87. Robertson DE, Smith W, Craft I. Reduction of ectopic pregnancy by ultrasound methods. Lancet 2:1524, 1987

88. Lecuru F, Querleu D, Buchet-Bouverne B, Subtil D: The effect of tubal injection of methotrexate on fertility in the rabbit. Fertil Steril 57:422, 1992

89. Ribic-Paucelj M, Novak-Antolic Z, Urhovec I: Treatment of ectopic pregnancy with prostaglandin E$_2$. Clin Exp Obstet Gynecol 16:106, 1989

90. Lindblom B, Hahlin M, Kallfelt B, Hamberger L: Local prostaglandin F$_{2a}$ injection for termination of ectopic pregnancy. Lancet 1:776, 1987

91. Lindblom B, Emk L, Hahlin M, Kallfelt B, Lundorff P, Thornburn J: Nonsurgical treatment of ectopic pregnancy. Lancet 1:1403, 1988

92. Egarter CH, Husslein P: Treatment of tubal pregnancy by prostaglandins. Lancet 1:1104, 1988

93. Egarter C, Fitz R, Spona J, et al: Treatment of tubal pregnancy with prostaglandins in a multicenter study. Gegurtshilfe Frauenheilkd 49:808, 1989

94. Vejtorp M, Vejerslev LO, Ruge SW: Local prostaglandin treatment of ectopic pregnancy. Hum Reprod 4:464, 1989

95. Robertson DE, Moye MAH, Hansen JN, et al: Reduction of ectopic pregnancy by injection under ultrasound control. Lancet 2:974, 1987

96. Timor-Tritsch I, Baxi L, Peisner DB: Transvaginal salpingocentesis: a new technique for treating ectopic pregnancy. Am J Obstet Gynecol 160:459, 1989

97. Lang P, Weiss PAM, Mayer HO: Local application of hyperosmolar glucose solution in tubal pregnancy. Lancet 2:922, 1989

98. Lund JJ: Early ectopic pregnancy: Comments on conservative treatment. J Obstet Gynecol Br Commonwealth 62:395, 1955

99. Ohel G, Katz M, Blumenthal B: Complete abortion of early ectopic pregnancy. Int J Gynecol Obstet 17:596, 1980

100. Mashiach S, Carp HJA, Serr DM: Nonoperative management of ectopic pregnancy: a preliminary report. J Reprod Med 27:127, 1982

101. Adoni A, Milwidsky A, Hurwitz A, Palti Z: Declining b-hCG levels: an indication for expectant approach to ectopic pregnancy. Int J Fertil 31:40, 1986

102. Carp HJA, Oelsner G, Serr DM, Mashiach S: Fertility after nonsurgical treatment of ectopic pregnancy. J Reprod Med 31:119, 1986

103. Derricks-Tan JSE, Scholz C, Tamber H: Spontaneous recovery of ectopic pregnancy: a preliminary report. Sur J Obstet Gynecol Reprod Biol 25:181, 1987

104. Garcia AJ, Aubert JM, Sama J, Josimovich JB: Expectant management of presumed ectopic pregnancies. Fertil Steril 48:395, 1987

105. Sauer MV, Anderson RE, Vermesh M, et al: Spontaneously resolving ectopic pregnancy: preservation of human chorionic gonadotropin bioactivity despite declining steroid hormone levels. Am J Obstet Gynecol 161:1673, 1989

106. Fernandez H, Rainborn JD, Papiernik E, Bellet D, Frydman R: Spontaneous resolution of ectopic pregnancy. Obstet Gynecol 71:171, 1988

107. Letterie GS, Wroble J, Jiyazawa K: Expectant management of persistant ectopic pregnancy. J Reprod Med 34:250, 1989

108. Carson SA, Stovall TG, Ling FW, et al: Spontaneous resolution of ectopic pregnancies delineated by low human somatomammotropin (HCS). Fertil Steril 55:629, 1991

109. Goldstein DP: Treatment of unruptured ectopic pregnancy with methtrexate with folinic acid rescue (MTX-FA). Presented at the 34th annual clinical meeting of the American College of Obstetricians and Gynecologists. New Orleans, May 1986

Ambulatory Gynecology, Second Edition,
edited by David H. Nichols and Patrick J. Sweeney.
J. B. Lippincott Company, Philadelphia, © 1995.

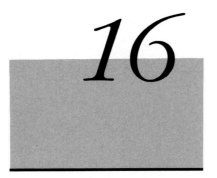

16

Surgical Management of Ectopic Pregnancy

Kristen L. Stoops and Alan H. DeCherney

There has been a marked decline in mortality associated with ectopic pregnancy in this country over the last 20 years. Present rates are down by a factor of seven, compared with those in 1970, and are less than one in 1000.[1] This decline, however, coincides with a fourfold increase in the overall incidence of eccyesis.[2] Decreasing mortality concomitant with increasing incidence of ectopic pregnancy has resulted from the development of techniques that allow for early diagnosis and successful treatment of this disorder.

Early diagnosis has been greatly facilitated by the advent and refinement of radioimmunoassay (RIA) of the β-subunit of human chorionic gonadotropin (hCG-β). During the first month of a normal gestation, the serum β-hCG level doubles about every 48 hours. In the event of ectopic pregnancy, the profile of serial hCG-β titers demonstrates suboptimal increases. The RIA technique is highly accurate and extremely sensitive, permitting detection of pregnancy within 10 days of conception.

Transvaginal ultrasound has also proved useful in the diagnosis of ectopic pregnancy. Enhanced resolution is achieved by the close proximity of the probe to the pelvic organs and the use of higher frequencies than those used in transabdominal ultrasound. As a result, gestational structures, cardiac activity, and free fluid in the cul-de-sac are more readily visualized. These two diagnostic tools—serial serum β-hCG levels and transvaginal ultrasound—are typically used in concert to rule out or affirm the existence of ectopic pregnancy.

The importance of early diagnosis cannot be overstated. The ability to diagnose extrauterine gestations before rupture occurs greatly reduces the risk of excessive blood loss and mortality. The surgeon is afforded the opportunity to effect treatment on a timely rather than emergent schedule. Under these circumstances, surgical options for the treatment of tubal ectopic pregnancy may include linear salpingotomy or salpingostomy, which may be performed either laparoscopically or at the time of laparotomy. In cases of extensive tubal damage, salpingectomy or segmental tubal resection, with the option of concurrent or future anastomosis, may be indicated. The opportunity to select from conservative procedures that have the effect of preserving tubal tissue and patency may enhance the patient's likelihood of future reproduction. Selection of a particular surgical approach should be based on several factors, including history of previous ectopic pregnancy, the patient's desire for future childbearing, the location on and extent of damage to the involved fallopian tube, and the status of the contralateral tube.

The relevance of the tremendous increase in the incidence of ectopic pregnancy over the past 2 decades must be analyzed in the context of the reproductive viability of patients with a history of this disorder. Representative studies show that roughly 50% of patients experiencing ectopic pregnancy have a history of one or no conception.[3] Only about 30% of patients studied whose first pregnancy was ectopic later produced a live infant without the use of assisted reproductive technology. Furthermore, several studies show that the likelihood of a second occurrence of ectopic pregnancy ranges from about 8% to 27%.[3-5] As these findings suggest, although tubal pregnancy may be symptomatic of inherent compromised fertility, its surgical treatment may further jeopardize fertility and therefore should be judiciously pursued. Prior tubal surgery increases the risk of ectopic implantation, with the degree of risk being dependent on the type of surgery performed and the extent to which the fallopian tube has been damaged.[5-9]

Irrespective of location within the genital tract, surgical treatment is the usual practice in the management of extrauterine gestations. The options for surgical management of tubal pregnancy and their respective indications and contraindications, surgical techniques, and implications for future fertility are addressed.

TUBAL ECTOPIC PREGNANCY

Factors Influencing the Selection of Appropriate Surgical Therapy

Radical surgical treatment of tubal ectopic pregnancy includes salpingectomy, salpingo-oophorectomy, or hysterectomy. Conservative therapy includes all procedures that attempt to preserve a part or all of the affected tube (eg, salpingostomy or salpingotomy performed either laparoscopically or through laparotomy, and mid-tubal resection, either with or without reanastomosis). Numerous factors must be considered by the surgeon in selecting the proper surgical approach for treatment of a given patient. The clinical status of the patient must be assessed to determine (1) the presence or absence of hemodynamic stability, (2) the extent of damage to the fallopian tube, (3) the condition of the contralateral tube, (4) the size of the conceptus, and (5) the location of the conceptus within the tube.[10] The presence and importance of any existing pelvic abnormalities must also be considered. Of primary importance is the selection of the most appropriate surgical procedure, which must also consider the patient's desire to preserve reproductive capability.

Laparoscopic assessment as a means of obtaining definitive information regarding the presence, location, and size of an ectopic pregnancy is advisable in most patients. The most obvious exceptions to this recommendation are those cases in which the patient is hemodynamically compromised.

Conservative Surgery

Hemodynamic stability is crucial in contemplating conservative therapy and is found to exist with increasing frequency because early diagnosis reveals the need for treatment before rupture occurs. Patients exhibiting acute symptoms may also be eligible for conservative therapy if hemodynamic compromise is not observed. The presence of a hemoperitoneum associated with a relatively slow rate of bleeding (ie, less than about 500 mL) is generally not associated with hemodynamic instability. In contrast, the patient who presents in shock requires emergency treatment, which often excludes the possibility of conservative surgical management, irrespective of the patient's desire for future reproduction.

Although tubal rupture is typically thought to require more radical surgical treatment (ie, salpingectomy), linear salpingostomy has been used in selected cases in which the extent of damage due to rupture is relatively limited. As reported by DeCherney and coworkers, the surgical technique for cases exhibiting rupture differed only in the need for meticulous debridement at the location of rupture before microsurgical repair.[11] It should be noted, however, that this form of treatment for cases of ruptured tubal pregnancy is controversial and that several patients were determined ineligible for the study because of excessive tubal damage.

The location of the implantation site is of immediate consequence in selecting the appropriate surgical procedure. In a study including 654 ectopic pregnancies, Breen found that most (about 80%) tubal gestations occurred in the distal two thirds of the fallopian tube, in the infundibular and ampullary sections.[12] Implantation in the isthmic portion of the tube occurred at a rate of about 11% and in the fimbrial region, at a rate of about 5%. In cases in which diagnosis is made before rupture, ampullary and infundibular eccyesis are usually treated with salpingotomy, either laparoscopically or using microsurgical laparotomy. In cases of infundibular ectopic pregnancy, the "milking" or squeeze technique may also be used. The procedure involves the direct application of pressure to the tube beginning at a location just proximal to the dilated segment and progressing distally in an attempt to extrude the gestational products from the fimbrial end. An increased rate of recurrent ectopic pregnancy has been documented after use of this technique, however.[13]

Although it was generally presumed that tubal conceptuses were situated intraluminally, studies by Budowick and coworkers in 1980 and by Senterman and colleagues in 1988 demonstrated that a large fraction of ectopic gestations penetrate the mucosa of the fallopian tube, resulting in extraluminal growth.[14,15] The extent of damage to the tube was found to be correlated with the degree to which gestational growth had proceeded beyond the confines of the lumen. Statistically, minimal destruction of the mucosal and muscularis layers of the tube were associated with intraluminal gestations, whereas greater destruction was associated with gestations in which growth had traversed the tube, resulting in fetuses that were at once intra- and extraluminal. Conceptuses located almost entirely extraluminally were associated with a lesser degree of damage to the muscularis and mucosal layers except at the site of implantation. In contrast to ampullary ectopic pregnancies, in which the muscularis layer is more often intact and for which linear salpingotomy is usually appropriate, isthmic gestations may violate the smaller lumen early in the pregnancy, resulting in more advanced tubal destruction. As a result, salpingotomy may not be the best surgical choice for treatment of isthmic pregnancies. DeCherney and Boyers demonstrated tubal occlusion on postoperative hysterosalpingogram in three of four patients on whom linear salpingotomy had been performed for the treatment of isthmic pregnancy.[16] An alternative procedure for treatment of isthmic ectopic gestation is partial resection of the tube, with either concurrent or postponed anastomosis. Postponing the anastomosis may be desirable to allow tubal tissues to become less edematous and engorged. In instances of minimal tubal damage, however, this delay may not be necessary.

The size of an ectopic gestation directly affects the amount of damage to the tube and therefore is of primary importance in the decision to proceed with linear salpingostomy. Many studies have been performed in an attempt to set an upper limit on the conceptus size that would still allow safe and effective treatment using salpingostomy.[17-20] The values obtained range from 3 to 5 cm, with 6 cm as an absolute upper limit. The use of the laparoscope imposes additional restrictions on size. Vermesh and coworkers consistently effected successful treatment of gestations up to 4 cm in size using the laparoscope but only four of six patients with gestations of 5 cm were successfully treated laparoscopically.[19] A limit of 4 to 5 cm therefore seems reasonable, although for the surgeon who is less experienced in cases of laparoscopic salpingostomy, a more conservative limit of 3 cm may be advisable.

The status of the contralateral tube should also be considered. Studies show that in 50% of ectopic pregnancies, the contralateral tube is diseased and may be completely occluded.[21-23] It may be difficult to judge the condition of the contralateral tube during surgery. Segmental tubal resection, which can be performed in less time than salpingectomy and so may be appropriate even when the patient is in shock, may be considered together with the possibility of future anastomosis.

The presence of extensive pelvic adhesive disease requires special consideration in the selection of appropriate surgical therapy for tubal pregnancy, especially when contemplating a laparoscopic approach. Pelvic adhesions may severely limit accessibility of the fallopian tube to the laparoscope, and there exists a strong possibility that lysis of adhesions may result in bleeding in the region of the ectopic gestation. For these reasons, the presence of adhesive disease is generally considered a contraindication for laparoscopic salpingostomy, and laparotomy should be performed.

Conservative therapy may not be advisable for patients with a history of previous ectopic pregnancy. A 64% intrauterine pregnancy rate and 12%

repeat ectopic rate after conservative laparoscopic surgery for initial tubal pregnancy was reported by Pouly and colleagues.[24] After conservative surgery for a second ectopic gestation, they found that intrauterine pregnancy rates fell to 21% and the repeat ectopic rate increased to 46%. Radical therapy may thus be preferable to the nearly 50% likelihood of a third ectopic pregnancy.

Radical Surgery

For the patient who presents in shock, having sustained extensive blood loss due to rupture, there is usually little choice but to proceed with salpingectomy, regardless of the patient's desire to preserve fertility. Although there exists a general trend toward more conservative therapy, salpingectomy is still considered by some to be the usual surgical treatment for tubal pregnancy, regardless of location of the conceptus within the tube.[25] From a surgical perspective, the advantage of salpingectomy is a greater degree of certainty that hemostasis and complete removal of the products of gestation are achieved, as compared with conservative procedures. In the event that profuse uncontrollable bleeding should occur while attempting to affect conservative surgical therapy, salpingectomy may be the only alternative. When future childbearing is not desired, salpingectomy should be performed.

The presence of extensive tubal damage in cases of eccyesis that could otherwise be treated conservatively is a relative indication for performance of salpingectomy. Such patients are generally at high risk for subsequent ectopic implantation. Patients experiencing a repeat ectopic pregnancy after conservative surgery for the initial incidence should also be considered likely candidates for salpingectomy because of the unacceptably high risk for recurrence.[24]

Women contemplating or involved in attempts at in vitro fertilization (IVF) may also be best served by salpingectomy in the treatment of ectopic pregnancy. The reason is that salpingectomy may improve ovarian access for future IVF attempts and may reduce the risk of ectopic pregnancy as a result of attempted IVF.

Salpingectomy may be performed at the time of laparotomy or through the laparoscope. Often, the decision to perform a laparotomy is made after laparoscopic confirmation of the ectopic diagnosis. Reasons for opting to perform salpingectomy at laparotomy (as opposed to laparoscopically) include a gestation that is too large to be treated using the laparoscope (ie, one that exceeds 3 cm in diameter); a gestation that is situated in the cornua; and extensive bleeding that may be uncontrollable with a laparoscopic approach.

SURGICAL TECHNIQUES

Laparoscopic Salpingostomy

When using an operative laparoscope, which allows for the introduction of surgical instruments through the operating channel, subumbilical and suprapubic punctures are made for introduction of the laparoscope and accessory trocar, respectively. The accessory trocar permits passage of atraumatic grasping forceps, used in securing the conceptus (Fig. 16-1). A third puncture site may be required if a laser is used to permit placement of a smoke evacuator and to transmit instruments used to hold the bowel away from the surgical area. A triple-puncture technique is also required when using a nonoperative laparoscope. In this case, the third puncture site is used for introduction of operative instruments.

The pelvic cavity should be inspected laparoscopically for active bleeding after evacuation and irrigation of any existing hemoperitoneum. Vasopressin is then injected along the antimesenteric border before incision of the tube. In cases of ampullary ectopic pregnancy, the conceptus is stabilized distally with the atraumatic grasping forceps and a 2-cm incision is extended along the antimesenteric border, directly over the gestational bulge. If the conceptus is located in the ampullary-infundibular segment of the tube, the incision may extend over the gestation to the fimbria. The tubal incision may be made using a variety of different instruments, including harmonic scalpel; scissors; CO_2, argon and KTP-532 lasers; Nd:YAG laser with a sapphire tip; and pinpoint electrocautery. The CO_2 laser offers better precision because of shorter penetration depth than some other types of surgical lasers but for the same reason offers less in the way of hemostatic properties. Conversely, Nd:YAG and KTP-532 lasers have greater penetration depths and thereby provide less precision but more effective coagulation.[26]

Spontaneous extrusion of the gestational products often occurs on incision of the tube. The remainder of the trophoblastic material should be gently separated from the tubal bed at the implantation site. Efforts to remove persistent products of conception may lead to bleeding and because this tissue usually necroses, extensive debridement is

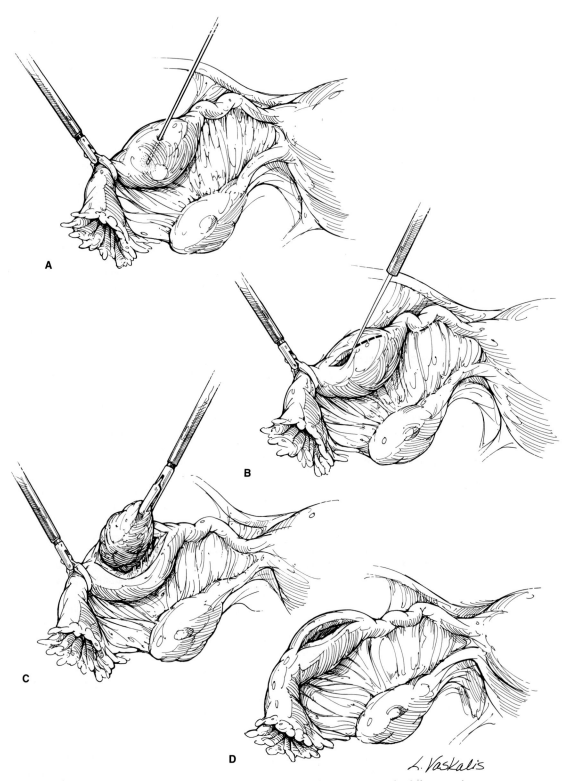

Figure 16–1. Laparoscopic salpingostomy. (**A**) An injection of pitressin into the fallopian tube.
(**B**) Incision of the fallopian tube to excise ectopic pregnancy. (**C**) Removal of ectopic pregnancy.
(**D**) Tube not closed to allow for healing by secondary intention.

generally not advisable. The implantation site is then irrigated and hemostasis is affected using laser coagulation or electrocautery.

If the gestational debris is larger than the operating channel of the laparoscope, scissors may be required to divide the tissue into smaller pieces in preparation for removal. An effort to remove segments of the conceptus whose dimensions exceed the diameter of the operating channel may dislodge the trophoblastic material from the grasping forceps, resulting in incomplete removal of gestational products. The tissue may then be lost in the pelvic cavity, where reimplantation has been known to occur.

With salpingostomy, the incision is allowed to heal by secondary intention, whereas salpingotomy implies closure with fine sutures. Both techniques offer similar results with regard to successful treatment of eccyesis and future fertility.[27] Therefore, salpingostomy is usually preferable because it implies a shorter time under anesthesia.

Salpingostomy at Laparotomy

This procedure is largely similar to that of laparoscopic salpingostomy, the most obvious difference being enhanced accessibility to the affected tube and surrounding area. Again, the hemoperitoneum is evacuated and a 2-cm incision is made along the antimesenteric border over the ectopic gestation. Pinpoint electrocautery or laser may be used to control bleeding, which often occurs from the edges of the incision. Fingertip pressure may be applied adjacent to the dilated portion of the tube to encourage extrusion. The remaining trophoblastic tissue is then gently removed, using suction or forceps. As in the laparoscopic procedure, excessive debridement of persistent gestational tissue is discouraged because of increased risk of bleeding.

Segmental Resection

This procedure involves the removal of the involved portion of the tube, leaving behind two discontinuous yet functional tubal segments. Using bipolar electrocautery forceps and proceeding from the distal to the proximal end of the effected segment, the tube, mesosalpinx, and blood vessels are fulgurated. By proceeding proximally along the length of the tube during fulguration, the conduction of electric current through the distal end of the tube and onto adjacent pelvic structures is avoided.

Scissors are then used to transect the distal and proximal ends of the diseased section of tube, and the intervening portion of the mesosalpinx is coagulated, cut, and removed.

Salpingectomy

Salpingectomy may also be performed at the time of laparotomy or through the laparoscope. From a procedural standpoint, often the only difference is the replacement of sutures (used during laparotomy) by coagulation methods during laparoscopy, although it is possible to suture through the laparoscope also.

To perform this procedure, the proximal isthmus of the tube is ligated. An additional ligature is placed at the level of the distal edge of mesosalpinx. This results in ligature at both ends of the vascular arc formed by the mesotubarian artery. Separate ligation may often be required for vessels that anastomose between the mesotubarian and ovarian plexus, particularly at the level of the ampulloisthmic junction. Especially when the laparoscope is used, ligature may be replaced by coagulation. The tube is then transected and removed. The proximal stump of the tube is closed with suture. The cut edges of the mesosalpinx may be covered by the two flaps of the broad ligament if they are pliable; this probably aids in the prevention of adhesion formation.

The question arises as to whether a cornual resection should be performed in conjunction with salpingectomy as a means of preventing future implantation in the tubal stump or in the interstitial region. Several reports have addressed this question.[28-31] The findings of Kalchman and Metzler indicate that protection against interstitial implantation is not guaranteed by systematic resection of the uterine cornua.[31] The number of cases of interstitial implantation after cornual resection appears to be sufficiently small as to render the additional surgery, with its inherent risk of rupture during uterine pregnancy, unwarranted.

For some time, gynecologists have contemplated the possible benefits of salpingo-oophorectomy over salpingectomy. Historically, this issue has been controversial. Ipsilateral oophorectomy is thought by some to enhance the possibility of future pregnancy by forcing all remaining ovulations to occur on the same side as the remaining tube.[32] This theory has not, however, been confirmed clinically. Studies show that there is little difference between salpingectomy and salpingo-oophorectomy with regard to subsequent intrauterine and repeat ectopic pregnancy rates.[21,34] Therefore, the performance of ipsilateral oophorectomy is generally restricted to women who have sustained severe impairment of ovarian blood supply.

POSTOPERATIVE MANAGEMENT

Because complete removal of all of the trophoblastic material is not ensured with conservative surgical approaches, hCG-β titers should be obtained on a weekly basis on all patients who have undergone this treatment until normal levels are reached. If the titers are decreasing and the patient is asymptomatic, management is generally limited to continued observation. If, however, the series of hCG-β values plateaus or increases, more aggressive treatment should be considered. The associated recurrence of pelvic mass or other symptoms may indicate the need for further surgical management. In most cases, salpingectomy at the time of laparotomy should be performed because of the strong probability that the remaining trophoblastic tissue is located extraluminally, and a second conservative procedure may be ineffective in removing the remaining products of conception.

The frequency of persistent ectopic pregnancy after laparoscopic salpingostomy ranges between 3% and 20%.[35,36] This complication may be more likely after the treatment of early ectopic pregnancy.[35] It is also more common after laparoscopic removal, as compared with incidence rates associated with removal at the time of laparotomy in cases of unruptured ampullary ectopic pregnancies.[37]

For situations in which titers have stabilized or increased but no other symptoms persist, treatment with methotrexate has proved effective.[38,39] Side effects associated with methotrexate therapy may include anemia or infection due to a decrease in red or white blood cell counts, stomatitis, gastrointestinal pain, and increased sensitivity to sunlight.

REPRODUCTIVE FUTURE AFTER SURGICAL THERAPY

Conservative Surgery

The reproductive future of patients after surgical treatment of ectopic pregnancy is influenced by factors that include postoperative tubal patency in the ipsilateral tube, the status of the contralateral tube,

the presence of additional risk factors for ectopic pregnancy, age, and history of infertility. Using postoperative hysterosalpingogram, tubal patency has been shown by several different investigators to range from 65% to 100%.[11,14,16,17,20,33,40-42] Unfortunately, patency does not always imply normal function. The condition of the contralateral tube must also be considered. If the contralateral tube is patent and without disease, intrauterine pregnancy may be accommodated by the traversal of gametes through this normal tube. Events of this type obscure the assessment of the potential of the ipsilateral tube for normal function. It is not uncommon, however, for the function of the contralateral tube to be impaired by conditions similar to those that gave rise to the index case.

More recent studies of pregnancy rates after laparoscopic linear salpingostomy determine intrauterine pregnancy rates of about 55% to 60%.[18,43,44] The same studies reveal recurrent ectopic pregnancy rates of about 14%. These results affirm the effectiveness of the laparoscopic approach, which has consequently replaced laparotomy as the standard treatment for uncomplicated tubal pregnancy.

Radical Surgery

A series of investigations performed during the decade from 1980 to 1990 is considered here in conjunction with our assessment of conception rates after radical surgery for ectopic pregnancy.[45-48] The findings of these studies indicate conception rates of 33.6% to 81.0%, with associated live birth rates (which were not available for all studies) ranging from 20.0% to 51.3%. These studies determined repeat extrauterine pregnancy rates of 5.8% to 12.8%. The intrauterine pregnancy rate after salpingectomy is thus similar to that observed after salpingostomy. This result has been confirmed many times, including a review by Oelsner of more than 2000 women for whom subsequent pregnancy rates were equivalent after salpingectomy and salpingotomy.[49]

NONTUBAL ECTOPIC PREGNANCY

Despite the fact that only a small percentage of all extrauterine pregnancies occur outside the fallopian tube, nontubal eccyesis presents a considerable challenge for the clinician. Diagnosis may be obscured by symptoms that mimic those associated with tubal pregnancy or by the absence altogether of abdominal symptoms. Definitive diagnosis may require laparoscopic visualization, and delayed diagnosis may result in rupture, separation, or hemorrhage, thereby complicating surgical therapy. Conservative surgical management of these cases is rarely appropriate. Surgical treatment most often involves excision of the conceptus and resection of tissue at the implantation site.

CONCLUSIONS

Times have changed dramatically in the past few years in regard to the surgical management of ectopic pregnancy. Only 5 years ago, the standard of care was salpingectomy. We have rapidly passed from this phase through an era of salpingostomy to salpingostomy through the laparoscope. Although linear salpingostomy through the laparoscope has some considerable disadvantages—in particular, retained products of conception—the rapid recovery time for the patient and the decreasing frequency of this complication with increased surgical experience makes it the treatment of choice in most ectopic pregnancies. This is facilitated by early diagnosis based on serial hCG-β testing and ultrasound.

The introduction of chemotherapy (methotrexate) into the arena of treatment modalities for ectopic pregnancy is helpful but also confusing. Questions remain as to the indications for its use and subsequent fertility. In cases of retained products of conception after linear salpingostomy, it is an ideal medication to use. Conversely, the treatment of ectopic pregnancy primarily with this modality remains questionable until there is better information regarding future fertility and long-term follow-up.

These changes in surgery for ectopic pregnancy continue to provide dynamic thinking with regard to this area of medicine.

REFERENCES

1. Centers for Disease Control: Morbidity and mortality weekly report. Ectopic pregnancy: United States, 1986. MMWR 38:41, 1989
2. Center for Disease Control and Prevention: Ectopic pregnancies—United States, 1988. MMWR 41:591, 1992
3. Kitchen JS, et al: Ectopic pregnancy: current clinical trends. Am J Obstet Gynecol 134:870, 1984
4. Schoen JA, Nowak RJ: Repeat ectopic pregnancy. Obstet Gynecol 45:542, 1975
5. Grant A: The effect of ectopic pregnancy on fertility. Clin Obstet Gynecol 5:861, 1962
6. Patton GW: Pregnancy outcome following microsurgical fimbrioplasty. Fertil Steril 37:150, 1982
7. Patton GW, Kistner RW: Atlas of infertility surgery, 2nd ed. Boston, Little, Brown, 1984
8. Gomel V: Tubal reanastomosis by microsurgery. Fertil Steril 28:59, 1977
9. Swolin K: Electromicrosurgery and salpingostomy: long term results. Am J Obstet Gynecol 121:418, 1974
10. Vermesh M: Conservatove management of ectopic gestations. Fertil Steril 51:559, 1989
11. DeCherney AH, Polan ML, Kort H, Kase N: Microsurgical technique in the management of tubal ectopic pregnancy. Fertil Steril 34:324, 1980
12. Breen JL: A 21 year survey of 654 ectopic pregnancies. Am J Obstet Gynecol 106:1004, 1970
13. Tinonen S, Nieminen U: Tubal regnancy, choice of operative method of treatment. Acta Obstet Gynecol Scand 46:327, 1967
14. Budowick M, Johnson TRB, Genadry R, et al: The histopathology of the developing tubal ectopic pregnancy. Fertil Steril 34:169, 1980
15. Senterman M, Rawle J, Tulandi T: Histopathologic study of ampullary and isthmic tubal ectopic pregnancy. Am J Obstet Gynecol 159:939, 1988
16. DeCherney AH, Boyers SP: Isthmic ectopic pregnancy: segmental resection as the treatment of choice. Fertil Steril 44:307, 1985
17. DeCherney AH, Romero R, Naftolin F: Surgical management of unruptured ectopic pregnancy. Fertil Steril 35:21, 1981
18. Pouly JL, Mahnes H, Mage G, et al: Conservative laparoscopic treatment of 321 ectopic pregnancies. Fertil Steril 46:1093, 1986
19. Vermesh M, Silva PD, Rosen GF, et al: Management of unrupture ectopic gestation by linear salpingostomy: a prospective, randomized clinical trial of laparoscopy versus laparotomy. Obstet Gynecol 73:400, 1989
20. Cartwright PS, Herbert CM, Maxson WS: Operative laparoscopy for the management of tubal pregnancy. J Reprod Med 31:589, 1986
21. Bender S: Fertility after tubal pregnancy. J Obstet Gynecol Br Emp 63:400, 1956
22. Vehraskari A: The operation of choice for ectopic pregnancy with reference to subsequent fertility. Acta Obstet Gynecol Scand 39(Suppl 3):1, 1960
23. Seigler AM, Wang CF, Westoff C: Management of unruptured tubal pregnancy. Obstet Gynecol Surv 36:599, 1981
24. Pouly JL, Chapron C, Manhes H, et al: Multifactorial analysis of fertility after conservative laparoscopic treatment of ectopic pregnancy in a series of 223 patients. Fertil Steril 56:453, 1991
25. Vermesh M, Silva PD, Sauer MV, et al: Persistent tubal ectopic gestation: patterns of circulation of β human chorionic gonadotropin and progesterone, and management options. Fertil Steril 50:584, 1988
26. Martin DC, Absten GT, Levinson CJ, Levinson CJ, Photopulos GJ: Intra-abdominal laser surgery, p 53. Memphis, Resurge Press, 1986
27. Tulandi T, Guralnick M: Treatment of tubal ectopic pregnancy by salpingotomy with or without tubal

sururing and salpingectomy. Fertil Steril 55:53, 1991

28. Flusher RW: Tubal pregnancy following homolateral salpingectomy. Am J Obstet Gynecol 78:355, 1959

29. Malkasian GD, Hunter JS, Remine WH: Pregnancy in the tubal interstitium and tubal remnants. Am J Obstet Gynecol 77:1301, 1959

30. Webster HD, Barclar DL, Fisher CK: Ectopic pregnancy: a 17 year review. Am J Obstet Gynecol 92:23, 1965

31. Kalchman GG, Meltzer MN: Interstitial pregnancy following homolateral salpingectomy. Am J Obstet Gynecol 19:1139, 1966

32. Jeffcoate TNA: Salpingectomy or salpingo-oophorectomy. Br J Obstet Gynaecol 135:74, 1955

33. Bruhat MA, Manhes H, Mage G, Pouly JL: Treatment of ectopic pregnancy by means of laparoscopy. Fertil Steril 33:411, 1980

34. Franklin, EW, Ziederman AM, Laemmle P: Tubal ectopic pregnancy: etiology and obstetric and gynecologic sequelae. Am J Obstet Gynecol 117:220, 1973

35. Seifer DB, Gutmann JN, Doyle MB, et al: Persistent ectopic pregnancy following laparoscopic linear salpingostomy. Obstet Gynecol 76:112, 1990

36. Seifer, Diamond MP, DeCherney AH: Persistent ectopic pregnancy. Obstet Gynecol Clin North Am 18:153, 1991

37. Seifer DB, Gutmann JN, Grant WD, et al: Comparison of persistent ectopic pregnancy after laparoscopic salpingostomy versus salpingostomy at laparotomy for ectopic pregnancy. Obstet Gynecol 81:378, 1993

38. Higgins KA, Schwartz MB: Treatment of persistent trophoblastic tissue after salpingostomy with methotrexate. Fertil Steril 45:427, 1986

39. Kenigsberg D, Porte J, Hull M, Spitz IM: Medical treatment of residual ectopic pregnancy: RU 486 and methotrexate. Fertil Steril 47:702, 1987

40. Johns DA, Hardie RP: Management of unruptured ectopic pregnancy with laparsocopic carbon dioxide laser. Fertil Steril 46:703, 1986

41. Schinfeld JS, Reedy G: Mesosalpingeal vessel ligation for conservative treatment of ectopic pregnancy. J Reprod Med 28:823, 1983

42. Smith HO, Toledo AA, Thompson JD: Conservative surgical management of isthmic ectopic pregnanices. Am J Obstet Gynecol 157:604, 1987

43. Vermesh M, Presser SC: Reproductive outcome after linear salpingostomy for ectopic gestation: a prospective 3 year followup. Fertil Steril 57:682, 1992

44. Mecke H, Semm K, Lehmann-Willenbrock E: Results of operative pelviscopy in 202 cases of ectopic pregnancy. Int J Fertil 34:93, 1989

45. Sherman D, Langer R, Sadovdky G, et al: Improved fertility following ectopic pregnancy. Fertil Steril 37:497, 1982

46. Paavonen J, Varjonen-Toivonen M, Komulainen M, Heinonen K: Diagnosis and management of tubal pregnancy: effect on fertility outcome. Int J Gynaecol Obstet 23:1291, 1988

47. Tuomivaara L, Kauppila A: Radical or conservative surgery for ectopic pregnancy? A follow-up study of fertility of 323 patients. Fertil Steril 50:580, 1988

48. Dubuisson JB, Aubriot EX, Foulot H, et al: Reproductive outcome after laparoscopic salpingectomy for tubal pregnancy. Fertil Steril 53:1004, 1990

49. Oelsner G: Ectopic pregnancy in the sole remaining tube and the management of the patient with multiple ectopic pregnancies. Clin Obstet Gynecol 30:225, 1987

Ambulatory Gynecology, Second Edition,
edited by David H. Nichols and Patrick J. Sweeney.
J. B. Lippincott Company, Philadelphia, © 1995.

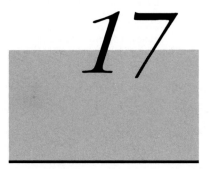

17

Menopause

Brian W. Walsh and Isaac Schiff

Menopause is defined by the permanent cessation of menses. This is but one aspect of the climacteric, during which time women undergo endocrine, somatic, and psychological changes over the course of several years. These changes are related both to aging and to estrogen depletion; it is difficult to quantify the respective effects of each. This chapter addresses the consequences of declining estrogen production in postmenopausal women as well as the possible beneficial value of hormonal replacement therapy.

AGING OF THE OVARY

The mean age of women at menopause is 51 years, with about 4% of women undergoing a natural menopause before age 40 years (Fig. 17-1).[1] The age at menopause is not influenced by prolonged periods of hypothalamic amenorrhea, number of pregnancies, or oral contraceptive use. Because the average age at menopause has not changed since antiquity, increases in life expectancy mean that American women live a third of their lifetime after ovarian failure.[2]

The aging process of the ovary appears to begin during fetal development. Although 7 million oogonia are present at 20 weeks gestation, only 700,000 remain at birth.[3] After birth, the number of oocytes continues to decline even before the onset of puberty.

For several years before menopause, estradiol and progesterone production decline, despite the occurrence of ovulatory cycles.[4] This waning of ovarian follicular activity reduces the negative feedback inhibition of estradiol on the hypothalamic–pituitary system, resulting in a gradual rise in follicle-stimulating hormone (FSH). The remaining ovarian follicles are increasingly less responsive to FSH; menopause occurs when the residual follicles are refractory to elevated concentrations of FSH.

Estrogen production by the postmenopausal ovary is minimal (Fig. 17-2). The major source of postmenopausal estrogens is adrenal androgens, particularly androstenedione, which undergoes aromatization by peripheral tissues to estrone. Typically, 2.8% of androstenedione is converted to estrone but higher rates are seen in obese women, who have more adipose tissue to aromatize andro-

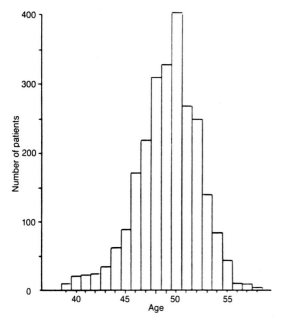

Figure 17–1. Age of menopause in 2000 women during a natural menopause. (Gambrell RD Jr: The menopause: benefits and risks of estrogen-progesterone replacement therapy. Fertil Steril 37:457, 1982. Reproduced with permission of the publisher, The American Fertility Society.)

gens.[5] This partly explains why obese women have fewer menopausal symptoms than thin women.[6] The mean concentration after menopause of estrone is 35 pg/mL, which is higher than the mean concentration of estradiol, 13 pg/mL.[7] This estradiol is produced by conversion from estrone.

The postmenopausal ovary continues to produce testosterone and androstenedione, primarily from stromal and hilar cells (Fig. 17-3). The mean concentration of testosterone in women after menopause (about 250 pg/mL) is minimally lower than that of premenopausal women. In contrast, the mean postmenopausal concentration of androstenedione (850 pg/mL) is about half that of premenopausal women (1500 pg/mL).[7] Because these postmenopausal androgens are no longer opposed by estrogens, they may lead to increased hair growth on the upper lip and chin.

VASOMOTOR FLUSHES

One of the most frequent and troublesome symptoms for women at the climacteric is vasomotor instability (flushes): about 80% of women experience

hot flushes within 3 months of a natural or surgical menopause. Of those women, 85% experience them for more than a year and 25% to 50% for up to 5.[8] Hot flushes lessen in frequency and intensity with advancing age, unlike other sequelae of menopause, which progress with time.

Definitions and Pathophysiology

Hot flushes are the subjective sensation of intense warmth of the upper body. They typically last for 4 minutes and range in duration from 30 seconds to 5 minutes.[9] They frequently follow a prodrome of palpitations or a sensation of pressure within the head and may be accompanied by weakness, faintness, or vertigo. They usually end in sweating and a cold sensation.

A vasomotor flush is the objective component of this phenomenon, characterized by a visible ascending flush of the thorax, neck and face. The first event is an increase in peripheral blood flow, particularly to the fingers, with peak skin temperature reaching a maximum 5 minutes later. This increase in blood flow appears to be limited to the cutaneous vasculature and does not involve blood flow to muscle; thus, blood pressure remains stable during a flush. The loss of body heat through the skin causes core body temperature to fall.[10] A rise in plasma luteinizing hormone (LH) is the final event, reaching its peak 12 minutes after the flush begins.

When hot flushes occur at night, they may awaken the patient from sleep. This was shown by simultaneously recording finger temperature and skin resistance as objective indices of vasomotor flushes while monitoring the stages of sleep, using a sleep polygraph (electroencephalogram, electromyelogram, and electrooculogram; Fig. 17-4).[11] The waking episodes were indeed temporally associated with the occurrence of hot flushes. The resultant poor quality of sleep may in turn lead to chronic fatigue, characterized by such symptoms as irritability, poor concentration, and impaired memory.

Etiology

Hot flushes result from the withdrawal of estrogens and not from hypoestrogenism per se. They therefore accompany menopause, whether it occurs naturally, surgically, or medically (ie, hypoestrogenism induced by the use of long-acting gonadotropin-releasing hormone agonists or by danazol). The discontinuation of exogenous estrogens may

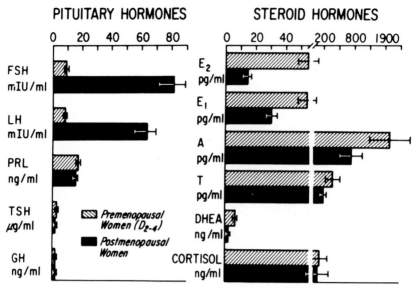

Figure 17–2.   Circulating concentrations of pituitary and steroid hormones in pre-menopausal (menstrual cycle, day 2 to 4) and postmenopausal women. (Yen SSC: The biology of menopause. J Reprod Med 18:28, 1977.)

also precipitate flushes: women with Turner's syndrome, who are hypoestrogenic, do not have hot flushes unless exogenous estrogens have been prescribed and are later withdrawn.[12]

Men also may have hot flushes but as a consequence of testosterone withdrawal. In fact, 73% of men who undergo orchiectomy for prostatic cancer have flushes.[13] Treatment with estrogens provides relief but the flushes may return if estrogen treatment is discontinued.[14] Androgens do not need to be converted to estrogen to suppress hot flushes be-

cause a nonaromatizable androgen, fluoxymesterone, is fully effective in relieving flushes.[15]

Obese women tend to be less troubled by hot flushes: women who experience minimal symptoms at menopause weigh considerably more than those who are severely symptomatic.[6] Obese women are relatively "protected" from hot flushes because they are functionally less hypoestrogenic for two reasons: (1) their increased adiposity allows greater peripheral conversion of adrenal androgens into estrogens, and (2) their sex hormone–binding globulin

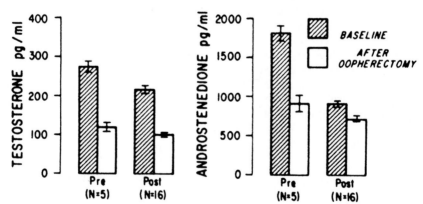

Figure 17–3.   Serum testosterone and androstenedione levels before and 6 to 8 weeks after bilateral oophorectomy. Five premenopausal (*Pre*) and 16 postmenopausal (*Post*) women were studied. (Judd HL, Lucas WE, Yen SSC: Effect of oophorectomy on testosterone and androstenedione levels. Am J Obstet Gynecol 118:793, 1974.)

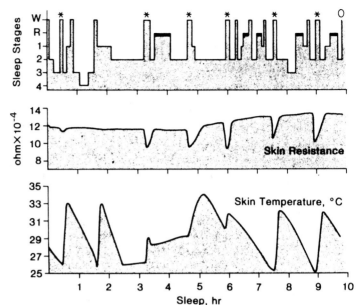

Figure 17–4. Sleepgram and recordings of skin resistance and temperature in a postmenopausal subject with severe hot flashes. Asterisks denote objectively measured hot flashes. (Erlik Y, Tataryn IV, Meldrum DR et al: Association of waking episodes with menopausal hot flushes. JAMA 245:1741, 1981.)

levels are typically lower and therefore a greater proportion of their estrogens are unbound and free to act on target tissues (Fig. 17-5).[5,16]

Vasomotor flushes are caused by an acute lowering of the hypothalamic thermoregulatory setpoint, precipitated by estrogen withdrawal. The presence of estrogen may stabilize the thermoregulatory center by maintaining hypothalamic opioid activity. The loss of estrogen at menopause may cause a hypothalamic "opioid withdrawal," leading to thermoregulatory instability. This hypothesis is supported by the observation that estrogen prescribed in physiologic amounts induces hypothalamic opioid activity.[17]

Estrogen's stabilizing effect on the hypothalamic thermoregulatory center may also be mediated by neurotransmitters such as norepinephrine (NE). As shown in Figure 17-6, the intraneuronal level of NE is regulated by the balance between the enzymes tyrosine hydroxylase (the rate-limiting step of NE synthesis from tyrosine) and monoamine oxidase (which irreversibly degrades NE to inactive metabolites).[18] After synthesis, NE is stored in prejunctional vesicles. When released into the synaptic cleft, NE binds to postjunctional receptors to propagate a response, either excitatory or inhibitory. This action is terminated by the rapid reuptake of NE back into the postjunctional neuron.

In animals, estrogen has multiple effects on NE neurons. Estrogen stimulates tyrosine hydroxylase activity, thereby increasing NE synthesis.[19] In addition, estrogen reduces monoamine oxidase activ-

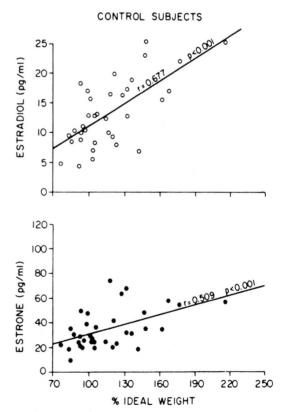

Figure 17–5. Correlation of plasma estradiol and estrone levels with percentage of ideal weight in postmenopausal women. (Judd HL, Davidson BJ, Frumar AM, et al: Serum androgens and estrogens in postmenopausal women. Am J Obstet Gynecol 136:859, 1980.)

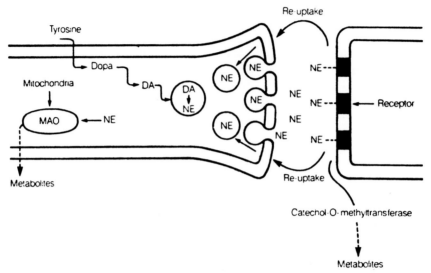

Figure 17–6. Schematic representation of an adrenergic junction. Tyrosine is converted by the enzyme tyrosine hydroxylase to 3,4 dihydroxyphenylalanine (DOPA); decarboxylated to dopamine (DA); hydroxylated to form norepinephrine (NE); and stored in vesicles. Upon release, NE interacts with adrenergic receptors. This action is terminated by re-uptake of NE into the prejunctional neurons. Norepinephrine is degraded into inactive metabolites by monoamine oxidase (MAO) and catechol-o-methyl transferase. (From Berkow R (ed): The Merck manual of diagnosis and therapy, ed 16, p 2652. Copyright 1992 by Merck & Co., Inc. Used with permission.)

ity and so retards NE degradation.[20] Both of these actions increase the intraneuronal level of NE. Estrogen also augments NE release and inhibits NE reuptake, thereby potentiating its effect on postjunctional receptors.[21,22] Lastly, estrogen appears to increase the number of α_2-hypothalamic postsynaptic receptors.[23] All of these actions serve to enhance α_2-adrenergic activity. Because this work has been performed in animals, it is not definitely known whether estrogen has the same effects in humans. Nevertheless, these findings suggest that estrogens enhance α_2-adrenergic activity and that estrogen withdrawal may lead to vasomotor flushes due to reduced α_2-adrenergic activity.

This hypothesis is supported by the finding that α_2-agonists such as clonidine, aldomet (after conversion to its active form, methylnorepinephrine), and lofexidine suppress hot flushes.[24–26] This also explains why estrogen treatment must be given for 2 to 4 weeks before hot flushes are maximally relieved; they do not act directly but must alter central NE metabolism.[27] This alteration of NE metabolism may persist for a short time after estrogen withdrawal, thereby explaining why hot flush relief continues for a few weeks after estrogens are discontinued.

Diagnosis

History and physical examination should be sufficient to make the diagnosis and exclude other conditions that may resemble hot flushes such as thyrotoxicosis, carcinoid tumor, pheochromocytoma, anxiety, diabetic insulin reaction, alcohol withdrawal, and diencephalic epilepsy. Menopause may be confirmed by demonstrating an elevated serum FSH. The finding of a low serum estradiol level is not diagnostic, however, because premenopausal women frequently have low levels during menses.

Treatment

Estrogens

Because hot flushes result from estrogen withdrawal, the most direct therapy is estrogen replacement, which is more than 95% effective.[27] By relieving hot flushes, particularly those occurring at night, estrogen replacement improves sleep quality; estrogen treatment reduces sleep latency and increases rapid-eye-movement sleep.[28] Moreover, symptoms that appear to result from chronic sleep disturbance are significantly improved by estrogen replacement; estrogen use decreases insomnia, irritability, and anxiety and improves memory.[29]

Treatment with estrogen does not produce immediate relief of hot flushes (Fig. 17-7).[27] Hot flush frequency is not reduced until after 2 weeks of treatment and treatment is not maximal until after 4 weeks. Thus, treatment for 1 month is necessary to evaluate the adequacy of a particular dose in relieving flushes. After 1 month, the dose may be increased because there appears to be a dose-response relation between estrogen dose and degree of hot-flush suppression. For example, 3 weeks of treatment with transdermal estradiol, 0.025 mg, reduces flushes by 40%; 0.05 mg by 53%; 0.10 mg by 83%; and 0.20 mg by 91%.[30]

Estrogen replacement is not a permanent cure for hot flushes: they return when treatment is discontinued. The patient should be advised of this when terminating estrogen therapy. The return of hot flushes may be minimized by slowly tapering the dose over several weeks or months.

Progestins

Women with endometrial cancer undergoing treatment with depo-medroxyprogesterone acetate (depo-MPA) were incidentally noted to have relief of their hot flushes. A clinical trial later found depo-MPA to have a dose-dependent effect, with 50 mg reducing flushes by 60%, 100 mg by 75%, and 150 mg by 85%.[31] In addition, hot flush frequency did not decline until after 2 weeks of treatment, and maximal suppression did not occur until after 4 weeks. This temporal relation in hot flush relief and dose-dependency resembles that seen with transdermal estrogens. The use of depo-MPA is associated with a high incidence of irregular vaginal bleeding and a prolonged but unpredictable duration of action. For that reason, oral MPA, which has a considerably shorter and more predictable half-life than the depot form, is more commonly given. Treatment with 20 mg daily for 1 month reduces flushes by 70%, compared with a 15% reduction seen with placebo treatment.[32] A lower dose of MPA, 10 mg daily, reduces flush frequency by 87% and is better tolerated by patients.[33]

The mechanism of action of progestins is unknown. It is hypothesized that they too may act by central neurotransmitters because they raise the hypothalamic thermoregulatory set-point during the luteal phase of ovulatory women. Progestins are useful in patients for whom estrogen is contraindicated but they may cause irregular vaginal bleeding in addition to abdominal bloating, constipation, breast tenderness, and mood changes.

α-Adrenergic Agonists

Women treated with antihypertensive medicines were incidentally noted to have fewer hot flushes. It is hypothesized that they act by central effects on hypothalamic neurotransmitters to stabilize the thermoregulatory center. They may also act directly on the peripheral vasculature to block cutaneous vasodilation. Clonidine, an α-adrenergic agonist, significantly lowers hot flush frequency by 30% to 40% when used at doses of 0.1 and 0.2 mg twice daily. At these dosages, patients frequently complain of dizziness and dry mouth.[34] For that

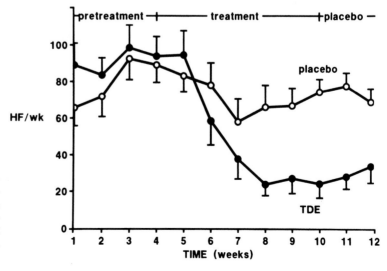

Figure 17–7. Change in subjective hot flashes recorded by postmenopausal women treated with transdermal estrogen (TDE) and placebo. (Haas S, Walsh B, Evans S, et al: The effect of transdermal estradiol on hormone and metabolic dynamics over a six-week period. Obstet Gynecol 71:671, 1988.)

reason, the initial dosage should be 0.05 mg twice daily, increasing to 0.1 mg twice daily if hot flushes persist and if there are no side effects. Similarly, another α-adrenergic agonist, lofexidine, reduces hot flushes by as much as 66%.[26] The initial dosage of lofexidine, 0.1 mg twice daily, was increased by increments of 0.1 mg (up to a maximum of 0.6 mg) every 2 weeks until flushes were abolished or until side effects (dry mouth, fatigue, headache) were intolerable. Aldomet, 250 mg three times daily, also reduces hot flushes by 20%.[25] Because the use of α-adrenergic agonists is limited by their side effects, hypertensive patients are the best candidates for this nonhormonal treatment.

Bellergal

Bellergal, a preparation of ergotamine tartrate, belladonna alkaloids, and 40 mg phenobarbital, is 50% effective when given as one tablet twice daily.[35] It is unknown which of its components is responsible for its effect. This medicine should rarely be necessary because it has addictive potential and safer alternative treatments are available.

Other Agents

Tricyclic antidepressants and oxazepam have been proposed for the treatment of hot flushes. Because they have not been compared with placebo, their therapeutic efficacy is unproved. Comparison with placebo is important because many investigators have shown placebo to significantly reduce hot flushes.

OSTEOPOROSIS

Definition and Etiology

Osteoporosis is the progressive reduction in bone mass without qualitative abnormalities. It affects trabecular bone earlier than cortical bone, and its major consequence is fracture. The most frequent sites of fracture are the vertebral bodies, distal radius, and femoral neck. It develops when the rate of bone resorption exceeds the rate of bone formation.

Primary osteoporosis results from estrogen deficiency and constitutes 95% of all cases. Estrogen receptors are present in bone and therefore estrogen may act on bone directly.[36] Estrogen may also act by any of the following mechanisms:

1. By decreasing the sensitivity of bone to parathyroid hormone without changing the amount of circulatory parathyroid hormone
2. By increasing calcitonin; this is consistent with the facts that:
   A. High-estrogen states, such as oral contraceptive use and pregnancy, are associated with elevated calcitonin[37]
   B. Men, who have greater bone mass than women, have higher calcitonin levels[38]
   C. Calcitonin levels decline with age and menopause and rise with estrogen replacement by directly increasing intestinal calcium absorption[39,40]

Secondary osteoporosis, which constitutes a minority of cases, may result from any of the following disorders: glucocorticoid or heparin use, renal failure, hyperthyroidism (endogenous or iatrogenic), primary hyperparathyroidism, hyperadrenalism, dietary calcium deficiency, or upper intestinal surgery.

Incidence

At all ages, women have less bone mass than men. Both sexes achieve peak bone mass at age 30 years and progressively lose bone mass at a rate of about 1% to 2% per year after age 40 years.[41] In women, this rate increases to 3.9% per year for the 6 years that follow menopause (Fig. 17-8).[42]

Individuals with a lower peak bone mass are more likely to develop significant osteoporosis. Thus, women are at higher risk than men, whites and Orientals more at risk than blacks, and thin women more at risk than those who are obese.[43,44] The greater bone mass of obese women may be due to their increased weight, which mechanically stresses their axial skeleton. Their greater bone mass may also be due to their higher endogenous estrogen levels resulting from (1) increased peripheral aromatization of androstenedione to estrone, and (2) lower sex hormone–binding globulin levels, with greater free estradiol levels.[5,16]

The rate of bone loss varies greatly among individuals: women who smoke, drink alcohol, are sedentary, or consume low-calcium, high-protein, or high-phosphate diets lose bone mass more quickly.[45-48] Family history is also a significant risk factor.

Twenty-five percent of women beyond age 60 years show vertebral fractures on x-ray, as do 50%

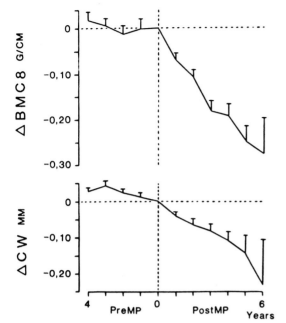

Figure 17–8. Mean (± standard error mean) changes in bone mass, measured as bone mineral content (g/cm) of the proximal (*BMC8*) forearm and mean cortical width (*CW*); millimeters of metacarpals 2, 3, and 4 of both hands. (**Δ**) Changes from the last premenopausal (*PreMP*) year. Broken horizontal line gives values for the last premenopausal year (*0*), and the broken vertical line indicates the last premenopausal year. (Falch JA, Oftebro H, Haug E: Early postmenopausal bone loss not associated with decrease in vitamin D. J Clin Endocrinol Metab 64:836, 1987.)

of women beyond age 75 years.[49,50] Twenty-five percent of women beyond age 80 years have a hip fracture, with the annual incidence being 1.3% per year after age 65 years and 3.3% per year after age 85 years.[51,52] One out of six women with hip fractures are not alive 3 months after the event.[53] The annual healthcare cost in the United States for these fractures is estimated to be $7 billion.

Diagnosis

Once osteoporosis has occurred, it may not be significantly reversed. Known risk factors for osteoporosis (age, weight, calcium and caffeine intake, alcohol and tobacco use, and urinary markers of bone turnover) do not identify 30% of women with low bone mass.[54] Thus, several radiologic techniques are used to detect early losses of bone mass

before significant osteoporosis has developed. The identification of early bone loss may permit treatment to be initiated before a fracture occurs. Because osteoporosis affects trabecular bone earlier than cortical bone, those modalities that measure trabecular bone preferentially are the most informative.

Single-photon absorptiometry of the distal radius is inexpensive, easy to perform, and requires only 5 mrem of radiation. Because the distal radius consists of 75% cortical bone and 25% trabecular bone, measurement at this site may not detect early bone loss. In skilled hands, it has an accuracy within 5% and a precision of 2% to 4%.[55]

Dual-photon absorptiometry of the second to fourth vertebral body offers an advantage because this site consists of 60% cortical bone and 40% trabecular bone. It is more expensive, requires 5 to 15 mrem, and has an accuracy within 5% to 7%, with a precision of 2% to 5%.[55]

Computed tomography scanning of the vertebral body measures 5% cortical bone and 95% trabecular bone and may detect changes over an interval as brief as 6 months.[56] It has the greatest radiation exposure (200 mrem) and expense and has a precision of 1% to 3%.

The most recent modality to be developed, quantitative digital radiography, has become the technique of choice. It provides high-resolution images, with excellent precision (1% to 2%) and lower radiation exposure (1 to 3 mrem).[57] Quantitative digital radiography requires fewer than 8 minutes per study, which is considerably shorter than the 20 to 45 minutes needed for dual-photon absorptiometry.

Measurement of a woman's bone density today does not predict her bone density in the future. To identify those women who will be "fast bone losers" (ie, greater than 3.1% loss per year of forearm bone mineral content), a nonradiologic method has been proposed.[58] A single measurement of a fasting urinary calcium to creatinine ratio greater than 270 mmol/mol, fasting urinary hydroxyproline to creatinine ratio greater than 11.2 mmol/mol, serum alkaline phosphatase greater than 120 g/L *and* a fat mass index less than 0.222 (calculated from height and weight) correctly identifies 79% of the fast losers and 78% of the slow losers. Because the predictive value of a positive test is only 53%, reliance on this method misses a substantial proportion of women who would benefit from estrogen replacement.

Patients found to have osteoporosis or osteoporosis-related fractures should undergo history and physical examination to exclude an underlying etiology. Measurement of serum calcium, phosphate, alkaline phosphatase, creatinine, sedimentation rate, thyroid studies, or serum protein electrophoresis may assist in identifying any of those disorders but will all be normal in patients with primary osteoporosis.

Prevention

Because established osteoporosis cannot be significantly reversed, the emphasis of medical management should be on prophylaxis rather than on treatment. Stopping smoking, reducing dietary phosphates, and particularly, exercising regularly all act to conserve bone mass.

Estrogens

Estrogens clearly prevent the loss of bone mass and thereby reduce the incidence of osteoporotic fractures. They decrease bone resorption (Fig. 17-9),[59] increase intestinal calcium absorption, and reduce renal calcium excretion.[60] Low doses of estrogen appear to be as effective as higher ones: 0.625 mg and 1.25 mg of conjugated equine estrogens (CEE) are equally effective in both preventing bone loss and reducing the incidence of fractures (Fig. 17-10).[61] Although ethinyl estradiol and mestranol are also effective, conjugated estrogens and estradiol are preferred because they have a lesser impact on the liver.[62]

Because bone loss is irreversible, estrogen treatment should be initiated as soon as possible after menopause to maximize the amount of bone preserved. Treatment should be taken for at least 6 years to substantially reduce the lifetime risk of fracture (Fig. 17-11).[61] Because there is no method that identifies all patients who will develop osteoporosis, most postmenopausal women are potential candidates for this therapy. Measurement of baseline bone density may be helpful for patients for whom the decision to initiate estrogen replacement is difficult. A normal bone density does not rule out the future development of osteoporosis, however.

Progestins

Progestins used alone also reduce the urinary loss of calcium but preservation of bone mass has not yet been demonstrated.[63] Appropriate doses are MPA, 10 mg daily, or depo-MPA, 150 mg intramuscularly, every 3 months.[64,65] Combined with estrogen, progestins may act synergistically to increase bone mass. A proposed mechanism is that progesterone may block glucocorticoid receptors located on bone, preventing endogenous glucocorticoids from exerting their inhibitory effects on bone metabolism.[66]

Many women cannot take or choose not to take

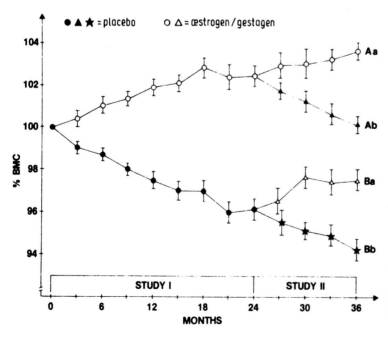

Figure 17–9. Bone mineral content (BMC) as a function of time and treatment in 94 (*study I*) and 77 (*study II*) women soon after menopause. (Christiansen C, Christiansen MS, Transbol I: Bone mass in postmenopausal women after withdrawal of estrogen/gestagen replacement therapy. Lancet 1:459, 1981.)

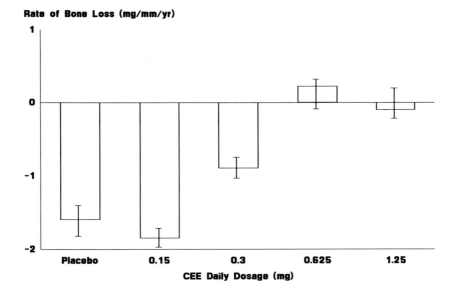

Figure 17–10. Mean annual change (± standard error mean) in bone mass in women treated daily with placebo or 0.15, 0.3, 0.625, and 1.25 mg of oral conjugated equine estrogens (CEE). Bone mineral content measured by single-photon absorptiometry at the midpoint of the third right metacarpal. (Adapted from Lindsay R, Hart DM, Clark DM: The minimum effective dose of estrogen for prevention of postmenopausal bone loss. Obstet Gynecol 63:759, 1984.)

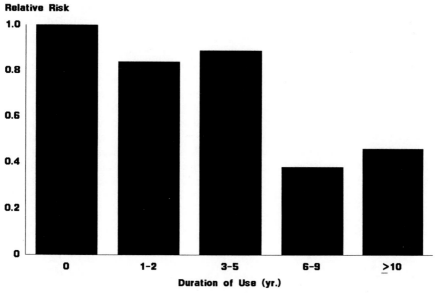

Figure 17–11. Relative risk for hip or forearm fracture according to duration of postmenopausal estrogen use. (Adapted from Weiss NS, Ure CL, Ballard JH, et al: Decreased risk of fractures of the hip and lower forearm with postmenopausal use of estrogen. N Engl J Med 303:1195, 1980.)

hormonal treatment and are therefore at risk for developing osteoporosis. For those women, multiple alternate therapies have been proposed. Six such treatments have been evaluated for efficacy in preventing or reversing osteoporosis: calcium, fluoride, diphosphonates, calcitonin, Vitamin D, and thiazides.

Calcium

The efficacy of calcium in preventing postmenopausal bone loss has been controversial. One well-designed study found that oral calcium supplementation in early postmenopausal women with adequate dietary calcium intakes did not prevent bone loss (Fig. 17-12).[67] Calcium use may prevent bone loss in selected patients, however, as shown in a 2-year clinical trial of 300 healthy postmenopausal women given either placebo or 500 mg of calcium carbonate or calcium citrate maleate.[68] Calcium treatment did not prevent bone loss in (1) women who had undergone menopause within the preceding 5 years and (2) women who consumed more than 400 mg calcium per day. For women who were 6 or more years after menopause *and* who consumed less than 400 mg of calcium, calcium supplementation did prevent bone loss. Calcium citrate maleate was more effective than calcium carbonate, possibly because of better gastrointestinal absorption. Thus, it appears that calcium supplementation may reduce age-related bone loss occurring in women many years after menopause who have low dietary-calcium intakes. Although calcium supplementation cannot prevent the estrogen-related bone loss occurring shortly after menopause, it may have a role in permitting a lower dose of estrogen (ie, 0.3 mg CEE) to be used.[69] Caution should be used in patients with a history of renal stones.

That calcium may prevent age-related bone loss was also suggested in a study of 37 healthy premenopausal women between ages 30 and 42.[70] Half of these women were instructed to increase their dietary calcium intake by an average of 610 mg/day; age- and weight-matched controls maintained their usual diet. After 3 years, vertebral bone density was unchanged in the women who had raised their calcium intake but was 3% lower in controls. It should be noted that the increase in dietary calcium was accompanied by increased consumption of calories (by 28%), fat (by 38%), and protein (by 60%). In addition, the increased calcium group gained 4.2 kg versus 3.4 kg for the control group over the 3 years. Thus, the prevention of age-related bone loss seen in this study may be because of increased body fat, resulting from higher caloric consumption. The possibility does exist, however, that increasing dietary calcium after peak bone mass is achieved in the third decade may reduce age-related bone loss and perhaps lessen the incidence of osteoporotic fractures later in life.

Fluoride

Fluoride stimulates bone formation and increases cancellous bone mass as much as twofold.[71] There is a suspicion, however, that the bone formed is structurally abnormal and weak and more likely to fracture. The effect of fluoride treatment on the incidence of osteoporotic fractures was evaluated in 200 osteoporotic postmenopausal women.[72] They were randomized to treatment with sodium fluoride, 75 mg daily, or to placebo. Although fluoride treatment increased vertebral bone density by 35%, it did not reduce the incidence of vertebral fractures. Most worrisome was that the incidence of nonvertebral fractures was threefold higher in the fluoride group. This was attributed to a fluoride-induced loss of cortical bone, suggested by a 4% decrease in density of the radial shaft. Thus, fluoride increases cancellous bone at the expense of cortical bone. Not only is the additional cancellous bone structurally weak (which will not prevent vertebral fractures) but the loss of cortical bone in-

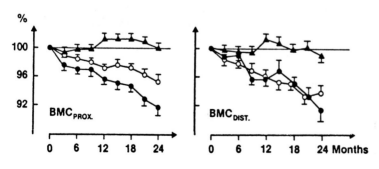

Figure 17–12. Bone mineral content of the proximal (BMC_{prox}) and distal (BMC_{dist}) radius of postmenopausal women treated with percutaneous estrogens (▲), calcium (●) and placebo (○). (From Riis B, Thomsen K, Christiansen C: Does calcium supplementation prevent postmenopausal bone loss? N Engl J Med 316:173, 1987.)

creases the risk of fracture of nonvertebral bones. Fluoride does not appear to be effective in the prevention or treatment of osteoporosis.

Diphosphonates

Etidronate, a diphosphonate, has been used to treat Paget's disease of bone because it retards both osteoblastic and osteoclastic activity, which are both abnormally high in this condition. When etidronate is given in low doses, however, the anti-osteoclastic activity predominates, so that bone mass may increase. Two clinical trials evaluated the effect of etidronate on vertebral bone density and fracture rates.[73,74] Both studies administered etidronate, 400 mg daily for 2 weeks, which was prescribed four times per year. Etidronate significantly increased vertebral bone density by 2% per year over the 2 to 3 years of observation and substantially decreased the incidence of vertebral fractures. Watts and coworkers found that 2 years of treatment with etidronate lowered vertebral fracture rates by 50% for the entire cohort and by 70% for women with the least amount of bone mass at the start of treatment.[73] Storm and associates noted that after the first year of treatment, the incidence of new vertebral fractures was more than 80% lower in the etidronate users.[74] These studies indicate that short-term intermittent cyclic therapy with etidronate can reverse postmenopausal vertebral bone loss and the incidence of fractures. The diphosphonates may offer promise as (1) an alternative to estrogen in the prevention of osteoporosis; (2) an adjunct treatment for women who demonstrate bone loss while taking estrogen; and (3) a primary treatment for women with established osteoporosis. Because the duration of these studies was short (2 and 3 years) and etidronate remains present in bone for many years, the long-term safety and efficacy of etidronate needs to be established before routine use.

Calcitonin

Calcitonin is a peptide hormone secreted by the C cells of the thyroid gland. Its main physiologic role is to protect against hypercalcemia, primarily by inhibiting bone resorption. It exerts this action by binding to high-affinity receptors on osteoclasts and markedly inhibiting osteoclastic activity. Treatment with calcitonin increases bone mass to a variable extent; the greatest increases are seen in women with the highest rates of bone turnover.[75] Calcitonin is available in the United States only in an injectable form. The usual dose is 50 to 100 U daily or every other day. It appears to have a direct anal-gesic effect in patients with acute fractures. About 10% to 20% of patients experience headache, nausea, and flushing. A calcitonin nasal spray has been developed and may be better tolerated than the injectable forms.

Vitamin D

The physiologic action of the biologically active form of vitamin D (1,25-dihydroxyvitamin D_3) is to increase the efficiency of intestinal calcium absorption. A clinical trial in 3200 elderly women evaluated the effect of 18 months of treatment with vitamin D, 20 µg (800 IU)/day. Vitamin D significantly decreased the incidence of new hip fractures by 43% and of nonvertebral fractures by 32%.[76] Lower doses of vitamin D have been studied in other clinical trials and have generally not been found to be effective. Because higher doses carry a risk of hypercalciuria and even hypercalcemia, this agent should be prescribed with caution.

Thiazide Diuretics

Because thiazide diuretics reduce the urinary excretion of calcium, they have been proposed as another modality to prevent osteoporosis. Two studies suggest that thiazides may indeed prevent osteoporotic fractures.[77,78] Lacroix and colleagues prospectively followed 9500 elderly men and women for 4 years and identified 242 cases of hip fracture.[77] After controlling for the greater body weight and lower incidence of tobacco use of thiazide users, they found the relative risk of hip fracture in thiazide users was significantly reduced to 0.68 (confidence interval: 0.49 to 0.94). Dose and duration of thiazide use were not analyzed. Felson and coworkers analyzed 176 cases of hip fracture and 672 age-matched controls from the Framingham study cohort.[78] High-dose thiazide use reduced the risk of hip fracture (relative risk: 0.31; confidence interval: 0.11 to 0.88) but past use had no effect. Surprisingly, low-dose thiazide use appeared to increase the risk of hip fracture (relative risk: 2.23; confidence interval: 1.26 to 3.94), which may be a spurious finding. Clearly, a clinical trial is necessary to define the optimal thiazide dose and minimum treatment duration that preserves bone mass and to determine how long any benefit persists after discontinuation of treatment. It should also be recognized that thiazides may have the potentially deleterious effects: increased plasma cholesterol, triglycerides, glucose and uric acid levels; decreased high-density lipoprotein levels; and potassium depletion, which may predispose to arrhythmias. If the efficacy of thiazide diuretics in preventing fractures is confirmed by clinical trials and this benefit outweighs the risks of thiazide use, thiazides may be particularly useful in the medical treatment of hypertensive postmenopausal women.

GENITAL ATROPHY

Pathogenesis

The tissues of the lower vagina, labia, urethra, and trigone derive from a common embryonic origin, the urogenital sinus, and are estrogen-dependent.[79] After the loss of estrogen at menopause, the vaginal walls become pale (because of diminished vascularity) and thin, typically only three or four cells thick. The vaginal epithelial cells contain less glycogen, which before menopause had been metabolized by lactobacilli to create an acidic pH, thereby protecting the vagina from bacterial overgrowth. Loss of this protective mechanism leaves the thin, friable tissue vulnerable to infection and ulceration. The vagina also loses its rugae and becomes shorter and inelastic.

Patients may complain of symptoms secondary to vaginal dryness, such as dyspareunia and vaginismus, which may compromise sexual satisfaction and lead to diminished libido. Women may also present with symptoms secondary to vaginal ulceration and infection such as vaginal discharge, burning, itching, or bleeding.

The urethra and urinary trigone undergo atrophic changes similar to that of the vagina. Dysuria, urgency, frequency, and suprapubic pain may occur in the absence of infection. Presumably, this occurs because the markedly thin urethral mucosa allows urine to come in close contact with sensory nerves. In addition, the menopausal loss of the resistance to urinary flow by thick, well-vascularized urethral mucosa has been hypothesized to contribute to urinary incontinence.[80]

Diagnosis

Atrophic vaginitis is usually diagnosed by its typical appearance. The presence of atrophy may be confirmed by a vaginal cell maturation index, obtained by scraping the lateral vaginal wall at the level of the cervix. The exfoliated cells may then be classified by degree of maturation, with a small proportion of superficial cells indicating a high degree of vaginal atrophy. If any atypical lesions are pre-sent, they should undergo biopsy to establish a diagnosis. If a discharge is present, it should be evaluated for pathogens such as *Candida*, *Neisseria gonorrhoeae*, *Chlamydia*, *Trichomonas*, and *Gardnerella*. If *Candida* species are found, the patient should be screened for diabetes because the low glycogen content of unestrogenized vaginal epithelial cells does not ordinarily support their growth.

Atrophic urethritis–trigonitis is diagnosed by ruling out the presence of infection. Urethroscopy is usually not necessary but would reveals a pale atrophic urethra.

Treatment

Estrogen is the most effective therapy, with the dose required generally being lower than that needed to treat hot flushes or osteoporosis. Thus, treatment of those conditions usually relieves genital atrophy. If atrophy is the only indication for estrogen treatment, daily use for a minimum of 2 to 12 weeks is needed to reverse the atrophic changes. Once atrophy is relieved, therapy may be tapered to two to three times per week. Usual daily oral doses are CEE, 0.3 or 0.625 mg; estrone, 0.3, 0.625, or 1.25 mg; or micronized estradiol, 1 or 2 mg.[81] Transdermal estradiol, 0.05 mg twice weekly, is also effective. Estrogens may also be administered vaginally, such as CEE, 0.3 mg, or micronized β-estradiol, 0.2 mg.[82,83] Although most of the estrogen acts locally, some of it is rapidly absorbed into the systemic circulation and could stimulate endometrial growth.[84] Thus, a progestin should generally be given intermittently with vaginal estrogens for patients with an intact uterus and repeated for as long as the patient has withdrawal bleeding.

If estrogens are contraindicated, synthetic mucopolysaccharides or water-soluble lubricants may relieve dyspareunia. Vaginal stenosis may be improved by the use of graduated vaginal dilators.

ATHEROSCLEROSIS

Cardiovascular disease (CVD) is the leading cause of death among women in industrialized countries: more than 50% of postmenopausal women succumb to CVD. Estrogens have been hypothesized to protect against atherosclerosis because the incidence of CVD is low before menopause. Premenopausal women have about a fifth the CVD mortality of men but after menopause, the incidence of CVD in women exponentially rises to approach that of men

(Fig. 17-13).[85] One explanation is that a premenopausal woman's estrogen confers protection, which is lost at menopause. This is supported by the observation that women who undergo a premature surgical menopause (ie, bilateral oophorectomy) and do not use estrogen replacement have twice the incidence of CVD than age-matched premenopausal controls. If they use estrogen replacement, however, their incidence of CVD is the same as premenopausal women of the same age. Premature natural menopause, in contrast, has not been found to increase CVD risk when controlled for age, smoking, and estrogen use.[86]

Epidemiologic Studies

Epidemiologic studies have compared the incidence of CVD among postmenopausal estrogen users and nonusers. Retrospective case–control studies provided inconsistent results, although most found estrogen use to be associated with less CVD.[87–89] Prospective cohort studies, which have fewer sources of bias, generally showed that estrogen use reduced CVD.[90–93] One notable exception is the Framingham study, which demonstrated an adverse effect or no effect of estrogen treatment, depending on how CVD was defined and which multiple regression model was used.[94,95] In contrast, the Nurses' Health study (the largest cohort study, following 48,000 postmenopausal women for up to 10 years) identified 405 cases of nonfatal myocardial infarction (MI) or fatal coronary heart disease.[96] The relative risk of coronary heart disease with estrogen use was significantly reduced to 0.89 (95% confidence interval: 0.78 to 1.0) for "ever" use (i.e. history of estrogen use in the past) and 0.56 (confidence interval: 0.40 to 0.80) for current use (i.e. estrogen use at the time of the last survey). Even women at low risk for CVD (nonsmokers without diabetes, hypertension, obesity, or hypercholesterolemia) had significantly less CVD if they used estrogens. Adjustment for numerous cardiovascular risk factors did not alter these findings, arguing against any major physician bias to prescribe estrogens to healthier women.

Additional evidence for the benefit of estrogens was provided by a prospective study of more than 8000 postmenopausal women living in a moderately affluent retirement community in Southern California.[97] More than 1400 women died during 7 years of observation. The investigators found that all-cause

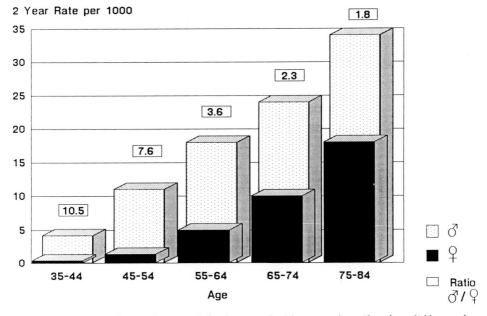

Figure 17–13. Incidence of myocardial infarctions (MI) by age and sex (female, *solid bar*; male, *stippled bar*): 26 years of follow-up, Framingham Study. Ratio of male to female MIs for each age group is noted at top of graph. (Adapted from Lerner DJ, Kannel WB: Patterns of coronary disease morbidity and mortality: a 26-year follow-up of the Framingham population. Am Heart J 111:383, 1986.)

mortality rates were 20% lower for those women who had ever taken postmenopausal estrogens compared with women who did not (relative risk of death: 0.80; confidence interval: 0.70 to 0.87). The greatest reductions in mortality were seen with current use and with long duration of use: current use for more than 15 years was associated with a 40% lower mortality. This reduction in mortality was *not* dependent on the dose of estrogen used: both high (ie, more than 1.25 mg daily) and low (ie, less than 0.625 mg daily) doses of oral CEE (the most common estrogen used) were associated with nearly equal reductions. This is an interesting observation because 0.625 mg and 1.25 mg of conjugated estrogens produce nearly equal increases in high-density lipoprotein (HDL) levels and decreases in low-density lipoprotein (LDL) levels.[98] Because few women in this cohort took progestins or parenteral estrogens, the effect of those hormones on mortality cannot be determined from this study.

Most of the reduced mortality in estrogen users observed in this study was because of fewer deaths from occlusive arteriosclerotic vascular disease.[97] Estrogen users were also found to have 20% less cancer mortality, observed for many malignancies including those of the breast (relative risk: 0.81). One possible explanation is that estrogen users may have greater health awareness or increased medical surveillance and therefore less extensive disease at the time of diagnosis. As expected, estrogen users had excess mortality from endometrial cancer (relative risk: 3.0).

Women who underwent menopause before age 45 years showed the greatest benefit from estrogen use. For women whose menopause occurred after age 54 years, estrogen treatment did not reduce mortality. Estrogen use also appeared to reduce mortality for women who smoke, have hypertension, or who had a history of angina or MI; their risk approached that of healthy women who did not use estrogen (Table 17-1). This is a significant finding because at one time, hypertension, tobacco use, and coronary disease were considered to be relative contraindications to estrogen replacement. This was based on the increased incidence of stroke and heart attack seen with high-dose oral contraceptives and with high-dose conjugated estrogens prescribed to men as secondary prevention of MI.[99] This does not appear to be a concern with the lower doses of estrogen prescribed for postmenopausal use.

The findings of these studies argue for offering estrogen replacement to nearly all postmenopausal women, particularly those who underwent menopause before age 45 years or have risk factors for CVD. The results further argue for continuous long-term treatment because increased duration of treatment is associated with further reductions in mortality. It should be remembered, however, that these studies are epidemiologic observations of estrogen users and nonusers and *not* clinical trials. Although investigators control for many potential confounding factors, the possibility exists that healthier women are more likely to seek and be prescribed estrogens. Definitive proof of the benefit of

Table 17–1

Relative Risks of All-Cause Mortalities by Selected Characteristics and History of Use of Estrogen Replacement Therapy[*]

	Use (Ever) of Estrogen Replacement Therapy	
	No	Yes
Elevated blood pressure		
No	1.00*	0.79†
Yes	1.54‡	1.15
Angina/MI history		
No	1.00*	0.81
Yes	1.62‡	1.02
Smoking		
Never	1.00*	0.74‡
Ever	1.28	1.05
Alcohol consumption		
No	1.00*	0.56‡
Yes	0.61‡	0.39‡
Quetelet's index (wt/ht² × 1000)		
35	1.14	0.92
≥35	1.00‡	0.72†
Exercise, h/d		
<0.5	1.00*	0.73‡
0.5–0.9	0.67‡	0.61‡
≥1.0	0.56‡	0.43‡
Age at last menstrual period		
<45	1.0*	0.71
45–54	0.81†	0.65‡
≥55	0.75*†	0.75†

(Data from Henderson et al.[97])

*Reference group.

†p<0.05.

‡p<0.001.

MI, myocardial infarction.

estrogen in reducing mortality would require a long-term, large-scale, placebo-controlled clinical trial.

Angiographic Studies

Evidence that women with pre-existing atherosclerosis may benefit from estrogen replacement was provided by Sullivan and colleagues.[100] These investigators had previously reported that estrogen users undergoing coronary catheterization are less likely to have coronary occlusion when compared with nonusers (relative risk: 0.44; confidence interval: 0.29 to 0.67).[101] In their most recent study, they retrospectively analyzed the all-cause mortality of women who had undergone catheterization over the preceding 10 years. Relatively few of their subjects were estrogen users, which was defined as estrogen use at the time of catheterization (5% of subjects) or estrogen use beginning sometime thereafter (another 5% of subjects). The adjusted 10-year survival of women with severe coronary stenosis who used estrogens was 97% but was only 60% for nonusers. For mild to moderate coronary stenosis, 10-year survival was 95% for users and 85% for nonusers. Although these findings suggest that women with coronary atherosclerosis may benefit from estrogen use, it should be recognized that this is a retrospective study with potential bias. The decreased mortality seen in estrogen users may have been partly a self-fulfilling prophecy because estrogen nonusers who lived the longest after catheterization had the greatest opportunity to begin estrogen treatment and to be classified as estrogen users.

Clinical Trials

The only clinical trials to reduce CVD by estrogen treatment have been performed in men. Early studies, enrolling men after MI, showed that estrogen treatment reduced serum cholesterol but not the incidence of a second event.[102,103] The Coronary Drug Project, consisting of 1101 MI survivors, was terminated when excess thrombotic events (particularly pulmonary emboli) occurred in the estrogen-treated group; CVD incidence was not reduced.[99] A similar observation was made in men with prostatic cancer treated with the estrogen (diethylstilbestrol), which increased CVD—possibly by causing excessive fluid accumulation, leading to congestive heart failure, or by increasing thromboembolism.[104] This adverse action of estrogen in men may have been the consequence of the highly potent estrogens used and may not reflect the action of physiologic levels of estrogen.

Mechanisms of Action of Estrogen

Because men and women have an equal incidence of CVD when matched for lipoprotein concentrations, the sex difference in CVD may be a consequence of the characteristic sex differences in serum lipoprotein concentrations.[105] Thus, premenopausal women appear to be protected against CVD by their typically lower LDL levels and higher HDL levels, compared with men of the same age (Fig. 17-14). Coincident with the loss of estrogen at menopause, however, female LDL levels rise to exceed those of men.[106] This loss of estrogen may directly cause this increase in LDL because estrogen replacement lowers LDL levels by 15% to 19% by increasing the clearance of LDL from the circulation (Fig. 17-15).[98] In contrast, HDL levels in women decline by only 5% at menopause.[106] Thus, the HDL-raising effect of oral estrogens (typically 16% to 18%) appears to be a pharmacologic action of the high portal estrogen concentrations presented to the liver after intestinal absorption.[98] Therefore, if endogenous estrogens protect against CVD, an effect on LDL rather than on HDL is the likely mechanism. In contrast, exogenous estrogens may protect by both raising HDL and lowering LDL.

An alternative explanation has been proposed for the sex difference in CVD because a semilogarithmic plot of female cardiovascular deaths against age shows that the rate of increase in the rate of CVD is constant throughout a woman's lifetime and is not accelerated after menopause. In comparison, male CVD shows a decline in the rate of increase after the onset of the "male climacteric," when testosterone levels wane (Fig. 17-16).[107] This decline in androgens may therefore be a major factor responsible for the lower female to male CVD ratio seen with increasing age. Androgens are known to adversely effect serum lipoproteins: both exogenous use (eg, testosterone enanthate and methyltestosterone) and endogenous increases in androgens (occurring during puberty) lower HDL levels.[108,109]

About half of the observed reduction in CVD of estrogen users (compared with nonusers) can be explained by higher HDL and lower LDL levels.[110] Thus, it is possible that estrogens may reduce CVD by means other than beneficial changes in lipoprotein levels. This is supported by the observation

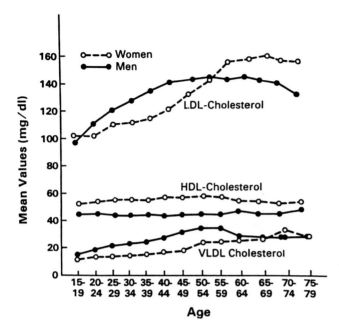

Figure 17–14. Trends by age and sex in lipoprotein cholesterol fractions, Framingham study. (Kannel WB: Risk factors for coronary disease in women. Perspective from the Framingham study. Am Heart J 114(2):413, 1987.)

that primates given an estrogen combined with norgestrel, an androgenic progestin, had substantially less atherosclerosis on autopsy compared with control animals, despite marked reductions in HDL levels induced by the norgestrel.[111] Multiple alter-

native mechanisms for the protective action of estradiol have been proposed; for example:

1. Estrogens may prevent the oxidation of LDL, to make it less atherogenic.

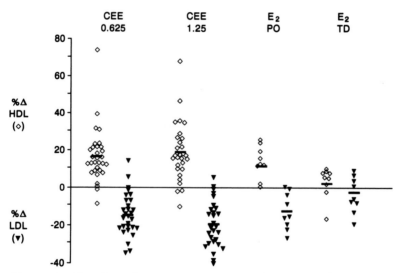

Figure 17–15. Effect of estrogen treatments on plasma LDL and HDL cholesterol concentrations. Each point represents the individual percentage change with estrogen as compared with placebo. The horizontal bar denotes the mean of the percentage changes. (From Walsh BW, Schiff I, Rosner B, Greenberg L, Ravnikar V, Sacks F: Effects of postmenopausal estrogen replacement on the concentrations and metabolism of plasma lipoproteins. N Engl J Med 325:1196, 1991.)

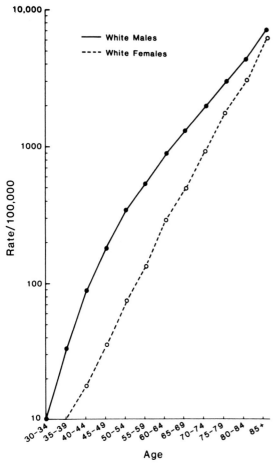

Figure 17–16. Age-specific mortality rates for ischemic heart disease by sex (whites only; United States, 1977). (Ross RK, Paganini-Hill A: Estrogen replacement therapy and coronary heart disease. Semin Reprod Endocrinol 1:19, 1983.)

2. Estrogen may alter prostaglandin metabolism, increasing prostacyclin levels and decreasing thromboxame levels; both of these actions promote vasodilation.[112]
3. Estrogens may act directly on vessel walls to induce vasodilation, which is biologically plausible because estrogen receptors have been located at multiple sites throughout the vascular system.[113,114]

Preliminary work has provided evidence for these hypotheses. The preponderance of evidence from epidemiologic studies indicates that estrogen use prevents the development of heart disease. There are, however, no long-term randomized studies of postmenopausal estrogen replacement to prove this beneficial effect of estrogen. Such a clinical trial is necessary to demonstrate conclusively that postmenopausal estrogen use reduces the incidence of CVD.

ESTROGENS

Pharmacology

Once the decision has been made to treat a postmenopausal woman with estrogen, the next issue is to decide how it should be prescribed. Many preparations are available: conjugated estrogens, synthetic estrogens, and micronized estradiol. All may be given orally or parenterally, continuously or cyclically. Because oral estrogens have been prescribed for more than 30 years, most of the demonstrated long-term benefits of estrogen are based on the experience with oral use. As time passes, the benefits of parenteral estrogens are becoming apparent. The most common estrogens taken orally are CEE, 0.625 mg; micronized β-estradiol, 1 mg; and piperazine estrone sulfate, 1.25 mg. At these doses, the mean peak serum estradiol level ranges from 30 to 40 pg/mL, similar to that of the premenopausal early follicular phase; the estrone level ranges from 150 to 250 pg/mL.[115] These doses are usually effective in relieving menopausal symptoms such as hot flushes and vaginal atrophy and in preventing osteoporosis. Generally, CEEs are twice as potent per unit weight compared with pure estrone preparations because up to 50% of CEE consists of the potent equine estrogens, equilin and 17 dihydroequilin sulfates, with the remainder being estrone sulfate.[116] These equine estrogens have a prolonged action, due partly to storage in and slow release from adipose tissue, and have been detected in the blood as long as 13 weeks after administration.[117]

Orally administered estradiol is rapidly converted in the intestinal mucosa to estrone. Oral estrogens are then presented to the liver, where 30% of an initial dose is conjugated with glucuronide on the first pass.[118] These conjugates undergo rapid renal and biliary excretion. The biliary conjugates are hydrolyzed by intestinal flora, allowing 80% to be reabsorbed and returned to the liver. They may then be reconjugated and excreted or may enter the systemic circulation. This enterohepatic circulation contributes to the prolonged effect of orally administered estrogens. Thus, patients with altered gut flora (eg, antibiotic therapy) may not sufficiently hydrolyze these conjugates, thereby preventing reabsorption; they may thus require higher doses for a therapeutic effect. Also, patients chronically maintained on phenytoin have enhanced glucuronidation and more rapidly excrete estrogens.[119] They too may require higher doses.

The concentration of estrogen in the portal circulation after oral ingestion is four to five times higher than that in the general circulation. Thus, hepatocytes are exposed to higher estrogen levels after oral estrogen administration than are cells of other organs. Estrogens given orally therefore have a more profound effect on hepatic metabolism than those given parenterally. Although many of these actions on the liver may potentially be deleterious, such as stimulating the production of renin-substrate and coagulation factors, some effects may be beneficial, such as increasing HDL production and increasing LDL catabolism.[98] Both of these effects on lipoproteins may reduce cardiovascular risk.

Synthetic estrogens are chemical derivatives of estradiol and are the estrogens used in oral contraceptives. Ethinyl estradiol (EE) results from the addition of a 17-ethinyl group, which impedes catabolism by the liver, leading to its long half-life of 48 hours. The other commonly used synthetic estrogen, mestranol, must undergo demethylation by the liver to become EE, its active form. Because this demethylation is only 50% complete, mestranol has only half the potency of EE.[120] These synthetic estrogens, when given orally, are more than 100 times as potent on a per-weight basis as natural estrogens in stimulating the production of hepatic proteins.[116] Because the minimum dose for therapeutic effect (eg, to reduce urinary calcium excretion [10 µg]) exceeds the lowest dose that markedly elevates hepatic globulins (5 µg), synthetic estrogens are not recommended for postmenopausal use.[121]

Parenteral estrogens may be given by vaginal, transdermal, or subcutaneous routes. Vaginal estrogens are absorbed and enter the systemic circulation, achieving a fourth of the circulatory level of an equal dose given orally.[122] They exert a potent local effect: 0.3 mg CEE given vaginally produces the same degree of epithelial maturation as 1.25 mg given orally.[82,123] The continued use of estrogen vaginally leads to increased circulatory levels due to enhanced transfer across a healthier, more vascularized epithelium.[118]

Twenty-five milligram subdermal estradiol pellets are effective but have variable life spans of 3 to 6 months and are difficult to remove. More convenient are transdermal skin patches applied twice weekly. They provide constant serum estrogen levels: the 0.05 mg patch produces a mean serum estradiol of 70 pg/mL and an estrone of 50 pg/mL, which is usually effective in relieving hot flushes and preventing bone loss.[27,124] Whether parenteral estrogens reduce the incidence of CVD has yet to be demonstrated.

Possible Side Effects

Estrogens may cause nausea, mastalgia, headache, and mood changes. More serious risks may be those that follow.

ENDOMETRIAL NEOPLASIA. Unopposed estrogen use (ie, without the addition of a progestin) may induce endometrial hyperplasia and ultimately, adenocarcinoma. Most of the carcinomas associated with estrogen use are of early stage and low grade and have not deeply invaded myometrium.[125] The adjusted 5-year survival is 94%, compared with 81% for estrogen nonusers,[126] possibly because of one or more of the following: (1) women prescribed estrogens are generally in better health than nonusers; (2) they are evaluated more frequently, allowing earlier diagnosis; or (3) only well-differentiated endometrial neoplasms retain estrogen receptors, by which exogenous estrogens can provide a stimulus.

Retrospective case–control studies find that unopposed estrogen use increases the risk of endometrial cancer two- to fourfold, thereby increasing the incidence from one in 1000 women (aged 50 to 74 years) per year to four in 1000 women per year. The increase in risk appears to be related to both the dose and duration (minimum, 1 to 2 years) of estrogen use (Fig. 17-17).[127] The relative risk of endometrial cancer is 1.2 with 0.625 mg conjugated estrogens daily and 3.8 with 1.25 mg daily.[128] This elevated risk persists for more than 6 years after discontinuation of therapy. Estrogen use increases equally the risk of both early (stages I and II) and extrauterine (stages III and IV) disease. Of interest is that women who used oral contraceptives for more than 12 months and later used unopposed postmenopausal estrogens did not have an increased risk of endometrial cancer. Thus, the risk of endometrial cancer associated with unopposed estrogen use is low for women using 0.625 mg CEE, particularly if they previously used oral contraceptives.[128]

Progestins can both prevent and reverse endometrial hyperplasia. Studd and coworkers, follow-

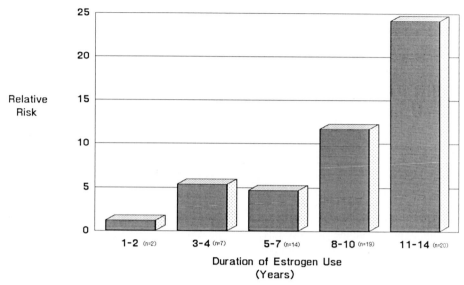

Figure 17–17.   Relative risk of endometrial cancer according to duration of postmenopausal estrogen use. (Adapted from Weiss NS, Szekely DR, English DR. et al: Endometrial cancer in relation to patterns of menopausal estrogen use. JAMA 242:261, 1979.)

ing 855 women using annual endometrial biopsies for up to 5 years, found an annual incidence of hyperplasia of 15% among women taking 1.25 mg of unopposed conjugated estrogen.[129] The addition of a progestin for 7 days per month reduced this incidence to 3%. Ten days per month of progestin treatment lowered the incidence to 2%; 13 days of treatment reduced this to essentially zero (Fig. 17-18). Based on this data, progestins are typically given for at least 13 days per month. Progestin treatment has also been successful in completely reversing established endometrial hyperplasia, as seen in 94%

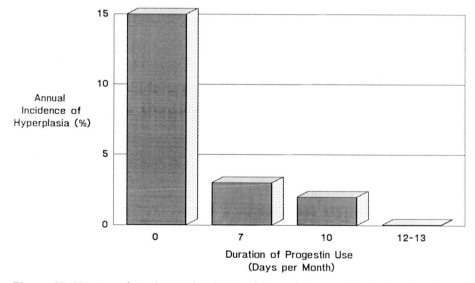

Figure 17–18.   Annual incidence of endometrial hyperplasia according to duration of progestin use per month. (Adapted from Studd JWW, Thorn MH, Patterson MEL, et al: The prevention and treatment of endometrial pathology. In Pasetto N, Paoletti R, Ambrus JL [eds]: The menopause and postmenopause, p 127. Lancaster, England, MTP Press, 1980.)

of 258 women treated with progestins.[130] Women who use estrogens combined with progestins have a significantly lower incidence of endometrial cancer (71 per 100,000) than do women who use estrogens alone (434 per 100,000) or no hormones (242 per 100,000).[131] Thus, women who use both estrogens and progestins are not considered to be at an increased risk of endometrial cancer.

Whitehead and associates provided biochemical and histologic evidence for the antihyperplastic effect of progestins on the endometrium.[132] They found that several progestins reverse the induction of estradiol and progesterone receptors produced by estrogen. In addition, progestins increase the activity of estradiol and isocitric dehydrogenases of the endometrium. The magnitude of these effects was more dependent on the duration of progestin therapy than on the dose. Specifically, 1 mg norethindrone (NET) appeared to be as effective as 10 mg; 150 μg of norgestrel was as effective as 500 μg.

OVARIAN NEOPLASIA. Estrogen replacement may possibly increase the risk of endometrioid cancer of the ovary, which comprises 10% to 20% of all ovarian malignancies; this has not been conclusively established.[133] It is not known whether progestin use reduces this risk, if it indeed exists.

BREAST NEOPLASIA. Whether postmenopausal estrogen use increases the risk of breast cancer has been actively debated. There is a suspicion, based on theoretic grounds, that estrogen use increases the risk of breast cancer because (1) breast cancer may be an estrogen-sensitive tumor, (2) estrogens may induce mammary tumors in rodents, and (3) women with prolonged endogenous estrogen exposure (eg, early menarche, late menopause, nulliparity) are at increased risk of breast malignancies. For this reason, more than 20 studies have been performed to resolve this issue. Nearly all found that postmenopausal estrogen replacement does not substantially increase the risk of developing breast cancer. The largest epidemiologic study consisted of 1960 cases of breast cancer with 2258 matched controls, identified through a breast-screening program with 280,000 participants.[134] The relative risk of breast cancer for all postmenopausal estrogen users (1.03) was not increased. There was a statistically significant increase in breast cancer risk with increasing duration of estrogen use: exposures of 10 to 14 years had a relative risk of 1.28; for more than 20 years, the relative risk was 1.47. This increase is of a small magnitude and averages 2% per year of estrogen use.

One study that has *not* found duration of estrogen treatment to increase the risk of breast cancer is the Nurses' Health study.[135] The investigators observed 722 cases of breast cancer in 23,000 postmenopausal women prospectively followed for up to 10 years. Past estrogen use, even for as long as 10 years, did not increase the risk of breast cancer but use within the preceding year modestly increased the risk of breast cancer (relative risk: 1.36; confidence interval: 1.11 to 1.67) in comparison with women who never used estrogens. This risk was not altered by the dose or duration of estrogen use. This elevated risk among estrogen users was confined to those women who regularly consumed alcohol; estrogen users who did not consume alcohol were *not* at increased risk. This raises the possibility that women who use postmenopausal estrogens may benefit from reducing their alcohol consumption. Of note is that estrogen users were more likely to have their cancer detected by mammography (41% versus 33%) and were 20% less likely to die from their cancer. Unfortunately, there were not enough progestin users to analyze the effect of this hormone on breast cancer risk. These results suggest that long-term past use of postmenopausal estrogens does not increase the risk of breast cancer but that current use may modestly increase this risk. For women taking estrogens, self-breast examination and mammography are especially important. Because death rates from CVD are more than four times that from endometrial and breast cancer combined, any adverse carcinogenic effect of estrogen would be outweighed by its reduction of CVD.

The possibility that the addition of a progestin may protect the breast as it does the endometrium has been suggested. Gambrell analyzed 69 cases of breast cancer and found 11 to be among combined estrogen and progestin users (incidence, 66.8 per 100,000 women-years) and 28 among estrogen-only users (incidence, 142 per 100,000 women-years), a difference that was *not* statistically significant ($p = 0.08$).[136] Thus, the benefit of progestins in preventing breast cancer remains unproved. Moreover, this hypothesis is contrary to the observation that the mitotic activity of the breast increases during the luteal phase (peak endometrial mitosis is during the follicular phase) and that progesterone induces mammary duct growth in rodents.[137,138] Because there is no good evidence that progestins reduce the risk of breast cancer but may adversely affect lipoproteins and thus increase cardiovascular mortality, the use of progestins in women without a uterus is unnecessary and possibly detrimental.

GALLBLADDER DISEASE. During the first year of use, estrogen treatment increases the risk of cholelithiasis by 20% (95% confidence interval: 0.7 to 2.1).[139] Cholelithiasis probably occurs because estrogens increase the hepatic excretion of LDL cholesterol and reduce the amount of chenodeoxy-cholic acid in bile, which keeps cholesterol in aqueous solution.[140,141]

THROMBOEMBOLIC DISEASE. Estrogen replacement increases the activity of the coagulation and fibrinolytic systems.[142] This may be clinically relevant only for women taking oral contraceptives, particularly those with the highest estrogen content, which are associated with increased risk of thromboembolic disease.[143] This appears to be a dose-response relation because the incidence of thromboembolic disease is not increased by estrogen replacement.[143]

HYPERTENSION. Estrogen replacement generally may modestly lower blood pressure in many women but occasionally may induce or exacerbate hypertension in others.[144,145] This idiosyncratic reaction to oral estrogens may be mediated by an increase in the hepatic production of renin substrate or by the production of an aberrant form.[146] Regardless, this elevation in blood pressure is usually reversible on discontinuation of estrogen.

GLUCOSE TOLERANCE. Although oral contraceptives are associated with impaired carbohydrate metabolism, the lower doses used for estrogen replacement have not been linked to impaired glucose tolerance.[147,148] Postmenopausal women with diabetes showed no change or an improvement of their disease with estrogen use, evidenced by lower glucose levels or reduced insulin requirements.[149] This is consistent with the observation that estrogen appears to increase the binding of insulin to its receptor.[150] Moreover, animal models show that estrogen improves experimentally-induced hyperglycemia.[151]

Contraindications

Absolute contraindications to postmenopausal estrogen replacement are:

1. Endometrial cancer, *unless* tumor was confined to uterus at time of diagnosis and there is no apparent recurrence for 2 years
2. Known or suspected breast cancer, unless benefits are believed to significantly outweigh the risks

3. Undiagnosed genital bleeding
4. Active liver disease
5. Active thromboembolic disease or a history of estrogen-related thromboembolic disease

Relative contraindications are:

1. Chronic liver dysfunction: the liver's ability to metabolize estrogen is impaired, leading to excessive levels of estrogen; this may be compensated by using smaller and less frequent doses
2. Poorly-controlled hypertension
3. History of thromboembolic disease: although postmenopausal estrogens have not been found to cause thrombosis, the possibility exists that they may do so in this group, which is at increased risk for having a second thrombotic event
4. Preexisting uterine leiomyomata or active endometriosis: estrogen use may prevent the involution of these conditions, which would be expected after menopause
5. Acute intermittent porphyria: estrogens may precipitate attacks

PROGESTOGENS

Progestins are primarily used to reduce the risk of endometrial stimulation induced by estrogen replacement. They may also be used to relieve hot flushes in patients who are not candidates for estrogen replacement.

Available Preparations

Progesterone and its derivatives may be absorbed by oral, vaginal, rectal, and intramuscular routes. Although convenient, oral absorption is highly variable, with a threefold difference between patients.[152] For this reason, variable clinical effects may be seen among patients given the same oral dose. After absorption, oral progestins are presented to the liver in high concentration, where they may alter the hepatic metabolism of serum lipoproteins. These progestins are then rapidly metabolized by the liver to deoxycorticosterone.[153]

Medroxyprogesterone acetate, 10 mg, is the most commonly used progestin in the United States and is effective against hyperplasia, with minor effects on serum lipids. For those patients unable to tolerate this dose, 5 mg may be used. The 5-mg dose in most cases offers similar protection against hyperplasia, except for the individual who poorly absorbs oral MPA.[154] Medroxyprogesterone acetate given intramuscularly in its depot form is well-absorbed but has a highly variable duration of effectiveness and frequently causes irregular vaginal bleeding. The usual dose is 50 to 150 mg intramuscularly every 1 to 3 months; the 50-mg dose is usually adequate to relieve hot flushes, whereas the 150-mg dose is as effective as 0.625 mg CEE in reducing urinary calcium excretion to premenopausal levels.[31,65] Megestrol acetate (MA), 40 to 80 mg daily, is also effective in suppressing hot flushes and reducing urinary calcium excretion to premenopausal levels. Micronized progesterone, 200 to 300 mg, is also active against hyperplasia without significantly altering serum lipids.[155]

19-Nortestosterone derivatives are the potent progestins used in oral contraceptives and have partial androgenic properties, with an adverse action on serum lipids. Norethindrone (norethisterone) was initially used in doses of 2.5 to 5 mg but 1 mg (as is used in low-dose oral contraceptives) is equally effective against hyperplasia but has a lesser impact on lipids. D,L Norgestrel, known for its more potent androgenic properties, was similarly used in 0.5 mg doses but it appears that 0.15 mg is equally effective.[132] Because only the L-isomer is biologically active, 0.15 mg of D,L norgestrel is equivalent to 0.075 mg levonorgestrel. In the near future, less androgenic 19-nortestosterone–derived progestins used in Europe will become available in the United States: desogestrel, norgestimate, and gestodene.

Adverse Effects

Progestins may produce abdominal bloating, mastalgia, headaches, mood changes, and acne. More importantly, all progestins, particularly the 19-nortestosterone derivatives (eg, norgestrel and NET) negatively affect serum lipids, especially by lowering HDL levels. Medroxyprogesterone acetate, 10 mg, was found by two studies to reduce HDL by 9% and 16%—differences that could not be shown to be statistically significant given the small number of patients studied (8 and 11, respectively).[156,157] Norgestrel, 500 µg (equivalent to 250 µg levonorgestrel), decreases HDL by 17% to 20% and NET, 10 mg, lowers HDL by 20% to 36%.[156,158,159] These particular doses of norgestrel and NET may be higher than necessary because 150 µg of norgestrel and 1 mg of NET are equally effective against hyperplasia.[132] The effect of these lower doses on lipids is unknown.

The net effect of a hormonal regimen on lipids depends on the particular estrogen and progestin used as well as the dose, route, and frequency of administration. Generally, progestins may negate wholly or partially the beneficial effect of estrogen on HDL and LDL. This may compromise the possible reduction in CVD observed with estrogen replacement. Moreover, the protective effect of progestins against breast cancer is unproved. Therefore, the use of progestins may be justified only for those women with an intact uterus for whom prevention of endometrial cancer is needed.

TREATMENT REGIMENS

Before initiating hormonal therapy, the patient should be evaluated by a history and physical examination, including blood pressure, breast and pelvic examination, stool guaiac, and Pap smear. Mammography should be performed (and repeated yearly) to prevent prescribing estrogens to a patient with pre-existing subclinical cancer of the breast. Serum cholesterol should be measured at least once every 5 years, provided it remains below 200 mg/dL. If serum cholesterol exceeds 200 mg/dL, follow-up should be arranged as outlined in Tables 17-2 and 17-3. An endometrial biopsy should be performed before treatment if there is a history of abnormal vaginal bleeding or if the patient is at increased risk of having a preexisting endometrial hyperplasia. The endometrium should be sampled if a patient bleeds at any time other than during the expected interval between days 11 to 20 of the cycle or if the bleeding is heavy. This may be accomplished by endometrial aspiration or, if adequate tissue cannot be obtained, by fractional dilation and curettage. Patients receiving unopposed estrogens for an extended time should undergo biopsy before therapy is instituted and yearly thereafter, regardless of bleeding, because the annual incidence of hyperplasia is 30%.[160]

The most commonly used schedule of hormone replacement in the United States for women with intact uteri is cyclic, using CEE, 0.625 mg given daily, and MPA, 10 mg given for the first 13 calendar days of each month. On this regimen, many patients experience withdrawal bleeding, typically between the 9th and 20th days of the month. For those patients who have previously undergone hysterectomy, no progestin is needed.

The schedule may be modified by substituting another estrogen for CEE or another progestin for MPA. Appropriate doses of other oral estrogens would be 1 mg of micronized β-estradiol and 1.25

Table 17–2

Initial Classification and Recommended Follow-up Based on Total Cholesterol in Adults without CHD*

Cholesterol (mg/dL)	Classification	Follow-up
< 200	Desirable	Repeat within 5 years**
200 to 239	Borderline-high	With fewer than two CHD risk factors: repeat in 1–2 years
		With two CHD: do lipoprotein analysis (see Table 17-3)
≥ 240	High	Do lipoprotein analysis (see Table 17-3)

*CHD, coronary heart disease; LDL, low-density lipoprotein, HDL, high-density lipoprotein.

**Do lipoprotein analysis if HDL <35 mg/dL.

Risk factors: male gender, postmenopausal female not taking estrogen, family history of premature coronary disease, cigarette use, hypertension, diabetes mellitus, HDL cholesterol, <35 mg/dL.

(From Report of the National Cholesterol Education Program Expert Panel Detection, Evaluation, and Treatment of High Blood Cholesterol Adults. JAMA 1993;269(3): 3015.)

Table 17–3

Classification and Treatment Decisions Based on LDL-Cholesterol*

Classification (mg/dL)	Initiation Level (mg/dL)**	Minimal Goal (mg/dL)
Dietary Treatment		
Without CHD and with fewer than two risk factors	≥ 160	< 160
Without CHD and with two risk factors	≥ 130	< 130
With CHD	> 100	≤ 100
Drug Treatment		
Without CHD and with fewer than two risk factors	≥ 190	< 160
Without CHD and with two risk factors	≥ 160	< 130
With CHD	≥ 130	≤ 100

*LDL, low-density lipoprotein; CHD, coronary heart disease.

**In men under 35 years of age and premenopausal women with LDL levels between 190–219 mg/dL, drug therapy should be delayed except in high-risk patients such as those with diabetes.

(From the Report of the National Cholesterol Education Program Expert Panel on Detection, Evaluation, and Treatment of High Blood Cholesterol in Adults. JAMA 1993;269(3):3015.)

mg of piperazine estrone sulfate. Parenteral estrogens such as transdermal estradiol are particularly useful for those women whom one desires to bypass the hepatic effects of oral estrogens, such as those with a prior history of hepatic dysfunction, thrombosis, or hypertension. The typical starting dose of transdermal estradiol is 0.05 mg applied twice weekly. After one month's time, many patients do not demonstrate an adequate clinical response to this dose and need to be increased to 0.10 mg; rarely is it necessary to use a dose higher than 0.10 mg.

To avoid withdrawal bleeding, continuous rather than cyclic treatment may be used.[161] Conjugated equine estrogens, 0.625 or 1.25 mg as needed to control symptoms, are given continuously with NET, 0.35 mg. The dose of NET is serially increased by 0.35 mg until all bleeding is abolished, up to a limit of 2.1 mg. Most patients initially have irregular vaginal bleeding. Many women discontinue treatment since the incidence of bleeding after 6 months is as great as 40%. Higher doses of NET are required to induce amenorrhea if 1.25 mg CEE is used. These higher doses of NET are associated with abdominal bloating and mastalgia, which may cause the patient to discontinue therapy. The effect of this regimen on serum lipids is unknown. NET, 0.35 mg, is available in the United States only as Micronor (Ortho Pharmaceutical, Raritan, N.J.) a progestin-only oral contraceptive. Medroxyprogesterone acetate, 2.5 to 5 mg, may substitute for NET in this schedule. If a patient develops vaginal bleeding after being amenorrheic on this regimen, an endometrial biopsy should be performed: two women with irregular bleeding out of a group of 41 women treated with continuous estrogen and progestin were found to have endometrial adenocarcinoma.[162]

Transvaginal-ultrasound monitoring has been used to screen postmenopausal women for endometrial pathology. This technique uses a high-frequency ultrasound transducer placed in the vagina, where it is in close anatomic proximity to the uterus, providing high-resolution imaging. This method is superior to transabdominal scanning because it overcomes difficulties in scanning women who are obese, have excessive bowel gas, or inadequate bladder filling because of discomfort or incontinence.[163] This allows measurement of endometrial thickness, which has been found to be accurate within 1 mm of actual thickness seen by pathology examination.[164] Two large series evaluated postmenopausal vaginal bleeding by transvaginal ultrasound before diagnostic dilation and curettage in 205 and 215 women, respectively.[165,166] The endometrium of women with endometrial can-

cer had a mean thickness of 18 + 16 mm; for women with endometrial atrophy, 3 + 1 mm. Both studies found no cases of endometrial cancer in women with endometrial thickness of less than 9 mm. Because 70% of women with postmenopausal vaginal bleeding have endometrium less than 5 mm thick, a substantial number of dilation and curettage procedures can be avoided.

CONCLUSIONS

Estrogen replacement offers significant benefits to many postmenopausal women, particularly those whose menopause occurred before age 45 years. Women at high risk for atherosclerosis or who already have CVD may also benefit from estrogen use. The increased risk of endometrial and breast cancer occurring with estrogen replacement appears to be small in comparison with its protective effect against CVD. The benefits and risks as they pertain to each individual patient should be reviewed with her in detail. She must ultimately decide whether to initiate therapy and give her informed consent.

REFERENCES

1. McKinlay S, Jeffreys M, Thompson B: An investigation of the age of menopause. J Biosoc Sci 4:161, 1972
2. Amundsen DW, Diers CJ: The age of menopause in classical Greece and Rome. Hum Biol 42:79, 1970
3. Schiff I, Wilson E: Clinical aspects of aging of the female reproductive system. In Schneider EL (ed): The aging reproductive system, p 9. New York, Raven Press, 1978
4. Sherman BW, West JH, Korenman SG: The menopausal transition: analysis of LH, FSH, estradiol, and progesterone concentrations during menstrual cycles of older women. J Clin Endocrinol Metab 42:629, 1976
5. Grodin JM, Siiteri PK, MacDonald PC: Source of estrogen production in postmenopausal women. J Clin Endocrinol Metab 36:207, 1973
6. Erlik Y, Meldrum DR, Judd HL: Estrogen levels in postmenopausal women with hot flushes. Obstet Gynecol 59:403, 1982
7. Vermeulen A: The hormonal activity of the postmenopausal ovary. J Clin Endocrinol Metab 42:247, 1976
8. Thompson B, Hart SA, Durno D: Menopausal age and symptomatology in general practice. J Biosoc Sci 5:71, 1973
9. Chang RJ, Judd HL: Elevation of skin temperature of the finger as an objective index of postmenopausal hot flushes: standardization of the techniques. Am J Obstet Gynecol 135:713, 1979

10. Mashchak CA, Kletsky OA, Artal R: The relation of physiological changes to subjective symptoms in postmenopausal women with and without hot flushes. Maturitas 6:301, 1985

11. Erlik Y, Tataryn IV, Meldrum DR, et al: Association of waking episodes with menopausal hot flushes. JAMA 245:1741, 1981

12. Yen SSC: The biology of menopause. J Reprod Med 18:28, 1977

13. Frodin T, Alund G, Varenhurst E: Measurement of skin blood-flow to assess hot flushes after orchiectomy. Prostate 7:203, 1985

14. Huggins C, Stevens RE, Hodges CU: Studies of prostatic cancer. II. The effects of castration in advanced carcinoma of the prostate. Arch Surg 43: 209, 1941

15. DeFazio J, Meldrum DR, Winer JH, et al: Direct action of androgen on hot flashes in the human male. Maturitas 6:8, 1984

16. Davidson BJ, Gambone JC, Lagasse LD: Free estradiol in postmenopausal women with and without endometrial cancer. J Clin Endocrinol Metab 52:404, 1981

17. D'Amico JF, Greendale GA, Lu JK, Judd HL: Induction of hypothalamic opioid activity with transdermal estradiol administration in postmenopausal women. Fertil Steril 55:754, 1991

18. Berkow R (ed): The Merck manual of diagnosis and therapy, p 2472. Rahway, NJ, Merck Sharp & Dohme Research Laboratories, 1987

19. Beattie CW, Rodgers CH, Soyka LF: Influence of ovariectomy and ovarian steroids on hypothalamic tyrosine hydroxylase activity in the rat. Endocrinology 91:276, 1972

20. Luine VN, McEwen BS: Effect of estradiol on turnover of type A monamine oxidase in brain. J Neurochem 28:1221, 1977

21. Paul SM, Axelrod J, Saadvedra JM, et al: Estrogen-induced efflux of endogenous catecholamines from the hypothalamus in vitro. Brain Res 178:499, 1979

22. Nixon RL, Jamowsky DS, David JM: Effects of progesterone, estradiol, and testosterone on the uptake and metabolism of ^{3}H-norepinephrine, ^{3}H-dopamine, and ^{3}H-serotonin in rat synaptosomes. Res Commun Chem Pathol Pharmacol 7:233, 1974

23. Johnson AE, Nock B, McEwen B, et al: Estradiol modulation of noradrenergic receptors in the guinea pig brain assessed by tritium-sensitive film autoradiography. Brain Res 336:153, 1985

24. Clayden JR, Bell JW, Pollard P: Menopausal flushing: double-blind trial of a nonhormonal medication. Br Med J 1:409, 1974

25. Hammond MG, Hatley L, Talbert LM: A double-blind study to evaluate the effect of methyldopa on menopausal vasomotor flushes. J Clin Endocrinol Metab 58:1158, 1984

26. Jones KP, Ravnikar VA, Schiff I: Effect of lofexidine on vasomotor flushes. Maturitas 7:135, 1985

27. Haas S, Walsh B, Evans S, et al: The effect of transdermal estradiol on hormone and metabolic dynamics over a six-week period. Obstet Gynecol 71:671, 1988

28. Schiff I, Regestein Q, Tulchinsky D, et al: Effects of estrogens on sleep and psychological state of hypogonadal women. JAMA 242:2405, 1979

29. Campbell S, Whitehead M: Estrogen therapy and the postmenopausal syndrome. Clin Obstet Gynecol 4:31, 1977

30. Steingold KA, Laufer L, Chetkowski RJ, et al: Treatment of hot flushes with transdermal estradiol. J Clin Endocrinol Metab 61:627, 1985

31. Morrison JC, Martin DC, Blair RA, et al: The use of medroxyprogesterone acetate for the relief of climacteric symptoms. Am J Obstet Gynecol 138: 99, 1980

32. Schiff I, Tulchinsky D, Cramer D, et al: Oral medroxyprogesterone acetate in the treatment of postmenopausal symptoms. JAMA 244:1443, 1980

33. Albrecht BH, Schiff I, Tulchinsky D, et al: Objective evidence that placebo and oral medroxyprogesterone acetate therapy diminish menopausal vasomotor flushes. Am J Obstet Gynecol 139:631, 1981

34. Laufer LK, Erlik Y, Meldrum DR, et al: Effect of clonidine on hot flashes in postmenopausal women. Obstet Gynecol 60:483, 1982

35. Lebherz TB, French LT: Nonhormonal treatment of the menopausal syndrome. A double-blind evaluation of an autonomic system stabilizer. Obstet Gynecol 33:795, 1969

36. Komm BS, Terpening CM, Benz DJ, et al: Estrogen binding, receptor mRNA, and biologic response in osteoblast-like osteosarcoma cells. Science 241:81, 1988

37. Lindsay R, Sweeney A: Urinary cyclic AMP in osteoporosis Scott Med J 21:231, 1976

38. Hillyard CJ, Stevenson JC, MacIntyre I: Relative deficiency of plasma calcitonin in normal women. Lancet 1:961:1978

39. Deftos LJ, Weisman MH, Williams G, et al: Influence of age and sex on plasma calcitonin in human beings. N Engl J Med 302:1351, 1980

40. Stevenson JC, Abeyasekera G, Hillyard CJ, et al: Calcitonin and the calcium-regulating hormones in postmenopausal women: effect of estrogens. Lancet 1:693, 1981

41. Heanly RP: Estrogens and postmenopausal osteoporosis. Clin Obstet Gynecol 19:791, 1976

42. Horsman A, Simpson M, Kirby PA: Nonlinear bone loss in oophorectomized women. Br J Radiol 50:504, 1977

43. Smith DM, Nance WE, Kang KW: Genetic factors in determining bone mass. J Clin Invest 52:2800, 1973

44. Dalen N, Hallberg D, Lamke B: Bone mass in obese subjects. Acta Med Scand 197:353, 1975

45. Daniell HW: Osteoporosis and the slender smoker. Arch Intern Med 136:298, 1976

46. Aloia JF, Cohn SH, Ostuni JA, et al: Prevention of involutional bone loss by exercise. Ann Intern Med 89:356, 1978

47. Matkovic V, Kostial K, Simonovic I, et al: Bone status and fracture rates in two regions of Yugoslavia. Am J Clin Nutr 32:540, 1979

48. Licata AA, Bou E, Bartter FC, West F: Acute effects of dietary protein on calcium metabolism in patients with osteoporosis. J Gerontol 36:14, 1981

49. Alffam PH: An epidemiologic study of cervical and intertrochanteric fractures of the femur in suburban population. Acta Orthop Scand 65:1, 1964

50. Iskrant AP: The etiology of fractured hips in females. Am J Public Health 58:485, 1968
51. Gordon G, Vaughan C: Clinical management of the osteoporoses. Acton, MA, Publishing Sciences Group, 1976
52. Lindsay R, Dempster DW, Clemens T, et al: Incidence, cost and risk factors of fracture of the proximal femur in the USA. In Christiansen C, et al (eds): Osteoporosis, p 311. Denmark, Aalborg Stoftsbogturkkeri, 1984
53. Gallagher JC, Nordin BE: In: van Keep PA, Lavritzen C, eds. Aging and estrogens. Basel, Karger WI FR946F v. 2 Oestrogens and calcium metabolism. 2:98, 1973
54. Slemenda CW, Hui SL, Longcoe C, Welman H, Johnston CC: Predictors of bone mass in perimenopausal women: a prospective study of clinical data using photon absorptiometry. Ann Intern Med 112:96, 1990
55. Dequeker JV, Johnston CC (eds): Noninvasive bone measurements. Oxford, IRL Press, 1981
56. Cann CE, Genant HK, Ettinger B: Spinal mineral loss in oophorectomized women. Determination by quantitative computer tomography. JAMA 244:2056, 1980
57. Kelly TL, Slovik DM, Schoenfeld DA, et al: Quantitative digital radiography vs dual photon absorptiometry of the lumbar spine. J Clin Endocrinol Metab 67(4):839, 1988
58. Christiansen C, Riis BJ, Rodbro P: Prediction of rapid bone loss in postmenopausal women. Lancet 1:1105, 1987
59. Christiansen C, Christiansen MS, Transbol I: Bone mass in postmenopausal women after withdrawal of estrogen/gestagen replacement therapy. Lancet 1:459, 1981
60. Lobo RA, Brenner PF, Mishell DR: Metabolic parameters and steroid levels in postmenopausal women receiving lower doses of natural estrogen replacement. Obstet Gynecol 62:94, 1983
61. Weiss NS, Ure CL, Ballard JH, et al: Decreased risk of fractures of the hip and lower forearm with postmenopausal use of estrogen. N Engl J Med 303:1195, 1980
62. Lindsay R, Hart DM, Aitken JM, et al: Long-term prevention of postmenopausal osteoporosis by estrogens. Lancet 1:1038, 1976
63. Lindsay R, Hart DM, Purdie D, et al: Comparative effects of estrogen and a progestagen on bone loss in postmenopausal women. Clin Sci Mol Med 54:193, 1978
64. Mandel FP, Davidson BJ, Erlik Y, et al: Effect of progestins on bone metabolism in postmenopausal women. J Reprod Med 27(Suppl 8):511, 1982
65. Lobo RA, McCormack W, Singer F, et al: Depomedroxyprogesterone acetate compared with conjugated estrogens for the treatment of postmenopausal women. Obstet Gynecol 63:1, 1984
66. Manolagas SC, Anderson DG: Detection of high-affinity glucocorticoid binding in rat bone. J Endocrinol 76:379, 1978
67. Riis B, Thomsen K, Christiansen C: Does calcium supplementation prevent postmenopausal bone loss? N Engl J Med 316:173, 1987
68. Dawson-Hughes B, Dalial GE, Karll EA, Sadowski L, Sahyoun N, Tannenbaum S: A controlled trial of the effect of calcium supplementation on bone density in postmenopausal women. N Engl J Med 323:878, 1990
69. Ettinger B, Cann L, Genant K: Menopausal bone loss: effects of conjugated estrogen and/or high calcium diet. Maturitas 6:108, 1984
70. Baran D, Sorensen A, Grimes J, et al: Dietary modification with dairy products for preventing vertebral bone loss in premenopausal women: a three year prospective study. J Clin Endocrinol Metab 70:264, 1990
71. Briancon D, Meunier PJ: Treatment of osteoporosis with fluoride, calcium, and vitamin D. Orthop Clin North Am 12:629, 1981
72. Riggs BL, Hodgson SF, O'Fallon WM, et al: Effect of fluoride treatment on the fracture rate in postmenopausal women with osteoporosis. N Engl J Med 322:802, 1990
73. Watts NB, Harris ST, Genant HK, et al: Intermittent cyclical etidronate treatment of postmenopausal osteoporosis. N Engl J Med 323:73, 1990
74. Storm T, Thamsborg G, Steiniche T, Genant HK, Sorensen OH: Effect of intermittent cyclical etidronate therapy on bone mass and fracture rate in women with postmenopausal osteoporosis. N Engl J Med 322:1265, 1990
75. Civitelli R, Gonnelli S, Zacchei F, et al: Bone turnover in postmenopausal osteoporosis. Effect of calcitonin treatment. J Clin Invest 82:1268, 1988
76. Chapuy MC, Arlot ME, Duboeuf F, et al: Vitamin D_3 and calcium to prevent hip fractures in elderly women. N Engl J Med 327:1637, 1992
77. Lacroix AZ, Wienpahl J, Wallace RB, et al: Thiazide diuretic agents and the incidence of hip fracture. N Engl J Med 322:286, 1990
78. Felson DT, Sloutskis D, Anderson JJ, Anthony JM, Kiel DP: Thiazide diuretics and the risk of hip fracture: results from the Framingham study. JAMA 165:370, 1991
79. Iosif CS, Batra S, Ek A, Astedt B: Estrogen receptors in the human female lower urinary tract. Am J Obstet Gynecol 141:817, 1981
80. Zinner NN, Sterling AM, Ritter RC: Role of urethral softness in urinary incontinence. Urology 16:115, 1980
81. Carr BR, MacDonald PC: Estrogen treatment of postmenopausal women. Adv Intern Med 28:491, 1983
82. Mandel FP, Geola FL, Meldrum DR, et al: Biologic effects of various doses of vaginally administered conjugated equine estrogens in postmenopausal women. J Clin Endocrinol Metab 57:133, 1983
83. Gordon WE, Hermann HW, Hunter DC: Safety and efficiency of micronized estradiol vaginal cream. South Med J 72:1252, 1979
84. Schiff I, Tulchinsky D, Ryan KJ: Vaginal absorption of estrone and 17 β-estradiol. Fertil Steril 28:1963, 1977
85. Lerner DJ, Kannel WB: Patterns of coronary disease morbidity and mortality: a 26-year follow-up of the Framingham population. Am Heart J 111(2):383, 1986

86. Coldnitz GA, Willett WC, Stampfer MJ, et al: Menopause and the risk of coronary heart disease in women. N Engl J Med 316:1105, 1987

87. Pfeffer RI, Whipple GH, Kurosaki TT, et al: Coronary risk and estrogen use in postmenopausal women. Epidemiology 107:479, 1978

88. Ross RK, Paganini-Hill A, Mack TM, et al: Menopausal estrogen therapy and protection from death from ischemic heart disease. Lancet 1:858, 1981

89. Bain C, Willett WC, Hennekins CH, et al: Use of postmenopausal hormones and risk of myocardial infarction. Circulation 64:42, 1981

90. Hammond CB, Jelousek FR, Leck L, et al: Effects of long term estrogen replacement therapy. Am J Obstet Gynecol 133:525, 1979

91. Bush TL, Cavan LD, Barrett-Connor E: Estrogen use and all-cause mortality. JAMA 249:903, 1983

92. Burch JC, Byrd, BF, Vaughn WK: The effects of long-term estrogen on hysterectomized women. Am J Obstet Gynecol 118:778, 1974

93. Petitti DB, Wingerd J, Pellegrin F, et al: Risk of vascular disease in women: smoking, oral contraceptives, noncontraceptive estrogens and other factors. JAMA 242:1150, 1979

94. Wilson PWF, Garrison RJ, Castelli WP: Postmenopausal estrogen use, cigarette smoking, and cardiovascular morbidity in women over 50. N Engl J Med 313:1038, 1985

95. Eaker ED, Castelli WP: Coronary heart disease and its risk factors among women in the Framingham study. In Eaker E, ed. Coronary heart disease in women. New York, Haymarket Doyma, 1987

96. Stampfer MJ, Colditz GA, Willett WC, et al: Postmenopausal estrogen therapy and cardiovascular disease: ten-year follow-up from the Nurses' Health Study. N Engl J Med 325:756, 1991

97. Henderson BE, Paganini-Hill A, Ross RK: Decreased mortality in users of estrogen replacement therapy. Arch Intern Med 151:75, 1991

98. Walsh BW, Schiff I, Rosner B, Greenberg L, Ravnikar V, Sacks F: Effects of postmenopausal estrogen replacement on the concentrations and metabolism of plasma lipoproteins. N Engl J Med 325:1196, 1991

99. The Coronary Drug Project Research Group: Findings leading to discontinuation of the 2.5 mg/day estrogen group. JAMA 226:652, 1973

100. Sullivan JM, Vander Zwagg R, Hughes FP, et al: Estrogen replacement and coronary artery disease. Arch Intern Med 150:2557, 1990

101. Sullivan JM, Vander Zwagg R, Lemp GF, et al: Postmenopausal estrogen use and coronary atherosclerosis. Ann Intern Med 108:358, 1988

102. Stamler J, Katz LN, Pick R, et al: Effects of long-term estrogen therapy on serum cholesterol-lipid-lipoprotein levels and mortality in middle aged men with previous myocardial infarction. Circulation 22:658, 1980

103. Oliver MF, Boyd GS: Influence of reduction of serum lipids on prognosis of coronary heart disease: a five year study using estrogen. Lancet 2:499, 1961

104. DeVogt HJ, Smith PH, Davone-Macaluso M, et al: Cardiovascular side effects of diethylstilbestrol, cyproterone acetate, and medroxyprogesterone acetate used for treatment of prostatic cancer. J Urol 135:303, 1986

105. Gordon T, Castelli WP, Hjortland MC, et al: High density lipoprotein as a protective factor against coronary heart disease. Am J Med 62:707, 1977

106. Matthews KA, Meilahn E, Kuller LH, Kelsey SF, Caggiula AW, Wing RR: Menopause and risk factors for coronary heart disease. N Engl J Med 321:641, 1989

107. Heller RF, Jacobs HS: Coronary heart disease in relation to age, sex, and the menopause. Br Med J 1:472, 1978

108. Bagatell CJ, Knopp RH, Vale WW, Rivier JE, Bremner WJ: Physiologic testosterone levels in normal men suppress high-density lipoprotein cholesterol levels. Ann Intern Med 116:(12 pt 1):967, 1992

109. Kirkland RT, Keenan BS, Probstfield JL, et al: Decrease in plasma high-density lipoprotein cholesterol levels at puberty in boys with delayed adolescence: correlation with plasma testosterone levels. JAMA 257:502, 1987

110. Bush TL, Barrett-Connor E, Cowan LD, et al: Cardiovascular mortality and non-contraceptive estrogen use in women: results from the Lipid Research Clinic's Program Follow-Up Study. Circulation 75:1002, 1987

111. Adams MR, Clarkson TB, Koritnik DR, Nash HA: Contraceptive steroids and coronary artery atherosclerosis in cynomolgus macaques. Fertil Steril 47(6):1010, 1987

112. Steinleitner A, Stanczyk FZ, Levin JH, et al: Decreased in vitro production of 6-keto-prostaglandin by uterine arteries from postmenopausal women. Am J Obstet Gynecol 161:1677, 1989

113. Harder DR, Coulson PB: Estrogen receptors and effects of estrogen on membrane electrical properties of coronary vascular smooth muscle. J Cell Physiol 100:375, 1979

114. McGill HC: Sex steroid hormone receptors in the cardiovascular system. Postgrad Med April 64, 1989

115. Lobo RA, Mishell Dr, Budoff PW, et al: Estrogen replacement therapy. In Symposium Proceedings, p 9. San Francisco, Abbott Pharmaceuticals. May 9–10, 1984

116. Mashchak CA, Lobo RA, Dozono-Takano R, et al: Comparison of pharmacodynamic properties of various estrogen formulations. Am J Obstet Gynecol 144:511, 1982

117. Whittaker PG, Morgan MR, Dean PD: Serum equilin, estrone, and estradiol levels in postmenopausal women receiving conjugated equine estrogens. Lancet 1:14, 1980

118. Siddle N, Whitehead M: Flexible prescribing of estrogens. Contemp Ob-Gyn 22:137, 1983

119. Englund DE, Johansson EDB: Plasma levels of oestrone, oestradiol, and gonadotropins in postmenopausal women after oral and vaginal administration of conjugated equine estrogens. Br J Obstet Gynaecol 85:957, 1978

120. Schwartz U, Hammerstein J: The estrogenic potency of ethinyl estradiol and mestranol—a comparative study. J Acta Endocrinol 72:118, 1973

121. Mandel FP, Geola FL, La JK, et al: Biologic effects of various doses of ethinyl estradiol in postmenopausal women. Obstet Gynecol 59:673, 1982

122. Deutsch S, Ossowski B, Benjamin I: Comparison between degree of systemic description of vaginally and orally administered estrogens at different dose levels in postmenopausal women. Am J Obstet Gynecol 139:967, 1981

123. Geola FL, Fumar AM, Tataryn IV, et al: Biological effects of various doses of conjugated equine estrogens in postmenopausal women. J Clin Endocrinol Metab 51:620, 1980

124. Stevenson JC, Cust MP, Gangar KF, Hillard TC, Lees B, Whitehead MI: Effects of transdermal versus oral hormone replacement therapy on bone density in spine and proximal femur in postmenopausal women. Lancet 336:256, 1990

125. Chu J, Schweid AI, Weiss NS: Survival among women with endometrial cancer: a comparison of estrogen users and nonusers. Am J Obstet Gynecol 143:569, 1982

126. Elwood JM, Boyes DA: Clinical and pathologic features and survival of endometrial cancer patients in relation to prior use of estrogens. Gynecol Oncol 10:173, 1980

127. Weiss NS, Szekely DR, English DR, et al: Endometrial cancer in relation to patterns of menopausal estrogen use. JAMA 242:261, 1979

128. Rubin GL, Peterson HB, Lee NC, Maes EF, Wingo PA, Becker S: Estrogen replacement therapy and the risk of endometrial cancer: remaining controversies. Am J Obstet Gynecol 162:148, 1990

129. Studd JWW, Thorn MH, Patterson MEL, et al: The prevention and treatment of endometrial pathology. In Pasetto N, Paoletti R, Ambrus JL (eds): The menopause and postmenopause, p 127. Lancaster, England, MTP Press, 1980

130. Gambrell RD, Massey FW, Castaneda TA: The use of the progestagen challenge test to reduce the risk of endometrial cancer. Obstet Gynecol 55:732, 1980

131. Gambrell RD: Clinical use of progestins in the menopausal patient. J Reprod Med 27:531, 1982

132. Whitehead MI, Townsend PT, Pryse-Davies J, et al: Effects of estrogens and progestins on the biochemistry and morphology of the postmenopausal endometrium. N Engl J Med 305:1599, 1981

133. Weiss NS, Lyon JL, Krishnamurthy S, et al: Noncontraceptive estrogen use and the occurrence of ovarian cancer. Journal of the National Cancer Institute 68:95, 1982

134. Brinton LA, Hoover R, Fraymeni JF: Menopausal oestrogens and breast cancer risk: an expanded case-control study. Br J Cancer 54:825, 1986

135. Colditz GA, Stampfer MJ, Willett WC, Hennekens CH, Rosner B, Speizer FE: Prospective study of estrogen replacement therapy and risk of breast cancer in postmenopausal women. JAMA 264:2648, 1990

136. Gambrell RD: Role of progestins in the prevention of breast cancer. Maturitas 8:1569, 1986

137. Anderson JJ, Ferguson DJP, Raab GM: Cell turnover in the "resting" human breast: influence of parity, contraceptive pill, age, and laterality. Br J Cancer 46:376, 1982

138. Dulbecco R, Henahan M, Armstrong B: Cell types and morphogenesis in the mammary gland. Proc Natl Acad Sci USA 79:7346, 1982

139. Kakar F, Weiss NS, Strite SA: Noncontraceptive estrogen use and risk of gallstone disease in women. Am J Public Health 78(5):564, 1988

140. Bennion LJ: Changes in bile lipids accompanying oophorectomy in premenopausal women. N Engl J Med 297:709, 1977

141. Heuman R, Larsson-Cohn U, Hammar M, et al: Effects of postmenopausal ethinyl estradiol treatment on gallbladder bile. Maturitas 2:69, 1979

142. Caine YG, Bauer KA, Barzegar S, et al: Coagulation activation following estrogen administration to postmenopausal women. Thromb Haemost 68(4): 392, 1992

143. Stampfer MJ, Goldhaber SZ, Manson JE, et al: A prospective study of exogenous hormones and risk of pulmonary embolism in women (Abstract 2689). Circulation 86(4):1, 1992

144. Mashchak CA, Lobo RA: Estrogen replacement therapy and hypertension. J Reprod Med 30 (Suppl):805, 1985

145. Crane MG, Harris JJ, Windsor W: Hypertension, oral contraceptive agents, and conjugated estrogens. Ann Intern Med 74:13, 1971

146. Shionoiri H, Eggena P, Barrett JD, et al: An increase in high-molecular weight renin substrate associated with estrogenic hypertension. Biochem Med 29:14, 1983

147. Spellacy WN: Carbohydrate metabolism in male infertility and female fertility-control patients. Fertil Steril 27:1132, 1976

148. Spellacy WN, Butri WC, Birk SA: Effect of estrogen treatment for one year on carbohydrate and lipid metabolism in women with normal and abnormal glucose tolerance test results. Am J Obstet Gynecol 131:87, 1978

149. Cantilo E: Successful responses in diabetes mellitus of the menopause provided by the antagonistic action of sex hormones on pituitary activity. Endocrinology 28:20, 1941

150. Ballejo G, Saleem TH, Khan-Dawood FS, et al: The effect of sex steroids on insulin-binding by target tissues in the rat. Contraception 28:413, 1983

151. Paik SG, Michelis MA, Kim YT, et al: Induction of insulin-dependent diabetes by streptozotocin: inhibition by estrogens, potentiation by androgens. Diabetes 31:724, 1982

152. Whitehead MI, Townsend PT, Gill DK, et al: Absorption and metabolism of oral progesterone. Br Med J (Clin Res) 280:825, 1980

153. Ottoson U-B, Carlstrom K, Dambes J-E, et al: Conversion of oral progesterone into deoxycorticosterone during postmenopausal replacement therapy. Acta Obstet Gynecol Scand 63:577, 1984

154. Gibbons WE, Lobo RA, Moyer DU, et al: A comparison of biochemical and morphological events mediated by estrogen and progestin on the endometrium of postmenopausal women. Am J Obstet Gynecol 154:456, 1986

155. Whitehead MI, Siddle N, Lane G, et al: The pharmacology of progestogens. In Mishell DR (ed): Menopause, physiology and pharmacology, p 326. Chicago, Year Book Medical Publishers, 1987

156. Silfverstolpe G, Gustafson A, Samsoie G, et al:

Lipid metabolic studies in oophorectomized women: effect on serum lipids and lipoproteins of three synthetic progestagens. Maturitas 4:103, 1982

157. Tikkanen MJ, Nikkila EA, Kuusi T, et al: Different effects of two progestins on HDL. Atherosclerosis 40:365, 1981

158. Hirvonen E, Malkonen M, Manninen V: Effects of different progestins. N Engl J Med 304:560, 1981

159. Ottosson UB, Johansson BG, Von Schoultz B: Subfractions of high-density lipoprotein cholesterol: a comparison between progestagens and natural progesterone. Am J Obstet Gynecol 151:746, 1985

160. Schiff I, Sela HK, Cramer D, et al: Endometrial hyperplasia in women on cyclic or continuous estrogen regimens. Fertil Steril 37:79, 1982

161. Magos AL, Brincat M, Studd JWW, et al: Amenorrhea and endometrial atrophy with continuous oral estrogen and progestin therapy in postmenopausal women. Obstet Gynecol 65:496, 1985

162. Leather AT, Savvas M, Studd JW: Endometrial histology and bleeding patterns after 8 years of continuous combined estrogen and progestogen therapy in postmenopausal women. Obstet Gynecol 78(6):1008, 1991

163. Mendelson EB, Bohm-Velez M, Joseph N, Neiman HL: Endometrial abnormalities: evaluation with transvaginal sonography. Am J Roentgenol 150(1):139, 1988

164. Nasri MN, Coast GJ: Correlation of ultrasound findings and endometrial histopathology in postmenopausal women. Br J Obstet Gynaecol 96 (11):1333, 1989

165. Grandberg S, Wikland M, Karlsson B, Norstrom A, Friberg LG: Endometrial thickness as measured by endovaginal ultrasonography for identifying endometrial abnormality. Am J Obstet Gynecol 164(1 pt 1):47, 1991

166. Klug PW, Leitner G: Comparisons of vaginal ultrasound and histologic findings of the endometrium. Geburtshilfe Frauenheilkd 49(9):797, 1989

167. Expert Panal: Summary of the second report of the National Cholesterol Education Program expert panel on detection, evaluation, and treatment of high blood cholesterol in adults. JAMA 269(23):3015, 1993

Ambulatory Gynecology, Second Edition,
edited by David H. Nichols and Patrick J. Sweeney.
J. B. Lippincott Company, Philadelphia, © 1995.

18

Geriatric Gynecology

David H. Nichols and May Wakamatsu

Women in the United States live a third of their lives after menopause. Many women in their sixth and seventh decade are busy with careers, recreational activities, and travel. They not only expect but are beginning to demand a better quality of life.

The number of women older than 65 years in the United States, estimated at 20 million in 1970, will grow to 65 million by the year 2030. Life expectancy at birth in a developed nation in the year 2000 is estimated to be 80 years, with maximum life expectancy remaining at 95 years. There have been no significant or relevant changes in the human body and its architecture in the past thousands of years but massive changes in the environment in which we live have taken place, permitting this increased lifespan. Thus, continuation, preservation, or reestablishment of quality of life are becoming significant issues in the delivery of health care. Matters pertaining to the quality of life in the aging female are truly international in scope, and failure to provide remedial help—or even more important, to have prevented the need for it—permits the development of an enormous burden of cost to be borne

by the public. Failure to provide this relief in a cost-effective manner not only deprives womankind of welcome relief but also often fills hospitals and nursing-home facilities with patients who have been ostracized by society and to whom their longevity becomes not a blessing but a nightmare.

The population distribution, gradually favoring the elderly, provides a larger number of older persons for whom to care. This change in demographics is taking place coincident with the climate of cutting health costs. The challenge lies in providing a better but cost-effective quality of life for the mature woman.

COST-EFFECTIVENESS AND QUALITY OF LIFE

To decrease health costs, many surgical procedures are performed on an outpatient basis and in-hospital procedures are accompanied by a required shortened length of stay, making it even more challenging to care for the elderly. Many elderly live alone and when discharged from the hospital have no one to help them during their postoperative convalescence. Visiting-nurse services can help to facilitate the nursing aspects of home care but even these resources are limited in terms of time and money.

PREVENTIVE HEALTH CARE

Cost-effective changes that are taking place to improve quality of life include instituting preventative health care measures. A regular routine of health screening tests, such as mammography, is becoming standard. More women are starting hormone-replacement therapy when they become menopausal, which decreases the degree of osteoporosis and consequently, the number of women suffering from hip fracture and myocardial infarctions later in their lives. As more attention is directed toward women's health problems, more women are being counseled to live healthier life-styles, specifically by following cholesterol-lowering diets and increasing daily exercise. Both measures also help to decrease the incidence of fractures and heart disease.

If started in childhood, a balanced diet (including an abundance of fresh fruits and vegetables, fiber, and naturally occurring vitamins, supplemented with calcium and vitamin D) may lead to a lifetime of healthful nutritional habits. High-quality prenatal care and careful and improved management during labor, delivery, and the postpartum phase reduces the incidence of obstetric damage to the pelvic soft tissues, preventing some of the problems in pelvic support that otherwise require reconstruction later in life. Timely episiotomy, properly repaired for the patient older than 25 years or the patient with impaired elastic tissues, minimizes soft-tissue obstetric damage.[1]

Some gynecologic problems not discussed in other chapters that are more prevalent among elderly women but certainly not specific to them must be considered.

PROBLEMS

Besides the health problems that arise simply from aging, women undergo additional life changes of menopause. With the onset of menopause, the endogenous supply of estrogen essentially becomes insignificant. Estrogen lack contributes to relatively rapid changes in women's physiology and anatomy, which then become manifest as clinical problems.

In the Roman Empire, the average life expectancy of a woman was 23 years; by the turn of the century in the United States, it was only 40 years. During this century, however, a woman's life expectancy has doubled, and a 50-year-old woman has the potential of reaching 80 years or more. Despite the increase in lifespan, the average age of the menopause has remained 51.4 years. Thus, a woman can expect to live a third of her life in a postmenopausal, estrogen-deprived environment.[2]

Genital Atrophy

Atrophy of the genitourinary tract epithelium is a common problem faced by all women to some degree. Without estrogen, the vulvar and vaginal epithelium become thin and glands become inactive, leading to increased sensitivity and dryness. For those women who are sexually active, dyspareunia may significantly decrease the quality of life. This symptom may not be volunteered by the patient and usually requires direct inquiry from the health care provider.

Diagnosis of atrophy can usually be made easily, given the appropriate clinical setting and examination. The vulvar and vaginal epithelium appear thinned and whitened, with loss of labial folds and loss of vaginal rugae. A watery, blood-tinged vaginal discharge may be noticed. In severe cases of atrophy, vaginal agglutination may be present. Any suspicion of neoplastic change can be ruled out by cytologic screening, colposcopy when the former is abnormal, and if morphologically suspicious, the performance of a colposcopically directed biopsy establishes the diagnosis.

The treatment of choice for atrophy is replacement of estrogen. This can be accomplished with oral hormone-replacement therapy if the patient is an appropriate candidate, with vaginal estrogen cream, or both. Some patients on oral hormone-replacement therapy may still complain of the symptoms of atrophy and may benefit from vaginal estrogen applications in addition to oral therapy. A usual dose to ameliorate vaginal atrophy symptoms is estrogen vaginal cream, 1 g at bedtime once a week. This dose has been shown to have insignificant systemic effects, so concomitant therapy with a systemic progesterone agent is not necessary. Lubricating agents may relieve some of the dryness symptoms for patients in whom estrogen therapy is contraindicated (ie, breast or uterine cancer patients).

Genital Prolapse

The pelvic floor, which supports the uterus, bladder, and rectum, is often weakened by childbirth, repetitive stresses, trauma, and age. Weaknesses are occasionally of congenital origin, and a positive family origin and a positive family history may often be elicited. Because the genitourinary structures are estrogen-dependent tissues, prolapse that was previously mild may become symptomatic or severe when women become postmenopausal. The three most common structures to prolapse are the uterus, bladder, and rectum, respectively labeled uterine prolapse, cystocele, and rectocele. These conditions commonly occur together because the events resulting in the pelvic-floor relaxation generally affect the supports of all three organs. Degrees of prolapse vary from mild and asymptomatic, which may only be noted by the examiner, to severe or procidentia, in which the entire vagina protrudes.

Signs and Symptoms

In patients with mild to moderate prolapse, symptoms range from none to complaints of mild low backache, dyspareunia, pelvic "heaviness," and a "feeling that things are falling out." These symptoms may worsen during late afternoon or evening after the patient has been on her feet all day and may regress when the patient is recumbent and the contributing effects of gravity are reduced. With more advanced prolapse, patients may complain of severe pelvic pain, disabling low back pain, difficulty walking, dyspareunia or apareunia, and notice a "bulge" coming from the vagina. Bladder prolapse (cystocele) may cause a feeling of inability to empty completely (causing the patient to void frequently) or precipitate frequent urinary tract infections, secondary to abnormally high postvoid residual urine volume with stasis. Hypermobility of the urethra (urethrocele) often accompanies the cystocele, resulting in coincident stress urinary incontinence. Rectocele, even when severe, may be entirely asymptomatic but complaints of difficulty evacuating the rectum and occasionally needing to "splint" the rectum by placing fingers in the vagina to help evacuation may be elicited.

Diagnosis

PHYSICAL EXAMINATION. Diagnosis of prolapse is made by examination in the office. If one is suspicious of cystocele, the patient should not empty her bladder, as is usually routine before being examined. In the dorsal lithotomy position, before any examining maneuver is performed, any structure that is prolapsing in this resting position should be noted and manually replaced. Before any instrument is placed into the vagina, the patient is asked to "bear down" or perform Valsalva's maneuver and again, any prolapsing structures and the order in which they appear should be noted. Initial appearances of cystocele and rectocele indicate primary damage to the lower supporting tissues, whereas the appearance of cervix or vaginal vault first indicates primary damage to the upper suspensory tissues. Occasionally, a cystocele or rectocele may occlude the entire vaginal opening and determination of the type of prolapse is impossible until a disassembled speculum is used, using the posterior speculum blade to alternately retract the anterior then posterior vaginal walls, so that the opposite wall can be seen in its entirety. When the anterior vaginal wall is retracted in this manner, usually uterine or vault prolapse can be observed, especially if the patient bears down as by Valsalva's maneuver. With one finger in the vagina, after the speculum has been removed, the patient is asked to voluntarily contract her pubococcygeal muscles and the external anal sphincter. The strengths and symmetry are observed and noted.

It is helpful to examine the patient who has prolapse when she is standing because this is the position in which the patient performs most of her daily activities, adding the pull of gravity to the prolapse. Occasionally, a prolapse that does not seem significant to the examiner when the patient is supine becomes obviously significant when the patient is examined standing and straining. This is most easily accomplished by having the patient stand facing the examiner, with one foot on a low stool or step at the foot of the examination table (Fig. 18-1). The patient can steady herself by placing a hand on the examining table. Most patients are cooperative and have no objection to this examination.

Nonsurgical Treatment

Treatment of genital prolapse should really begin with its prevention by including careful obstetric care and delivery; education about activities such

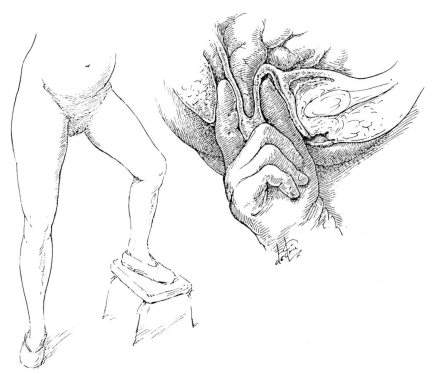

Figure 18–1.   Examination of the patient in a standing position permits the thumb in the vagina to note and replace any descent of the vaginal vault, whereas the index finger introduced into the rectum permits evaluation of any possible rectocele. When the patient strains, any enterocele present is evidenced by palpation of a bowel-filled sac prolapse dissecting the rectovaginal septum. (Reproduced with permission of Cine-Med, Inc. from Nichols DH: Repair of enterocele and prolapse of the vaginal vault. In Barber H (ed): Goldsmith's Practice of Surgery, Philadelphia, JB Lippincott, 1981.)

as heavy lifting, which may put the patient at risk for prolapse; teaching pelvic floor–strengthening exercises (Kegel) before prolapse occurs; and starting hormone replacement therapy (if not inappropriate) when postmenopausal.

If the prolapse and symptoms are mild, pelvic floor–strengthening exercises may be therapeutic. It is important to emphasize to the patient that quantity and quality of the exercises is crucial to success. It is helpful to check the patient in the office to make certain that she is using the correct muscles. Those patients who mistakenly contract their abdominal or gluteal muscles must be carefully instructed as to how to voluntarily contract the pubococcygei muscles. The patient is instructed to do a series of 15 Kegel contractions six times a day, holding each contraction for 3 to 5 seconds. In postmenopausal patients, oral or vaginal estrogen therapy should be started to combat the inevitable atrophy of the support structures.

If moderate prolapse is present with coincident urinary and rectal symptoms, therapy by qualified physical therapists with special training in the treatment of problems of the pelvic floor may be helpful. Biofeedback mechanisms can be used to help patients learn the correct muscles to use in pelvic floor exercises and to increase the strength of these muscles. Intermittent intravaginal electrostimulation may help to strengthen the pelvic floor muscles and has been shown to help stress urinary incontinence as well as bladder instability problems in many patients.

In many cases of moderate or severe prolapse, if exercises, physical therapy, and estrogen therapy do not resolve symptoms sufficiently, either a pessary or surgery is necessary. A pessary may be effective in providing temporary support of a prolapsed uterus, bladder, or rectum but is not a good long-term solution. Often, the vaginal wall gradually stretches until the largest pessary available can no longer be retained within the vagina and for many patients, surgery may be the best solution. (For a full discussion of the use of pessaries, please see Chapter 20).

FUNCTIONAL GYNECOLOGIC DISORDERS OF THE ELDERLY

Because the genitourinary organs are estrogen-dependent and subject to the aging process, functional disorders of the bladder and the anorectal complex increase in postmenopausal older women. These types of problems, particularly those relating to incontinence, have been overlooked in the past and their prevalence underestimated because of the social stigmata attached. Patients have been reluctant to initiate discussion of these problems, even with health care providers with whom they already have an established relationship and feel comfortable. Fecal or flatulence incontinence has been overlooked even more than urinary incontinence. Studies show, however, that of women with urinary incontinence, 30% have concomitant fecal or flatulence incontinence. It is important that health care providers specifically inquire about voiding and bowel function problems. Studies show that 30% to 60% of community-living women have problems with incontinence. The wide range is probably a function of the definition of incontinence that was used and the type of community sampled. In institutionalized patients, as many as 90% of older patients may have incontinence problems. Urinary or fecal incontinence may seriously detract from a patient's quality of life. Patients are often embarrassed about "accidents" or worried about having one, so go out socially only if toilet facilities are readily available or sometimes never go out because they do not want to take a chance. Previously active, healthy, social people may become reclusive, isolated from friends and family. Among the institutionalized patients in the United States, it is estimated that 100,000 women at any one time have long-term indwelling catheters. Long-term indwelling catheters invite complications, which include urinary tract infection, bacteremia, stones, and death from infection. It is evident that that the monetary cost and quality-of-life cost of incontinence is enormous in the United States alone—estimated in 1983 as more than $8 billion per year.[3,4]

Eighty-one percent of women older than 60 are sexually active; 65% at age 70 and older. This percentage drops to a quarter or less after the age of 75 because of failing health or a situation in which her partner has died. For the sexually active, frequency tends to decline with passing years. Although there are wide variations in behavior, someone who made love about twice a week during the first years of marriage may drop to twice a month after age 65. Desire may outlast sexual activity; a Duke University study found that half of seniors in their 80s and 90s are still interested in having sex. Interest and activity levels in previous years strongly predict sexual life after age 60 years. Those who could take it or leave it early in life are more apt to call it quits, whereas folks who relished erotic activity during youth and mid-life are more likely to have a sexually exciting old age.[5]

For women, sexual interest may be heightened by the drop in estrogen production that accompanies menopause. Libido increase as naturally produced testosterone, previously overshadowed by estrogen, becomes the older woman's dominant sex hormone. This effect is canceled out by hormone-replacement therapy, which maintains the premenopausal status quo. Generally, it takes longer for older women to achieve physical excitement. The vagina lubricates more slowly in preparation for intercourse; it is also smaller and less elastic. About one in three sexually active women older than 65 years finds intercourse painful and many use lubricants or estrogen creams to avoid discomfort. When these normal but potentially disturbing changes begin, some couples abandon their sex lives rather than considering how they might adapt—which may mean how to vary their techniques of making love or by seeking outside advice and counseling. Research indicates that in most cases, the man stops initiating relations and the woman acquiesces. A regression may evolve from no intercourse to no hugging, kissing, or cuddling, to not sleeping in the same bed, to not sleeping in the same room. This premature end to sexual relationships could be avoided if couples knew more about sexual aging and were willing to be flexible.[5] The male tendency to reach orgasm more slowly is well suited to the longer time a woman requires to become aroused. There are no more birth control hassles, children are no longer likely to burst into the bedroom at inopportune moments, and both have a lot more time than they used to. Elderly women fully retain their capacity for multiple orgasms and older men can have an orgasm without obtaining an erection. Participation may be hindered by ill health and coincident medical disease such as diabetes and arthritis, discomfort from the latter being minimized by taking pain medication before coitus and experimenting to find positions of maximum comfort. Medications may present unexpected difficulties—antihypertensive drugs may suppress libido, and antidepressants and tranquilizers may decrease desire and inhibit orgasm.[5]

OSTEOPOROSIS AND CARDIOVASCULAR DISEASE

Although osteoporosis and cardiovascular disease are not gynecologic problems per se, these two medical problems become significant health problems for postmenopausal women as they age. Preventing disease should be the goal of the primary-care physician in the ambulatory setting, so a patient's risk for osteoporosis and cardiovascular disease should be assessed.

It is well established that estrogen deficiency results in symptomatic osteoporosis in about 20% of women. Annually, 1.5 million fractures in the United States are associated with osteoporosis; 250,000 of those fractures are hip fractures. The 1-year case–fatality rate for persons with hip fracture is 15% to 20% and for those who survive, many cannot live independently after hip fracture.[6]

Before the sixth decade, the incidence of myocardial infarction in men is three times greater than in women. By age 65, the incidence of myocardial infarction in men and women is equal.[7] Estrogen-replacement therapy decreases both the risk of symptomatic osteoporosis and the risk of myocardial infarction in postmenopausal women. In the context of a patient's other gynecologic problems associated with aging, such as prolapse and incontinence, when discussing hormone replacement therapy, risk factors for osteoporosis and cardiovascular disease must also be considered.

SURGICAL CONSIDERATIONS FOR THE GERIATRIC PATIENT

General Considerations

Surgical morbidity and mortality are higher in the elderly group when emergency surgery is compared with elective surgery, a phenomenon conferred by associated diseases rather than old age itself.[8-10] Elderly people are not at an increased risk if they have no chronic illnesses.[11] Therefore, when a surgically correctable pelvic disorder that subtracts significantly from the quality of life has been identified, it is far safer that it be approached as a well worked-up, carefully evaluated elective procedure (providing time for identification, analysis, and correction of all risk factors) than as an emergency procedure when the depth of such an evaluation is precluded. Physical status rather than age is the more important factor in determining mortality.[11] Although patients of any age are at a greater risk of morbidity and mortality when they undergo an emergency procedure, elderly patients are particularly at risk, presumably because of their diminished physiologic reserve.[8,11-13] Procedures performed on an emergency basis in the elderly are associated with three to four times the mortality when performed as elective procedures.[12]

Several studies in both this country and abroad show that postoperative stay is not prolonged for the elderly but because more extensive evaluation before surgery is often necessary, their preoperative hospitalization may be prolonged. Although structural and functional changes in each organ system associated with aging may not affect basal function, they often adversely affect the capacity of the organ system to respond to *stress* and thus reduce the margin of error.[18]

Although healthy elderly individuals may exhibit normal cardiovascular function at rest, age-related changes in the cardiovascular system lead to a diminished cardiovascular reserve and response to stress, reflected by changes in cardiac output, vascular resistance, baroreceptor reactivity, and the response of the sympathetic nervous system.[14] The decreased elasticity and increased thickness of the major blood vessel walls rather than age-related alterations in the receptors themselves provide the most likely explanation for the depressed baroreceptor response in the aged population.[14] The elderly are less able to improve oxygen delivery to their tissues during periods of hypoxemia by increasing their heart rate and cardiac output. Tachycardia, one of the early clinical signs of hypoxia, may be absent in the elderly. Although all of these factors diminish cardiovascular reserve and the intraoperative margin of error, with meticulous management, age per se should not be a contraindication for surgery.[14] Similarly, kidney and pulmonary reserve of the elderly under stress may be compromised.

Pierson and associates studied coincident disease in women older than 75 years undergoing gynecologic surgery and compared them with a control group of patients younger than 55 years of age.[15] The incidence of major medical problems was 76% in the elderly group and 28% in the control group. Most common problems in the elderly group were hypertension (52%), arteriosclerotic heart disease (38%), and diabetes (20%). In the control group, the most common problem was varicose veins. Operative risk rises in proportion to the number and severity of the medical problems. The risk of surgery may not be justified if the patient's medical status is associated with a more dismal prognosis than the underlying surgical problem itself.[14,16,17] With the recent focus on women's health, more women are interested and motivated to live a healthier life.

Indications

For patients beyond the age of 65 years, the principal indications for major gynecologic surgery are:[18]

1. Postmenopausal bleeding
2. Prolapse of the uterus with cystocele and rectocele
3. Adnexal mass
4. Primary or recurrent urinary stress incontinence
5. Post hysterectomy prolapse of the vaginal vault
6. Carcinoma of the endometrium
7. Carcinoma of the ovary
8. Carcinoma of the vulva

Preoperative and Postoperative Evaluation of the Surgical Patient

Testing

Preoperative laboratory work should be carefully arranged in anticipation of hospitalization, so that abnormalities can be studied and corrected if necessary. A preoperative electrocardiogram should be routine in every patient older than the age of 40 years.

If the patient has a history of urinary incontinence that is significant, requiring the use of sanitary protection, or if urinary incontinence has appeared after replacement of the prolapsed vaginal vault manually or by a pessary, a competent urodynamic assessment should be considered (see Chap. 19). The routine use of intravenous pyelography is not cost-effective and it is generally employed only if the patient has had previous pelvic major surgery performed by another surgeon. The arithmetic of the expense of routine intravenous pyelography is astonishing. In the United States,

there are about 700,000 hysterectomies performed per year. If each patient were to have a preoperative intravenous pyelogram, for which a charge of $200 would be made, the cost ($200 × 700,000) would be $140 million. Of these 700,000, one out of every 40,000 develops a severe reaction to the contrast dye and 20 per year die of the reaction. If each patient who had a preoperative intravenous pyelogram would get a postoperative test as well to check on "silent" injury, the expense to the public would be another $140 million for a total of $280 million per year and 20 deaths. Clinically indicated intravenous pyelography to evaluate costovertebral backache, hematuria, or the effects of previous pelvic surgery should be performed as necessary preoperatively but there seems to be little place for routine prehysterectomy intravenous pyelography.

Preoperative Considerations

Generally, the vaginal route for surgery is far less stressful on the patient than is the abdominal because the duration of surgery is shorter, the depth of anesthesia is not so great, and the patient usually can be given a conduction anesthetic, which is less likely to disturb her blood pressure. Ileus and intestinal obstruction occur less frequently because there is less handling of the bowel, and postoperative atelectasis is reduced because of easier respiratory excursions in the absence of abdominal incisional pain.

Of the invasive gynecologic malignancies in the patients older than 65 years of age, 70% of the patients with carcinoma of the vulva are in this age group, with 40% having adenocarcinoma of the endometrium, 35% having carcinoma of the ovary, and 25% having carcinoma of the cervix.

Infection may be particularly troublesome in the elderly because it is more difficult to recognize. The hyperthermal response of infection may be less than in the younger patient. Older patients generally experience less pain, which contributes to the paucity of localizing symptoms. Leukocytosis is less prevalent than in younger patients.

A study of 795 patients 90 years of age and older undergoing surgery at the Mayo Clinic demonstrated immediate higher morbidity and mortality after *emergency* procedure but *overall* excellent survival at the end of 2 and 5 years, comparable with the rate expected.[19] A preoperative and therefore pre-existing central nervous system deficit was the most powerful predictor of poor outcome and survival in the elderly, in contrast to cardiac and respiratory diseases, which had little impact on short-term morbidity or mortality.[19,20] The nervous system in the elderly, subject to blood supply inadequacy, decreased hemostatic reserve, and specific disease, cannot adapt well to acute stress or sudden change. Good antiseptic and surgical techniques are obligatory because nosocomial infections are more likely, especially with the use of urinary catheters and intravenous drainage tubes. The kidney in the elderly has a greater tendency to fail. Once renal shutdown occurs, reversion to normal function is difficult. Postoperative urinary output requires assiduous monitoring. One must watch for symptoms of adult respiratory distress syndrome if marked shock has occurred. Myocardial infarction may produce few of the usual symptoms, especially in patients who are obese. The only early signs may be tachycardia, falling blood pressure, pulmonary edema, arrhythmia, premature contractions, auricular fibrillation, and congestive heart failure. Consultation with a cardiologist and appropriate use of cardiac monitoring are essential components of this necessary vigilance for the older surgical patient.[21]

The gynecologic surgeon quickly learns that biologic age is more important than chronologic age. Essential to good medical care for the elderly is an understanding of chronic medical diseases, preventive measures, remedial therapy, and social influences of prolonged illness.[18] Infection is the principal cause of postoperative morbidity and mortality, despite current use of prophylactic antibiotic therapy.[18]

When considering surgery as a solution to the patient's needs, one must adhere to the following goals: relief of symptoms, reestablishment of normal anatomic relations, and restoration of function. One must be certain that the proposed surgery is clearly warranted, that the patient's medical condition is adequate to withstand the stress of surgery, and that the risk–benefit ratio favors benefit. The operation should be one with which the surgeon is thoroughly familiar and one that he is convinced will truly improve the quality of the patient's remaining years of life. The patient and her family must be given an informed consent form, with adequate time to discuss it among themselves and to raise any questions or doubts that should be clarified. The patient's primary-care physician, internist, and cardiologist, if necessary, should be asked for their written opinions concerning the patient. There also should be a preoperative consultation with a representative of the department of anesthesia, outlining the choice of anesthesia and the necessity for any significant ancillary consultations that might be desirable.

It is good to relate the possible complications that should be considered, so that the patient and her family might participate in the informed decision-making complex of having surgery. They should be given information regarding the anticipated length of the operative procedure and the likelihood that transfusion may be required, so that autologous blood can be set aside if desired.

Postoperative Considerations

If present in the older woman, special risks must be identified; significant postoperative complications as a consequence of these risks impose a greater likelihood of risk than intraoperative complication.

The surgeon should be comfortable in the diagnosis and treatment of postoperative complications, so that they may be addressed promptly and effectively. As Lee has pointed out in personal communication, it is not so much the complication that produces mortality but a complication of a complication.

Most elderly patients have lost much of their sense of thirst and tend to live in a state of hemoconcentration. During anesthesia, they are hydrated intravenously, producing a hemodilution of their concentrated blood, which appears during postoperative testing to be a drop in hemoglobin and hematocrit. When over the next 3 or 4 postoperative days the patient resumes her original and usual reduced oral fluid intake (intravenous hydration having been discontinued), the hemoconcentration gradually returns and there appears to be a coincident increase in hemoglobin and hematocrit. This phenomenon must be considered when evaluating a patient's postoperative laboratory data.

If the patient has been on significant medication that affects her daily life, this should be continued to the morning of surgery and reinstituted as soon as practical postoperatively. For new medications, it should be remembered that the elderly patients often have an exaggerated response to any medication that they have been given, and it is safer to opt for low-range doses, so that the patient's need and response can be appropriately titrated.

The patient should be told who will be seeing her daily postoperatively and if she has a catheter in place, how long to expect it to remain and what to do about its care.

The surgeon should plan daily postoperative rounds for the patient, spend enough time with her to answer all of her questions, and be compassionate in understanding her special needs, forgetfulness, and occasional episodes of confusion. The patient and her family must be given specific instructions regarding postoperative care, the conditions under which to call the surgeon's office for advice (eg, hemorrhage, fever, unusual pain, obstipation, urinary burning), and told when to come in for postoperative examination. It is most desirable for the surgeon or member of the surgeon's staff to contact the patient within the first few days after discharge to inquire about her general welfare, answer any questions that may be verbalized, and give information that is relevant to her continued care. An arrangement should be verbalized for postoperative examination, for which the patient should be sent an appropriate reminder card.

The open area of a contracting wound decreases more slowly in older patients, and wound breakdown is increased. Although healing time may be prolonged, procedures can be safely performed, with a reasonable expectation of benefit if allowances for these factors are made during postoperative care. The strength of postoperative collagen is greater in the younger patient than in the elderly but after 4 postoperative months, there actually may be more collagen in the wounds of the older patient, as noted in animal experiments. Provided that allowances in additional time for postoperative healing are understood and agreed on by the patient, the results of surgery need not be compromised. Surgical healing proceeds but at a slightly slower rate.[22]

SUMMARY

With the massive increase in the number of elderly patients in our population, it is essential that gynecologists and other health care providers prepare for the prevention, diagnosis, and treatment of significant disorders in the urogynecologic system. The risks and benefits of surgical treatment in addition to alternate means of therapy must be thoroughly explained to the patient and her family. When these disorders are surgically correctable and a surgical decision has been reached, the patient must be given the benefit of the correct operation (preceded by careful analysis of the risk–benefit ratio) performed expertly by an experienced operator and followed by appropriate postoperative care. The duration of hospitalization should be no longer than necessary, so that the entire treatment plan may be cost-effective, with the unlikely need for fu-

ture reoperation. In this manner, appropriate care may be affordable to the patient and to the public. This also significantly improves the quality of life during the senior years, providing the opportunity for longevity to be a blessing rather than an endurance contest.

REFERENCES

1. Nichols DH: Episiotomy. In Nichols DH (ed): Gynecologic and obstetric surgery, p 1048. St. Louis, Mosby-Year Book, 1993
2. Barber HK: The graying of the baby boom: are we prepared? Female Patient 17:11, 1992
3. Brazda JF: Washington report. Nation's Health March 1983:3
4. Resnick NM, Yalla SV, Laurino E: The pathophysiology of urinary incontinence among institutionalized elderly persons. N Engl J Med 320:1, 1989
5. Elias M: Late-life love. Harvard Health Letter 18:1, 1992
6. Star VL, Hochberg MC: Osteoporosis: treat current injury, retard future loss. Intern Med 14:32, 1993
7. Herbst AL, Mishell DR Jr, Stenchever MA, Droegemueller W: Comprehensive gynecology, 2nd ed, p 1245. St. Louis, Mosby-Year Book, 1992
8. Greenburg AG, Saik RP, Pridham D: Influence of age on mortality of colon surgery. Am J Surg 150:65, 1985
9. Palmberg S, Hirsjarvi E: Mortality in geriatric surgery: with special reference to the type of surgery, anesthesia, complicating disease, and prophylaxis of thrombosis. Gerontology 25:103, 1979
10. Reiss R, Deutsch AA, Eliashiv A: Decision making process in abdominal surgery in the geriatric patient. World J Surg 7:522, 1983
11. Amaral JF, Greenburg AG: The physiologic stress of surgery. In Nichols DH (ed): Gynecologic and obstetric surgery, p 77. St. Louis, Mosby-Year Book, 1993
12. Greenburg AG, Salk RP, Coyle JJ, Peskin GW: Mortality and gastrointestinal surgery in the aged: elective vs emergency procedures. Arch Surg 116:788, 1981
13. Lilly MP, Engeland WC, Gann DS: Responses of cortisol secretion to repeated hemorrhage in the anesthetized dog. Endocrinology 112:681, 1983
14. Polacek DJ, Buchbaum HJ: Surgery in the aged. In Buchbaum HJ, Walton LA (eds): Strategies in gynecologic surgery, p 181. New York, Springer-Verlag, 1986
15. Pierson RL, Figge PK, Buchbaum HJ: Surgery for gynecologic malignancy in the aged. Obstet Gynecol 46:523, 1975
16. Goldman L: Cardiac risks and complications of noncardiac surgery. Ann Intern Med 98:504, 1983
17. Hirsh RA: An approach to assessing perioperative risk. In Goldman DR, Brown FH, Levy WK, et al (ed.): Medical care of the surgical patient, p 31. Philadelphia, JB Lippincott, 1982
18. Piscitelli JT, Parker RT: Primary care in the post-

menopausal woman. Clin Obstet Gynecol 29:343, 1986

19. Hosking MP, Warren MA: Preoperative evaluation and prognosis after surgery in elderly patients. Geriatric Med Today 9:19, 1990

20. Hosking MP, Warren MA, Lobdell CM, et al: Outcomes of surgery in patients 90 years of age and older. JAMA 261:1909, 1989

21. Graber EA, Feldman GB: Special problems of geriatric patients. Contemp Ob/Gyn 83, 1987

22. Stromberg BV: Wound healing in the elderly. Geriatric Medicine Today 8:93, 1989

Ambulatory Gynecology, Second Edition,
edited by David H. Nichols and Patrick J. Sweeney.
J. B. Lippincott Company, Philadelphia, © 1995.

Gynecologic Urology

Veronica T. Mallett and David A. Richardson

A thorough understanding of the genital urinary problems affecting women becomes increasingly important as the population ages. It is well known that in the United States the human female has a longer life expectancy and that the number of elderly females is growing and constitutes an ever larger proportion of our population. With advancing age, the number of chronic illnesses increases, including the problem of urinary dysfunction. Urinary dysfunction is not unique among women but data indicate that women are more likely to be affected. Probably the most devastating of the urinary infirmities affecting women is the condition of urinary incontinence. Precise figures are not easy to obtain; however, in one study of 515 females older than the age of 45 years, 22% complained of incontinence.[1] In another study of 1955 noninstitutionalized men and women aged 60 years or older, the prevalence of incontinence among women was 37.7%—twice that of men.[2] Despite the prevalence of this disorder, fewer than half of those individuals in the community discuss their condition with their primary care provider. The social and psychologi-

cal impact of this disorder can be devastating, leading to embarrassment, depression, and social isolation of the affected individual.

The purpose of this chapter is to provide the practicing physician with a basic understanding of the pathophysiology of some of the major urogynecologic disorders and to provide a practical approach to the diagnosis and treatment of these disorders in an ambulatory setting.

ANATOMY AND NEUROPHYSIOLOGY

There are several factors that act in concert to maintain continence. Most of these factors involve the urethral-closure mechanism and detrusor muscle function. Understanding the structure of the lower urinary tract and its integral relation to the pelvic floor is essential to understanding the physiology and treating the pathologic conditions affecting this region. An intricate discussion of the anatomy is beyond the scope of this text. What is provided is a basic overview of the neurophysiology and anatomic structure of the bladder, urethra, and their pelvic floor attachments.

Bladder

The bladder's major function is to act as a reservoir, relaxing to receive urine during filling and contracting to evacuate urine during the emptying phase. It consists of the detrusor musculature and its underlying mucosa in addition to the vesical trigone, which lies within the dorsal wall of the bladder. The wall of the bladder is made up of three layers: an outer adventitial layer, a middle connective-tissue layer, and an inner muscular layer. The muscular layer is a meshwork of muscle fibers, which when contracted act to reduce the volume of the bladder lumen. The urinary trigone consists of a triangular-shaped area of smooth muscle that has as its base the two ureteral orifices and at its apex, the internal urethral meatus. At the level of the internal urethral meatus is the trigonal ring, an area of trigonal musculature surrounding the internal meatus in the region of the vesical neck. It is thought by Delancey and others that this structure is important in vesical neck closure.[3] Because of its anatomic configuration, the trigone undergoes less distention during filling.

Urethra

The urethral wall comprises three layers: a mucosal epithelium, smooth muscle coat, and periurethral striated muscle. The smooth muscle coat has both inner longitudinal fibers and outer circular fibers. Delancey, in a study of urethral anatomy, expressed the striated urogenital sphincter topographically as a percentage of urethral length (Fig. 19-1).[4] He further described the striated sphincter as being divided into three muscles. The sphincter urethrae is circular in orientation and surrounds the urethral lumen from about 20% to 60% of its length. The second portion of the sphincter, the compressor urethrae, occupies the distal third of the urethra (60% to 80% of its length), lying adjacent to the urethral lumen. The third portion (urethrovaginal sphincter) lies immediately beneath the compressor urethrae. The urethrovaginal sphincter originates in the vaginal wall, whereas the compressor urethrae originates near the ischiopubic ramus. These muscle fibers are separate only in their lateral projections. All three portions function together to constrict the urethra when contracted in its upper portion and compress its ventral wall in the lower portion, providing a backup to the continence mechanism. The periurethral striated muscle has both fast-twitch and slow-twitch fibers, which provide both resting tone and the ability to reflexively increase urethral pressure by muscular contraction during increases in abdominal pressure. This ana-

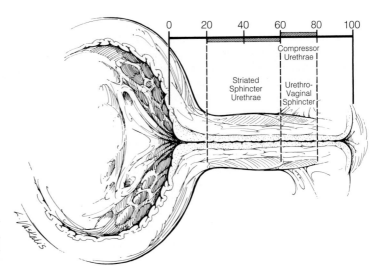

Figure 19–1. Topographic representation of the periurethral muscles, expressed as a percentage of total urethral length.

tomic configuration and the urethral attachments described below act in concert to maintain continence.

Urethral Attachments

The urethra and vagina are not separate structures. They are fused in the distal two thirds of the urethra and held together by the endopelvic fascia. The endopelvic fascia envelopes the periurethral tissues and anterior vaginal wall, which attach to the arcus tendineus and medial border of the levator ani. This attachment of the periurethral tissue and vagina to the levator ani muscles allows contraction of the muscle to elevate the urethrovesical junction, just as relaxation of the pelvic floor results in downward descent of the urethrovesical junction.

Continence is maintained during increases in abdominal pressure by transmitting intraabdominal-pressure increases to both the bladder and proximal urethra. If there is a downward axial rotation of the urethra during stress, the urethra receives less pressure than the bladder and under sufficient force, incontinence results. This downward axial mobility can occur from separation of the urethra and vagina from the lateral attachments or relaxation of the levator ani muscles. Surgical therapies to remedy stress incontinence are directed toward improving pressure transmission by preventing urethral mobility.

Central Nervous System Control

The voiding act involves a complex interaction of the cerebral cortex, brain stem, and sacral micturition region of the spinal cord. The central nervous system innervation is discussed as a whole, with specific references to clinical evaluation of the different control regions. The purpose of grouping central nervous system (CNS) control is to provide an overall picture of the complex interaction required for normal micturition and to emphasize the interrelatedness of the different areas of control.

Impulses originate in the frontal lobe of the cerebral cortex and terminate in the brain stem, with input from the cerebellum. This interaction coordinates voluntary control of micturition. If affected by abnormalities such as Parkinson's disease, brain tumors, and trauma, the patient is not able to voluntarily suppress a detrusor contraction, resulting in an abnormal cystometrogram.

Additional impulses originate in the pontine portion of the brain stem and travel to the sacral micturition area. Normal functioning of the pontine portion of the CNS system provides for a detrusor contraction sufficient for emptying. Abnormalities that alter the function of this neuronal complex, including spinal cord trauma, spinal cord tumors, and multiple sclerosis, result in poor emptying and increased residual urine. The net effect of the input provided by the cerebral cortex brain stem circuit and the brain stem spinal cord circuit is to coordinate the ability to suppress a detrusor contraction as well as to provide a contraction sufficient for complete emptying. The cystometrogram is the primary means to assess integrity of these systems.

Coordination of detrusor and urethral muscular activity during voiding is provided by afferent nerves of the detrusor muscle that travel to the sacral micturition area. Injuries to the circuit at this level result in failure of the urethra to relax during voiding and associated voiding difficulties. Surface electromyography (EMG) or complex electrodiagnostics of the pelvic floor and spinal cord may indicate damage to this circuitry, revealing a condition known as detrusor sphincter dyssynergia. As with the other circuitry described, spinal cord tumors and trauma and multiple sclerosis can affect the integrity and function of this circuit.

In addition to the circuitry, there is both peripheral and central innervation of the periurethral striated muscles, originating in the pudendal region of the sensorimotor cortex. These motor fibers terminate by synapsing on the pudendal nucleus in the sacral micturition region of the sacral spinal cord. This allows innervation of the pelvic floor musculature.

Additionally, signals originate in the sensorimotor cortex of the frontal lobe and terminate in the pudendal area of the sacral micturition area. The test for integrity of the central and peripheral innervation of the periurethral striated muscles is external EMG of the anal sphincter. Interruption of this pathway interferes with the coordination of bladder contraction and concurrent periurethral muscle relaxation.

AUTONOMIC NERVOUS SYSTEM

Parasympathetic Innervation

Parasympathetic innervation originates in sacral segments S_2–S_4 and travels to the detrusor muscle and urethra through the pelvic nerve. The detrusor muscle is under parasympathetic control by the neurotransmitter acetylcholine. When the parasympathetic receptors are stimulated, the bladder contracts and contraction of urethral smooth muscle is inhibited.

Sympathetic Innervation

Sympathetic innervation originates in spinal cord segments T_{10}–L_2 and travels to the detrusor muscle and urethra by the hypogastric nerve. α-Receptors from the sympathetic nervous system, when stimulated, cause contraction of the urethral sphincter and smooth muscle of the urethra and produce relaxation of the detrusor muscle. Urethral and detrusor muscle relaxation is under sympathetic nervous control by β-receptors.

APPROACH TO PATIENTS WITH INCONTINENCE

Multiple conditions cause urinary incontinence in the female. Successful management of this condition depends on obtaining the correct diagnosis. The primary purpose of an appropriate urologic investigation is to differentiate between genuine stress incontinence and the unstable bladder (detrusor instability) and to rule out other less common causes. The basic evaluation of patients with urinary incontinence includes:

• History
• Physical examination
• Urethral mobility test
• Urinary diary
• Urinalysis and culture
• Simple cystometrogram

History

The history of any patient with a complaint of incontinence must include inquiries regarding the urologic, gynecologic, neurologic, and psychiatric conditions, and current medications and any current medical disorders—specifically, the presence of diabetes, thyroid disease, and hypertension. Past medical, surgical, and obstetric histories and past methods to alleviate incontinence should be included.

Urologic Symptoms

Stress incontinence is the loss of urine with increases in abdominal pressure (ie, coughing, lifting, laughing, sneezing, or straining). Inquiries regarding onset and relation to menopause and pregnancy should be made. Frequency of urinary incontinence, events precipitating leakage, and severity of leakage (ie, drips versus large amounts) should be elicited. In a group of patients with genuine stress incontinence, 70% to 100% complain of stress incontinence; however, more than half of patients with other urologic disorders also complain of this symptom.

Urgency is a strong desire to void. Urge incontinence is the loss of urine associated with the strong desire to void. The symptom of urgency is present in up 90% of women with unstable bladder. These symptoms can be associated with both genuine stress incontinence and the unstable bladder.

Urinary frequency is a nonspecific symptom, defined as voiding at least every 2 hours. It occurs in patients with either stress urinary incontinence or an unstable bladder. Many times, however, patients have developed a habit of frequent voiding. Other patients consume large amounts of fluids. Occasionally, undiagnosed patients with diabetes mellitus or diabetes insipidus can be identified.

Nocturia is the passage of urine more than two times nightly. This symptom is nonspecific and nonsensitive. The chance of detrusor instability or mixed incontinence increases with the number of urologic symptoms. Nocturia can be related to patients' sleep habits, fluid consumption, or medications taken. Occasionally, patients with nocturnal diuresis can be identified.

Enuresis is the involuntary loss of urine while sleeping (bed-wetting). A relatively rare complaint, it may be seen in patients with stress urinary incontinence but is more commonly reported by women with an unstable bladder.[5]

There are numerous other symptoms the physician should be aware of. Among these are dysuria, postvoid dribbling, and postvoid fullness. Dysuria (painful urination) is usually not associated with conditions of incontinence. It is important, however, to differentiate between internal and external dysuria. Internal dysuria may be the result of an underlying cystitis, which can closely mimic genuine stress incontinence if untreated. External dysuria may be the result of an undiagnosed vaginitis, an easily treated cause of dysuria.

Postvoid dribbling is a symptom that should be regarded essentially as normal and the patient taught mechanisms of dealing with this. Postvoid fullness may occasionally be related to outflow obstruction, especially in the estrogen-deprived female.

Other infrequently elicited symptoms are continuous incontinence, incontinence during intercourse, and hematuria. Occasionally, patients have continuous incontinence, suggesting urinary tract fistula, congenital damage to the urinary tract, or low-pressure urethra. Incontinence during intercourse is an embarrassing symptom, often not elicited unless the physician asks directly, but may be the patient's primary concern. Hematuria may either be gross (frank blood in the urine) or microscopic. It requires further investigation if present after urinary tract infection has been ruled out.

Patients with lower urinary tract disease present with a variety of symptoms. Unlike many areas of medicine, urologic complaints do not lend themselves to diagnosis by history alone. This was demonstrated amply by Cardozo and Stanton in a group of 200 patients with genuine stress incontinence and unstable bladder. Patients were assigned to diagnostic categories based on history alone, and the misdiagnosis rate was found to be in the range of 20% to 40%.[6] Jarvis and coworkers, in a study of 100 consecutive incontinent women using history and physical alone, found the diagnosis to be confirmed in only 65 women.[7] In Quigley's study of 1277 patients whose only complaint was urge incontinence, 29% had genuine stress incontinence.[8] The reasons for this are many and should not be unexpected, considering the many patients with nonspecific and mixed symptoms. For example, the symptoms of urgency may be caused by a urinary tract infection, unstable bladder, urethral diverticula, urethritis, or genuine stress incontinence. Similarly, urinary tract symptoms may arise from nonurologic conditions such as diabetes, thyroid disorders, or CNS disturbances.

GYNECOLOGIC HISTORY

The gynecologic history is important to exclude the presence of related gynecologic pathology. Symptoms of prolapse, pressure, dragging, or a sensation that "everything is falling out" are commonly seen in incontinent patients. The presence of other conditions, including multiple myoma, endometriosis, dyspareunia, and dysmenorrhea, can impact on treatment modalities selected for treating the incontinence. A radical vulvectomy or Wertheim hysterectomy can significantly change urethral vesicle

dynamics. If a patient has had any previous anti-incontinence procedure, the type of surgery, the duration of its effectiveness, and complications occurring during the surgery should be identified. If possible, copies of the previous surgical records should be obtained. If the procedure has failed, it is important to note if the incontinence is the same or worse and whether other symptoms are present.

NEUROLOGIC HISTORY

Back problems, trauma, previous stroke, parkinsonism, diabetic neuropathy, degenerative nerve diseases, occult spina bifida, multiple sclerosis, and other CNS disturbances can produce symptoms related not only to urinary incontinence but also to fecal incontinence. Patients with neurologic disease may lose awareness of a full bladder or wetness or lose the ability to control the flow of urine. Other symptoms predicting neuropathy include limb weakness or visual-type disturbances and autonomic dysfunction such as excessive sweating or poor regulation of blood pressure.

PSYCHIATRIC HISTORY

It is difficult for physicians to determine whether psychiatric disturbances cause bladder problems or whether the chronic disease brought to the surface unresolved issues that the patient may need help in resolving. Patients with severe stress incontinence may be embarrassed, depressed, have a lowered self-esteem, and feel isolated from the world. Any number of life events may trigger vesicle instability (ie, death in the family, loss of job, marital difficulties, or recognition of previous abuse).

MEDICATION HISTORY

Many commonly prescribed medications affect the bladder and lower urinary tract (Table 19-1). For example, any antihypertensive medication with an α-blocking mechanism can lead to a lowered urethral pressure. Caffeine significantly lowers urethral pressure and increases fluid volume, doubly stressing the continence mechanism. Inquiries should be made regarding amount and forms of caffeine intake. Diuretics, dantrolene, and Triavil can all cause urinary frequency. Levodopa and levopropoxyphene are known to cause frequency, retention, and incontinence.

Table 19–1
Drugs That Lower the Continence Mechanism

Agent	Comment
Phenoxybenzamine (Dibenzyline); prazosin (Minipress)	α-Adrenergic blocker that can decrease sphincter tone in proximal urethra
Loop diuretics (furosemide, ethacrynic acid, bumetamide)	Cause rapid diuresis, leading to polyuria and frequency; may over-stress continence mechanism in immobile patients
Phenothiazine derivatives	These drugs have α-blocking activity, which may lead to incontinence; however, these drugs may also cause urinary retention
Caffeine	Excessive amounts of caffeine may lower urethral pressure
Phenytoin	In large amounts, may cause incontinence

PAST MEDICAL HISTORY

Any past medical history of diabetes, hypertension, and pulmonary disorders causing chronic cough may impact on the incontinence mechanism. Resnick, in his study of urinary incontinence in the elderly, made a point that there are many transient causes of incontinence in the elderly, which when properly treated can resolve patient symptomatology.[8a] He devised a mnemonic—DIAPPERS—to help recall the categories of external problems that can lead to incontinence.

D Delirium (or any confusional state)
I Lower urinary tract infection
A Atrophic urethritis/vaginitis
P Pharmaceutical
P Psychological
E Endocrine disorders (hypercalcemia, hyperglycemia, and hypothyroidism)
R Restricted mobility (inability to reach the toilet and undress before voiding.
S Stool impaction

CLINICAL EXAMINATION

The physical examination should be complete and include an evaluation of estrogen status, pelvic relaxation, muscle tone, and a neurologic evaluation. The external genitalia, vagina, and urethra should be examined for any signs of estrogen deprivation, atrophic vaginitis, urethritis, or loss of vaginal rugae. After this, the urethra should be palpated for a diverticulum and milked to elicit the presence of pus or tenderness. Patients should be examined in both the dorsal lithotomy and standing positions to uncover any effect gravity may have on perineal supports (ie, cystocele, rectocele, enterocele, or uterine prolapse). The patient should be instructed to perform Valsalva's maneuver in both the lithotomy and standing positions and the result should be noted. Pubococcygeus and levator ani muscle tone should be evaluated by placing two fingers in the vaginal fornix and instructing the patient to tighten her pelvic floor muscle (or any command that leads to contraction of the pubococcygeus) and to hold the contraction for as long as she can. Symmetry of the contraction, strength, and duration of the response should be noted. A woman with good perineal strength is usually able to contract for greater than 6 seconds. A bimanual examination is performed to rule out any gynecologic pathology. Rectovaginal examination is included to assess anal tone and the degree and presence of a rectocele or enterocele in both the dorsal lithotomy and standing positions.

NEUROLOGIC EXAMINATION

The basic neurologic examination includes assessment of lower limb strength and sensation and deep tendon reflexes. Perineal sensation (S_2, S_3, S_4) is easily assessed using the back of a cotton-tipped swab stroked on the buttock and thigh. Rectal reflex is tested by stroking the perianal region and watching for the wink or contraction of the rectal sphincter.

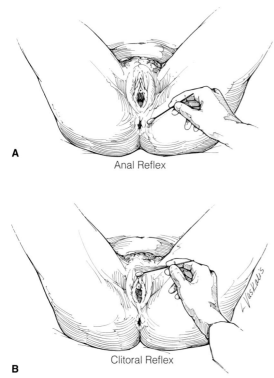

A

Anal Reflex

B

Clitoral Reflex

Figure 19–2. Anal and clitoral reflex. (**A**) Perianal stroking with a cotton-tipped swab causes contraction of the anal sphincter. (**B**) Clitoral tapping with a cotton-tipped swab causes constriction of the pelvic floor.

The bulbocavernosus reflex is elicited by tapping or lightly touching the clitoris with a cotton-tipped swab, which produces a contraction of the anal sphincter (Fig. 19-2). These reflexes may be normally absent in the older patient and may be difficult to obtain in the obese patient.

ASSESSMENT OF URETHRAL MOBILITY

The assessment of urethral mobility can be performed by inspection and palpation, bead-chain cystourethrogram, cotton-tipped swab testing, or ultrasound. It cannot be overemphasized that urethral mobility does not diagnose stress urinary incontinence. Documentation of urethral mobility is valuable because most operative procedures are designed to stabilize the urethra and prevent downward axial mobility. Lack of urethral mobility is associated with significantly higher surgical failure

rates, whether patients have normal or low urethral pressure.

Inspection and palpation are usually reliable; however, error may occur in two ways. The first is by confusing descent with the presence of redundant periurethral vaginal tissue. The second is by not appreciating descent of the urethral vesical junction during stress. This often occurs in the evaluation of young nulliparous women.

Bead-chain cystourethrography was popular in the 1960s and 1970s. The procedure involved the introduction of radiopaque dye into the urethra and visualization of the bladder and urethra statically and dynamically, with a beaded chain to aid in the delineation of the urethra, bladder, and urethral base. The urethrovesical junction normally resides posteriorly and superiorly to the lower edge of the symphysis. In patients with anatomic disruption, the junction descends below this level.

It was quickly learned that static radiographic measurements were poor predictors of incontinence. The test originally was to be used to differentiate between anterior and posterior defects in the urethral vesical angles. The results were not reproducible and were variable to interpretation. Stage, in a study of 172 incontinent females, found that urethrography without the bead chain was of minor value in differentiating between stress and urge incontinence. More than half of the women with stress incontinence had no suspension defect or posterior suspension defects not typically associated with stress incontinence.[9] With newer, more reliable methods to distinguish between stress and urge incontinence, bead-chain cystourethrography is no longer considered primary in the diagnosis of urethral mobility and incontinence.

The degree of urethral mobility can easily be assessed in the physician's office by performing a cotton-tipped swab test. A lubricated cotton-tipped swab is introduced into the urethra with the patient in the dorsal lithotomy position. The resting angle from the horizontal is then measured, using an orthopedic goniometer. The patient is asked to cough, strain, or bear down and the change in the urethral axis is measured (Fig. 19-3). Additional useful information obtained during the cotton-tipped swab test is the degree of downward deviation from the horizontal when the patient is asked to tighten her pelvic floor muscles. This deviation indicates elevation of the pelvic floor, pelvic floor muscle strength, and attachment of the urethra to the lateral pelvic side walls.

The cotton-tipped swab test is unreliable in dif-

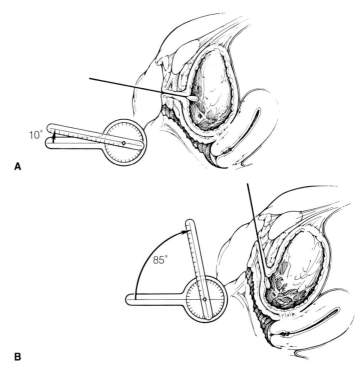

Figure 19–3. Cotton-tipped test. (**A**) Resting angle is measured in the horizontal position, using an orthopedic goniometer. (**B**) Straining angle is measured during strong Valsalva.

ferentiating genuine stress incontinence from detrusor instability. Walters and Diaz compared the cotton-tipped swab measure in women with stress incontinence and in women with other types of urinary dysfunction. It was found that no difference existed between the two incontinent study groups.[10] There were, however, differences between continent patients and those with stress incontinence. Montz and Stanton investigated 100 patients, using cotton-tipped swab measurements and video cystourethrography, and found poor sensitivity and specificity in diagnosing patients with stress incontinence.[11]

Major improvements in the resolution of ultrasonic images and the invention of vaginal and rectal ultrasound probes have facilitated the use of the ultrasound in the evaluation of the urethra, bladder, rectum, and pelvic floor. Investigators in the use of the ultrasound as a diagnostic modality predict a role for the use of ultrasound in diagnosing and assessing pelvic floor defects and urethral mobility. Benson and associates used the vaginal probe ultrasound to assess urethral mobility, anorectal angle, and urethral descent in both normal women and women with incontinence. They found a greater degree of urethral mobility in the stress-incontinent

woman.[12] Other researchers (Chang and colleagues and Vierhout and Janssen) have used the transrectal approach to visualize the urethra and bladder. Both state that this approach is superior to abdominal and transvaginal ultrasound in the ability to visualize the structures dynamically without obstructing mobility.[13,14] All authors mentioned make claims regarding the use of the ultrasound as being equivalent to cystography in diagnosing mobility and descent, although there is no data presented to support this claim.

URINARY DIARY

The physician should obtain a 24-hour urolog and a 7-day voiding diary. Variables in the diary should include times voided, volumes voided, volumes at which the patient experiences urinary leakage, number of leakage episodes throughout the day or week, and total 24-hour urinary volume (Fig. 19-4). The purpose of the voiding diary is to assess severity of the incontinence problems and correlate previous historical symptoms. The 24-hour volume measurements identify the infrequent voider and the high-output voider. These diaries are useful not

INSTRUCTIONS FOR 24-HOUR VOIDING DIARY

1. Choose a 24-hour period to keep this record when you can conveniently measure every voiding.

2. Begin your diary with the first voiding upon arising and end with the first voiding of the next morning.

3. Record time of all voidings and episodes of leakage.

4. Estimate severity of leakage:

    1 - Few drops
    3 - Change underwear or pad
    5 - Change outerwear or pad soaked

5. Describe the activity you were performing at the time of leakage, and if you were not actively doing anything, record whether you were sitting, standing or lying down.

PLEASE COMPLETE THIS PRIOR TO YOUR VISIT TO OUR CLINIC.

EXAMPLE:

ENTER TIME OF VOID OR LEAK	AMOUNT OF URINE VOIDED (cc)	SEVERITY OF LEAKAGE	WHAT WAS GOING ON WHEN YOU LEAKED?
8:OO am	200 cc		
9:15 am		1- FEW DROPS	COUGHED HARD
9:45 am		3 -CHANGED PANTS	STRONG URGE,HEARD WATER RUNNING
11:30 pm	150 cc		

A

Figure 19–4. (**A–C**) Urinary diaries with instruction. Use of a "flying nun's hat" on the toilet seat facilitates accurate measurement.

only in quantifying and characterizing the nature of the incontinence but also in charting response to the therapeutic intervention, whether a surgical or nonsurgical approach is selected.

SIMPLE CYSTOMETROGRAM

The simple cystometrogram is an essential part of the work-up of incontinence. The cystometrogram answers four basic questions.

1. Can the patient empty her bladder completely?
2. Does the patient have normal bladder function?
3. Is there evidence of an unstable bladder?
4. Can the urinary leakage be documented?

The patient is asked to obtain a clean-voided urine specimen. In the dorsal lithotomy position, the patient is catheterized and residual urine is measured. Residual urine should be obtained before the beginning of the cystometrogram. A value of less than 50 mL is considered normal. Higher values alert the physician to the possibility of outlet obstruction, multiple sclerosis, occult spina bifida, spinal cord trauma, or some autonomic dysfunction. Although not a guarantee of normal detrusor function, residual urine measurement is an easily performed and often forgotten first step in ruling out urinary tract dysfunctions.

After the residual urine has been obtained, the bladder is filled with saline using a 60-mL catheter-tip syringe (Fig. 19-5). The volume at first bladder

24-HOUR URINARY DIARY

DATE: _____

NAME: _____

ENTER TIME OF VOID OR LEAK	AMOUNT OF URINE VOIDED (CC)	SEVERITY OF LEAKAGE 1 - 2 - 3 - 4 - 5	WHAT WAS GOING ON WHEN YOU VOIDED?

1 - Few drops
3 - Change underwear or pad
B 5 - Change outerwear or pad soaked

Figure 19–4. *(Continued)*

sensation (90 to 150 mL), fullness (350 mL), and maximum capacity (400 to 600 mL) is noted. Loss of urine or a rise in the fluid level of the syringe during the filling phase, despite a patient's efforts to suppress a detrusor contraction, is indicative of an unstable bladder. Fluid is removed until the patient is comfortably full and the catheter removed.

In the absence of increased intra-abdominal pressure (respiration, coughing, or bearing down), a sudden elevation of water height occurring simultaneously with the sensation of urgency is diagnostic of the unstable bladder. Because of the difficulty distinguishing artifact from detrusor contractions, false-positive results may occur. Simple supine cystometrogram detects only 50% of the unstable bladders, yielding many false-negative results. The standing cystometrogram is more sensitive with the addition of the provocative maneuvers. If a patient has significant complaints of urge, frequency, and

urge incontinence and an unstable bladder is not diagnosed, the patient should undergo further urodynamic evaluation.

A stress test is performed with a comfortably full bladder. The patient is asked to cough and bear down in the sitting position to observe the presence of urinary leakage. If leakage is not visualized, the test is performed in the standing position. Provocative maneuvers (heel bouncing, sound of running water, or laughter) may elicit a detrusor contraction.

It is imperative to document leakage at some point in this examination. Inability to do so requires that other methods of documentation be undertaken (ie, the perineal pad test or Pyridium pad test) to determine whether the leakage is indeed urine. Timing of the leakage is critical. If the patient loses urine simultaneously with a cough, it is considered to be a positive stress test. If the loss of urine is

SEVEN DAY VOIDING LOG

Name _____

	6am	7am	8am	9am	10am	11am	12am	1pm	2pm	3pm	4pm	5pm	6pm	7pm	8pm	9pm	10pm	11pm	12am	# Times Void At Night	Pads Used During Day
Monday																					
Tuesday																					
Wednesday																					
Thursday																					
Friday																					
Saturday																					
Sunday																					

INSTRUCTIONS   ENTER

E When you **empty** your bladder

S When you **leak with** **cough, sneeze, exercise**

U When you **leak with** a strong **urge**

C

Figure 19–4. *(Continued)*

delayed, the physician is required to rule out a detrusor contraction provoked by the coughing. After the testing is completed, the patient is given prophylactic antibiotics to prevent the development of an infection.

PESSARY TEST

An adjunct to the stress test is the pessary test. Women with mild to moderate pelvic relaxation may have marked stress urinary incontinence; however, as the prolapse increases in size, incontinent patients may note a cessation of symptoms. The mechanism of continence in these women with severe prolapse is essentially urethral obstruction or urethral kinking.[15] The pessary test is designed to uncover occult or masked incontinence. After the placement of a pessary large enough to reduce the prolapse without obstructing the urethra, the patient is observed for leakage with stress. If leakage occurs, the test is positive and an anti-incontinence procedure should be included in the operative plan. Bergman and coworkers evaluated 67 women who had severe prolapse but no incontinence. With pessary correction, 35% showed signs of incipient stress incontinence and reduced pressure–transmission ratio.[16]

PERINEAL PAD TEST

Perineal pad weighing has been proposed by some authors as a useful method to document incontinence and quantify the severity of the leakage. The patient is provided with a pre-weighed pad and instructed to drink 500 mL of fluid. Thirty minutes later, she is instructed to perform a variety of maneuvers to increase abdominal pressure, including laughing, coughing, running in place, washing

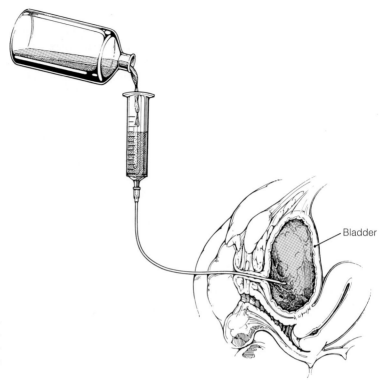

Figure 19–5. Simple cystometrogram. Usually performed in the supine position, with careful observation of the water height in the syringe.

hands, or picking up objects from the floor. Jorgensen found that this test had lower false-negative rate than stress-test and voiding cystourethrography.[17]

LABORATORY TESTS

The most important laboratory test result is negative urinalysis and culture because all the symptoms of incontinence could be caused by a lower urinary tract infection. Asymptomatic bacteriuria and urinary tract infection are common in women of all ages and increase in frequency with age. It is embarrassing, costly, and dangerous to perform complicated urodynamic evaluation, only to find later that the positive findings were caused by an undocumented bladder infection. The presence of pyuria or hematuria in the absence of a documented urinary tract infection requires further work-up.

Additional laboratory tests include those for thyroid-stimulating hormone and T4 to rule out thyroid disorder if an unstable bladder is diagnosed. If the patient has any voiding abnormalities or conditions suggesting overflow incontinence, blood urea nitrogen and creatinine levels should be attained to assess renal function and rule out acute renal failure secondary to outflow obstruction. Serum calcium levels should be obtained because hypercalcemia is a notable cause of incontinence in the elderly.

URODYNAMIC TESTING

Patients older than age 50 years, who are more likely to have detrusor instability or mixed incontinence; patients with previous failed incontinence surgery; or patients with no anterior vaginal relaxation or a straining angle on cotton-tipped swab of less than 30° benefit from multichannel subtracted urodynamic testing. Additionally, patients with a gynecologic malignancy treated with radical pelvic surgery or those with continuous incontinence, a laboratory finding of hematuria, or inconclusive findings in the office evaluation (eg, high residual urine, lack of filling sensation, or high or low capacity) should have further testing before an operative intervention is planned.

Urodynamic testing is a series of measurements that provide a dynamic representation of bladder and urethral physiology using pressure, flow, and surface EMG measurements. The type of equipment purchased (Fig. 19-6) determines the complexity of data obtained. The following is an overview of the information provided in a standard multichannel setup. A brief overview of voiding cystourethrography and urethrocystoscopy is also provided.

Uroflowmetry

Uroflowmetry is primarily used to determine whether the patient is voiding normally and to rule out outlet obstruction (Figs. 19-7 and 19-8). A normal flow rate is less than 20 mL/second. Maximum flow rates of more than 15 mL/second are indicative of obstruction and warrant further investigation if the patient's history and examination dictate. If there is significant concern regarding voiding difficulties, instrumented uroflowmetry should be obtained. The use of instrumented uroflowmetry allows simultaneous measure of the intraurethral

pressure, intravesical pressure, intra-abdominal pressure urethral closure pressure, true detrusor pressure, and flow rate. This enables the physician to determine whether the patient is voiding with a detrusor contraction (using Valsalva's maneuver) or simply relaxing the urethral sphincter. This data may help predict which patients may develop postoperative urinary retention.

Cystometry

Cystometry is used to measure bladder pressure during filling and to diagnose an unstable bladder, atonic bladder, or noncompliant bladder (Fig. 19-9). True detrusor pressure is defined as the pressure generated only by the detrusor muscle. It is determined by subtracting intra-abdominal pressure (as measured by a rectal or vaginal transducer) from bladder pressure. The measurement of detrusor pressure requires at least two channels on the uro-

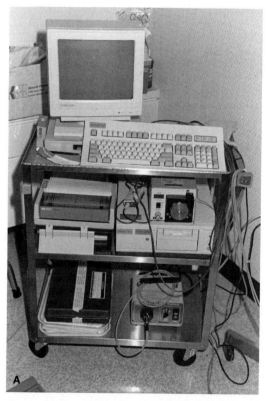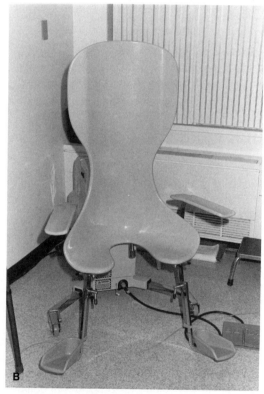

Figure 19–6.   (A) Urodynamic machines come in all shapes and sizes. Shown is an example of the Surgitek urodynamic machine. (B) Birthing chair; useful for positioning the patient for urodynamic testing.

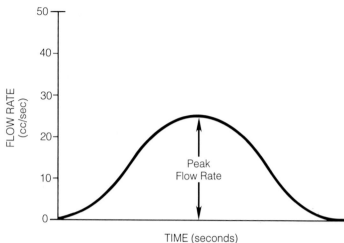

50 — 40 — 30 — 20 — 10 — 0 —

FLOW RATE (cc/sec)

Peak
Flow Rate

TIME (seconds)

Figure 19–7. Non-instrumental uro-flowmetry. Peak flow should be more than 10 mL/second.

dynamic machine. Single-channel measurements may confuse increase of abdominal pressure on using Valsalva's maneuver with detrusor activity. The patient's bladder is filled, using a microtip transducer and normal saline at a rate of 75 to 100 mL/minute in the sitting position. The patient is asked

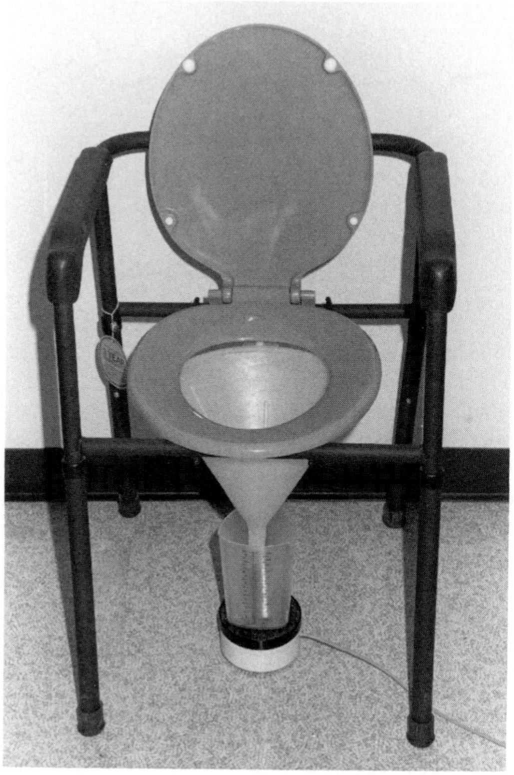

Figure 19–8. Uroflowmetry chair. Patient voids on commode while rate and volume are recorded.

to report first sensation and fullness, as with the simple cystometrogram. Careful observation of the perineum and simultaneous measurement of abdominal and intravesical pressure allow determination of the true detrusor pressure. A rise in true detrusor pressure associated with urge and leaking is diagnostic of an unstable bladder. If documentation of unstable detrusor activity fails during the simple cystometrogram, the patient is asked to stand and cough repetitively, heel bounce, or listen to the sound of running water, as described in the section on simple cystometrogram. Absence of a detrusor contraction during filling in the sitting and standing position is indicative of a stable bladder.

Profilometry

Urethral profilometry is the measure of urethral pressure over the length of the urethra (Fig. 19-10). The simplest way to perform this test is to manually and slowly withdraw the pressure transducer from the bladder out to the urethral meatus. Sophisticated equipment automatically coordinates the chart speed and speed of an automatic device that pulls the pressure transducer, generating a curve from which functional length and urethral closure pressure can be derived. Functional length is that length of urethra over which urethral pressure exceeds bladder pressure when measured simultaneously. Total urethral length is the true anatomic urethral length that adds the additional distance as the catheter is being withdrawn. In women whose incontinence is a result of anatomic disruption, functional length is usually shorter than the continent female.

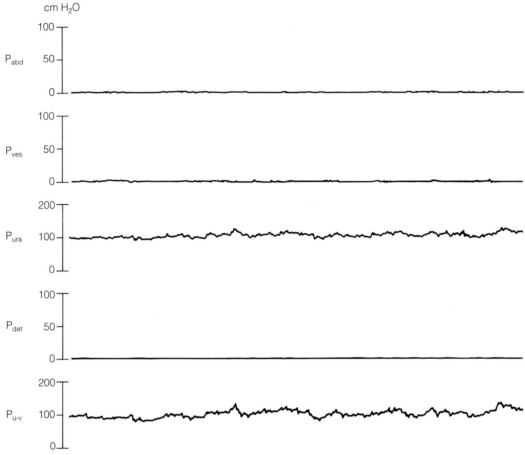

cm H₂O

P_abd

P_ves

P_ura

P_det

P_u-v

Figure 19–9.   Normal cystometrogram. Note the absence of detrusor contractions during bladder filling. (P_{abd}) abdominal pressure; (P_{ves}) vesical pressure; (P_{ura}) urethral pressure; (P_{det}) true detrusor pressure (vesical pressure minus abdominal pressure); (P_{u-v}) urethral closure pressure.

In both the incontinent and continent female, functional length is longer in the supine position than the erect position.

Closure pressure is the value calculated by subtracting bladder pressure from urethral pressure, reflecting the urethral pressure generated to resist urine flow. Pressure below 20 cm H_2O is an indicator of poor urethral function and is associated with higher than average surgical failure rate. Urethral closure pressure profile depicts urethral closure pressure along urethral functional length. A cough pressure profile may be performed to obtain pressure transmission ratio. During this procedure, the catheter is gradually withdrawn through the urethra while the patient repeatedly coughs (Fig. 19-11). If the urethrovesical junction is adequately supported, coughing generates pressure increases in both bladder and urethra, the area under the pressure curve remains positive, and pressure transmission is said to be 100%. If the patient is incontinent, there is little or no area of positive pressure and the patient leaks. Richardson, in a study of 145 women, found the cough profile to have a high specificity (92%) but a relatively low sensitivity (41%). In the population studied, there were many women with stress incontinence who also had a normal cough urethral pressure profile. The authors interpreted these findings to be a caution against using this test as a single indicator of the condition or as the only test verifying success or failure of therapeutic intervention.[18]

Pressure transmission ratio is calculated by dividing the change in maximum urethral closure pressure by the change in bladder pressure and then multiplying times 100. In the normal continent female during coughing, the urethra receives the

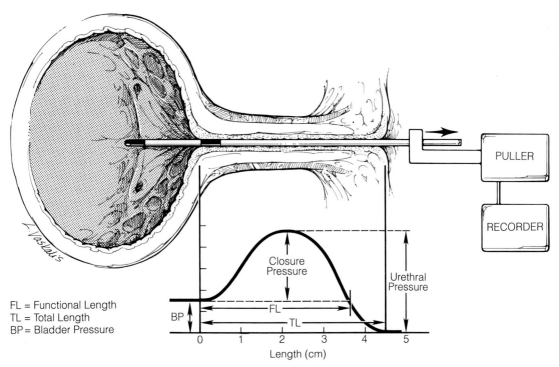

FL = Functional Length
TL = Total Length
BP = Bladder Pressure

Figure 19–10.   Urethral profilometry. *Functional length* is that length of the urethra in which urethral pressure exceeds bladder pressure. *Closure pressure* is the difference between bladder pressure and urethral pressure.

same force as the bladder because of good pressure transmission. In the incontinent female, the bladder receives more pressure than the urethra because of the axial rotation of the urethra. Once bladder pressure exceeds urethral pressure, urine flows through the urethra and incontinence results.

Voiding Cystourethrogram and Videocystourethrography

The voiding cystourethrogram is a radiologic test useful in obtaining a dynamic view of the bladder and urethra during voiding. It demonstrates nicely the pathology of the urethrovesical junction, allowing radiographic visualization of urethral diverticula and presence of anatomic defects in the bladder base. Use of the cystourethrogram in combination with a video recording device and a multichannel instrumented uroflowmeter allows dynamic observation of the bladder and urethra, while simultaneously recording the associated pressure generated during voiding. The patient's bladder is filled with radiopaque iodine and first sensation, fullness, and

intravesical and detrusor pressure are recorded in addition to flow rate. Measurement of these parameters are recorded alongside the radiographic image on the television monitor. Visualization of the anatomic and pressure abnormalities allows precise assessment of a voiding dysfunction and dysfunction of the lower urinary tract. Drawbacks to this form of evaluation are dose of radiation, patient discomfort, cost, and unproved overall benefit.

Urethrocystoscopy

Urethrocystoscopy is useful for evaluation of urethral inflammation, urethral diverticula, interstitial cystitis, and to rule out other intrinsic maladies of the bladder or urethra. Usually well tolerated by the patient, use of this diagnostic tool also requires some training but it is easily learned and easily performed in the office setting. In the past, urethrocystoscopy was thought to be useful in the diagnosis of genuine stress incontinence when funneling of the bladder neck was observed. The study by Vesi and colleagues found an open bladder neck in nearly

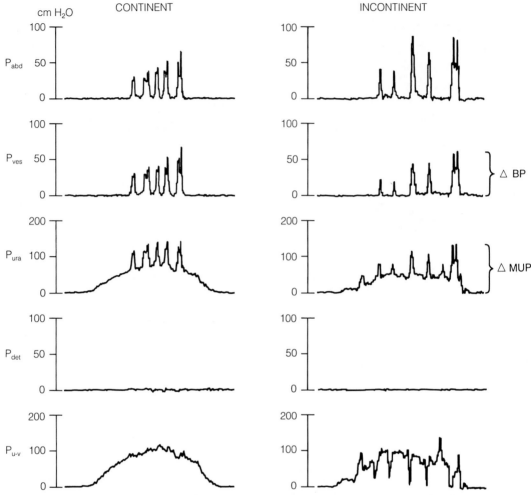

Figure 19–11. Cough pressure profiles. Continent patient maintains positive area under closure pressure curve ($P_{u\text{-}v}$). Incontinent patient fails to maintain a positive area and leaks. The change in closure pressure during coughing is reflected by calculation of pressure transmission ratio (PTR). (*BP*) bladder pressure; (*MUP*) maximum urethral pressure; PTR = $\triangle$MUP/$\triangle$BP × 100%.

50% of the asymptomatic postmenopausal women, thus challenging the validity of this finding in the diagnosis of genuine stress incontinence.[19]

Scotti, in a comparison study of urethrocystoscopy and urodynamics, found urethrocystoscopy to be a relatively insensitive predictor of genuine stress incontinence and thus cautions against its singular use to diagnose this condition.[20]

TREATMENT OF INCONTINENCE

The two conditions most commonly causing incontinence are the unstable bladder (also known as detrusor instability) and genuine stress incontinence.

Once the work-up has been completed and the condition diagnosed, deciding on treatment involves a discussion with the patient, wherein the physician outlines the various treatment options. Familiarity with all of the easily available option is essential to good patient care. The following section provides an overview of the commonly used modalities for the treatment of incontinence.

UNSTABLE DETRUSOR

The terminology accepted by the International Continence Society defines the unstable detrusor as "one that is shown objectively to contract, spontaneously or on provocation, during filling phase while the patient is attempting to inhibit micturition"(Figs. 19-12 and 19-13).[21] If there is an associated neurologic disorder, the condition is called detrusor hyperreflexia. The incidence of the unstable bladder increases with age, occurring less than 5% of the time in the very young, progressing to as much as 38% in the elderly, and reaching nearly 80% in the institutionalized incontinent patient.[22] Coexistent genuine stress incontinence and detrusor instability (mixed incontinence) occurs in about 30% of patients with genuine stress urinary incontinence (GSUI).

Detrusor instability may result from a variety of etiologies, including cerebrovascular accident, neurologic disorders, outlet obstruction, and local irritation or infection. The most common causes are

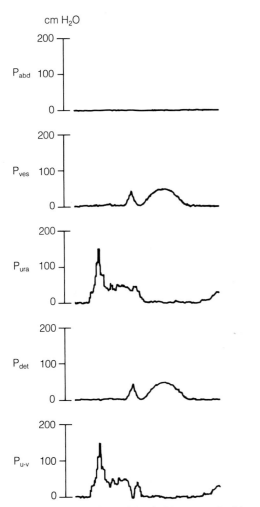

Figure 19–12. Unstable bladder, provoked by catheter movement.

idiopathic and psychogenic. The symptom complex associated with this condition includes urgency, frequency, urge incontinence, and nocturia. Symptoms of stress incontinence may accompany this disorder, thus history alone is not diagnostic. A history of childhood or adult-onset enuresis is highly predictive of the presence of this disorder but is uncommonly reported. The classic presentation is that of a postmenopausal female who complains of a sudden strong urge to void, followed by an involuntary loss of urine if she is not able to void immediately. The physical examination is generally not useful except in the evaluation of other conditions. The condition may be strongly suspected, however, based on the history, physical examination, and simple cystometrogram just described, with the addition of the appropriate laboratory examinations and urinary diary. If performed, urodynamic testing reveals uninhibited detrusor contraction with involuntary loss of urine and an inability to inhibit that contraction during a standing cystometrogram with provocative maneuvers. Uroflowmetry may reveal a normal or obstructed voiding pattern, with incomplete emptying.

Treatment alternatives for the unstable bladder include behavioral interventions, pharmacologic therapy, and electrical stimulation.

Behavioral Intervention

Treatment regimens for unstable bladder are based on the premise that the patient has lost cortical control mechanism learned during childhood and must be taught to regain that control. The primary behavioral intervention is the bladder drill. The purpose of the bladder drill is to gradually increase the interval between voiding, increase the volume the patient can hold, and to decrease or stop urgency and leaking. The patient is given a rigid, timed voiding schedule, to which she must agree to adhere. She is instructed that she is to void at a certain interval, initially every half hour or every hour, depending on the severity of urgency and leakage documented on her urinary diary. She is to void at the prescribed time, even if she does not need to urinate. If she feels the urge to void before that interval, she must wait. The patient is asked to keep a urinary diary. Once this has been mastered, the prescribed interval is increased by 15 minutes and progressively increased until the interval between voiding is down to every 2 to 3 hours. Use of this method of therapy is well known and found to be effective, with cure rates in the range of 75% to 85%.[23]

Another form of behavioral therapy is biofeed-

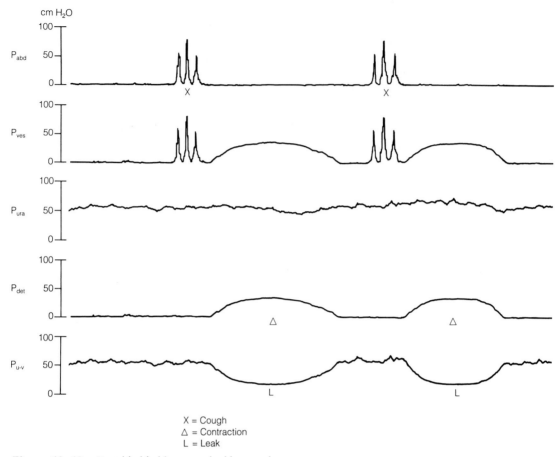

X = Cough
△ = Contraction
L = Leak

Figure 19–13.   Unstable bladder, provoked by cough.

back, which uses auditory or visual feedback for the patient. This feedback may be instituted on the first teaching session or on an ongoing basis. It is useful in conjunction with the cystometrogram to teach the patient to recognize low-level detrusor contractions and to suppress the urge associated with them. This requires additional expense, however, and may not be practical for physicians in an ambulatory setting.

Drug Therapy

There are many agents available for the treatment of unstable bladder (Table 19-2). The mainstay of therapy includes drugs that have some anticholinergic effects. Others that are less commonly used and less well studied include the antispasmodics, antidepressants, calcium-channel blockers, and antiprostaglandins.

Anticholinergic drugs used in the treatment of unstable bladder do not act specifically on the bladder and thus produce an array of anticholinergic side effects. The most intolerable of these is dryness of the mouth. Others include constipation, tachycardia, drowsiness, confusion, and blurred vision. Anticholinergic agents are contraindicated in patients with closed-angle glaucoma. The major drugs in this anticholinergic class are methantheline bromide (Banthine), 50 mg four times daily, and Pro-Banthine, 30 mg four times daily. Effectiveness with these medications in relieving the unstable bladder approached 82% in one study by Walter; however, the drug was reported by some to be equivalent to placebo.[24] Despite a failure to demonstrate an overall success with the drug, it is used widely among practitioners.

Oxybutynin chloride is the most widely prescribed medication for the medical treatment of an unstable bladder. It has antispasmodic and local anesthetic effect and has both anticholinergic and

Table 19–2
Drugs for the Treatment of Unstable Bladder

Classification	Drug	Dosage	Comments
Anticholinergics	Propantheline bromide Banthine	15–30 mg bid to tid 150 mg qid or bid	Relatively inexpensive but contraindicated in patients with narrow-angle glaucoma
Spasmolytics	Oxybutynin chloride	5–10 mg tid	Oxybutynin can be given 2.5 mg tid to qid, with similar results
	Flavoxate hydrochloride	200 mg qid	No benefit seen in randomized controlled studies
Tricyclic agents	Imipramine	25–50 mg bid 10–25 mg bid to tid in elderly	Side effects may be particularly problematic in the elderly
Calcium-channel blockers	Terodiline Nifedipine	25 mg bid 10 mg tid	Studied extensively in Europe— has both anticholinergic and calcium-channel-blocking activity; side effects include xerostomia and decreased visual acuity; not yet FDA approved
Prostaglandin synthetase inhibitors	Indomethacin Ibuprofen Mefanic acid	50–100 mg bid 600–800 mg tid 250–500 mg tid	In vitro studies suggest theoretic benefit in preventing bladder contraction; no good clinical trials demonstrating efficacy

smooth muscle–relaxant properties. Several studies show it to be superior or equal in efficacy to the anticholinergics.[25] Side effects are similar to those of the anticholinergics in frequency and severity.

Tricyclic antidepressants (specifically, imipramine) have gained urologic acceptance for the treatment of enuresis in children. It is not known how it produces its effect but it has significant success in the treatment of unstable bladder.[26] Its use in the elderly is somewhat restricted by its multiple side effects, specifically orthostatic hypotension, conduction disturbances, and altered mental status.

Electrical Stimulation

Increasingly, physicians are using electrical stimulation for the treatment of unstable bladder. Evidence obtained in a study by Lindstrom suggests that electrical stimulation activates inhibitory nerve fibers in the sympathetic hypogastric nerve while simultaneously exciting the neurons in the pelvic nerve, leading to reflex detrusor inhibition.[27] Fall reported on a series of 40 women with incontinence, 20 of whom had detrusor instability.[27a] Nine women with detrusor instability were cured after withdrawal of stimulation for longer than 6 months but in most cases, continuous or intermittent stimulation was necessary to maintain continence.

Eriksen, in a study of 71 women with stress, motor-urge, and mixed stress and urge incontinence, found 55 of the women were treated successfully using an anal electrode.[28] Although recurrent use of electrical stimulation may be required, patient acceptance with the newer devices is improved and may lead to a lasting cure.

GENUINE STRESS INCONTINENCE

Stress incontinence is defined as an involuntary loss of urine from the bladder through the urethra by a sudden increase of intra-abdominal pressure without a detrusor contraction. Patients with this condition present with complaints of loss of urine with coughing, sneezing, laughing, exercise. Once diagnosed, discussion with the patient should include a brief description of the various treatment options. For women with severe stress incontinence, surgery is generally accepted to be the best choice. For women with mild to moderate stress incontinence, the management must be individualized. There are some patients for whom surgery is unwanted and inappropriate—for example, women who simply do not want surgery, women who are not medically stable, or those who desire further

Table 19–3
Guidelines for Nonsurgical Management of Incontinence

Decrease bladder volume
    Timed voiding
    Fluid management
Increase urethral pressure
    Try α-agonist
    Avoid α blockers
    No caffeine
Improve pressure transmission
    Estrogen
    Pessary
    Pelvic-floor exercises
        Exercises alone
        Cones
        Biofeedback
        Electrical stimulation

childbearing, the effect of which is unknown and may adversely affect a repair. Before the surgeon and the patient choose the surgical option, they should be aware of the many nonsurgical approaches available to address this multifactorial disease. The nonsurgical options discussed include decreasing bladder volume, increasing urethral pressure, and improving pressure transmission (Table 19-3).

Bladder Volume

Earlier in the chapter, the value of the urinary diary was discussed as was the impact the information can have on treatment. If one identifies the infrequent voider, simply decreasing the interval of the void may decrease the incontinent episodes. The urinary diary may also identify the over-drinker. Changing the patient's fluid-intake habits may provide an easy cure. From the diary, events that trigger incontinence can be identified. Occasionally, one realizes that the incontinence is occurring only during a specific type of exercise (ie, leaking during aerobics or jogging). If this is the case, the simplest and least invasive solution is to change the type of exercise being performed. Swimming is an excellent alternative, providing an excellent cardiovascular and total body workout while allowing the woman to be free from embarrassment should incontinence occur.

In addition to modification of behavior in the over-drinker and infrequent voider, the urinary di-ary can be used in the implementation of the bladder drill. Fantl, in a study of 123 noninstitutionalized women, found implementation of the bladder drill to be effective in 57% of the incontinent females, with similar success in both the patient with detrusor instability and the patient with urethral sphincter incompetence (genuine stress incontinence).[28a] Overall quantity of urine lost was reduced by 54% across both groups. A recommendation resulting from these findings is the need to include the bladder drill as a noninvasive first step in the treatment of incontinence.

Urethral Pressure

Urethral pressure is generated under resting conditions by the interaction of urethral smooth muscle, periurethral striated muscle, and a combination of collagen–vascular–elastic tissue components. The smooth muscle component is under α-adrenergic control. Stimulation of these receptors with sympathomimetic drugs may increase outlet resistance and significantly decrease urinary leakage in many patients. Stewart reported 23% were cured and 36% markedly improved in patients treated with Ornade.[29] Collste studied 24 women in a double-blind placebo controlled study using phenylpropanolamine (PPA). Fourteen patients preferred PPA, four preferred placebo, and six found both ineffective. Closure pressure was significantly increased, and this correlated to an improvement of symptoms.[30] Different agents that have been employed include ephedrine, pseudoephedrine, phenylpropanolamine, and propadrine. Table 19-4 lists specific dosages for these agents.

Conversely, α-adrenergic–blocking medications lower outlet resistance. Prazosin hydrochloride has been shown to be associated with incontinence. Elimination of this medication may result in a cure. In addition, the use of a moderate amount of caffeine not only acts as a diuretic, increasing the urinary volume, but effectively lowers urethral pressure, thus altering the urethral continence mechanism.

Improved Pressure Transmission

There are three nonsurgical methods of increasing pressure transmission to the urethra: insertion of a pessary, estrogen, and pelvic floor muscle retraining.

Table 19–4

Over-the-Counter and Prescription Medications
With α-Adrenergic Properties

Drug	Dosage
Pseudoephedrine (Sudafed)	15–30 mg tid
Phenylpropanolamine (Ornade)	50–75 mg tid
Phenylpropanolamine HCl	
(Dexatrim)	50 mg tid
(Contac S-R)	75 mg bid
(Appedine)	25 mg tid
Imipramine (Tofranil)*	10–15 mg tid

*Has both α-adrenergic and anticholinergic properties.

Use of a pessary can improve pressure transmission to the urethra by elevating the urethrovesical junction, thereby placing the urethra back into an intraabdominal position. The problem is trying to find a pessary large enough to elevate the urethrovesical angle without obstructing the urethra or causing vaginal discomfort. For a select group of women, the pessary is a reasonable alternative to surgery or a good temporizing mechanism to allow increased continence while undergoing a pelvic floor muscle-strengthening program. Use of the pessary is not without side effects. Many women discontinue use secondary to pain, vaginal discharge, difficulty voiding, vaginal erosion, inability to hold the pessary in place, and impaction.

Estrogen Use

It is well known that vaginal and urethral tissues are sensitive to hormonal manipulation. Hilton, in a study of 10 women, found that there was a significant reduction of symptoms of stress incontinence, urgency, and difficulty voiding with the use of estrogen, despite there being no significant increase in closure pressure or functional length.[31] Hilton found overall improvement in pressure transmission, however. Fantl, in a 1988 comparison study of estrogenized and nonestrogenized women, found no direct effect of estrogen supplementation on urethral function, despite a decrease in nocturia and urine volume lost.[32] Initially, estrogens are best administered vaginally. Response occasionally does not occur until after 2 months of therapy.

Pelvic Floor Muscle Retraining

Strengthening of the pelvic floor muscle can increase urethral pressure and improve pressure transmission. If the vaginal attachments to the levator ani muscles have not been torn, tightening of the pelvic floor muscle raises the urethrovesical junction into an intraabdominal position. If the muscles are tightened during increases in intra-abdominal pressure, improved pressure transmission results. Strengthening may be augmented with vaginal cones, biofeedback, and electrical stimulation. The success of any pelvic floor muscle retraining depends on patient education, compliance, and motivation to avoid surgery.

An effective Kegel exercise program involves (1) identification of the muscles, (2) strengthening the muscle, and (3) teaching the patient how to use her muscles under stress. The physician should feel the muscle contraction and assess the baseline muscle strength so that some documentation of improvement can be made (Fig. 19-14). Learning may be facilitated by having the patient feel the contraction in her vagina and visualize the pelvic floor with a mirror while she contracts the levator ani muscles. Rapid contraction of the pelvic floor is designed to strengthen fast-twitch fibers, and sustained contraction of the pelvic floor is designed to strengthen slow-twitch fibers. A combination of exercises is necessary to attain a satisfactory result. Of primary importance is teaching the patient how to use her muscles under stress. She must be taught to automatically contract during any increase in abdominal pressure. To facilitate learning of muscle use during daily activity, the patient must be instructed to exercise in a variety of settings (ie, she must practice contracting with coughing, lifting, and laughing). The patient must be monitored consistently over time, and at least 2 months of exercises are usually required to see results. Ferguson and coworkers, in a study of a 6-week pelvic exercise program, showed significant increase in muscle strength and decrease in urinary incontinence in the 20 patients studied; however, a year later, only 50% were still exercising and only 25% were still improved. Three patients elected surgical intervention.[33]

Vaginal Cones

Vaginal cones were designed by Plevnik to improve the ability of the muscle to contract. The cones are of equal shape and volume but of increasing weight, from 20 to 100 g. Patients begin with the heaviest cone they can retain without voluntarily holding the

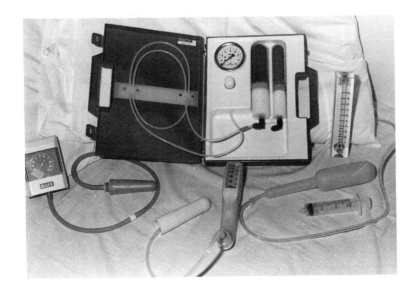

Figure 19–14. Perineometers, useful for measuring baseline muscle strength and assessing patients' progress. Patient is asked to squeeze her pelvic floor muscles and hold, and the pressure generated during the squeeze is recorded.

cone and retain this cone for 15 minutes twice daily. Once the patient feels comfortable, she is instructed to graduate to a heavier weight. Peattie and colleagues demonstrated a 70% cure rate among 30 premenopausal women awaiting surgery using this method.[34]

Electrical Stimulation

Electrical stimulation with rectal or vaginal probes has been used successfully to facilitate storage and prevent urine leakage with stress. Use of the stimulator mimics Kegel exercises and might be described as an electrical "Kegeler"(Fig. 19-15). Tan-

agho and Schmidt found prolonged stimulation in dogs produced muscle hypertrophy. Stimulated fibers showed increased glycolytic activity, thus increasing fatigue resistance.[35] Eriksen and Eik-Nes demonstrated in 55 women that anal electrical stimulation with stress, urge, and mixed incontinence could cure 68% of patients. At 2 years, success was reduced to 56% and 36% had undergone surgery[36]; however, in the high compliance group, 72% remained cured at 2 years. A variety of modalities exist to deliver the electrical stimulation therapy. Eriksen and Plevnik used chronic intermittent stimulation;[36a,36b] however, Godec reported success using acute maximal stimulation, with 17 of 20 pa-

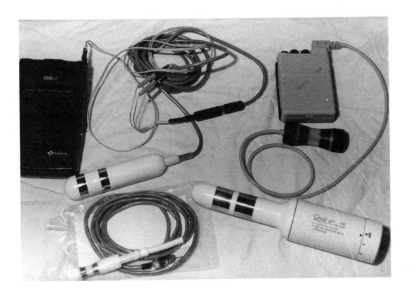

Figure 19–15. Multiple devices for electrical stimulation.

tients reporting relief or improvement.[37] Newer modalities promise to be more user-friendly and convenient to encourage compliance.

Biofeedback

Biofeedback may also be used in patients with stress incontinence to facilitate correct exercising and compliance (Fig. 19-16). Burgio compared the effectiveness of pelvic floor exercise, using verbal feedback, with a biofeedback device. The biofeedback group had a 50% reduction of leakage.[38] As with any type of exercise, patient compliance and physician involvement vary considerably. Response to any form of conservative therapy is best with younger patients who have had no previous surgery for the condition, have a mild form of stress incontinence, and are motivated. Active involvement of the physician may not be practical for the busy office practitioner but by training existing office personnel to be supportive, patient compliance can be improved and thus outcome.

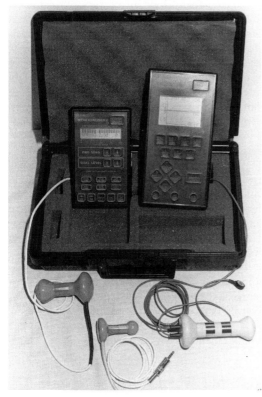

Figure 19–16. There are many devices available for biofeedback that provide auditory or visual feedback for a correctly performed contraction. Verimed myoexerciser shown here.

DISORDERS PRODUCING SENSORY COMPLAINTS

Conditions occurring in the urinary tract that cause dysuria, frequency, or urgency are cystitis, urethritis, urethral syndrome, urethral diverticulum, and interstitial cystitis. The diagnosis and treatment of these disorders follow.

The most common of the conditions yielding a sensory complaint is that of cystitis. Bacterial infection of the urinary tract is the most common human bacterial infection, occurring 10 times more often in females than in males, except in the neonate. Its prevalence increases with age, occurring in almost 10% of women older than the age of 50 years. Predisposing factors include poor toilet hygiene, introital colonization through sexual activity, compromise of the immune defense, shortened urethra, and any factor leading to compromise of the vesical defense (ie, infrequent or incomplete voiding). Most of these infections are related to sexual intercourse.

The condition is classically confirmed by the presence of 100,000 urine colony count on a clean-catch specimen. Stamm, in a study of colony counts after suprapubic aspiration of women with acute dysuria, demonstrated that the traditional criterion of a more than 10^5 colony count identified only 51% of women whose urine contained coliform.[39] He concluded that the best diagnostic criterion is 10^2 colony count.

For most patients experiencing their first infection, 80% to 85% of the time the pathogen is *Escherichia coli*, sensitive to all antibiotics. The remaining pathogens include *Staphylococcus saprophyticus*, *Pseudomonas*, *Klebsiella*, and other species.

Use of antibiotics in the preceding 3 months changes the bacterial flora and may lead to resistant strains and colonization with *Klebsiella* or *Candida* species or enteroccoci and other bacteria.[40] Therapy may be of a variety of lengths. Single-dose therapies are almost comparable in efficacy but may result in a higher recurrence rate. Greenberg, in a randomized trial of single dose, 3-day, and 7-day therapy with trimethoprim–sulfamethoxazole, found single-dose–therapy patients to have a significantly higher rate of recurrence (Table 19-5).[41]

Recurrent infection is defined as reinfection with different bacterial strains rather than a persistence of the same bacteria. Infection with a different bacteria is the cause of recurrent infection in most cases. Bacterial persistence within the kidney or elsewhere in the urinary tract is rare indeed. The

Table 19–5
Efficacy of Antibiotic Treatment for Bacterial Infection of the Urinary Tract

Agent	Cured in 3 Days (%)	Cured in 4 Weeks (%)
Cefadroxil, 100 mg as a single dose	47	25
Cefadroxil, 500 mg bid for 3 days	68	58
Cefadroxil, 500 mg bid for 7 days	83	70
TMP-SMX, 320–1600 mg as a single dose	91	65
TMP-SMX, 160–800 mg bid for 3 days	96	88

knowledge that almost all recurrent infections are reinfection is key to the concept that recurrence is treated with prophylaxis, not with more or stronger antimicrobial agents. The regimen most commonly used is 100 mg nitrofurantoin after intercourse and at first episode of dysuria.

Acute urethritis usually results from an infection of the urethra with either *Chlamydia*, gonorrhea, or the trichomonads. The resulting symptom complex is classically characterized by dysuria, urgency, and frequency, with accompanying pyuria, with or without bacteriuria. The microscopic appearance of the urine may give a clue to the nature of the infection when traditional culture shows no growth. Treatment with an appropriate antimicrobial covering both gonorrhea and *Chlamydia* species usually results in cure.

Urethral syndrome is characterized by chronic symptoms of urgency, frequency, and dysuria, without obvious and distinct cause. The multiple causes ascribed to this symptom complex include infection, vaginitis, hypoestrogenism, allergy, obstruction, and psychiatric disturbances. The leading theory regarding etiology and pathogenesis of the chronic urethritis is that the condition results from inflammation and infection in the periurethral and Skene's glands. Complaints should be assessed with urinalysis to detect pyuria, with chlamydial culture, and with urethroscopy. Wet-mount and vaginal culture should be performed to rule out infection with *Candida* species or bacterial vaginosis. If the patient has a positive culture, the patient should first receive antibiotic treatment. Stamm and coworkers studied 42 women with urethral syndrome and found 11 of 42 positive for *Chlamydia trachomatis*. Additionally, all patients who were both culture- and pyuria-positive responded to antimicrobial therapy; however, there was no effect in patients who were pyuria-negative.[42]

If the initial investigation and treatment fail to result in a cure, urethroscopy should be performed.

Urethroscopic findings include redness and exudate, which eventually lead to the formation of inflammatory fronds and cysts. Urethroscopy and culture should be combined with a urinary diary and simple cystometrogram. The patient with the sensation of urgency without dysuria and normal cystometrogram is most liking voiding at first sensation. Therapy in that case should be directed at behavioral intervention, using bladder drills. For patients who fail to respond to either of the described modalities, there are a variety of treatments available for this condition. Dilation and urethral massage may be performed. This treatment modality is thought to be effective by expelling inspissated mucous and debris from the infected periurethral glands. Suburethral trigger-point injection of steroids is also used to combat inflammation and promote healing. Other treatment modalities include cryosurgery, laser surgery, topical antibiotics, and surgical removal of the glands, none of which have been studied in controlled trials.

Hypoestrogenic urethritis is a condition resulting from estrogen depletion and atrophic changes. Women with this condition also complain of frequency, urgency, nocturia, and dysuria. Physical examination reveals an atrophic urethra and vagina, which is often pale or red and friable. Urethral caruncle and urethral prolapse are also common. Endoscopically, the urethra is pale and friable, with or without stenosis. In addition to the symptoms of dysuria and frequency, difficulty voiding may accompany this condition. Treatment with vaginal estrogen cream usually ameliorates symptoms but urethral dilation may periodically be required.

Urethral Diverticulum

Urethral diverticulum is an out-pouching of the wall of the urethra, occurring anywhere along its length. Although diverticula may be asymptomatic, the most common presenting symptoms are dysuria, frequency, urgency, and postvoid dribbling. Other symptoms include incontinence, recurrent urinary tract infection, pain, and postvoid dribbling. Diagnosis is easiest if there is a visible mass sub- or periurethral, from which pus is expressed with pressure. Confirmation and localization of the diverticulum is performed with the use of urethrocystoscopy and voiding cystourethrogram.

Surgical correction is warranted after treatment of acute infection in patients with large diverticula that are symptomatic. Small diverticula may initially be treated with urethral dilation and antibiotics or marsupialized and drained before surgical excision. Multiple methods of surgical correction are available. The procedure selected depends on location of the diverticula, presence of multiple diverticula, age, and symptoms of the patient.

Interstitial Cystitis

Interstitial cystitis is an uncommon disease of the bladder, leading to painful progressive fibrosis and contraction of the urinary bladder. Ninety percent of all reported cases occur in women. The pathogenesis of the condition is unclear, with multiple etiologic entities proposed, ranging from infectious agents, genetic abnormalities, allergies, lymphatic obstruction, and collagen vascular disease. A theory proposed by Parsons is that the condition results from a defective bladder surface coat of GAG glycoaminosglycans.[43] In its most severe form, there is greatly diminished bladder contraction and visible scarring of the bladder lining. There appears, however, to be a subgroup of patients who are younger and have symptoms of interstitial cystitis without the diminution of bladder capacity under anesthesia.

The patients suffer a symptom complex of frequency, nocturia, small urinary volume when voiding, and a feeling of pain and pressure with the least volume of urine in the bladder. Dyspareunia is commonly reported. Painful vulvar syndrome and endometriosis have been associated with interstitial cystitis.[44] Diagnostic criteria include:

1. Urinary frequency
2. Pain relieved by voiding
3. Negative urine culture
4. Typical cystoscopic appearance

The typical cystoscopic appearance is that of small, discrete submucosal hemorrhages early in the disease, followed by linear cracking and the classic Hunner's ulcer. Random biopsies in the presence of these finding are helpful to rule out carcinoma in situ and to confirm the presence or absence of mast cells. Those women with mast cells may represent an entirely different population of patients than those women with an absence of mast cells. Mast cells are thought to be released secondary to some unidentified allergen and are associated with the release of histamine, which is thought to be related to the pain of interstitial cystitis. This may imply some useful role of antihistamines. Histologic manifestations include nonspecific inflammation of the bladder and submucosa, with vasodilation and edema.

The mainstay therapy in our clinic includes the use of bladder pillar block and triamcinolone steroid injection, followed by bladder distention and instillation of dimethyl sulfoxide. The patient is usually given several of these treatments in the office and prescribed amitriptyline for home use. Bladder drills are later employed once the pain and frequency are under control. The individual components of the common therapies are discussed below.

Dimethyl sulfoxide has anti-inflammatory effects and breaks down and blocks conduction of peripheral nerves.[45] In addition to those effects, it also provides some local analgesia and has bacteriostatic and vasodilating effects. Barker found that satisfactory symptomatic relief was achieved in 80% of patients completing therapy, with no significant side effects.[46]

Elmiron (sodium pentosanpoly sulfate) is being studied for the treatment of patients with interstitial cystitis. Its mechanism of action is unclear but it appears to be that of protecting the surface mucin lining of the bladder (GAG layer). The glycosaminoglycan in the bladder help prevent bacterial adherence to the bladder. When heparin (a glycosaminoglycan) is instilled into the lumen of a mucous-deficient bladder, the heparin binds to the surface and prevents microbial adherence to the bladder lining. Pentosanpolysulfate works similar to heparin and has the advantage of being in the oral form—3% to 6% of which is excreted in the urine—yet it has virtually no anticoagulant properties. Parsons found that 80% of patients had decreased pain, urgency, and nocturia; however, Holmbertzen, in a placebo-controlled study, found no clinical or statistical effect of the drug.[47,48]

Amytrptyline is useful in patients with interstitial cystitis to aid in the relief of symptoms of urgency and pelvic pain. Hanno and colleagues reported decreases in the pain and daytime frequency as well as complete relief in eight of 25 patients treated with medication alone.[48a]

Other therapies include hydrodistension under anesthesia, thought to result in nerve plexus stretching and thus increasing bladder capacity. Parsons reported that bladder drills significantly decrease symptoms by 50% in up to 70% of those treated.[49] Less common therapies include electrical stimulation, bladder infiltration with steroids, transurethral resection, instillation of silver nitrate, and laser surgery of the bladder.

Whichever therapy is chosen for the patient, a great deal of intensive psychological counseling is necessary to adequately control the pain. We have seen several women who, with careful exploration of their past, revealed history of sexual or physical abuse. In these women, the symptoms do not resolve when only medical therapy is instituted. Whatever the therapy, this clinical entity is debilitating and difficult to treat.

CONCLUSION

The National Institutes of Health sponsored the first consensus conference on incontinence in 1988. Subsequently, the institute has published guidelines mandating physician knowledge and education about diagnosis and treatment options for incontinence and other urinary infirmities affecting adults. This chapter provides the general gynecologist an overview of the diagnosis and nonsurgical treatments for most causes of incontinence and an overview of a few of the most common urinary tract infirmities affecting women. It is not designed to be all-inclusive because there are entire textbooks written on the subject. What has been provided is the basic knowledge necessary for the practicing physician to begin to address this under-investigated and under-addressed area.

REFERENCES

1. Hording U, Pedersen K, Sidenius K, et al: Urinary incontinence in 45-year-old women. Scand J Urol Nephrol 20:183, 1986
2. Diokno AC, Brock BM, Brown MB, Herzog AR: Prevalence of urinary incontinence and other urological symptoms in the non- institutionalized elderly. J Urol 136:1022, 1986
3. Delancey JOL: Correlative study of paraurethral anatomy. Obstet Gynecol 68:91, 1986
4. Delancey JOL: Anatomy of the female bladder and urethra. In Ostergard D, Bent A (eds): Urogynecology and urodynamics, 3rd ed, p 11. Baltimore, Williams & Wilkins, 1991
5. Whiteside CG, Arnold EP: Persistent primary enuresis: a urodynamic assessment. Br Med J 1:364, 1975
6. Cardozo L, Stanton SL: Genuine stress incontinence and detrusor instability: a clinical and urodynamic review of 200 cases. Br J Obstet Gynaecol 87:184, 1980
7. Jarvis GJ, Hall S, Millar DR, et al: An assessment of urodynamic examination in incontinent women. Br J Obstet Gynaecol 87:893, 1980
8. Quigley GJ: The epidemiology of urethral-vesical dysfunction in the female patient. Am J Obstet Gynecol 151:220, 1985
8a. Resnick NM: Urinary incontinence in the elderly. Hospital Practice, Nov 1986
9. Stage P, Fischer-Ramussen W, Hansen R: The value of colpo-cysto-urethrography in female stress and urge incontinence and following operation. Acta Obstet Gynecol Scand 65:402, 1986
10. Walters MD, Diaz K: Q-tip test: a study of continent and incontinent women. Obstet Gynecol 70:208, 1987
11. Montz FJ, Stanton SL: Q-tip test in female urinary incontinence. Obstet Gynecol 67:258, 1986
12. Benson JT, Sumners JE, Pittman JS: Definition of normal female pelvic anatomy using ultrasonic techniques. J Clin Ultrasound 19:275, 1991
13. Chang HC, Chang SC, Kuo HC, Tsai TC: Transrectal sonographic cystourethrography: studies in stress urinary incontinence. Urology 36:488, 1990
14. Vierhout ME, Janssen H: Supine and sitting rectal ultrasound of the bladder neck during relaxation, straining, and squeezing. Int Urogynecol J :141, 1991
15. Richardson DA, Bent AE, Ostergard DR: The effect of uterovaginal prolapse on urethral vesical pressure dynamics. Am J Obstet Gynecol 146:901, 1983
16. Bergman A, Kooning PP, Ballard CA: Predicting postoperative urinary incontinence development in women undergoing operation for genitourinary prolapse. Am J Obstet Gynecol 158:1171, 1988
17. Jorgensen L, Lose G, Andersen JT: One hour pad-weighing test for objective assessment of female incontinence. Obstet Gynecol 69:39, 1987
18. Richardson DA: Value of cough pressure profile in the valuation of patients with stress incontinence. Am J Obstet Gynecol 155:808, 1986
19. Vensi E, Cardozo L, Studd J, et al: The urinary sphincter in the maintenance of female continence. Br J Med 292:166, 1986
20. Scotti R, Ostergard D, Guillaume A, Kohatsu K: Predictive value of urethroscopy as compared to urodynamics in the diagnosis of genuine stress incontinence. J Reprod Med 772, 1990
21. Abrams P, Blavias JG, Stanton SL, Andersen JT: Standardization of terminology of lower urinary tract function. Neurourol Urodyn 7:403, 1988
22. Starer P, Libow S: Lays measurement of residual urine in the evaluation of incontinent nursing home residents. Arch Gerontol Geriatr 7:75, 1988
23. Frewen WK: A reassessment of bladder training

in detrusor dysfunction in the female. Br J Urol 54:372, 1982

24. Walter S: Detrusor hyperreflexia in female urinary incontinence treated pharmacologically. Urol Int 33:316, 1978

25. Holmes DM, Montz FJ, Stanton SL: Oxybutynin versus probanthine in the management of detrusor instability: a patient-regulated variable dose trial. Br J Obstet Gynaecol 96:607, 1988

26. Castleden CM, Duffin HM, Gulati RS: Double blind study of imipramine and placebo for incontinence due to bladder instability. Age Ageing 15:299, 1986

27. Lindstrom S, Fall M, Carlson CA, Erlandson BE: The neurophysiology basis of bladder inhibition in response to intravaginal electrical stimulation. J Urol 129:405, 1983

27a. Fall M: Does electrostimulation cure urinary incontinence? J Urology 131:664, 1981

28. Eriksen BC, Bergman S, Mjolnerod OK: Effects of anal electrical stimulation with the "Incontan" device in women with urinary incontinence. Br J Obstet Gynaecol 94:147, 1987

28a. Fantl JA, Hurt WG, Dunn W: Detrusor instability syndrome: the use of bladder retraining drills with and without anticholinergics. Am J Obstet Gynecol 140:885, 1981

29. Stewart BH: Stress incontinence: conservative therapy with sympatho-mimetic drugs. J Urol 115:558, 1976

30. Collste L: Phenopropanolamine in the treatment if female stress urinary incontinence. Urology 30:358, 1987

31. Hilton P: The use of intravaginal estrogen cream in genuine stress incontinence. Br J Obstet Gynaecol 90:940, 1983

32. Fantl JA, Wyman J, Anderson MS, Matt D, Bump R: Postmenopausal urinary incontinence: comparison between non-estrogen supplemented and estrogen supplemented women. Postmenopausal urinary incontinence: comparison between non-estrogen supplemented and estrogen-supplemented women. Obstet Gynecol 71:823, 1988

33. Ferguson KL, McKey PL, Bishop KK, Kloen P, Verheul JB, Dougherty MC: Stress urinary incontinence: effective pelvic muscle exercises. Obstet Gynecol 75:671, 1990

34. Peattie AB, Pelvnik S, Stanton SL: Vaginal cones: a conservative method of treating genuine stress incontinence. Br J Obstet Gynaecol 95:1049, 1988

35. Tanagho EA, Schmidt RA: Electrical stimulation in the clinical management of the neurogenic bladder. J Urol 140:1331, 1988

36. Eriksen BC, Eik-Nes SH: Long term electro-stimulation of the pelvic floor: primary therapy in female stress incontinence: Urol Int 44:90, 1989

36a. Eriksen BC, Eik-Nes SH: Longer-term electrostimulation of the pelvic floor: primary therapy in female stress incontinence? Urologica Internationalis 44(2):90, 1979

36b. Plevnik S, Janez J: Maximal electrical stimulation for urinary incontinence. Urology 14(6):638, 1979

37. Godec C, Cass A: Acute electrical stimulation for urinary incontinence. Urology 12:340, 1978

38. Burgio KL: Urinary incontinence in the elderly: bladder sphincter biofeedback and toilet skills training. Ann Intern Med 104:507, 1985

39. Stamm W, Counts GW, Running KM, Finn S, Turck M, Holmes K: Diagnosis of coliform infection in acutely dysuric women. N Engl J Med 307:463, 1982

40. Stamey T: Recurrent urinary tract infections in female patients: an overview of management and treatment. Rev Infect Dis 9(Suppl 2):S195, 1987

41. Greenberg RN, Reilly PM, Luppen KL, Weinandt WJ, Ellington LL, Bollinger MR: Randomized study of single dose, three day, and seven day treatment of cystitis in women. J Infect Dis 153:277, 1986

42. Stamm WE, Wagner K, Amsel R, et al: Causes of acute urethral syndrome in women. N Engl J Med 303:409, 1980

43. Parsons CL, Schmidt JD, Pollen JJ: Successful treatment of interstitial cystitis with sodium pentosanpolysulfate. J Urol 130:51, 1983

44. Sircus SI, Sant GR, Ucci AA: Bladder detrusor endometriosis mimicking interstitial cystitis. Urology 32:339, 1988

45. Sant GR: Intravesical fifty percent dimethyl sulfoxide (Rimso-50) in the treatment of interstitial cystitis. Urology 29:17, 1987

46. Barker SB: Prospective study of intravesicle dimethyl sulfoxide in the chronic inflammatory bladder disease. Br J Urol 59:142, 1987

47. Parsons CL: Successful treatment of interstitial cystitis with pentsanpoly sulfate. J Urol 138:513, 1987

48. Holm-Bertzen M: A prospective double-blind, placebo controlled, multi-center trial of sodium pentosanpoly sulfate in the treatment of interstitial cystitis and related painful bladder disease. J Urol 138:503, 1987

48a. Hanno P, Levin PM, Mon IC, et al: Diagnosis of interstitial cystitis. Br J Urol 66(3):265, 1990

49. Parsons CL: Interstitial cystitis: successful management by increasing voiding intervals. Urology 37:207, 1991

Ambulatory Gynecology, Second Edition,
edited by David H. Nichols and Patrick J. Sweeney.
J. B. Lippincott Company, Philadelphia, © 1995.

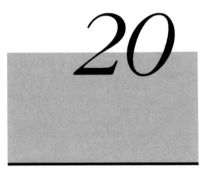

The Vaginal Pessary

David H. Nichols and Peter Julian

USES OF A VAGINAL PESSARY

A properly fitted pessary can provide support for dropped, sagging, or prolapsed pelvic tissues in a symptomatic patient who cannot yet undergo surgery; hold in anteversion a symptomatic retroverted uterus; or restore temporarily a defective vaginal depth and the proper angle of the vaginouterine axis in a patient experiencing habitual abortion. In a patient with a mild genital prolapse or uterine retroversion in association with a backache, the use of a properly fitted vaginal pessary may indicate the amount of relief that can be expected from restorative surgery. It may be used as a test for the results one might anticipate from surgery for urinary incontinence and may be helpful after an unsuccessful prolapse repair by providing a window for emotional, physical, and social spacing before another surgical repair experience.[1]

The patient who wears a pessary must be regularly examined, the pessary removed and cleaned, and the vagina inspected for infection or ulceration. If the latter are found, the pessary is temporarily removed and an intravaginal sulfa cream prescribed in addition to a course of intravaginal estrogen.

When the vagina has healed, the pessary is replaced.

Active pelvic inflammation contraindicates the use of a pessary; as a foreign body, it increases pelvic congestion and discomfort. Fixed retroversion of the uterus and pain after insertion are also contraindications to the use of a pessary.

The patient and her family should understand that a pessary is often a temporary treatment (unless life expectancy is shortened) because the patient may demonstrate vaginal stretching and coincident levator atrophy or neuromuscular disability over a long period of time, requiring placement with a pessary of larger size. Ultimately, such a patient is no longer be able to retain a pessary.

Diagnosis of Backache and Pelvic Pressure

Most multiparas and a few nulliparas have some degree of genital relaxation, and many have coincident symptomatic low backache. The gynecologist must decide whether such a backache is the result of the genital prolapse or of some nongenital problem (eg, urologic trouble, lumbosacral strain, sacroiliac disorder, intervertebral disk disorder, or osteoarthritis).

The backache that is of gynecologic origin and is related to the displacement of pelvic structures characteristically is absent in the morning, coming on during the day, grows worse as the day progresses, and eases when the woman lies down, when the pull of gravity on the displaced pelvic structures has been relieved. In contrast, a chronic backache of orthopedic origin characteristically is most severe in the morning when the patient first arises because it is related to the looseness of the back muscles and the joint instability that develops during sleep. Because the joint instability causes pain, the supporting muscles gradually develop a degree of spasm throughout the day, progressively reducing the instability of the back and the consequent pain so that by evening, the patient is more comfortable.

The patient whose backache has both gynecologic and orthopedic origins is a diagnostic challenge because it may be difficult to identify which factor is the primary contributor to the pain. The use of a carefully chosen and properly fitted vaginal pessary restores the pelvic architecture temporarily and may relieve traction on pelvic structures, facilitating the diagnosis. If pain is relieved the patient may be a good candidate for restorative surgery.[2]

The gynecologist should check the vagina during the first week that the pessary is in place. If properly fitted, the pessary should remain in place for another 2 to 4 weeks before being removed. By noting the amount of pain relief that the patient experiences after the pessary has been put in place, the gynecologist can separate a complex backache into its components and decide how much of the pain results from an orthopedic problem and how much results from a uterine malposition. If the symptoms return after removal of the pessary, appropriate pelvic reconstructive surgery is likely to be successful. If symptoms are unrelieved by a properly fitted pessary, they are probably of orthopedic origin and gynecologic reconstructive surgery is not likely to be helpful.

Any necessary surgery should be performed without undue delay. Even those tissues being supported by a pessary slowly lose their muscle tone as they age, at which time the patient may no longer be able to retain a pessary. In addition, as years pass, the patient's general health may deteriorate, increasing the risks of surgery. Finally, *prolonged* use of a pessary for genital prolapse in the ambulatory patient may injure the pelvic nerves and, by interfering with innervation of the pelvic muscles, further compromise the function of the pelvic floor and even lead to paravaginal anesthesia, decreased anal sphincter tone, increased severity of the prolapse, and both urinary and fecal incontinence.

Temporary Correction of Malpositions of the Uterus and Vagina

Pessaries may be used to correct a symptomatic uterine retroversion. Together with improvement in the patient's posture, the wearing of a pessary may relieve dyspareunia and backache. Poor abdominal pressure transmission is often associated with current or future urinary incontinence among genital prolapse patients with large cystocele.[3] In some instances of urinary stress incontinence associated with rotational descent of the bladder neck, a properly fitted pessary may support the vesicourethral junction and give some indication of the success to be expected from future surgery. The Smith or Hodge pessary may restore urinary continence when worn by the patient with urinary stress incontinence by (1) stabilization of the urethra and vesicourethral junction, and (2) enhancement of urethral resistance through increased urethral length and closure pressure.[4] A pessary may be used temporarily for this purpose as well as for restoration of pelvic comfort in patients for whom surgery is inconvenient.

If urinary incontinence develops in a prolapse patient after insertion of a pessary and if such a patient is to receive surgical repair of her prolapse, she requires the addition of a supplemental surgical procedure at the vesicourethral junction to prevent postoperative incontinence (eg, the addition of a coincident vesicourethral sling procedure).

Obstetric Indications for Use of a Pessary

There are several obstetric indications for the use of a pessary. For example, a pessary may support an enlarging uterus in the pelvis of a pregnant patient with symptomatic genital prolapse.[5] When the enlarging uterus and its contents have become larger than the pelvic inlet (ie, when the cork is bigger than the neck of the bottle), the pessary should be removed. The obstetrician may reinsert the pessary after delivery and allow it to remain in place until the uterus has returned to its normal size. Pessary support of the postpartum uterus may permit faster resolution of subinvolution by improving circulation and reducing venous congestion.

In cases of habitual abortion, in which the axis of the uterus parallels the axis of the vagina, a properly fitted pessary may reposition these axes at right angles to one another, so that increases in intra-abdominal pressure are no longer transmitted directly through the cervix in the axis of the vagina. When successful in reestablishing a normal cervicovaginal angle, such a pessary should be left in place until the patient has reached term; however, it should be removed from time to time during pregnancy, so that the pessary can be cleaned, the vagina inspected, and the pessary replaced. Spontaneous rupture of the membranes and labor may occur within 24 hours of planned removal of the pessary at term.

TYPES OF PESSARIES AND THEIR USES

Several types of pessaries are in use (Fig. 20-1). Because vaginal size not only varies normally but also may change during the aging process, each type of pessary comes in a variety of sizes to fit the configuration of the individual vagina. Modern pessaries are made of Lucite or a softer plastic, and many are notched for easy insertion. A properly fitted pessary causes no symptoms and does not interfere with bowel or bladder function. If the patient finds the pessary uncomfortable or if it interferes with any vital function, the size or design of the pessary is improper for the patient; the pessary should be promptly removed and replaced with one that is more appropriate.

An intravaginal tampon is the simplest of pessaries and may be used for symptomatic relief of minor degrees of prolapse. Retrodisplacement of the uterus is best treated by the Smith, Hodge, or Risser type. The Smith type has a rounded form and is used in the woman with a well-defined pubic notch. The Hodge type, although similar, has a broad, almost flat, and squared, slightly concave anterior surface, which avoids excessive urethral compression. The Risser type has a larger weight-bearing zone to accommodate the needs of the patient with greater vaginal width.

The ring pessary is useful for patients with uterine or vault prolapse, either for determining whether surgery will relieve symptoms or for providing support if surgery is contraindicated or the patient wants more children. Unlike pessaries that fill the vagina, a properly fitted ring pessary should not interfere with coitus. The donut pessary fills the vagina and forms a cradle beneath the cervix or vaginal vault (Fig. 20-2). An inflatable donut-type ring is helpful for elderly women who are not sexually active because such a pessary exerts its pressure over a wide surface of vagina and, thus, reduces the risk of ulceration, which is normally increased in the thinning, aging vagina; however, because of the large surface area in contact with the vagina it may stimulate a vaginitis with leukorrhea and over a long period, initiate an unwelcome vaginal odor. The inflatable ball pessary may be used when other types fail because it can be expanded after insertion by pumping air into the pessary with a hand-held pump, which can then be detached from the pessary. The pessary can be deflated and removed for cleaning and reinserted.

The cube or bee-cell pessary has a large surface area, although it is sometimes the easiest of all pessaries to insert and remove (except in the impaired patient); the large surface area of the pessary is prone to stimulate vaginitis and excess vaginal discharge and odor. One advantage of the six-sided bee-cell pessary is that the patient can remove, cleanse, and reinsert it herself after douching if she is able and so wishes. Many patients consider this an improvement over the rubber donut. For the patient who cannot change and clean the spheric or cylindrical pessary herself, an attendant must learn these procedures. All pessaries that affect a larger surface area are associated with an increased vaginal discharge, however, and should be removed, cleaned, and replaced bi-monthly.

The Gehrung type is an arch-like pessary, designed to raise the bladder floor vaginal apex and thin out a rectocele. It is prone to dislodgement and change in position must be checked frequently.

All modern pessaries are of plastic and most are foldable, which aids considerably in their insertion. A well-lubricated pessary is compressed and inserted into the vagina.

A ring pessary supports the prolapse without occluding the vagina. The ring pessary with support is advantageous if there is a large cystocele present.

The Gellhorn pessary is helpful for the treatment of genital prolapse in women who refuse surgery or in whom surgery is contraindicated. Available in a variety of sizes, ranging from 1 to 5 inches in diameter, this pessary resembles a large collar button and comes with a small drainage canal down the center of its stem. Its retention, like that of other pessaries, requires some competence in the tissues of the pelvic diaphragm.

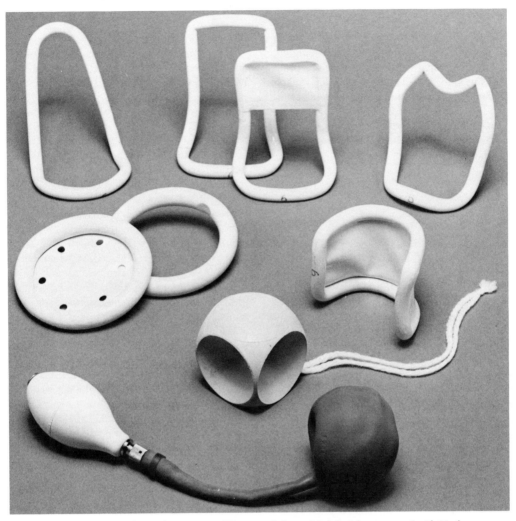

Figure 20–1. Commonly used pessaries. (*Top row,* left to right) Smith pessary; Smith-Hodge pessaries, with and without crossbard; Risser pessary. (*Middle row*) Ring pessaries (*left*); Gehrung pessary for cystocele (*right*). (*Bottom row*) Inflatable pessary and Bee-Cell pessary. (Courtesy Milex Products, Inc., 5915 Northwest Highway, Chicago, Illinois 60631)

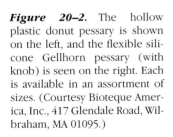

Figure 20–2. The hollow plastic donut pessary is shown on the left, and the flexible silicone Gellhorn pessary (with knob) is seen on the right. Each is available in an assortment of sizes. (Courtesy Bioteque America, Inc., 417 Glendale Road, Wilbraham, MA 01095.)

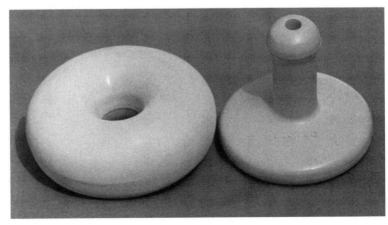

345

The Gellhorn pessary, although occluding the vagina and precluding coitus, is the pessary most frequently used for massive prolapse. It is available in a foldable form, with a knob on the end of the stem, to increase the ease with which it can be removed (see Fig. 20-2). It requires strong pubococcygeal support if it is to be retained during a patient's lifting and straining.

PROCEDURE FOR PESSARY INSERTION

Before insertion of the pessary, a complete pelvic examination is performed, the general health and condition of the vagina carefully assessed, cytology is obtained, and the state of the pubococcygei and remainder of the levator ani estimated by asking the patient to voluntarily contract the pelvic muscles. The gynecologist estimates the vaginal width as a guide toward selecting the correct size of pessary. Necessary cytologic smears are obtained, and any vaginal surface abnormalities thoroughly studied before pessary insertion.

The Smith-Hodge pessary is particularly useful in treating acquired symptomatic uterine retroversion. In a gentle pelvic examination, the physician replaces the uterus in an anterior position, notes the direction and depth from the posterior fornix to the back of the pubis, and chooses the appropriate length and width of the pessary. The physician then grasps the pessary in one hand, its large concavity toward the patient's head, and uses the index finger of the opposite hand to depress the perineum. The pessary is inserted sideways until it reaches the vault of the vagina; then it is turned as the vaginal finger depresses the topmost rim of the pessary behind the cervix. The middle finger is used to advance the rounded tip of the pessary into the posterior fornix behind the cervix, with the curve in a cranial direction (Fig. 20-3). The flattened anterior portion is placed behind the pubis.

When the Smith-Hodge pessary is properly seated, the cervix lies in its center and an examining finger can slip between it and the vaginal wall on all sides. After inserting the pessary, the physician should ask the patient to sit on the edge of the examining table for a few moments and then to walk around the room to see whether the pessary becomes either dislodged or uncomfortable. If it does, it must be removed and the patient refitted with a better size.

The Smith, Hodge, Risser, and ring pessaries are notched at each end. The physician need only halve the width temporarily by compressing the pessary from side to side during insertion. Once behind the pubis, the pessary expands to its original width.

Reexamination should be performed within 48 hours to determine the need for size change if the pessary is uncomfortable and thereafter, every month or two.[6] If infection or inflammation is apparent, the pessary should not be reinserted until the abnormality has been corrected, estrogen and local antibiotics given as necessary, and the patient advised to stay off her feet as much as possible until the pessary has been replaced. If the patient is proficient in removing her own pessary at bedtime and replacing it on arising, infection and ulceration are unlikely. The patient then can pursue a program of annual visits, having been cautioned to report any abnormal urogenital symptoms, such as bleeding or pain, that might develop between visits.

To remove the pessary, the index finger should be inserted beneath the pessary, breaking any suction that may be present, and the pessary removed by gentle traction.

The gynecologist should ask the patient to stand and strain, walk around a bit and sit, and the position and fit of the pessary then rechecked.

To place the Gellhorn pessary, the physician depresses the perineum and then inserts the disk into the vagina with the flat of the disk in the sagittal plane. When the pessary is all the way inside, the physician rotates and positions it so that the stem is directed caudally, with the knob always in the axis of the vagina to keep it in place and to facilitate removal (Fig. 20-4).

The gynecologist should be able to painlessly sweep a fingertip between each edge of the pessary and the vaginal wall.

The patient's time can be conserved if she is taught to remove, clean, and replace the pessary herself. She can remove it at night (when gravity is no longer pulling on the prolapse) if she wishes and replace it in the morning when she arises. If the patient is disinterested in doing this on a daily basis, she might be taught to take it out weekly or monthly to clean it and replace it. This will save many trips to the physician's office for the sole purpose of a pessary change.

If the patient is unable to do this, her physician should examine her monthly, removing the pessary, confirming that it is the correct size, checking the vagina for signs of inflammation or irritation, and

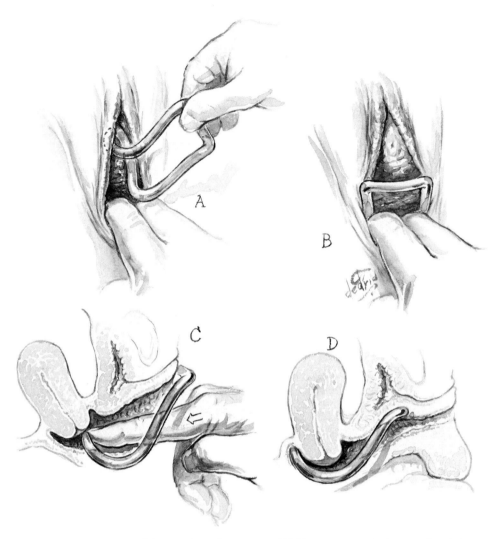

Figure 20–3. Insertion of the Smith-Hodge pessary. (**A**) The perineum is depressed and the pessary introduced. (**B,C**) The fingers gently carry the round portion of the pessary to a spot behind the cervix. (**D**) The proper position of the fitted pessary is noted in sagittal section. The round portion rests comfortably in the posterior fornix, and the flattened anterior portion is beneath the vesicourethral junction. When the patient strains, the pessary is supported by the posteroinferior surface of the pubis.

finally, cleaning and replacing the pessary. If it is cracked or defective in shape it should be exchanged for a new one. Discoloration alone is not a reason for replacement.

Whichever type of pessary has been chosen, the physician should show the patient a diagram that illustrates in sagittal section the pessary's position in the vagina so that should it become necessary to remove the pessary on short notice, the patient knows how to hook her finger into it and take it out by applying traction and pressing it against her perineum.

The patient should also be aware that in some patients, the pelvic floor is so weak that a pessary is expelled spontaneously with exertion or during a bowel movement. The physician should advise patients who wear a pessary to report promptly either discomfort or pessary expulsion.

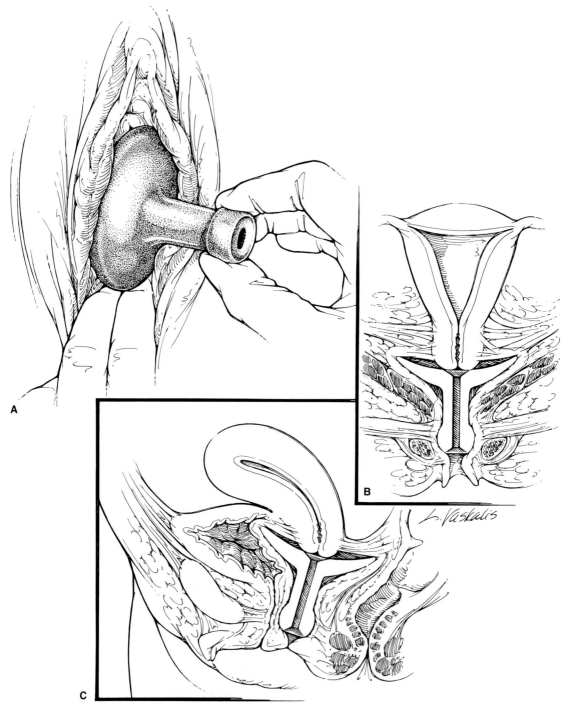

Figure 20–4. Insertion of a Gellhorn pessary. (**A**) The perineum is depressed and the disk portion of the pessary is inserted. (**B**) It should rest comfortably and be retained above the pelvic diaphragm. (**C**) Notice in sagittal section that the properly fitted pessary elevated the vaginal vault and uterus to a position once again within the pelvis and at the same time relieved some of the distention of the cystocele and rectocele. (From Nichols DH: Gynecologic and obstetric surgery. St. Louis, Mosby-Year Book, 1993, with permission.)

COMPLICATIONS OF PESSARY USE

Complications of pessary use, although infrequent, are more common among those in whom the presence of the pessary has long been forgotten or ignored. These problems include vaginitis, vaginal discharge, bleeding, abscess, ulceration of the vagina, urinary obstruction, and rarely fistula formation. A long-forgotten pessary (eg, in a patient with major cerebral deterioration or dementia) may erode into rectum or bladder at a point of pressure, creating a troublesome fistula that requires surgical repair. Carcinoma has been reported. Shnaub reports an incidence of 2.6% of cervical cancers and 30% of vaginal cancers in a series of 2500 patients treated in France since 1971.[7] Ninety-three of the 96 tumors occurred at the site of contact of the vagina with the pessary, implicating chronic inflammation as probably etiologic in these cases. Most of these pessaries had presumably been in place for a long time without periodic inspection. The most common reasons for discontinuing pessary include vaginitis and discharge, vaginal bleeding, poor retention of the pessary, new urinary or rectal continence problems, vaginal neoplasia, apareunia, inability to accept or tolerate hormone replacement, and the inconvenience of necessary periodic trips to the physician's office for checking of pessary position and inspection of the vagina. Appropriate surgical reconstruction is the therapeutic alternative to pessary use.[8]

The accomplished gynecologist should be expert not only in the nonsurgical management of genital prolapse but also in the choice and performance of appropriate surgical options as well.

REFERENCES

1. Brubaker L: The pessary: an important gynecological option. Menop Med 2:1, 1994
2. Zeitlin MP, Lebherz TB: Pessaries in the geriatric patient. J Am Geriatr Soc 40:635, 19923.
3. Bergman A, et al: Predicting postoperative urinary incontinence development in women undergoing operation for genitourinary prolapse. Am J Obstet Gynecol 158:1171, 1988
4. Bhatia NN, et al: Urodynamic effects of a vaginal pessary in women with stress urinary incontinence. Am J Obstet Gynecol 147:876, 1983
5. Dewhurst J: Integrated obstetrics and gynecology for postgraduates, 3rd ed, p 636. Boston, Blackwell, 1981
6. Wood NJ: The use of vaginal pessaries for uterine prolapse. Nurse Pract 17:31, 1992
7. Schnaub S, Sun XS, Maingon PH, et al. Cervical and vaginal cancer associates with pessary use. Cancer 69:2505, 1991
8. Nichols DH: Gynecologic and obstetric surgery, p 440. St. Louis, Mosby-Year Book, 1993

Ambulatory Gynecology, Second Edition,
edited by David H. Nichols and Patrick J. Sweeney.
J. B. Lippincott Company, Philadelphia, © 1995.

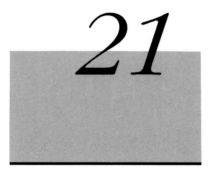

Transvaginal Sonography

Ilan E. Timor-Tritsch and Ana Monteagudo

On entering the office of an obstetrician–gynecologist, the patient usually undergoes a conversation about the reason for the office visit, a speculum examination of the vagina and the cervix, and finally, a bimanual examination of the pelvic organs. If the physician's digital examination does not detect a suspicious or obvious finding, the patient is reassured that everything is okay. Nothing could be more uncertain regarding our patients than these words. This is especially true if the patient is somewhat overweight or if it is hard to palpate the adnexal region secondary to guarding or anxiety. On how many occasions might the physician write this sentence in the patient's chart: "A fullness was felt in the adnexa"? Is "fullness" a diagnosis? A structure? Or is it really a term indicating that, "I do not have the slightest idea what it is"? To clarify the ignorance, tests are ordered and usually, off-site imaging procedures are called on to rule out a list of diseases. Most of the time, however, the answer is straightforward and the question could have been answered with the patient still on the examination table by using a simple diagnostic procedure: transvaginal sonography (TVS).

The introduction of ultrasonography as a diagnostic tool in obstetrics and gynecology was probably one of the most important advances of the past 20 years. Along the same line (although some may disagree slightly) the diagnostic and therapeutic use of TVS has unilaterally changed the practice of this specialty in the last decade. With proper training and some experience, the modern obstetrics–gynecology provider can significantly increase office effectiveness by including TVS in the diagnostic algorithm and even in the therapeutic regimen. If trends regarding the use of sonography in the office and the emergency room continue, the time is coming soon when every single obstetrics–gynecology office and emergency room will operate one or more ultrasound machines equipped with transvaginal probes.

From the outset, the distinction between an imaging laboratory and an office using TVS must be made. The imaging laboratory is equipped with sophisticated equipment and operated by expert imaging specialists. The private office of an obstetrician–gynecologist typically uses dedicated, smaller, and less expensive units, equipped mainly

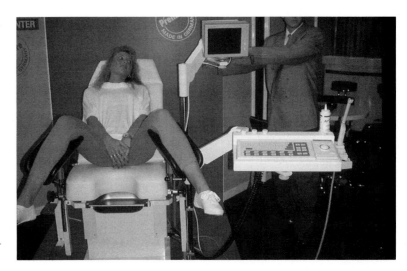

Figure 21–1. Transvaginal sonography equipment.

with transvaginal probes in addition to one general-purpose transabdominal probe, operated by the obstetrician–gynecologist (Fig. 21-1). The main purpose is to enhance the bimanual pelvic examination with instantly available imaging of the pelvic contents.

The objectives of this chapter are to elaborate on (1) the factors that enable the introduction of ultrasound equipment into the office setting, and (2) the major applications and impact of office-based ultrasound.

WHY ADOPT THE TECHNIQUE OF TRANSVAGINAL SONOGRAPHY?

Among the many reasons to use this technique, the most important are picture quality, ease of operation, and dynamic use of the transvaginal probe.

Picture Clarity

Picture clarity is not only the most important property of TVS but it is also the one that catches the eye of the uninitiated observer. Once the theoretic basis of the clear pictures are understood by the obstetrician–gynecologist, it is relatively easy to capture his or her interest and attention regarding the use of the technique.

Transvaginal probes usually employ higher frequencies than do transabdominal ultrasound probes, yielding greater picture clarity and excellent resolution, which does not change significantly with further magnification of the picture on the screen. Sound waves generated by a typical 3.5-MHz transabdominal ultrasound probe penetrate somewhat deeper into the body to reach the pelvic organs through the abdominal wall but deeper penetration is achieved at the cost of resolution.[1-3] Even dynamic focusing—available on more modern machines—cannot completely match the resolution of a picture obtained using a higher-frequency transvaginal ultrasound probe, creating a trade-off situation of resolution and depth of penetration when choosing between these probes.

Ease of Operation

It is relatively easy to use a transvaginal ultrasound probe. Obstetrics–gynecology residents, ultrasound technicians, and other professionals who had no previous experience in ultrasound scanning mastered the technique with relative ease and speed and became proficient within a short time.[4] In learning the technique of TVS, previous experience using transabdominal scanning is helpful but not necessary. The typical response of most residents and private practitioners who mastered TVS technique was, "We can hardly understand how we could manage to practice office gynecology without transvaginal sonographic examination of the patient."

Indeed, it is easy to become dependent on the use of TVS once it is incorporated in the office routine.

Dynamic Use of the Transvaginal Probe

During a traditional bimanual pelvic examination, the physician obtains information about the pelvic organs or any pathology by using both the vaginally inserted fingers and the abdominally placed second hand.[2,3] The organ of interest is placed between the two examining hands, and size, consistency, texture, location, and mobility can be ascertained. No matter how experienced the examiner, information about the internal morphologic structure of organs can only be obtained by means of the transvaginal probe. The correctly performed transvaginal sonographic examination always combines the use of the vaginally inserted probe with the abdominally placed second hand, enabling the examiner to move structures in and out of the "site" of the probe. In addition to looking at the organs that are moved in and out of the focal range of the vaginal probe, the examiner can also touch organs that are in question with the tip of the probe. Thus, under direct visual examination, information can be obtained about sensation of pain and its origin.

Because the uterus, the ovaries, or a questionable pelvic mass can easily be moved by the push–pull motion of the transvaginal probe, the sliding of the organs created by the movement of the probe can be used as a test of the presence or absence of adhesions in the pelvis. This test was previously described as the "sliding-organs sign."[2] Additionally, if pelvic fluid is detected, a sudden brisk tugging movement on any fluid collection can create movement of the floating particles; therefore, more accurate information about the nature of the fluid can be obtained.

A commercially available "finger-tip probe" can be placed on the index finger so that an examination combining a pelvic bimanual examination and TVS can be performed at the same time. Another way to achieve a combined pelvic and ultrasound examination is to slide one examining finger alongside the regular transvaginal probe to simultaneously touch and see the structure in question.

An additional advantage of the transvaginal probe is its use in obese patients or in patients who for any reason guard their abdominal muscles. In these cases, one can almost replace inadequate bimanual examinations with the transvaginal probe to reach adequate clinical decisions.

PERFORMING TRANSVAGINAL SONOGRAPHIC EXAMINATION

Almost all textbooks on TVS have extensive descriptions of the scanning technique.[3,5–7] The following description is an abbreviated version of the most important aspects of transvaginal scanning.

Preparing the Equipment and the Transducer

The ultrasound equipment and a hard copy–producing device (eg, thermal printer) should be made ready before the examination (before the transducer probe is inserted into the vagina). The patient's identification and other pertinent data (eg, the date of her last menstrual period) should be entered using the keyboard. Even if the physician does not plan to perform a TVS examination, it is advantageous to routinely enter the patient's identification data before the patient is placed on the examining table. Thus, if during the examination there is need of TVS examination, the equipment is ready to be used. It is also advantageous to have a foot pedal to freeze the screen and activate the printing devices because the examiner uses both hands to examine the patient by TVS.

The transducer tip is covered with ultrasound coupling gel and placed into the digit of a clean rubber glove or a condom. A small amount of KY gel (Johnson & Johnson, New Brunswick, NJ) or coupling gel is then applied to the top of the covered probe, easing its insertion. Infertility patients who are close to mid-cycle should be scanned using saline or water or the patient's natural secretions to avoid exposure of the sperm to the possible untoward effects of coupling gels. After completing the examination, the probe is cleaned with a tissue, using alcohol or a disinfectant solution. Because most disinfectant solutions work within 5 to 10 minutes, this time can be used to generate the patient's report. It is wise to contact the manufacturer for recommended solutions for keeping the probes clean. It is important that the examiner wear gloves while performing a TVS examination.

Proper Scanning Technique

To obtain the proper necessary images in different planes, directions, and depths, a variety of maneuvers with the probe may be employed:

Rotating the handle along the probe's longitudinal axis

Tilting or angling the probe in different directions

Pushing and pulling the probe in and out to align the focal region with the region of interest in the pelvis

In addition to maneuvering the probe, a variety of images can be obtained by manipulating the field of view. This can be done by using mechanical sector scanners and electronic probes. Most machines offer different types of zooming features. If the field of view in the zoom-in mode can be moved across the entire field, this is called "pan-zooming" and is considered to be the best type of zoom feature available. It is advantageous to begin by using the widest panoramic view and then to gradually "home-in" to the region of interest for better definition.

It is possible to steer the field of view from side to side. This feature is available on an increasing number of machines and is enabled by using the "track ball." Using this electronic or mechanical steering, side-to-side movement and angling of the probe within the vagina can be avoided—maneuvers that usually cause discomfort to patients.

Focusing

Focusing can be achieved electronically if a solid-state electronic probe is used or—in the case of mechanical probes—by electronically filtering and selectively enhancing different frequencies of the emitting crystal. Mechanical probes, with annular-array crystal configurations that are focused at different depths, have been developed, creating a wide focal range. In some probes, electronic or mechanical steering of the scanning plane can also be achieved. It is of utmost importance that the operator be completely familiar with the actual orientation of the planes and the scanning angles to avoid confusion in localizing structures in the pelvis.

Scanning Routine

We suggest that a relatively strict and rigid scanning routine should always be followed. This consists of the following general steps:

1. Scan the cervix first, when the probe is advanced into the vagina. A quick but thorough look at the bladder can also be performed at this time (looking at the bladder often provides important information).

2. Localize the uterus because it is the largest structure in the midline. It should be evaluated in the longitudinal and the transverse plane (Fig. 21-2). The cervix should also be scanned by gently pulling out the probe and directing it toward the cervix or by using any of the mechanical or electronic means to move the scanning plane. If the patient is pregnant, the pregnancy should be scanned and evaluated.

3. Next, focus on the adnexa. The ovaries should be sought, usually between the lateral aspect of the uterus and the large vessels on the respective sides in the pelvis (Fig. 21-3). An attempt should be made to see whether the fallopian tubes can be seen; however, one should always remember that normal tubes are not seen by sonography in the pelvis. If one detects a tube, it is usually because of the presence of surrounding pelvic fluid or some fluid, blood, or a gestation within the tubes. At this time, the right and left adnexa should be evaluated for possible adnexal masses. If such masses are found, a detailed sonographic description is mandatory.

4. The last target is the cul-de-sac. The probe should be tilted as far as possible posteriorly and the cul-de-sac evaluated in the transverse and in the longitudinal position. If fluid is seen, its measurement in the three customary planes should be made (Fig. 21-4).

ORIENTATION, IMAGE PLANES, AND SCREEN DISPLAYS

Although TVS produces obvious and clear images, the orientation confuses most operators. It seems that orientation is the hardest to teach and the hardest to explain in a manner that is well understood by novice sonographers or sonologists. Once this aspect is mastered, however, the steepest part of the learning curve is conquered. On-screen orientation at the time of TVS means that the sonologist or sonographer is aware *at all times* which scanning plane is displayed on the screen and most importantly, which is true left, right, caudad, cephalad, anterior, and posterior on the monitor.

Conventional imaging plans are coronal, sagittal, and transverse. Using TVS, however, these scanning planes can be used only if one relates the scanning planes to the pelvis itself.

Longitudinal applies to a dimensional direction along the longest axis of the body. Using TVS,

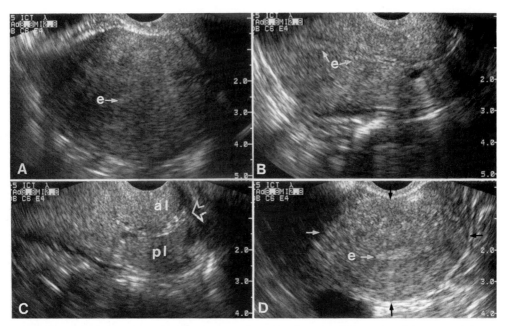

Figure 21–2. This anteverted uterus is scanned in sagittal images. (**A**) Fundus; (**B**) Corpus; (**C**) Cervix; and (**D**) Cross-section of the body. (*e,* endometrium; *al,* anterior cervical lip; *pl,* posterior cervical lip; *open arrow,* external cervical os; *small arrows* on panel D, boundaries of the uterine body)

however, longitudinal means that the scanning plane is placed across the longest dimension of the scanned organ (ie, the longitudinal image of the ovary). Most of the time, this scanning plane is not synonymous with the traditional longitudinal plane of the pelvis.[8,9]

Two planes can usually be applied to the longitudinal axis of the body: the sagittal and the coronal planes. In contrast, only one plane—the transverse (or cross-sectional) plane—can be applied to the two short axes of the body (anteroposterior and laterolateral). This is also true if a pelvic organ is scanned. For example, the uterus and other organs in the pelvis can be imaged cross-sectionally. Be-

cause of the restricted movement of the probe in the vagina, with TVS, only a mid-sagittal or mid-coronal plane can be obtained. As opposed to transabdominal sonography, in which the sagittal plane of the linear probe can be successively moved laterally in a parallel fashion, TVS is able to move this sagittal plane only in a radial fan-like fashion. The apex of this fan is the tip of the transducer. The ovaries, the uterus, and the tubes assume (most of the time) different positions in the pelvis. Their longest dimensions point in different directions, which are hard to describe using the classic transabdominal scanning planes. It is therefore customary to apply a different connotation to the TVS

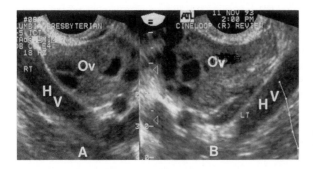

Figure 21–3. The right and the left ovary (*Ov*) are depicted on panels **A** and **B** above the right and left hypogastric vessels (*H$_V$*).

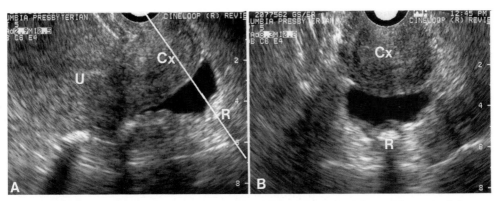

Figure 21–4. In the cul-de-sac, a small amount of fluid is evident. (A) Sagittal image of the lower part of the uterine body (*U*) and the cervix (*Cx*). (B) The cornual section of the cervix seen along the white line in **A** (*R*, rectum).

terms for scanning pelvic organs using the "organ-oriented" approach.[8,9] Therefore, if the "longitudinal (axis) of the ovary" is mentioned, this does not necessarily mean that it lies parallel to the longitudinal axis of the pelvis, it merely describes the fact that the image represents the longest possible measurement of the ovary.

The display of image planes is also a critical issue of TVS. Traditionally, transabdominal ultrasound images are displayed with the apex of the image at the top of the screen. Thus, the anterior aspect (ie, the abdominal wall) of the patient is displayed on the top of the screen, and the posterior

aspect (ie, the back) is at the bottom of the image. On a sagittal scan of the patient, the direction of the patient's head is displayed at the left, and the direction of the feet at the right of the monitor. If a transverse scan is displayed, the patient's right side is on the left side of the screen, and the patient's left side is displayed on the right side of the screen.

Transvaginal ultrasound images are displayed in two ways: with the apex of the "pie" pointing upward and with the apex of the fan pointing downward (Fig. 21-5). The apex of the "pie" represents the footprint of the transducer. If the apex is on top of the screen, on a sagittal (longitudinal) plane, the

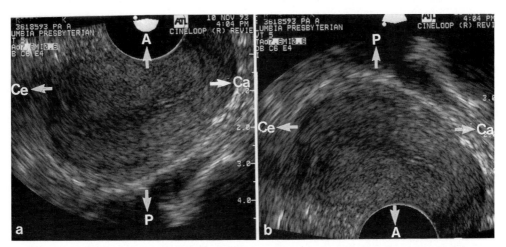

Figure 21–5. Orientation of transvaginal scans: (**A**) The apex of the "pie" points upwards. Therefore, anterior (*A*) is up, posterior (*P*) is down, cephalad (*Ce*) points to the left, and caudal (*Ca*) to the right of the image. (**B**) The European method of scanning—the apex of the "pie" points downwards. Therefore, anterior (*A*) is down, posterior (*P*) is up, cephalad (*Ce*) is on the left, and caudal (*Ca*) is on the right of the image.

filling bladder is seen on the upper left side of the monitor. The fundus of an anteverted uterus appears to be pointing to the left of the screen on the same side that the bladder is displayed. The cervix points toward the upper right side of the picture. On a cross-sectional (horizontal or coronal) plane, the patient's right ovary is seen on the left and her left ovary on the right side of the monitor.

Almost all machines offer a left–right as well as an apex-invert switch. These can be activated or deactivated as desired. The operator should be fully aware of their meaning, however. More information regarding the display of TVS images and the controversies surrounding this issue has been published.[10,11] It is important to realize that there is an urgent need for standardization in this area. At this time, most operators in the United States display the footprint of the transvaginal probe pointing toward the upper part of the monitor.

INCORPORATING TRANSVAGINAL SONOGRAPHY INTO THE GYNECOLOGIC BIMANUAL EXAMINATION

After the proper patient history is obtained, patients usually undergo the customary abdominal examination and a bimanual pelvic examination. Presenting signs and symptoms usually determine the priority level of the diagnostic algorithm. The more urgent problems provide the opportunity to efficiently use the on-site transvaginal ultrasound examination. Sonographic scanning of the pelvis is an established method for work-up of almost any problem in the gynecologic or obstetric practice. Even though the primary bimanual examination of the pelvis is important, this examination can be supplemented by a more objective imaging technique. Usually, sonographic imaging (and TVS in particular) requires the transfer or the referral of the patient to an outside imaging laboratory. Valuable time can thus be wasted. If the necessary equipment is available in the physician's office (or in the emergency room area) and the provider is proficient in performing TVS, the evaluation of the pelvis can be accomplished in a matter of minutes. Instantaneous access to real-time pictures of the pelvis saves time and is highly accepted by the patients, who appreciate a comprehensive gynecologic examination. In most cases, adequate treatment of the disease can be instituted at the end of the scanning.[12–16]

In a recent article, routine preoperative trans-

vaginal ultrasound examination of gynecologic patients by resident and attending physicians was evaluated.[17] Transvaginal sonography was quickly learned by the resident and attending physicians. The authors also disclosed that the diagnostic capability of TVS (before scheduled surgical cases) was better than the bimanual pelvic examination and increased precision of preoperative diagnosis in the patient population studied.

There are several important advantages to using TVS in the office and the emergency room setting:

1. The diagnosis in most cases that present in an office setting or in the emergency room can be established at the time of the initial contact with the patient.
2. The scans can be performed in a relatively short time, therefore causing no significant discomfort or inconvenience to the patient.
3. Scheduling is improved because a final solution to the patient's problems can be provided in fewer contacts.
4. Referrals to remote or off-site imaging laboratories can be avoided.
5. There are fewer missed diagnoses than with a bimanual examination.
6. Patient compliance is high.

Within several years, most obstetrics–gynecology offices and emergency rooms probably will use TVS as an integral part of the examination of the female patient.[18]

DOCUMENTING A SCAN IN THE OFFICE

There is a basic difference between the documentation required after transvaginal sonographically enhanced bimanual examination in an office or emergency room setting and that required for the examination performed in an imaging laboratory where only this kind of service is provided. In an office or an emergency room setting, one should be able to obtain an annotated thermal print. After the documentation of positive findings, a detailed note should be inserted in the patient's chart to describe the findings. Lack of findings, however, do not require taking pictures of normal organs, and a simple sentence of "no apparent pathology was seen during TVS" is usually sufficient.

Motivated by the multitude and the magnitude of problems in image documentation, several solutions have been proposed, all based on the use of electronic devices. High-resolution monitors, fast data storage, and high-capacity optical disks linked to super-fast computers with large memory capacity are just a few. The primary goals are fast storage and fast retrieval. It is worthwhile to explore these solutions because they simplify data acquisition and retrieval and provide proper documentation.

TRAINING

Training is most important for individual obstetricians and gynecologists who desire to use TVS in their office settings. Just as surgery or laparoscopy is not performed without proper previous training, it is inconceivable that TVS should be used without proper training.

Several training methods are available. Theoretic courses are in abundance. It is a good idea to follow a good course for several days because the theoretic grounds for the use of TVS are described. Courses are usually accredited through the American College of Obstetricians and Gynecologists, The American College of Radiologists, or The American Institute of Ultrasound in Medicine.

An increasing number of basic textbooks and monographs are available in English and several other languages. Dedicated imaging journals address TVS issues on an ongoing basis and several articles can be found in specialty journals. Videotape lectures and soon CD-ROM will also be available.

The most important training is still that provided by residency and fellowship programs. Directors of obstetric and gynecologic departments and residency program coordinators should provide a formal and detailed training in general ultrasonography and in TVS in particular. Conversely, residents and fellows must be receptive and willing to become proficient in this exceptional diagnostic modality as an integral part of their clinical diagnostic skills. Once the years of fellowship and residency are over, it is increasingly difficult and expensive to learn the necessary skills in the aforementioned courses and hands-on training sessions.

LIMITATIONS OF TRANSVAGINAL SONOGRAPHY

There are only a few limitations to performing TVS. The imperforate hymen or patient refusal are the only two absolute contraindications for TVS. Some of the relative contraindications include the fear of introducing infections in pregnant patients with ruptured membranes and virginal introitus. The progressively decreasing transducer size may be a good solution to examining elderly patients with relative stricture of the vagina and for virginal patients. Although perineal scanning is an alternative, one should be aware that it does not replace vaginal scanning but merely represents a replacement of TVS for special cases. It should be noted that bleeding in the first or second trimester of pregnancy does not constitute a contraindication to transvaginal scanning. If it is appropriate to bimanually examine these patients, TVS does not pose additional risk. Transvaginal sonography can safely be used in patients suspected of placenta previa because the axis of the cervix and that of the vaginal probe safely prevent introduction of the probe into the cervical canal.

CLINICAL APPLICATIONS OF TRANSVAGINAL SONOGRAPHY

Although detailed discussion is precluded by the scope of this chapter, the following is a list of applications in obstetrics and gynecology and in interventional ultrasonography in which the use of TVS has been widely accepted and documented.

Obstetric and Gynecologic Uses:

The diagnosis of intrauterine pregnancy
Early and reliable diagnosis of early pregnancy failure
Scanning for fetal central nervous system malformations throughout the entire pregnancy
Comprehensive malformation work-up in the early second trimester
Doppler color-flow studies of fetal blood vessels and the fetal heart
Detection of malformations, beginning in the first trimester
Early diagnosis of amnionicity and chorionicity in multifetal pregnancies
Diagnostic and management support for infertility
Diagnosis and management of ectopic pregnancy
Accurate scanning of the uterus and the ovaries
Early detection of ovarian and endometrial cancer, including morphologic and color-flow studies

Interventional Uses:

Aspiration of certain ovarian cysts
Multifetal pregnancy reduction
Aspiration and drainage of pelvic fluid collections

Aspiration of ova for in vitro fertilization–embryo transfer (IVF/ET)

Treatment of ectopic gestations by puncture and injection of potassium chloride or methotrexate, including tubal pregnancies, cornual pregnancies, and cervical pregnancies

Chorionic villus sampling

Early amniocentesis

Summary

Transvaginal sonography has unilaterally changed the practice of obstectrician–gynecologists in the last decade and become a valuable scanning method for the obstetric and gynecologic patient. The easily obtained crisp pictures are easy to interpret and may therefore be employed as an adjunct to the bimanual examination at the time of the initial obstetric–gynecologic examination. It is our belief that in the near future it will become the gold standard of office practice.

REFERENCES

1. Timor-Tritsch IE, Bar-Yam Y, Elgali S, Rottem S: The technique of transvaginal sonography with the use of a 6.5 MHz probe. Am J Obstet Gynecol 158:1019, 1988
2. Timor-Tritsch IE, Rottem S, Thaler I: Review of transvaginal ultrasonography: a description with clinical application. Ultrasound Quarterly 6:1, 1988
3. Zimmer EZ, Timor-Tritsch IE, Rottem S: The technique of transvaginal sonography. In Timor-Tritsch IE, Rottem ST (eds): Transvaginal sonography, 2nd ed, p 61. New York, Elsevier, 1991
4. Timor-Tritsch IE, Greenidge S, Admon D, Reuss LM: Emergency room use of transvaginal ultraso-nography by obstetric and gynecologic residents. Am J Obstet Gynecol 166:866, 1992
5. Goldstein SR: Endovaginal ultrasound, 2nd ed. New York, Alan R. Liss, 1991
6. Fleischer AC, Kepple DM (eds): Transvaginal sonography: a clinical atlas. Philadelphia, JB Lippincott, 1992
7. Nyberg DA, Hill LM, Bohm-Velez M, Mendelson EB: Transvaginal ultrasound. St. Louis, Mosby-Year Book, 1992
8. Rottem S, Thaler I, Goldstein SR, Timor-Tritsch IE, Brandes JM: Transvaginal sonographic technique: targeted organ scanning without resorting to "planes." J Clin Ultrasound 18:243, 1990
9. Dodson MG, Deter RL: Definition of anatomical planes for use in transvaginal sonography. J Clin Ultrasound 18:239, 1990
10. Bernaschek G, Deutinger J: Current status of vaginosonography: a world-wide inquiry. Ultrasound in Ob Gyn 2:352, 1992
11. Timor-Tritsch IE: Standardization of ultrasonographic images: let's all talk the same language! Ultrasound in Ob Gyn (Opinion) 2:311, 1992
12. Goldstein SR: Incorporating endovaginal ultrasonography into the overall gynecological examination. Am J Obstet Gynecol 162:625, 1990
13. Timor-Tritsch IE: Is office use of vaginal sonography feasible. Am J Obstet Gynecol 162:983, 1990
14. Goldstein SR: How ultrasound enhances the bimanual exam. Contemporary Ob/Gyn 37:102, 1992
15. Timor-Tritsch IE: Office and emergency room use of transvaginal sonography. In Timor-Tritsch IE, Rottem S (eds): Transvaginal sonography, 2nd ed, p 493. New York, Elsevier, 1991
16. Timor-Tritsch IE: Transvaginal sonography in gynecologic practice. Curr Opin Obstet Gynecol 4:914, 1992
17. Frederick JL, Paulson RJ, Sauer JV: Routine use of vaginal ultrasonography n the preoperative evaluation of gynecologic patients. An adjunct to resident education. J Reprod Med 36:779, 1991
18. Timor-Tritsch IE: Office use of transvaginal sonography: ostriches in the sand (editorial). Ultrasound Obstet Gynecol 3:157, 1993

Ambulatory Gynecology, Second Edition, edited by David H. Nichols and Patrick J. Sweeney. J. B. Lippincott Company, Philadelphia, © 1995.

Hysteroscopy

Charles M. March

Intrauterine pathology has been found in up to 10% of infertile couples and in as many as a third of those with recurrent pregnancy loss. Although defects have been found in 13% of asymptomatic patients undergoing elective sterilization, up to 62% of patients who are infertile have been reported to have abnormalities.[1,2] Second-trimester and early third-trimester losses are likely to be caused by congenital anomalies and submucosal myomas. Abnormal uterine bleeding is a frequent indication for office visits and for minor and major surgical procedures.

For many decades, gynecologists used only hysterosalpingography, curettage, and the confusing palpatory sensations afforded by the tip of a uterine sound or curette to detect intrauterine pathology. Over the past 3 decades, the superiority of direct inspection of the uterine cavity over blind endometrial curettage to diagnose and treat abnormal bleeding has been documented.[3,4] Inadequate illumination and the lack of suitable uterine-distending media hindered the advancement of hysteroscopy, however.

Cold-light fiber optics solved the problem with illumination. Hysteroscopy emerged as a valuable procedure having many applications only after the feasibility of using a highly viscous dextran solution to provide uterine distention and a clear view (even in the presence of blood and cellular debris) was demonstrated by Edstrom and Fernstrom.[5]

Both hysterography (HSG) and hysteroscopy are used to study the uterus (Table 22-1). Hysteroscopy not only permits confirmation of the nature of a lesion suggested by HSG but also allows the surgeon to localize the lesion and to plan therapy. These two studies should be considered complementary rather than competing. Hysteroscopy is the first choice for patients who are likely to have uterine pathology. As a screening procedure, however, HSG is preferred for those physicians who do not have office hysteroscopy available. Moreover, information about the fallopian tubes, which can only be obtained by the HSG, makes this procedure especially important for infertile patients.

INSTRUMENTATION

Hysteroscopes may be contact or panoramic, and panoramic may be rigid or "flexible." Telescopes have outer diameters between 2.7 and 4.0 mm. The

Table 22–1
Comparison of Hysterosalpingography and Hysteroscopy

	Hysteroscopy	*Hysterosalpingography*
Inspection	Direct	Indirect
Diagnosis	Definitive	Presumptive
Localization	Accurate	Vague
Type of procedure	Diagnostic, therapeutic	Diagnostic
Organs studied	Uterus	Uterus, tubes
Cost	Moderate	Low
Radiation	None	Minimal

telescope may have a 0° viewing angle and thus provide a "straight on" view or may have a foreoblique lens, which provides a view that is 12°, 15°, 25° or 30° off the horizontal. Some telescopes have a focusing knob that allows it to be used as a contact device. Others provide magnification. Diagnostic sheaths are between 3.3 and 4.5 mm in diameter. For operative hysteroscopy, 7- or 8-mm sheaths are available. These larger sheaths allow the placement of one or two accessory instruments. A hysteroscope with channels that are completely isolated from each other can provide true continuous rinsing of the cavity.

Some operating sheaths have a modification at the distal end, the Albarron bridge, which allows the accessory instrument to be deflected toward a lesion or structure. This modification is especially valuable for patients whose tubal ostia are placed eccentrically and who wish to have transcervical sterilization or tubal cannulation.

The microcolpohysteroscope provides a magnified view of the endocervix and uterine cavity and may be useful in evaluating patients with cervical intra-epithelial neoplastic lesions that extend into the canal.[6] If the full extent of the lesion can be seen, the most abnormal areas may undergo biopsy under direct vision, thereby reducing the need for conization.

The hallmarks of contact hysteroscopy are simplicity and convenience.[7] Neither a light source nor distending medium is necessary. The 6-mm telescope is favored because it requires less cervical dilation. A biopsy–grasping forceps that fits over the 6-mm endoscope can be used to removed an embedded intrauterine device (IUD). A focusing device that increases the depth of field is a mandatory attachment.

Because the contact hysteroscope does not pro-

vide a panoramic view, most physicians find its use more difficult to master than that of the panoramic hysteroscope. Complete inspection of the cavity requires discipline and patience. Gentle pressure against the mucosa permits a good view, even if the patient is bleeding. Its simplicity of use and maintenance makes the contact hysteroscope a valuable and convenient diagnostic tool that may also be used for vaginoscopy, cystoscopy, and amnioscopy.

"Flexible" hysteroscopes are not truly flexible but are steerable.[8] The outer diameter varies between 3.5 and 4.8 mm and the distal end can be deflected over an arc of 130° to 160°. By rotating the entire instrument, it is possible to view all of the uterine cavity. The 1-mm media channel can be used to deliver either CO_2 or 5% glucose in water. The larger flexible hysteroscope can be used for surgery and has a 2-mm operating channel for biopsy forceps and microscissors. The view afforded by flexible hysteroscopes has a "ground glass" quality and thus is inferior to that obtained by a rigid telescope. The leading edge can be "maneuvered" around lesions, however; therefore, this hysteroscope can provide a view of structures partially obscured by a myoma or polyp. Moreover, this telescope affords the surgeon a parallel view of even the most eccentrically placed ostium, allowing the surgeon to cannulate tubes. Each hysteroscope has a role and instrument selection depends on the goals of the user and the needs of the patient.

Ancillary equipment includes an aspirating cannula, biopsy forceps, scissors, alligator forceps, and a fulgurating electrode. The aspirating cannula should be considered an essential rather than optional instrument. Because blood and cellular debris may be present before beginning the hysteroscopy or as a consequence of intrauterine surgery, a method of maintaining a clear view is important. Even though dextran media are not miscible with blood and continuous-flow instruments can irrigate the cavity well, an aspirating catheter permits pinpoint clearing of certain regions, especially the cornual recesses.

Scissors can be used to incise a septum, to lyse adhesions, or to excise a polyp or pedunculated myoma. Biopsy forceps should be used to document the histology of any lesion that is not excised. Alligator forceps can retrieve retained IUDs or other foreign bodies. Most of these instruments are flexible or semirigid. The latter are more durable.

Coagulation can be achieved using a flexible electrode or fiber to deliver laser energy from an Argon or Nd:YAG source. The latter can use a bare 600-mm fiber or one with a sapphire tip. If the latter is used, the tip *cannot* be cooled with gas.[9]

A four-pronged "cervical-sealing" tenaculum is also available. This instrument reduces the leakage of medium through a patulous cervix.[10] A simple bivalve speculum with only one arm between both blades permits it to be removed easily after insertion of the instruments, thereby reducing patient discomfort.

The urologic resectoscope has been modified for use by the gynecologist. This instrument has an inner sheath with an insulated tip and may be used "as is." Most gynecologic surgeons prefer to use the resectoscope as a continuous-flow instrument, however, because of its ability to clear the operative field of blood and cellular debris. A larger outer sheath that is 25 or 27 French has multiple perforations at its distal end. The medium is instilled through the inner sheath into the uterus and then flows out through perforations in the outer sheath. Either gravity or suction may be used to withdraw the medium from the uterus through the outer sheath.

The electrodes extend a maximum of 4 cm beyond the end of the outer sheath. The most common electrodes used in gynecologic surgery are the roller ball (or bar) and the loop. The roller electrodes are between 2 and 4 mm in diameter or width. The cutting loops available are generally between 5 and 7 mm in outer diameter. Another electrode available for gynecologic applications is the knife, useful in cutting septa and synechiae.

Some resectoscopes allow the outflow-sheath mechanism to be converted to use as an operating hysteroscope by use of a bridge. This bridge allows the surgeon to use a 7 French operating channel for insertion of semirigid instruments or a laser fiber.

MEDIA

Low Viscosity

Five-percent glucose in water is introduced by an intravenous infusion bag. The rate of flow is controlled by gravity or by increasing the infusion pressure with a hand pump, a blood pressure cuff, or automatic pumps. One disadvantage of this type of medium is that it mixes with blood, thus obscuring vision. These media are ideally suited for use in continuous-flow systems, however, and permit flushing the cavity of blood and cellular debris. Normal saline, Ringer's lactate, 3.3% sorbitol, or 1.5% glycine may also be used for hysteroscopy and have the same attributes and limitations as glucose in water.[11] Electrolyte-containing media cannot be used during electrosurgery.

Carbon Dioxide

A special insufflator is required (the CO_2 insufflator used for laparoscopy *must not* be used).[12] Carbon dioxide is instilled at a flow rate of 25 to 100 mL/minute at a maximum pressure of 200 mmHg. Because the refractile index of CO_2 is 1.00, the appearance of the tissue is more "true to life" than with other media.[13] There is also less magnification. A patulous cervix limits the ability to maintain adequate uterine distention. During prolonged procedures, up to 500 mL of CO_2 may be needed to compensate for both absorption and spill into the peritoneal cavity. Intraperitoneal CO_2 causes shoulder pain when the patient resumes an erect position. This dry medium is suited perfectly for office diagnostic procedures.

High Viscosity

Because dextran is immiscible with blood, it provides excellent visualization and is "forgiving" to the novice hysteroscopist. It is instilled using a 5-mm tubing attached to a 50-mL syringe. An alternative is installation using a CO_2-driven pump with special infusion tubing. Intermittent delivery of 5- to 10-mL volumes to enhance visualization results in less uterine cramping. This medium carmelizes quickly and thereafter is difficult to remove from instruments; thus, instruments *must* be rinsed immediately after the procedure with a copious amount of hot water. Although Rheomacrodex (a 10% solution of dextran, molecular weight 40,000 in 5% glucose in water) may be used, Hyskon Hysteroscopy Fluid (a 32% dextran solution, molecular weight 70,000 in 10% glucose in water) was developed specifically for use in hysteroscopy.[5] The excellent clarity and minimal equipment needed make Hyskon the medium of choice for operative hysteroscopy. Blood and cellular debris are layered against the uterine wall and are easy to remove with an aspirating catheter. Almost all examinations may be completed using 25 to 100 mL. During difficult operative procedures, larger volumes may be necessary but the total amount infused should not exceed 500 mL. Recent FDA guidelines restrict the use of Hyskon to 250 mL "non-recovered."

TECHNIQUE

Except during menses, hysteroscopy may be performed at any time during the menstrual cycle. Visualization is best, however, within 2 to 3 days after the cessation of menstrual flow. The endometrium is flat early in the proliferative phase, which facilitates visualization of the tubal ostia. In addition, the endometrium is less friable early in the cycle and the chance of misinterpreting polypoid endometrium as a true polyp is reduced, as is the risk of interrupting a pregnancy.

Hysteroscopy may be performed in the office. There are no special preoperative instructions or tests necessary. Patients who have a history of pelvic infection should have a cervical culture before surgery. Pelvic tenderness should be considered evidence of possible infection and may dictate postponing the procedure. For most patients, prophylactic antibiotics are not necessary. For brief procedures, premedication with 600 mg of ibuprofen is sufficient. For a longer operation, sedation consisting of meperidine, midazolam, or diazepan should be given. The use of these drugs mandates that the patient leave the office in the care of another person. If general or regional anesthesia is necessary, an outpatient surgical unit provides an adequate setting and the patient may be discharged in a few hours.

After the introduction of a paracervical block with 10 mL of 1% chloroprocaine without epinephrine into each uterosacral ligament, the uterine cavity is sounded. The cervix is then dilated to between 4 and 7 mm. A 4.5-mm sheath is used if the procedure is to be diagnostic only and a 7- or 8-mm sheath is available for operative procedures. Because the uterine walls are in apposition, the cavity

must be distended to ensure proper visualization. The hysteroscope is engaged in the external os and advanced into the uterine cavity only if the view is clear. After inspection of the endocervical canal and lower uterine segment, the hysteroscope is advanced into the cavity and the lateral walls, upper fundus, cornual recesses, and tubal ostia are inspected systematically. In addition, polyps may be excised and embedded IUDs removed. Resection of myomas or lysis of moderate or severe adhesions requires general or regional anesthesia. If a uterine division is found, simultaneous laparoscopy is necessary to differentiate the bicornuate from the septate anomaly.

CONTRAINDICATIONS

The only absolute contraindication to hysteroscopy is acute pelvic infection. Active uterine bleeding, pregnancy, a recent uterine perforation, and uterine cancer are relative contraindications. If Hyskon is used to distend the uterine cavity, a satisfactory examination can usually be accomplished, even if the patient is bleeding heavily. If low-viscosity media are used, a continuous-flow system is needed to flush the blood and cellular debris from the cavity. The contact hysteroscope may also be used in those with a recent uterine perforation. Although hysteroscopy may be used to diagnose and stage cancer, the potential for tumor dissemination has prevented its widespread use. This theoretic objection does not apply to contact hysteroscopy or CO_2 panoramic hysteroscopy. The contact hysteroscope has been used to detect retained products of conception after spontaneous or induced abortion.

INDICATIONS

The indications for hysteroscopy are discussed in this section. An outline of these indications is shown in Table 22-2.

Confirm Abnormal Hysterosalpingogram

Although a normal HSG obviates the need for hysteroscopy, the findings of abnormal roentgenograms must be confirmed.[14]

Table 22–2
Indications for Hysteroscopy

Intrauterine Pathology

Confirm abnormal HSG

Intrauterine adhesions

Congenital anomalies

Excessive bleeding
    endometrial carcinoma
    endometrial polyps
    leiomyomata uteri
    endometrial ablation

Tubal obstruction

Embedded foreign bodies

Reproductive Failure

Unexplained infertility

Recurrent abortion

Sterilization

Intrauterine Adhesions

Intrauterine adhesions can be diagnosed definitively and their extent classified. Lysis of adhesions under direct vision is safer and more complete than blind curettage or hysterotomy. Before beginning adhesiolysis, the extent of the disease is classified (Table 22-3).[15,16] Under hysteroscopic guidance, only scar tissue is incised and adjacent normal endometrium is not traumatized. This tissue becomes a source for endometrial regrowth over the freshly dissected surfaces. Each adhesive band is divided with miniature scissors. Restoration of uterine architecture to normal can be achieved even in those with complete uterine obliteration. Those who have extensive disease, however, should undergo simultaneous laparoscopy. The laparoscopist guides the hysteroscopist to reduce the risk of uterine perforation. The intensity of the light source for the laparoscope is reduced markedly, permitting the laparoscopist to detect dissection into the myometrium sooner because the light of the hysteroscope begins to shine through the uterine serosa at a single point. After the cavity's configuration has been restored, the uterus has a uniform glow. After adhesiolysis as large a loop IUD as possible is placed in the cavity and retained for 2 months; postoperative use of an IUD may reduce the chances that the raw, dissected surfaces will readhere.[17] Copper-bearing IUDs and the Progestasert IUD may have too small a surface area to prevent adhesion reformation, and those that contain copper may induce an excessive inflammatory reaction. If a loop IUD is not available, an 8 French Foley catheter with a 3-mL balloon may be used. The balloon is inflated, the catheter remains for 1 week, and a broad-spectrum antibiotic is prescribed during that time. Special silastic uterine splints are also available to maintain separation of the uterine walls.

Conjugated equine estrogens, 5 mg/day, are prescribed for 60 days, and medroxyprogesterone acetate, 10 mg, is added during the last 5 days of estrogen therapy.[17] This high-dose hormone regimen stimulates the endometrium maximally to promote reepithelialization of the previously scarred surfaces. The adequacy of therapy should be assessed by repeat hysteroscopy or by HSG after withdrawal bleeding. If the HSG is normal, complete resolution may be presumed. If the HSG is abnormal, hysteroscopy should be repeated.

After one hysteroscopic treatment, 90% of our patients have had a normal uterus. Although most of the others have needed only a second procedure to restore normal uterine architecture, a few women have needed three to six operations. Ninety-eight percent of those who had amenorrhea or hypomenorrhea now have normal menses. The importance of a postoperative study to verify normalcy of the cavity before permitting conception cannot be overemphasized. Severe obstetric com-

Table 22–3
Classification of Intrauterine Adhesions by Hysteroscopic Findings

Class	Findings
Severe	More than three fourths of uterine cavity involved; agglutination of walls or thick bands; ostial areas and upper cavity occluded
Moderate	A fourth to three fourths of uterine cavity involved; no agglutination of walls, adhesions only; ostial areas and upper fundus only partially occluded
Minimal	Less than a fourth of uterine cavity involved; thin or filmy adhesions; ostial areas and upper fundus minimally involved or clear

March CM, Israel R, March AD: Hysteroscopic management of intrauterine adhesions. Am J Obstet Gynecol 130:653, 1978.

plications have been reported in patients who conceived before having postoperative studies performed to document complete resolution of the adhesions.[18] It is likely that these women had persistent disease, causing the subsequent obstetric problems.

The results are excellent and surpass other types of therapy.[19,20] Seventy-five percent of our patients who wished to conceive and who had no other known infertility factors have done so, and more than 85% of the pregnancies have been successful. Two patients have had placenta previa and two required manual removal of the placenta. One patient had retained placental fragments, which were detected when a curettage was performed to stop hemorrhage 3 weeks after delivery. Her follow-up HSG had been abnormal but she conceived before another hysteroscopic procedure was performed. These results are superior to those achieved by outdated treatment modalities such as blind disruption of adhesions by a sound or curette.

Congenital Anomalies

Uterine anomalies are found in 1% to 2% of all women, in 4% of infertile women, and in 10% to 15% of women with recurrent abortion.[21] Abortion and obstetric problems such as premature labor and abnormal fetal presentations are the most common symptoms in patients with uterine anomalies.[22] Although two thirds of pregnancies in women with uterine duplications progress to term, abortion has been reported to occur in as many as 30% of pregnancies in women with septate uteri.[23]

Hysterography and hysteroscopy can be used to delineate uterine defects and serve as a baseline before treatment. Before metroplasty, a complete investigation is mandatory, so that other causes of recurrent abortion can be ruled out.

A uterine septum is not usually an indication for surgery in infertile patients because this defect has not been reported to cause infertility. Laparotomy and incision or excision of the septum was formerly the procedure of choice for women with this anomaly and a history of recurrent abortion. The procedures advocated by Tompkins and by Jones were the most popular.[24] Hysteroscopic treatment of septa has relegated these procedures to antiquity.

Hysteroscopy is used to assess the size of the septum and to incise it.[25] Simultaneous laparoscopy is needed to verify that the uterus is unified externally and also to provide guidance for the hysteroscopist. Flexible scissors are passed through the operating channel, and the central portion of the anteroposterior column of the septum is incised. If the septum is 3-cm or less wide at the top of the fundus, the incision is carried cephalad from the most inferior point of the septum and directed laterally as the most superior aspect of the uterus is approached. The fibroelastic band of tissue retracts immediately and does not bleed. The dissection is continued until the septum is incised completely and the uterine architecture is normalized.[26,27] Broader septa are treated differently. The incision is begun at the most inferior portion of the septum, and the scissors are directed superiorly along one lateral margin of the septum up to 0.5 cm from the junction with normal myometrium. Next, the other lateral margin in incised up to the same level and subsequently, each new lateral aspect is incised alternatively until only a short broad notch (Fig. 22-1E) remains between the tubal ostia. Finally, this notch is incised, beginning from one cornual recess and progressing to the other. This approach is used because bleeding usually occurs at the interface between myometrium and septum and if treatment of this portion is delayed until the end of the procedure, blood loss is minimized and excellent visualization ensured. The dissection is complete when both tubal ostia can be visualized simultaneously, even when the hysteroscope is high in the cavity, when the hysteroscope can move freely from one cornual recess to another, or when the laparoscopist observes that the entire uterus "glows" uniformly, even when the distal end of the hysteroscope is located in one cornual recess. A splint is not used.

If the cervix is septate also, it is not disturbed because this area is vascular and heavy bleeding may occur, because cervical incompetence may ensue and because the cervical portion of the septum does not hinder labor. The hysteroscope is placed in one horn and a uterine sound in the other. The sound is used to deflect the septum toward the hysteroscope and the scissors that incise it just above the internal os. After a perforation has been made between he two horns, the remaining upper portion of the septum is treated as described above.

Some have used a laser or a resectoscope to incise a septum. These instruments offer no advantage over scissor incision and cause more tissue damage.[28] We have evaluated patients who developed extensive intrauterine adhesions after laser incision of a uterine septum. In addition, anatomic results are significantly worse when a resectoscope is used.[29]

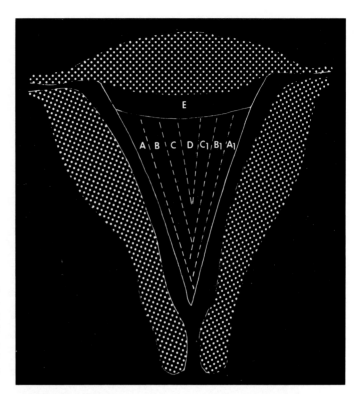

Figure 22–1. Diagram of surgical approach to wide uterine septum. Sequential incisions are made through all of area *A,* then *A₁, B, B₁, C, C₁,* and *D.* Finally, the residual notch (**E**) is incised. (March CM, Israel R: Hysteroscopic management of recurrent abortion caused by septate uterus. Am J Obstet Gynecol 156:834, 1987.)

The patient may be discharged a few hours after the procedure is finished. To epithelialize the area over the incised septum, conjugated estrogens, 1.25 mg daily, are prescribed for 25 days. Medroxyprogesterone acetate, 10 mg daily, is given during the last 5 days of the estrogen treatment. Office hysteroscopy or an HSG should be performed after the withdrawal menses. If normal, the patient may attempt to conceive immediately thereafter.

Preoperative and postoperative HSGs of a patient treated by hysteroscopic incision are shown in Figure 22-2. Outcomes are excellent in four series of hysteroscopic treatment of patients with uterine septa and histories of recurrent abortion.[27,29–31] In our initial series, the rate of abortion was reduced from 95% (pretreatment) to less than 15% (posttreatment; Table 22-4).[27] These results equal those of abdominal metroplasty.[32] A comparison of transfundal with transcervical techniques for incision of the septate uterus is shown in Table 22-5. These differences were demonstrated most clearly in a report by Fayez, who compared his personal results with both procedures.[33]

The multiple advantages of hysteroscopic therapy make it the method of choice for treating uterine septa. Because this method of treatment is so easy and safe, some have suggested that we expand the indications for treating patients with uterine septa. For example, it should be used before in vitro fertilization or gamete intrafallopian transfer and may be used before complex therapy such as ovulation induction with gonadotropins or even for patients with unexplained infertility. The value of hysteroscopic treatment of uterine septa for these "expanded" indications remains uncertain. Its value for those with reproductive failure is unquestioned, however.

Excessive Bleeding

Curettage and hysterectomy are used often as methods of controlling abnormal bleeding. Dilation and curettage are usually required when the patient has evidence of endometrial hyperplasia or if the biopsy is inadequate to exclude malignancy and in cases of profuse bleeding, hypovolemia, recurrent bleeding, and failed medical therapy. Curettage has no place in the long-term management of dysfunctional uterine bleeding, however. Recurrences of excessive bleeding occur in more than two thirds of patients with dysfunctional uterine bleeding treated by curettage alone. If the patient is anovulatory, intermittent progestational therapy prevents recur-

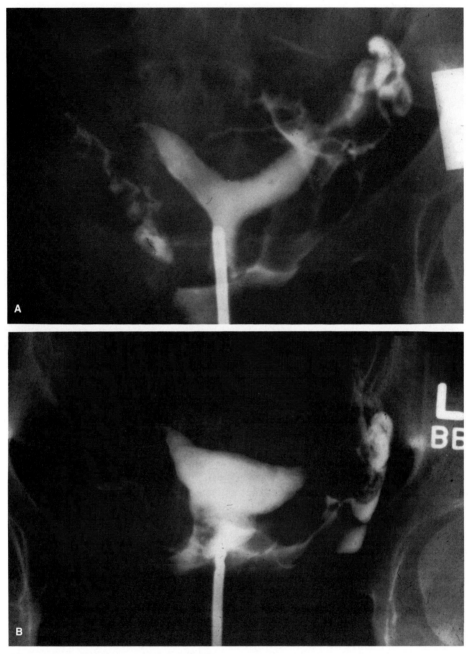

Figure 22–2. (**A**) Preoperative and (**B**) postoperative hysterogram on patient with septate uterus who underwent hysteroscopic treatment.

rences in most patients. For those with ovulatory menorrhagia, menstrual blood loss was unchanged 2 or more months after dilation and curettage.[34] Hysteroscopic examination of the endometrial cavity at the time of dilation and curettage helps to rule out the presence of a polyp or submucosal myoma.

Among 342 patients who underwent both hysteroscopy and curettage, uterine inspection and directed biopsy was six times more likely to demonstrate more advanced pathology than did curettage in the group of 71 women whose histologic findings were not in agreement.[4] Hysterectomy, the last re-

Table 22–4
Reproductive Outcome Before and After Hysteroscopic Metroplasty

	Preoperatively (n = 240)	Postoperatively (n = 63)
Term; survived	7	51
Premature; survived	5	4
Premature; neonatal death or stillbirth	16	0
Spontaneous abortion	212	8
Successful	12 (5%)	55 (87%)

March CM, Israel R: Hysteroscopic management of recurrent abortion caused by septate uterus. Am J Obstet Gynecol 156:834, 1987. Reproduced with permission of the publisher.

sort for the treatment of abnormal bleeding, is indicated when all other modalities fail or when there is associated pelvic pathology.

Endometrial Carcinoma

Although the standard method to differentiate stage I endometrial carcinoma from stage II disease is the fractional curettage, errors in staging occur 10% to 15% of the time. Contact hysteroscopy or CO_2 panoramic hysteroscopy is a safe and accurate method of differentiating these two stages and providing important information about the progression of the disease.[35]

Table 22–5
Comparison of Hysteroscopic and Abdominal Metroplasty

Abdominal	Hysteroscopic
Major surgery	Minor surgery
Inpatient procedure	Outpatient procedure
2 hours duration	30 minutes duration
Contraception, 3 months	Contraception, 1 month
Cesarean section needed	Vaginal delivery possible
Postoperative HSG (HSC)	Postoperative HSG (HSC)

HSC, hysteroscopy.

Endometrial Polyps

Endometrial polyps are frequently a cause of menometrorrhagia and often cannot be removed completely with polyp forceps or a curette.[3] Hysteroscopic excision using forceps or a loop electrode is an easily performed procedure, however. If scissors are used to excise the polyp, its base should be fulgurated or curetted to reduce the risk of recurrence. If curettage rather excision under hysteroscopic control is used for removal, the hysteroscope must be reinserted to verify that removal was complete.

Leiomyomata Uteri

Leiomyomas of the uterus are the most common solid pelvic tumor and they occur in 20% of women 35 years of age or older.[36] Infertility, first- or second-trimester abortion, premature labor, and abnormal presentations have all been associated with submucous myomas.[37]

Intramural and submucous myomas have the greatest impact on reproductive capability. The latter may hinder endometrial nutrition and afford a poor implantation site (resulting in abortion or infertility). Large intramural myomas may cause enlargement of the endometrial cavity (possibly resulting in poor sperm transport) and may occasionally occlude the intramural portion of the tube or both tubes. Both types, but particularly the submucous variety, may not allow normal uterine enlargement during pregnancy and thus lead to abortion and premature labor.

Intramural myomas are diagnosed usually by bimanual examination. The presence of submucous tumors may be suspected during curettage but an HSG or hysteroscopy is necessary for confirmation. Smooth, circular, or crescent-shaped defects persisting after the entire cavity is filled suggest submucous myomas. Occasionally, it is impossible to differentiate the defect caused by a myoma from that of an endometrial polyp or a gestational sac. The HSG also gives prognostic information because marked tubal disease would contraindicate conservative surgery unless the patient is interested in in vitro fertilization. An HSG may also demonstrate the filling of multiple channels in the tumor mass, which communicate with the endometrial cavity, and thus the diagnosis of adenomyosis can be made.

The definitive diagnosis of a submucosal myoma is made by hysteroscopy. Direct visualization can establish the nature of the defect more accurately and pinpoint the location, size, and relation to the tubal ostia and internal os.

Indications for myomectomy are (1) to conserve the uterus in a woman with large or symptomatic myomas, and (2) to improve reproductive potential. Before performing a myomectomy to improve reproductive potential, a complete infertility investigation must be performed to place the role of myomas in proper perspective. Additional infertility factors should be corrected if possible before surgery. Subsequent pregnancy rates are reduced if myomectomy is performed in patients with multifactorial infertility. Smaller myomas (less than 7 cm) may be resected or, if pedunculated, may be excised under hysteroscopic control. Three types of instruments have been used. A standard operating hysteroscope with scissors has been used to resect submucosal myomas. The line of resection follows that of the adjacent normal endometrial surface. This technique is most suitable for smaller myomas in the center of the endometrial cavity. After resection, the mass must be morcellated to permit removal through the cervical os.

Another approach is to use a resectoscope to shave the myoma to a point level with the normal endometrial surface.[38,39] This technique may be used for larger myomas and for those that are placed eccentrically. If multiple submucosal myomas are present and if these myomas occupy most of the endometrial surface or oppose one another, endoscopic resection is not advised. Much of the endometrial surface will be damaged by resection and the risk of synechiae formation is high. An alternative for moderately sized opposing-wall myomas is a two-stage procedure; that is, resecting the myomas at 2-month intervals so that one endometrial surface heals before the other side is traumatized.

After the induction of anesthesia and a pelvic examination, the uterine cavity is sounded and the cervix is dilated to 9 mm. The resectoscope and all tubing are filled with medium, the instrument is introduced into the endocervical canal, and systematic inspection of the cavity is performed. If the depth of myometrial involvement is thought to be great, a preoperative magnetic resonance imaging (MRI) scan should be performed. This helps to identify which myomas have an intramural component so large that transuterine resection would be of little value if only the intracavitary component were excised or which are dangerous if the resection were carried far into the uterine wall. Any large surface vessels are coagulated before beginning the resection. The resection is carried out beginning with that portion of the myoma that bulges most into the uterine cavity. The electrosurgical unit is set initially at 30 watts but more power is often needed for some tumors, especially those that are more fibrous. Only cutting current is used. The resecting loop is passed superior to the myoma and withdrawn back toward the insulated sheath. As the loop passes the tumor, it is activated and a piece of the myoma is excised. The loop should only be activated when it is completely in view and not in contact with adjacent normal endometrium or a tubal ostium. As fragments are resected, they should be pushed cephalad to the myoma to maintain a clear view. If the view becomes obscured, the fragments should be retrieved with polyp forceps.

As the resection progresses, some of the tumor that had been intramural commonly is extruded into the cavity and becomes available to the resecting electrode. The resection may be continued to a point even with the normal adjacent endometrium or even to just below this level *but no further*. If the resection is continued into the underlying muscle, marked hemorrhage may occur and the risk of uterine perforation is real. Moreover, deep dissection is usually not necessary. If a small intramural component is left in situ, uterine contractions over the ensuing weeks often cause that fragment to be extruded into the uterine cavity and subsequently aborted. This mechanism probably explains the high rate of success, even if a portion of the myoma remains. Myomas that are located on the most superior aspect of the uterus are more difficult to resect because access to them is limited. The easiest access to these myomas is with a quartz fiber transmitting energy from an Nd:YAG laser and delivered by a panoramic hysteroscope.

Operator caution is critical to endoscopic resection of submucosal myomas. Tumors that are attached to the region of the internal cervical os are more vascular and injury to large vessels may occur. Abdominal removal should be considered. Myomas that have a large intramural component (more than half of the uterine wall) may be resected but tend to cause recurrent symptoms shortly after surgery. If the MRI scan demonstrated that the submucosal myoma extends close to the uterine serosa, an abdominal approach should be used. The same approach is needed in patients who have symptoms related to other myomas that are intramural or subserosal. A combined approach of resection of myomas and endometrial ablation may be used in women with multiple or solitary submucosal myomas who do not wish to conserve fertility. Pretreatment with a gonadotropin-releasing–hormone (GnRH) agonist or danazol should be used before ablation to induce endometrial atrophy.

Since Neuwirth reported resecting of submucosal myomata with a resectoscope, the value of this technique has been proved by other investigators.[38–40] Long-term follow-up by Derman and coworkers has demonstrated a low recurrence rate.[41] Ninety percent of our patients have had no recurrence of bleeding over 1 to 10 years of follow-up. Most investigators were experienced hysteroscopists before undertaking resection of submucosal myomas using a resectoscope or laser. A thorough preoperative investigation and correction of anemia reduces the risk of complications. Although simultaneous laparoscopy has not been used at our center, it may be helpful, especially during a surgeon's early experience with this valuable approach to the symptomatic submucosal leiomyoma. In contrast to abdominal myomectomy, patients can attempt to conceive 1 month after surgery and can deliver vaginally. If a GnRH agonist is used before myomectomy, estrogen therapy should be used immediately after surgery to reduce the risk of adhesion formation over the atrophic endometrium. An HSG or repeat hysteroscopy should be performed before conception.

Endometrial Ablation

Laser photovaporization of the endometrium has been used to treat menorrhagia.[42] An Nd:YAG laser was used under hysteroscopic visualization. Before the procedure, all patients were given danazol, 800 mg/day for 2 to 3 weeks. An additional 2 weeks of danazol treatment followed the laser procedure. This regimen cured 203 of 210 patients, including many with organic lesions such as submucosal myomas. Similar results have been reported by Loffer, using a "nontouch" technique to destroy the endometrium.[43] Photovaporization causes varying degrees of uterine contraction, scarring, and adhesion formation, as shown by follow-up HSGs and hysteroscopy. DeCherney and coworkers, Townsend and coworkers, and Vancaille used a resectoscope to destroy the endometrium with cautery.[44–46] The instruments used are different but the techniques of endometrial destruction are similar. Preoperative endometrial sampling is mandatory to rule out the presence of any endometrial atypicalities. If the patient has more than minimal uterine enlargement or other symptoms related to leiomyomata, this procedure will not relieve all her complaints. The use of a drug to cause endometrial atrophy before surgery facilitates ablation and increases efficacy. We use leuprolide acetate for 2 months before surgery. Surgery is performed on an outpatient basis, under general or regional anesthesia. Because the results of endometrial ablation are similar irrespective of whether a resectoscope or a laser is used, we prefer to use the former: the instrument is readily available, is less costly, and the procedure may be performed more rapidly. A 2.5-mm roller electrode is used to coagulate the endometrium. The electrosurgical unit is set at 50 watts but occasionally 70 watts or more is needed. The end point is a series of overlapping yellowish-brown furrows. It is important that the thermal injury be conducted down to the basalis so that the endometrium does not regenerate. Although a loop electrode may be used to resect the endometrium, the depth of resection is more difficult to control; therefore, damage to uterine muscle may occur, with resultant hemorrhage and increased absorption of medium. A continuous-flow resectoscope is used. Both sorbitol and glycine provide a clear view. The ablation begins in the cornual regions and is carried inferiorly to just above the level of the internal os. Ablation below this point increases the risk of damage to large blood vessels. Medroxyprogesterone acetate, 150 mg, is given intramuscularly on the day of the procedure to maintain hypoestrogenism and therefore facilitate adhesion formation. During the 2 months after surgery, the uterine cavity is sounded intermittently to disrupt adhesions in the lower segment so that the process of endometrial obliteration proceeds from above and downward, thereby reducing the chance of developing hematometra. Endometrial ablation is an alternative to hysterectomy when other modalities have failed, are contraindicated, or are undesirable. The goal of endometrial ablation is relief of hypermenorrhea; thus, hypomenorrhea or even normal menses should be considered successful outcomes. About half of patients develop amenorrhea, a fourth have hypomenorrhea, 15% have normal menses, and there is a 10% failure rate. Therefore, any patient who demands amenorrhea should have a hysterectomy.

All patients must be willing to accept sterilization as a consequence of the surgery and although the risk of subsequent pregnancy is small, some have advocated simultaneous tubal sterilization. If the patient is at risk for pregnancy, a barrier method should be employed until long-term amenorrhea has been documented. When postmenopausal hormone replacement therapy is given to these patients, a progestin should be added to the estrogen to protect any remaining islands of endometrium from unopposed estrogen stimulation.

Tubal Obstruction

The etiology of proximal tubal obstruction remains obscure. In many cases, the presumptive diagnosis (made by hysterosalpingography) is proved to be incorrect when laparoscopy with transcervical hydrochromopertubation is performed. Most of these patients had spasm at the proximal uterotubal junction during the HSG. Others had anatomic damage at both the proximal and distal tubal regions or at only the proximal segments. Those with bipolar disease should probably undergo in vitro fertilization because the results of microsurgery remain poor. Those with salpingitis isthmica nodosa usually have a poor prognosis because the disease tends to be extensive, progressive, and predisposing to ectopic pregnancy. Tubal reimplantation or microsurgical tubocornual anastomosis was previously the only method of treating patients who had occlusion of the proximal fallopian tube. Although transcervical balloon tuboplasty (TBT) under fluoroscopic control is probably efficacious, treatment with hysteroscopy offers advantages.[47] Most TBT protocols require that patients have normal distal tubes. Therefore, laparoscopy is usually a prerequisite to TBT. During that laparoscopy, coaxial dilation of the proximal fallopian tube under hysteroscopic guidance is a convenient alternative to TBT because treatment is applied at the same time, thereby speeding treatment and reducing cost and discomfort.

As an adjunct to salpingography and to assess the tubal surface anatomy after relief of proximal obstruction or before salpingostomy, falloposcopy has emerged as a tool of the future. Although falloposcopy has been performed from the peritoneal side, falloposcopes have been passed into the tube after being guided up to the tubal ostium using a flexible hysteroscope.[48]

Embedded Foreign Bodies

The combination of ultrasound and alligator forceps can remove most "lost" or embedded IUDs. The first step is to provide a second method of contraception as soon as the possibility of an expelled or extrauterine device is encountered. After the next menstrual period, an attempt is made to retrieve the filaments from the endocervical canal. If they are not detected, the cavity is sounded in order "palpate" the device. If the device is felt, it is retrieved using an alligator forceps or hysteroscopy. If it cannot be felt, one or more imaging procedures should be used to localize the device, which is then removed by the appropriate surgical procedure. For those who have the capability of office hysteroscopy, it can readily be performed before ultrasound or HSG. Panoramic hysteroscopy permits the gynecologist to locate the device, assess the extent of perforation (if any), and remove it atraumatically under direct vision. If the device is properly in place and the patient wishes to retain it, the filaments may be retrieved and brought back into the endocervical canal and vagina. This approach is safer and less traumatic than blind approaches. If an embedded device is partially intracavitary, the base is grasped with forceps and the device, forceps, and hysteroscope are withdrawn as a single unit. If only a small portion of the device is visible, it may be partially extrauterine and may have involved the bowel. In these instances, simultaneous laparoscopy is advised.

UNEXPLAINED INFERTILITY AND RECURRENT ABORTION

Unexplained infertility and recurrent abortion continue to frustrate gynecologists and patients. Although it had been believed that direct inspection of the uterine cavity in women with normal hysterograms would provide important information about the preimplantation phase of the endometrium and thus provide clues to diagnosis and treatment, this hope was not realized. Although the correlation between the presumptive diagnosis of a uterine abnormality detected by HSG and the definitive diagnosis established by hysteroscopy is excellent, discrepancies occur.[49,50] If the properly performed hysterogram is normal, hysteroscopy is not necessary.[14] If any of the necessary elements of the radiographic study are absent (eg, long axis of the uterus parallel to the film plate; view of endocervical canal; view of uterus during the early filling phase; absence of uterine contractions, which obscure the upper fundus) or if a cavity defect is present, hysteroscopy is a mandatory step in the evaluation of the infertile woman, the patient with recurrent abortion, and those who have had only one second-trimester loss. Obviously, the iodine contrast media for HSG should not be introduced by a balloon catheter, which would obscure the uterine contour.

STERILIZATION

Electrocoagulation of the tubal ostia was described initially by Schroeder in 1954.[51] The most extensive clinical trials were performed in the early 1970s by Quinones and Lindemann and their coworkers, who demonstrated bilateral occlusion in 80% to 90% of cases.[52,53]

A subsequent collaborative study, however, revealed many pregnancies, including ectopic pregnancies, and a disproportionately high number of those were in the intramural portion of the tube.[54] It was suggested that excessive thermal injury to that segment of the tube facilitated recanalization.[55] Many serious complications (including bowel injuries and deaths) were reported and this method was abandoned.[54]

A variety of rigid and expandable plugs and chemical agents have been used; after a brief period of enthusiasm, all have fallen into disfavor, as has the use of formed-in-placed silicone plugs, which were studied extensively in the 1980s.[56-65]

POSTOPERATIVE CARE

Little care is needed after hysteroscopy. Those who have had only local anesthesia may leave the office after a brief rest period. If a parenteral narcotic or tranquilizer has been used, the patient may leave in the care of another person after an hour. If general anesthesia has been used, standard guidelines of the hospital or day-surgery unit are followed. Bleeding, usually light, should be expected for a few to 10 days. Mild cramping should persist for less than 1 day. Coitus may be resumed in 1 week and if the patient wishes to conceive, she may attempt to do so after 1 month, provided all adjunctive therapy has been completed and any necessary

postoperative inspection of the cavity proved it to be normal.

COMPLICATIONS AND MANAGEMENT

Complications have been infrequent in the more than 3000 hysteroscopies we have performed. Most have been mild; the frequency of complications can be reduced if strict guidelines are followed (Table 22-6).

Bleeding

In our series of more than 3000 procedures, bleeding occurred in 12 patients and was usually secondary to a laceration at the site of tenaculum placement. In two women, a branch of the uterine artery was severed and tamponade, using an intrauterine balloon, was used successfully to arrest the bleeding. In another patient, heavy bleeding necessitating transfusion occurred after IUD placement after incision of a uterine septum (splints are no longer used after hysteroplasty). Bleeding may also occur after extensive dissection of synechiae or resection of polyps or a submucous myoma. Almost all bleeding is caused by myometrial injury, not by incision of a septum, scar, polyp, or myoma.

Infection

Only two patients developed pelvic infection after hysteroscopy. Both had histories of salpingitis and one was found to have a positive cervical culture for *Neisseria gonorrhoeae* when she was admitted for intravenous antibiotic therapy. Broad-spectrum antibiotic therapy, including an agent effective

---

Table 22–6
Methods of Avoiding Complication During Hysteroscopy

Take a careful history and physical

Follicular phase timing

Advance telescope only in a clear field

Do not over-dilate

Monitor media volume

Use cautery/laser with care

Use laparoscopy liberally

against anaerobic organisms (eg, clindamycin or chloramphenicol) should be instituted immediately if symptoms of infection develop. Prophylactic antibiotic therapy for hysteroscopy is not necessary.

Uterine Perforation

This is a rare complication of hysteroscopy and usually occurs only in the most severe cases of intrauterine adhesions. If the dissection proves to be extremely difficult, laparoscopy should be performed simultaneously to reduce the chance of uterine perforation. Central perforations may be managed by observation only. Antibiotics are not used and hospitalization is unnecessary.

The use of electrocautery and lasers inside the uterus increases the potential sequelae of uterine perforation because bowel or bladder injury may occur, as may damage to large blood vessels. The surgeon must be careful to activate the electrosurgical electrode or fire the laser only when the view is clear and all of the electrode or laser fiber can be seen. If a resectoscope is used, the electrode should only be activated when it is being withdrawn toward the sheath, never "going away." For patients undergoing endometrial ablation, the endocervical canal and internal os should not be treated because of the risk of damage to large blood vessels. Treatment with a gonadotropin-releasing–hormone agonist before endometrial ablation reduces endometrial height and perhaps myometrial thickness and blood flow. Although no data are available to gauge the subsequent susceptibility to uterine perforation or injury from an electrosurgical or laser energy, Indman and coworkers demonstrated that uterine surface temperature may reach 81°C if 100 watts of laser energy is applied.[61]

Endometrial Dislocation

The subsequent development of endometriosis is probably only a theoretic complication. Avoidance of hysteroscopy during menses further reduces the risk.

Anesthetic Accidents

The rare anesthetic complications are related to the agents used rather than to the hysteroscopic procedure itself.

Complications Related to the Medium

Allergic reactions to dextran occur rarely. If a large amount of dextran enters the venous circulation, circulatory overload is possible.[62,63] Hyskon enters the vascular system and can draw almost 10 mL of fluid from the extravascular space for each mL of Hyskon absorbed. A symptom complex consisting of acute noncardiogenic pulmonary edema and disseminated intravascular coagulation occurred in 12 of our patients.[64] All received large volumes (600 to 800 mL) of Hyskon and had extensive dissection of their endometrial surfaces. To avoid these serious complications, it is advisable to limit the total amount of Hyskon used to 500 mL or less, even if this means that the procedure must be terminated prematurely and completed at a later date. After absorption of about 200 mL of Hyskon, platelet dysfunction results. Sixty grams of high-molecular-weight dextran prolonged bleeding time in 40% of patients and caused severe prolongation in 10% of patients.[65] Cronberg and coworkers showed that 300 mL of Hyskon can prolong bleeding time in healthy volunteers.[66] Dextran decreases levels of fibrinogen and factors V, VIII and IX.

Acute fluid overload has also been reported when large volumes of glucose in water, saline, or sorbitol have been used. If large volumes of glucose in water have been absorbed, hyperglycemia and hyponatremia may develop.[67] This same complication may occur if large amounts of sorbitol or glycine are absorbed. If low-viscosity media are used, intake and output must be recorded accurately at 15-minute intervals. Use of a urologic or neurosurgical drape with a pouch to catch the effluent facilitates assessment of fluid absorption. Only rarely should fluid absorption exceed 3000 mL. Treatment with furosemide should be considered when this amount of fluid has been absorbed or sooner in those with cardiovascular or pulmonary problems. The use of warm low-viscosity media reduces the occurrence of hypothermia. In some patients, potent diuretics have been used prophylactically. If fluid overload or pulmonary edema occur, treatment is identical to that used when these events are not preceded by intrauterine surgery.

Carbon dioxide acidosis and arrhythmias are probably only theoretic complications if the proper insufflator is used. Deaths have occurred, however, when the sheathed fiber used to deliver Nd:YAG energy had a sapphire tip that was cooled by gas delivered at a high rate of flow.[9] These tips should be cooled by the liquid medium being used to distend the cavity. If CO_2 is used as the uterine-distending medium, a bare fiber should deliver the laser energy. Air emboli can also occur if care is not taken to eliminate bubbles and to keep the tubing full of fluid during changeover from one bag to another.

LEARNING HYSTEROSCOPY

Although hysteroscopy is easier to learn than laparoscopy, a disciplined approach and patience are necessary. Books, postgraduate courses, and a preceptorship serve to prepare the novice for performing diagnostic hysteroscopy—first, under supervision and then, independently. After the physician becomes adept at recognizing normal and abnormal structures, excision of polyps and small pedunculated myomas in addition to lysis of minimal adhesions may be undertaken. Incision of septa, more extensive adhesions, and the management of larger myomas are procedures of moderate difficulty and risk. If all the cavity is obliterated by scar tissue or if a laser or resectoscope is to be used inside the uterus, an accomplished hysteroscopist should be in charge of the procedure.

SUMMARY

Hysteroscopy is safe and permits the cause of excessive bleeding to be diagnosed with unparalleled accuracy. The treatment of certain causes of bleeding, intrauterine adhesions, and uterine septa has been revolutionized. Transcervical sterilization may become a reality. The days of "doing without seeing" have passed.

REFERENCES

1. Cooper JM, Houck RM, Rigberg HS: The incidence of intrauterine abnormalities found at hysteroscopy in patients undergoing elective hysteroscopic sterilization. J Reprod Med 10:659, 1983
2. Valle RF: Hysteroscopy in the evaluation of female infertility. Am J Obstet Gynecol 137:425, 1980
3. Burnett JE: Hysteroscopy-controlled curettage for endometrial polyps. Obstet Gynecol 24:621, 1964
4. Gimpleson RJ, Rappold HO: A comparative study between panoramic hysteroscopy with directed biopsies and dilatation and curettage. Am J Obstet Gynecol 158:489, 1988
5. Edstrom K, Fernstrom I: The diagnostic possibilities of a modified hysteroscopic technique. Acta Obstet Gynecol Scand 49:327, 1970
6. Hamou J: Microhysteroscopy. J Reprod Med 26:375, 1981
7. Baggish MS: Contact hysteroscopy: a new technique to explore the uterine cavity. Obstet Gynecol 59:350, 1979
8. Lin BL, Miyamoto N, Tomatsu M, et al: Flexible hystero-fiberscope: the development of a new flexible hystero-fiberscope and its clinical application. Acta Obstet Gynecol Jap 39:649, 1987
9. Baggish MS, Daniell JF: Death caused by air embolism associated with neodymium:yttrium-aluminum-garnet laser surgery and artificial sapphire tips. Am J Obstet Gynecol 161:877, 1989
10. Gimpelson R: Preventing cervical reflux of the distention medium during panoramic hysteroscopy. J Reprod Med 31:7, 1986
11. Haning RV Jr, Harkins PG, Uehling DT: Preservation of fertility by transcervical resection of a benign mesodermal uterine tumor with a resectoscope and glycine distending medium. Fertil Steril 33:209, 1980
12. Lindermann H-J, Siegler AM, Mohr J: The hysteroflator 1000s. J Reprod Med 16:145, 1976
13. Lindermann H-J: The use of CO_2 in the uterine cavity for hysteroscopy. Int J Fertil 17:221, 1972
14. Fayez JA, Mutie G, Schneider PJ: The diagnostic value of hysterosalpingography and hysteroscopy in infertility investigation. Am J Obstet Gynecol 156:558, 1987
15. March CM, Israel R, March AD: Hysteroscopic management of intrauterine adhesions. Am J Obstet Gynecol 130:653, 1978
16. The American Fertility Society: The American Fertility Society classification of adnexal adhesions, distal tubal occlusion, tubal occlusion secondary to tubal ligation, tubal pregnancies, müllerian anomalies and intrauterine adhesions. Fertil Steril 49:944, 1988
17. March CM, Israel R: Intrauterine adhesions secondary to elective abortion: hysteroscopic diagnosis and management. Obstet Gynecol 48:422, 1976
18. Friedman A, DeFazio S, DeCherney A: Severe obstetric complications after aggressive treatment of Asherman's syndrome. Obstet Gynecol 67:864, 1986
19. March CM, Israel R: Gestational outcome following hysteroscopic lysis of adhesions. Fertil Steril 36:455, 1981
20. Jewelewicz R, Khalof S, Neuwirth RS, et al: Obstetric complications after treatment of intrauterine synechiae (Asherman's syndrome). Obstet Gynecol 47:701, 1976
21. Buttram VC, Gibbons WE: Müllerian anomalies: a proposed classification (an analysis of 144 cases). Fertil Steril 32:40, 1979
22. Stein AL, March CM: The outcome of pregnancy in women with müllerian duct anomalies. J Reprod Med 35:411, 1990
23. Heinonen PK, Saarikoski S, Pystynen P: Reproductive performance of women with uterine anomalies. Acta Obstet Gynecol Scand 61:157, 1982
24. Rock JA, Jones HW Jr: The clinical management of the double uterus. Fertil Steril 28:798, 1977
25. Daly DC, Walters CA, Soto-Albors CE, et al: Hysteroscopic metroplasty: surgical technique and obstetric outcome. Fertil Steril 39:623, 1983
26. Israel R, March CM: Hysteroscopic incision of the septate uterus. Am J Obstet Gynecol 149:66, 1984
27. March CM, Israel R: Hysteroscopic management

of recurrent abortion caused by septate uterus. Am J Obstet Gynecol 156:834, 1987

28. Candiani GB, Vercellini P, Fedele, et al: Argon laser versus microscissors for hysteroscopic incision of uterine septa. Am J Obstet Gynecol 164:87, 1991

29. DeCherney AH, Russell JB, Graebe RA, et al: Resectoscopic management of müllerian fusion defects. Fertil Steril 45:726, 1986

30. Daly DC, Maier D, Soto-Albors C: Hysteroscopic metroplasty: six years experience. Obstet Gynecol 73:201, 1989

31. Perino A, Mencaglia L, Hamou J, et al: Hysteroscopy for incision of uterine septa: report of 24 cases. Fertil Steril 48:321, 1987

32. Rock JA, Zacur HA: The clinical management of repeated early pregnancy wastage. Fertil Steril 39:123, 1983

33. Fayez JA: Comparison between abdominal and hysteroscopic metroplasty. Obstet Gynecol 68:399, 1986

34. Nilsson L, Rybo G: Treatment of menorrhagia. Am J Obstet Gynecol 110:713, 1971

35. Sugimoto O: Hysteroscopic diagnosis of endometrial carcinoma. Am J Obstet Gynecol 121:105, 1975

36. Miller NF, Ludovici PP: On the origin and development of uterine fibroids. Am J Obstet Gynecol 70:720, 1955

37. Buttram VC, Reiter RC: Uterine leiomyomata: etiology, symptomatology and management. Fertil Steril 36:433, 1981

38. Neuwirth RS: A new technique for an additional experience with hysteroscopic resection of submucous fibroids. Am J Obstet Gynecol 131:91, 1978

39. Hallez JP, Netter A, Cartin R: Methodical intrauterine resection. Am J Obstet Gynecol 156:1080, 1987

40. Valle RF: Hysteroscopic removal of submucous leiomyomas. J Gynecol Surg 6:89, 1990

41. Derman SG, Rehnstrom J, Neuwirth RS: The long-term effectiveness of hysteroscopic treatment of menorrhagia and leiomyomas. Obstet Gynecol 77:591, 1991

42. Goldrath MH, Fuller TA, Segal S: Laser photovaporization of endometrium for the treatment of menorrhagia. Am J Obstet Gynecol 140:14, 1981

43. Loffer FD: Hysteroscopic endometrial ablation with the Nd:YAG laser using a nontouch technique. Obstet Gynecol 69:679, 1987

44. DeCherney AH, Diamond MP, Lavy G, et al: Endometrial ablation for intractable uterine bleeding: hysteroscopic resection. Obstet Gynecol 70:668, 1977

45. Townsend D, Richart RM, Paskowitz RA, et al: "Rollerball" coagulation of the endometrium. Obstet Gynecol 76:310, 1990

46. Vancaille T: Electrocoagulation of the endometrium with the ball-end resectoscope. Obstet Gynecol 74:425, 1989

47. Novy MJ, Thurmond AS, Patton P, et al: Diagnosis of cornual obstruction by transcervical fallopian tube cannulation. Fertil Steril 50:434, 1988

48. Kerin J, Daykhovsky L, Segalowitz J, et al: Falloposcopy: a microendoscopic technique for visual exploration of the human fallopian tube from the uterotubal ostium to the fimbria using a transvaginal approach. Fertil Steril 54:390, 1990

49. Taylor PJ: Correlations in infertility: symptomatology, hysterosalpingography, laparoscopy and hysteroscopy. J Reprod Med 18:339, 1977

50. Siegler AM: Hysterography and hysteroscopy in the infertile patient. J Reprod Med 18:143, 1977

51. Schroeder C: Uber Den Avsbau und Die Leistungen der Hysteroskopie. Arch Gynaekol 156:407, 1954

52. Quinones RG, Aznar RR, Duran HA: Tubal electrocauterization under hysteroscopic control. Contraception 7:195, 1973

53. Lindemann HJ, Mohr J: Tubensterilisation per Hysteroskop. Sexualmedizin 3:122, 1974

54. Darabi KF, Roy K, Richart RM: Collaborative study on hysteroscopic sterilization procedures: final report. In Sciarra JJ, Zatuchni GL, Speidel JJ (eds): Risks, benefits and controversies in fertility control, p 81. Hagerstown MD, Harper & Row, 1978

55. March CM, Israel R: A critical appraisal of hysteroscopic tubal fulguration for sterilization. Contraception 11:261, 1975

56. Sciarra JJ: Hysteroscopic approaches for tubal closure. In Zatuchni GL, Lablock MH, Sciarra JJ (eds): Research frontiers in fertility regulation, p 270. Hagerstown MD, Harper & Row, 1980

57. Falb RD, Lower BR, Crowley JP, et al: Transcervical fallopian tube blockage with gelatin-resorcinol-formaldehyde (GRF), In Sciarra JJ, Droegemuller W, Speidel JJ (eds): Advances in female sterilization techniques, p 208. Hagerstown, MD, Harper & Row, 1976

58. Reed TP III, Erb R: Hysteroscopic tubal occlusion with silicone rubber. Obstet Gynecol 61:388, 1983

59. Loffer FD: Hysteroscopic sterilization with the use of formed-in-place silicone plugs. Am J Obstet Gynecol 149:261, 1984

60. Houck RM, Cooper JM, Rigberg HS: Hysteroscopic tubal occlusion with formed-in-place silicone plugs: a clinical review. Obstet Gynecol 62:587, 1983

61. Indman PD, Lovoi PA, Brown WW III, et al: Uterine surface temperature changes caused by endometrial treatment with the Nd:YAG laser. J Reprod Med 36:505, 1991

62. Zbella EA, Moise J, Carson SA: Noncardiogenic pulmonary edema secondary to intrauterine instillation of 32% dextran 70. Fertil Steril 43:479, 1985

63. Leake JF, Murphy AA, Zacur HA: Noncardiogenic pulmonary edema: a complication of operative hysteroscopy. Fertil Steril 48:497, 1987

64. Jederkin R, Olsfanger D, Kessler I: Disseminated intra-vascular coagulopathy and adult respiratory distress syndrome: life threatening complications of hysteroscopy. Am J Obstet Gynecol 162:44, 1990

65. Langdell RD, Adelson E, Furth FW, et al: Dextran and prolonged bleeding time. JAMA 166:346, 1958

66. Cronberg F, Robertson B, Nillson IM, et al: Suppressive effect of dextran on platelet adhesiveness. Thromb Diath Haemorrh 16:384, 1966

67. Carson SA, Hubert GD, Schriock ED, et al: Hyperglycemia and hyponatremia during operative hysteroscopy with 5% dextrose in water distention. Fertil Steril 51:341, 1989

Ambulatory Gynecology, Second Edition,
edited by David H. Nichols and Patrick J. Sweeney.
J. B. Lippincott Company, Philadelphia, © 1995.

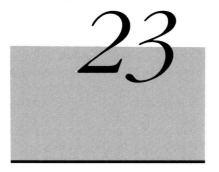

23

Colposcopy

Louis Burke

Coloscopy was first developed by Hinselmann in Germany in 1925. Investigators were curious then, as they are today, about the origin of cervical cancer. Hinselmann assumed that the primary focus of cervical cancer must be a minute ulceration, which, although undetectable by the naked eye, might be appreciated by suitably low-power magnification and illumination. He designed an instrument, which he called the *colposcope,* that directed sharply focused light on the cervix. The image of this focused light was viewed through binocular magnification. Thus, a new field of clinical investigation known as colposcopy was begun. Colposcopy therefore may be defined as the magnification of the gross appearance of the epithelium of the cervix, vagina, and vulva, using an instrument that is essentially a stereoscopic binocular microscope of low magnification (usually 10 to 40 times) and a strong light (Fig. 23-1).

Every colposcopic picture is a counterpart of a specific tissue pattern. Each tissue pattern is in turn determined by the nature of the surface epithelium and associated connective tissue stroma. The colposcope produces its effect by illuminating both surface epithelium and underlying stroma. When a sheet of epithelium composed of a particular cell population is interposed between the colposcopic light source and subjacent stroma, a characteristic visual impression is created. The visual image is a reflection of epithelial cell number, organization, and morphology. The image is also influenced by the vascular arrangement of the underlying stroma. Each of the many variations can therefore be modified by several possible changes in stromal vascular architecture and epithelial cellular morphology (Fig. 23-2).

INSTRUMENTATION AND TECHNIQUE

Each colposcope consists of a binocular low-power microscope having centered illumination from an incandescent or fiber optic source. It is usually mounted on the extension arm of an adjustable stand. Free movement of the focusing elements is possible. A green filter is inserted between the light source and the tissue to accentuate the color-tone differences between normal and abnormal patterns and to enhance the vascular pattern. Because red

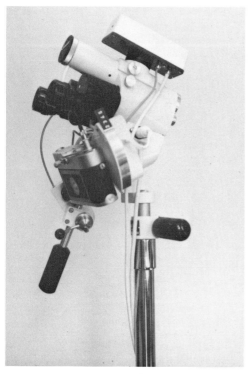

Figure 23–1. Leisegang IIIB colposcope with camera and flash unit attached.

light is absorbed, the vascular elements appear as black lines. Care should always be taken to place the colposcope in a location such that the light beam strikes the observed tissue at a right angle. The best focal-length distance of a lens for a working colposcope is between 12 and 25 cm. With a distance of 20 cm between the objective lens and the field of examination, punch biopsies and treatment can be performed under visual guidance of the colposcope. The diameter of a visualized field varies in different models between 20 and 23 mm with a magnification of 10. The binocular eyepieces are easily manipulated; they may be changed from 12.5 to 20 magnifications and may be adjusted for individual intraocular distances. Many colposcopes have the ability to alter the magnification by means of a series of lenses inserted between the ocular and the objective lenses. Some colposcopes have only three magnifications (eg, 6, 10, and 20), whereas others have as many as five, providing magnifications of 6, 10, 16, 25, and 40 times. Magnification is changed by the simple turning of the knob, without the need for refocusing. Most examinations, however, are adequately performed with a magnification of 12.5 to 13.5. Most single-magnification colposcopes come with a 25-mm objective lens and a magnification of 12.5 to 13.5.

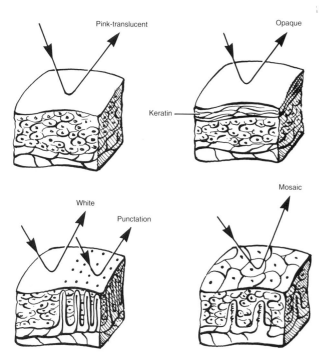

Figure 23–2. Tissue basis of colposcopy.

For colposcopic examination, the vagina and cervix are exposed as is usual for a gynecologic examination. Good colposcopic technique requires correct positioning of the patient and instrument. The patient must assume the dorsal lithotomy position. Inasmuch as she may have to maintain this position for as long as 25 to 30 minutes, the examination table should offer both maximal comfort and ease of inspection. Special knee and calf supports for the patient are useful. The usual stationary gynecologic table with conventional stirrups is acceptable for colposcopic examination. Such tables, however, may need to be elevated as much as 2 inches on wooden blocks for the physician to be able to perform the colposcopic examination without neck or back strain. Tables equipped with an automatic foot control for adjusting height are often helpful.

A warm vaginal speculum without lubricant should be introduced slowly into the vagina; the blades of the speculum must be partially separated soon after entry into the vagina to avoid traumatizing the exposed cervix. If necessary, a Pap smear can be taken concurrently with the colposcopic examination; however, because this may initiate bleeding and obliterate features of colposcopic interest, it is best for the smears to be taken before examination with colposcope.

The vagina and cervix should be inspected first, with the surface moistened with normal saline; a dry epithelial surface is nontransparent and gives a poor view of vascular patterns. Use of the green filter provides the best colposcopic impression of vascular patterns (Color Fig. 23-1). Inspection of the unprepared cervix and vagina should be followed immediately by scrutiny of the same areas with acetic acid. Acetic acid solution (3% to 5%) is applied to the cervix with moistened cotton balls. For reasons that remain obscure, acetic acid solution shrinks blood vessels, dissolves mucous, and causes an osmolar change in the intercellular space so that certain cells swell. Three-percent solution is the usual acceptable strength of the acetic acid. With weaker dilutions, the various lesions take longer to appear. Stronger solutions delineate the lesions more rapidly but are irritating to mucous membranes, especially after repeated application.

NATIVE EPITHELIA

The visible portion of the female genital tract is covered by stratified squamous epithelium, which lines the vagina and exocervix and is designated colposcopically as the *original* or *native* squamous epithelium. The endocervical canal is lined by a simple columnar epithelium, called the *original* or *native* columnar epithelium. The junction of these two tissue types, called the squamocolumnar junction, can appear at various locations on the cervix, depending on the age and estrogen activity of the woman in question (Fig. 23-3).

Native squamous epithelium shows little variation colposcopically from subject to subject. Under colposcopic illumination, it is uniformly pale pink and translucent and exhibits a feathery, vascular arrangement. Beneath the normal squamous epithelium is a flat capillary network between the lamina propria and the epithelium (Color Fig. 23-2).

Native columnar epithelium is unmistakable on colposcopy. Readily identified by its intense red hue, it is thrown up into many papillae. Each papillus has a complex vascular network consisting of uniformed coiled vessels having afferent and efferent loops. After being washed with diluted acetic acid, the columnar epithelium assumes a characteristic grape-like appearance (Color Fig. 23-3).

Colposcopic examination of the cervix is directed primarily toward investigation of tissue in the area in which the original squamous and original columnar epithelia come together. At this squamocolumnar interface, columnar epithelium is gradually transformed into squamous epithelium by the process of metaplasia. This dynamic area of change is known as the transformation zone. A clear understanding of the transformation zone is vital, not only to colposcopy but also to an understanding of the origin and development of cervical neoplasia.

TYPICAL TRANSFORMATION ZONE

The junction between original columnar and squamous epithelium is transitory. Presumably as result of a high plasma estrogen concentration and low pH conditions of the vagina, the original columnar epithelium is replaced by a metaplastic squamous epithelium. As the epithelium of the columnar layers become multilayered, the papillae fuse and the vascular structures of the individual papillae interconnect. The growth of metaplastic tissue pushes the vessels down, so that a vascular pattern similar to that of the original squamous epithelium develops. The process of metaplastic transformation results in the development of a new squamous epithelium, which is at first immature. When it becomes mature

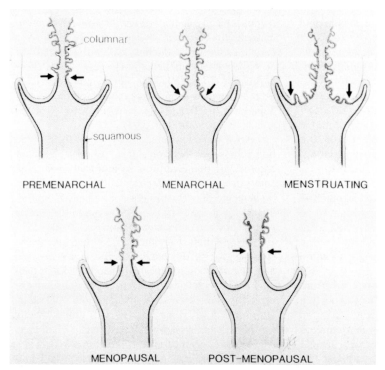

PREMENARCHAL   MENARCHAL   MENSTRUATING

MENOPAUSAL   POST-MENOPAUSAL

Figure 23–3. Location of the squamocolumnar junction at various times in a woman's life.

or glycogenated, it does not seem to be capable of neoplastic formation. There is evidence, however, that during the initial process of metaplasia, the cells are vulnerable to genetic change, resulting in the emergence of a new squamous epithelium, the cell population of which has somehow acquired neoplastic potential. Such epithelia exhibit the morphologic characteristics of precursors of squamous cancer of the cervix.

This process of epithelial succession from columnar to metaplastic to mature squamous epithelium probably occurs throughout a female's life. It is, however, most active in three phases of her life: during fetal existence, at menarche, and during her first pregnancy. The periods of most active metaplasia appear to correspond to the times at which high levels of estrogen are present. It appears that the estrogen causes the cervix to evert and allows a maximal amount of columnar tissue to be exposed to the vaginal environment. During menarche and a woman's first pregnancy, metaplasia is active in its early and immature form and therefore is at great risk of incorporating outside factors, which may stimulate it to develop an atypical metaplasia.

Squamous metaplasia occurs in sharply defined areas within the columnar epithelia. These areas can be of varying extension and can lie in the midst of normal columnar epithelium. Such islands of squamous cells overlying columnar epithelium

broaden, coalesce, and eventually join the peripheral edge of the original squamous epithelium. The coalescence of the papillae is seldom complete. Some islands of columnar epithelium often remain surrounded by metaplastic squamous epithelium. Sometimes the columnar epithelium persists in the deeper clefts in the stroma below the metaplastic squamous epithelium. This columnar epithelium has an outlet to the surface from which mucous can be expelled through small channels that persist in the metaplastic epithelium. These are called gland openings. If there is no outlet to the surface, retention cysts (or nabothian cysts) develop. The typical transformation zone can be identified by localization of the remnants of the original columnar epithelium, that is, islands of columnar epithelium that were bypassed in the metaplastic process, gland openings and nabothian cysts (Color Fig. 23-4).

ATYPICAL TRANSFORMATION ZONE

Under certain circumstances, the cause of which is unknown, the columnar epithelium undergoing metaplasia absorbs some oncogenic factor. This oncogenic factor may (1) be viral (herpesvirus, human papillomavirus); (2) come from the sperm (sperm DNA, histones); or (3) be due to some other factor.

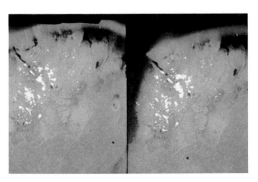

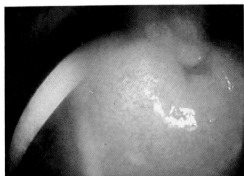

Color Figure 23–1.

Color Figure 23–2.

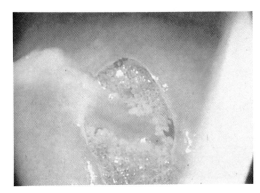

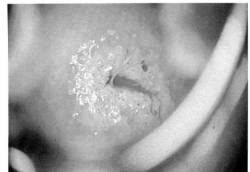

Color Figure 23–3.

Color Figure 23–4.

Color Figure 23–1. Colpophotograph taken with green–blue filter. The vascular changes of punctation and mosaic appear black. The abnormal epithelium also stands out in contrast to the normal epithelium.

Color Figure 23–2. Colpophotograph of the posterior cervical lip. Note the network blood vessels of the native stratified squamous epithelium.

Color Figure 23–3. Colpophotograph of the cervix after the application of 3% acetic acid. Note the papillae of columnar epithelium and the sharp squamocolumnar junction. Mucus can be seen streaming from the canal.

Color Figure 23–4. Colpophotograph of the cervix after the application of 3% acetic acid. Note the white, rimmed glands in the posterior cervix. The columnar epithelium has been transformed, and a well-developed transformation zone is present.

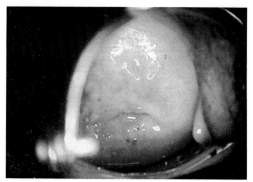

Color Figure 23–5.

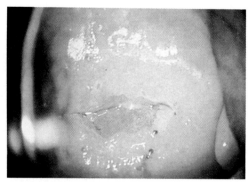

Color Figure 23–6.

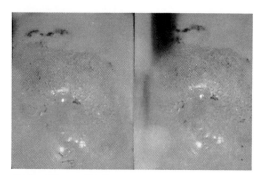

Color Figure 23–7.

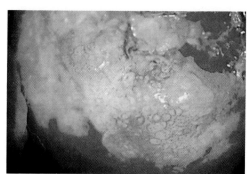

Color Figure 23–8.

Color Figure 23–5.   Colpophotograph of the cervix before the application of acetic acid. The patient has an abnormal smear consistent with CIN II, but no abnormality is noted. See Color Figure 16–6.

Color Figure 23–6.   The cervix after the application of 3% acetic acid. Note the sharply delineated aceto-white lesion between 3 and 4 o'clock. Biopsy revealed CIN II. The entire squamocolumnar junction is visible.

Color Figure 23–7.   Colpophotograph with green–blue filter. Note coarse punctation with greater than normal intercapillary distances. Biopsy revealed CIN III.

Color Figure 23–8.   Colpophotograph of the posterior cervical lip after the application of 3% acetic acid. Note the mosaic tiles of epithelium perforated with coarse vessels. Biopsy revealed CIN III.

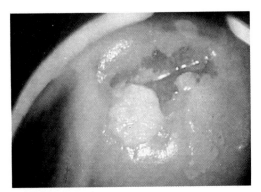

Color Figure 23–9.

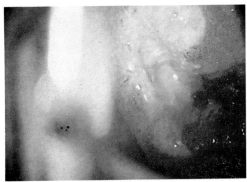

Color Figure 23–10.

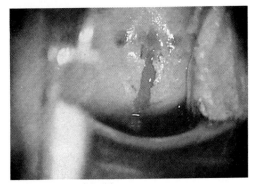

Color Figure 23–11.

Color Figure 23–9. Colpophotograph of a posterior cervix with leukoplakia. Note the raised, white, "corrugated" epithelium.

Color Figure 23–10. Cervix with raised, white epithelium. Note the presence of many atypical blood vessels at the top and the right side of the colpophotograph. Biopsy revealed invasive squamous-cell carcinoma.

Color Figure 23–11. Areas of an atypical transformation zone marked with Lugol's iodine stain before biopsy. Note that biopsy at 6 o'clock has gone through the marked area.

When the developing metaplastic cells incorporate these oncogenic factors, they start to grow in a manner different from that seen in a typical transformation zone. The individual papillae of the columnar epithelium do not coalesce or fuse. The atypical metaplastic epithelium completely fills the clefts and folds of the previous columnar epithelium. The central vascular network, under the influence of tumor angiogenesis factor, proliferates and remains in the thick stromal papillae, which are surrounded by metaplastic epithelium. The subepithelial vascular network undergoes profound alterations. The flat capillary network usually found beneath normal cervical epithelium becomes tortuous and compressed vertically by neoplastic epithelium; with extension close to the surface, it develops the atypical features called *punctation* and *mosaic structure*. Because of severe compression, some of the capillaries eventually disappear. This may result in an increase in the intercapillary distance. If the dividing cells produce keratin over the epithelium, a leukoplakic lesion develops. If there is epithelial proliferation with increased nuclear density but the vasculature does not penetrate the epithelium, the colposcopic picture is one of a white epithelium. Because this effect can be enhanced with the use of acetic acid, it is called aceto-white epithelium. Aceto-white epithelium is usually focal and can be seen only after the application of acetic acid and not with the naked eye. It is a transient phenomenon that is seen in the area of increased nuclear density. If neoangiogenesis has occurred, these new capillaries (called atypical blood vessels) can be seen running parallel underneath the surface epithelium. They appear as irregular vessels with abrupt courses and have been given various names, such as *commas, corkscrews, spaghetti, sausages,* and *large nondividing vessels.*

In summary, the transformation zone is said to be abnormal if any of the following are seen: acetowhite epithelium, punctation, mosaic, leukoplakia, abnormal blood vessels. These atypical colposcopic tissue patterns may occur singly or in combination; they may be unifocal or multifocal and almost invariably are sharply delineated from surrounding normal tissue. Their lateral margins rarely extend beyond the original squamocolumnar junction into the native squamous epithelium.

The colposcopic variations of atypia are found primarily within the transformation zone but may also be present in the vagina and on the vulva. Moreover, the same colposcopic characteristics that often signal a neoplastic change may also be found in nonneoplastic conditions such as metaplasia, infection, inflammation, and regeneration and repair after trauma, cautery, cryosurgery, or laser surgery. The presence of an abnormal transformation zone, although highly suggestive, does not prove that neoplasia exists. Thus, colposcopy cannot be performed in a vacuum but must be in concert with cytology; if cytologic examination suggests neoplasia, atypical colposcopic findings have greater significance. Colposcopic terminology is given in Table 23-1.

Table 23–1
Colposcopic Terminology

Normal Colposcopic Findings

Original squamous epithelium
Columnar epithelium
Transformation zone

Abnormal Colposcopic Findings

Atypical transformation zone
    Aceto-white epithelium
    Punctation
    Mosaic
    Leukoplakia (keratosis)
    Abnormal blood vessels
Suspect frank invasive cancer

Indecisive Colposcopic Findings

Vaginocervicitis
True erosion
Atrophic epithelium
Condyloma, papilloma

COLPOSCOPIC ATYPICALITIES

Acetowhite Epithelium

Acetowhite epithelium is the most common appearance of the atypical transformation zone. Whiteness of the abnormal epithelium presumably is related to the nuclear predominance of atypical cells. The significance of an acetowhite lesion is related to the intensity of its whiteness and to the sharpness of its borders. The whiter and more distinct a lesion, the greater is its histologic significance (Color Figs. 23-5 and 23-6).

Punctation and Mosaic

As columnar epithelium undergoes atypical metaplasia, the patterns of punctation and mosaic structure develop. As noted, the vascular networks within each columnar villus undergoes marked proliferation. Punctation and mosaic patterns are re-flections of this abnormal vascular change (Color Figs. 23-7 and 23-8). Since the processes of devel-opment of mosaic and punctation patterns from original columnar epithelium are basically similar, both changes frequently are found in the same focal lesion. Punctation and mosaic terminal vessels may show wide variations in size, shape, arrangement, and intercapillary distance, depending on the de-gree of associated histologic atypia. The greater the intercapillary distances, the more significant is the histology. Certain characteristics that indicate that punctation and mosaic patterns are likely to be in-nocuous are (1) an epithelium of normal color (the cells are not atypical and therefore not white and opaque), (2) a smooth surface that is level with orig-inal squamous epithelium, and (3) an indefinite or obscure lesion border. True punctation is generally found only within a well-demarcated area of white epithelium. Mosaic structure in the absence of white epithelium is uncommon in normal meta-plasia.

Leukoplakia

Leukoplakia, unlike the other abnormalities of the transformation zone, can be diagnosed without col-poscopy (Color Fig. 23-9). It is seen before the application of acetic acid and without the aid of low-power magnification. Under the colposcope, leukoplakia appears as a clearly demarcated white area with an irregular border and raised surface. Because of its considerable opacity, leukoplakia obscures the underlying vascular structure and thereby prevents analysis of the underlying tissue structure. It can thus cover areas of pathologic ep-ithelium. Localization of leukoplakia is important.

When it overlies normal squamous epithelium, it is usually of no great significance. When present within the transformation zone, however, espe-cially when surrounded by white epithelium, mo-saic, or punctation, it is disturbing. Although leu-koplakia is most often found in connection with benign lesions, the possibility of an underlying pre-cancerous lesion or even well-differentiated carci-noma must always be kept in mind. For these rea-sons, all keratotic areas require biopsy (Color Fig. 23-10).

Abnormal Blood Vessels

When the blood vessels appear not as punctation, mosaic, or delicately branching vessels but as irreg-ular vessels with abrupt courses, they are called atypical vessels.

GRADING OF COLPOSCOPIC LESIONS

All things being equal, the more abnormal the col-poscopic appearance, the greater the underlying histopathologic abnormality. By using the charac-teristics of the lesion (color, surface contour, speed and duration of acetowhite change, sharpness of the margin of the lesion, vascular patterns, inter-capillary distances, and the presence or absence of atypical blood vessels), it is possible for the colpos-copist with experience to differentiate the various forms of cervical intraepithelial neoplasia from each other and from invasive cancer (Table 23-2). Gynecologists practicing clinical colposcopy should guard against the temptation to make histo-

---

Table 23–2
Grading Colposcopic Lesions

Grade	Surface	Margin	Color	Time	Vessels	Pathology
I	Flat	Indistinct	White	Slow/short	Fine: normal ICD	Insignificant infection, repair HPV
II	Flat	Distinct	Whiter	Average/average	Dilated PN, mosaic, slight ↑ CD	Significant HPV, CIN I, CIN II
III	Raised	Sharp	Whitest	Fast/long	Coarse: marked ↑ CD, atypical BV	Highly significant CIN III, microinvasion–invasion

BV, blood vessel; CIN, cervical intraepithelial neoplasia; HPV, human papillomavirus; ICD, intercapillary distance; PN,

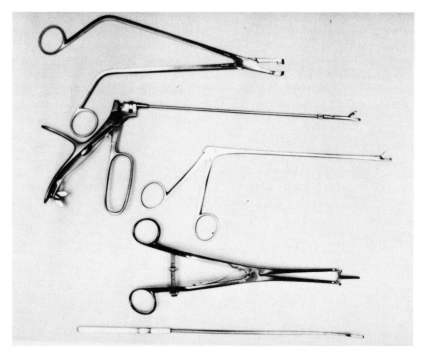

Figure 23–4.   Instruments used for cervical biopsy. *Top to bottom:* Tischler, Eppendorfer, and Younge-Kevorkian biopsy forceps; Kogan-Martin endocervical speculum; and Kevorkian endocervical curette.

logic diagnosis and should remember that acetowhite epithelium, punctation and mosaic structures, and areas of abnormal vasculature require biopsy for definitive confirmation of the true nature of the lesion.

BIOPSY

Colposcopy establishes the location and extent of foci of abnormal epithelium. Tissue sampling of specific abnormal areas can be performed easily under colposcopic guidance. A biopsy taken in the area of greatest colposcopic abnormality yields the diagnostic information necessary for implementation of appropriate therapy.

Carefully excised, well-preserved, well-oriented, and rapidly fixed specimens afford the best opportunity for accurate diagnosis. A variety of instruments may be used for punching out small sections of epithelium. The common instrument for removing small bites of tissue include the Eppendorfer, Kevorkian, Young, Tischler and Burke biopsy forceps (Fig. 23-4). The Eppendorfer, Kevorkian and

Table 23–3
Colposcopy in Gynecology

1. Used to supplement cytology
2. Used to direct biopsy
3. Used before cones and before hysterectomy for CIN III
4. Used for evaluation of the female offspring of mothers who took DES during pregnancy
5. Used for evaluation of lesions of the vagina
6. Used for evaluation of lesions of the vulva
7. Used in follow-up (carcinoma of the cervix, adenosis, CIN)

CIN, cervical intraepithelial neoplasia; DES, diethylstilbestrol.

Young instruments take small, relatively superficial samples. Unless the examiner stabilizes the cervix, they tend to slip off and the resulting sample is unsatisfactory. The Kevorkian and Young forceps have serrations on the posterior blade that aid in stabilizing the area requiring biopsy. The Tischler and Burke biopsy forceps have a projection on each blade that acts as a stabilizing tooth so that addi-

tional immobilization of the cervix is hardly ever necessary. The Tischler head is $5 \times 5 \times 4$ mm. The Burke biopsy forceps has a head that measures $5 \times 1 \times 3$ mm and thus, does not take as deep a biopsy as the Tischler forceps. This minimizes the possibility of excessive bleeding. Care should be taken so that the cutting edges of the biopsy forceps are not dulled by misuse. Forceps should not be au-

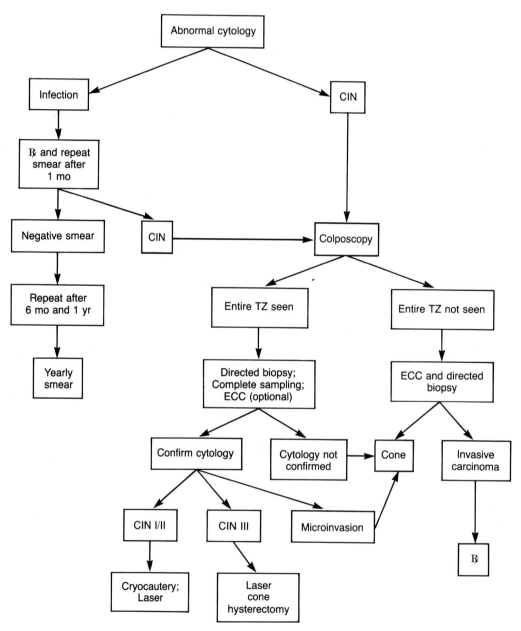

Figure 23–5. Algorithm for the investigation of abnormal smears. TZ, transformation zone; ECC, endocervical currettage.

toclaved; they should be soaked in dihaldehyde solution (Cidex) or sterilized with gas.

Sometimes the cervix or vagina must be stabilized for biopsy. A tonsil or iris hook can be used to tent the epithelium and thus facilitate the biopsy. It is advisable to obtain biopsy instruments of 15 cm in length when using colposcopes with fixed working distances of about 20 cm. If the biopsy instrument is longer than 15 cm, the area to undergo biopsy should be marked with dots of Lugol's solution and inspected after biopsy to ensure that the area designated as atypical has been removed (Color Fig. 23-11).

UNSATISFACTORY COLPOSCOPY

If the transformation zone and squamocolumnar junction are located within the endocervical canal and cannot be adequately visualized, the examination is termed an unsatisfactory colposcopic evaluation. Such an evaluation is most likely to occur in postmenopausal women or women who have undergone conization, cryocautery, or laser stenosis. If it occurs in conjunction with an abnormal cytologic examination, endocervical curettage is mandatory.

INDICATION FOR COLPOSCOPY

The various uses of colposcopy are listed in Table 23-3. The ability of the gynecologist to use this technique depends on many factors, the most important of which is his dedication to increasing his expertise. This depends on the liberal use of biopsy and the correlation of colposcopic findings with cytopathology. Colposcopy must be learned with an in-depth understanding of the underlying cytopathology. Only by constant review of cytology, colposcopy, and pathology can the gynecologist incorporate this technique into his armamentarium.

Figure 23-5 outlines a suggested schedule for evaluating an abnormal cytologic finding.

Selected Reading

Anderson M, Jordan J, Morse A, Sharp F: Integrated colposcopy. New York, Chapman & Hall, 1992

Barrasso R, Carpez F, Ionesco M, et al: Human papillomavirus and cervical intraepithelial neoplasia: the role of colposcopy. Gynecol Oncol 27:197, 1987

Burke L, Antonioli DA, Ducatman BS: Colposcopy: text and atlas. Norwalk, CT: Appleton & Lange, 1991

Coppleson M, Pixley EC: Colposcopy of the cervix. In Coppleson M, Monaghan JM, Morrow CP, et al (eds): Gynecologic oncology, 2nd ed. Edinburgh, UK: Churchill Livingstone, 1992

Gilardi EM, Vialetto P: The behavior of white epithelium: a short-term follow-up by chromocolposcopy. The Cervix and l.f.g.t. 11:11, 1993

Kishi Y, Inui S, Sakamoto Y: Colposcopic findings of gland openings of cervical carcinoma. Int J Gynaecol Obstet 25:223, 1987

Toplis PJ, Casemore V, Hallan N, et al: Evaluation of colposcopy in the postmenopausal woman. Br J Obstet Gynaecol 93:843, 1986

Ambulatory Gynecology, Second Edition,
edited by David H. Nichols and Patrick J. Sweeney.
J. B. Lippincott Company, Philadelphia, © 1995.

Cryosurgery

Steven E. Swift and Donald R. Ostergard

Cryosurgery is the technique of applying subfreezing temperatures to affect tissue destruction. It has been used in medicine in one form or another for more than 100 years and is a common office procedure in the practice of gynecology. It has a broad spectrum of application and is used to treat a variety of gynecologic pathology, from infections to preinvasive disease. It also has the benefit of being a safe and low-cost form of therapy that is effective if properly applied and requires little or no anesthesia or analgesia. Although most gynecologists are familiar with its application in preinvasive disease of the cervix, cryosurgery also plays a role in treating diseases of the vulva and urethra. This chapter will familiarize the reader with some of the technical aspects of cryosurgery and provide information on the uses and indications for cryosurgery in the practice of gynecology.

HISTORY

Cryotherapy in gynecology has a long history. One of the first formal reports on cryotherapy was that of Openchowski, who in 1883 used cold water circulating through the vagina to treat chronic cervicitis.[1] One of the next reports was by Fay and Henry, who in 1938 used circulating cold water in the vagina as palliative treatment in a patient with cervical cancer, a rectovesicovaginal fistula, and severe pain.[2] The treatment produced complete pain relief, a decrease in the tumor size, and partial healing of the fistulas. The patient died 9 months later of her disease but was noted to be pain-free for most of that time. Weitzer, in 1940, introduced a more reliable and consistent refrigerant in the form of solid carbon dioxide rods.[3] He used this technique on patients with cervicitis and reported cure rates of 90%. In 1942, Hall improved further on the applicator by developing a cryoprobe to deliver freon to the cervix.[4] The major advantage of this was the ability to rapidly defrost the applicator, thereby overcoming one of the major problems with cryosurgery. Previously, the time involved in allowing the body temperature to thaw the tissue to remove the applicator was unacceptably long.

In 1967, Crisp and coworkers first reported on the use of cryotherapy in patients with preinvasive disease and cancer of the cervix and vagina.[5] Twenty patients with carcinoma in situ (CIS) and stage I cervical cancer underwent cryotherapy and had definitive surgery 1 to 7 weeks postfreeze. In only one specimen was residual cancer identified. They also used this technique in patients with terminal malignant disease and were able to provide pain relief, decrease hemorrhage, and in some instances decrease tumor size. He was not able to increase longevity, however. In 1970, Crisp and associates treated 114 patients with preinvasive disease of the cervix with cryotherapy and reported no recurrences.[6] Their patients were diagnosed by cone biopsy and therefore, most of the abnormal tissue was removed before cryosurgery.

Townsend and Ostergard, in 1971, performed the first large study using cryosurgery in patients with preinvasive disease of the cervix diagnosed by colposcopy and biopsy.[7] They reported a 90% cure rate and showed that outpatient cryosurgery was an acceptable alternative to cone biopsy. Since then, there have been multiple studies demonstrating the efficacy of cryosurgery in treating cervical dysplasia.

From a historical perspective, cryosurgical techniques have also been attempted on the endometrium. Cahan, in 1964, conducted some preliminary studies on cryotherapy of the endometrium.[8] He treated six patients with menometrorrhagia and was able to decrease the bleeding in five of the six but did not report long-term follow-up. In the 1970s, Droegemueller attempted cryotherapy of the endometrium to treat dysfunctional uterine bleeding and as a sterilization technique.[9-11] His attempts likewise met with limited success because of difficulty in completely freezing the endometrial cavity and the difficulty that he found in effectively obliterating the endometrial cornu for sterilization. These uses for cryosurgery have been largely abandoned. Cryosurgery has evolved greatly over the past century from the use of ice water circulating in the vagina to the generation of cryoprobes. There have also been many proposed uses for cryotherapy in the field of gynecology, ranging from cancer therapy to sterilization. Although some of them have proved of little benefit, others are accepted treatment modalities and cryosurgery enjoys widespread use in the field of gynecology.

EFFECTS OF CRYOSURGERY

The effects of cryosurgery on tissue have been extensively studied and are well known. Tissue destruction is brought about by cellular disruption and avascular necrosis from the freezing process, and the histologic changes are so characteristic that they have been termed "cryonecrosis." Tissue repair and healing is accompanied by intense inflammation and hyalinization of the stroma. While these changes are characteristic follow-up cytology may be misinterpreted and misleading until the tissue has completely healed. Understanding the effects of cryosurgery on tissue destruction and repair gives a better appreciation of its role and allows avoidance of some of the common pitfalls that accompany its use.

Most studies agree that cellular death occurs at or around $-20°C$, the eutectic point of a sodium chloride solution. The primary effects are physical rupture of the cell wall by developing intra- and extracellular ice crystals in addition to changes in electrolyte balance and pH that occur with disruption of the phospholipid membrane. This leads to cellular dehydration, protein denaturation, and release of intracellular substances, which lead to further breakdown, dysfunction, and eventually cellular death (Fig. 24-1).[5,6,12-14,20] Avascular necrosis is also produced by small vessel obstruction and intracapillary sludging from the freezing process. Angiograms taken 1 hour after cryotherapy show no small-vessel filling in the area treated.[15] Larger vessels, however, are resistant to the effects of cryosurgery by their ability to draw heat or cold away from the tissue and therefore are not affected acutely. This limits the progression of the developing ice ball and explains the basic tenant of cryosurgery: the depth and extent of tissue destruction is inversely related to its vascularity.[16] There is also destruction of the afferent sensory nerve endings

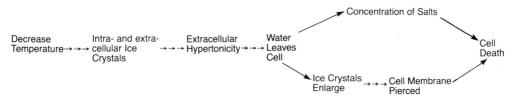

Figure 24–1. Mechanism of cellular destruction with cryosurgery.

and this explains the anesthetic effects of cryosurgery.

These properties make cryotherapy a safe and effective procedure. Localized lesions are effectively destroyed, whereas the surrounding tissue is spared. The effects on the vascular structures make it a relatively bloodless procedure, with only about half of the patients reporting post-treatment spotting. Also, its anesthetic properties make it well tolerated by patients who usually report only menstrual cramp–like discomfort.[17,20,21]

Although cryosurgery appears to be an ideal treatment modality, there are some potential adverse effects and complications that may arise during healing. The histologic changes that occur after cryosurgery during the repair process have been thoroughly documented and studied.[5,6,12–14,20] Twenty-four hours after freezing, there is resulting necrosis, with extensive edema and infiltration of the tissue, and a mucoid membrane develops overlying the treated area (Fig. 24-2). This area is sharply demarcated from the surrounding tissue, which shows little or no inflammation. Over the next several days to weeks, this membrane sloughs and is replaced by granulation tissue, which is responsible for the heavy serosanguineous discharge experienced by almost all patients. Subsequently, the squamous epithelium proliferates and re-epithelializes the lesion, so that by 1 month post-treatment, the cervix generally appears normal and the discharge abates. This may lead to the squamocol-

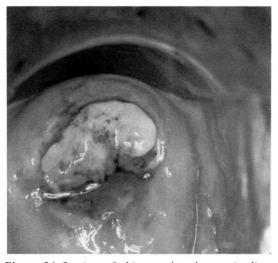

Figure 24–2. Area of white noted on the anterior lip of the cervix is the mucoid membrane that develops after cryosurgery (photograph taken 10 days after cryosurgery).

umnar junction migrating upward into the endocervical canal.

The underlying stroma is initially infiltrated with polymorphonuclear leukocytes and lymphocytes, and close inspection reveals that although the cells appear intact, they are mere ghosts, without metabolic activity. The endothelial cells slough into the vascular channels and contribute to the thrombosis. Over the next 3 to 4 weeks, the stroma is replaced by collagen and the vascular channels are re-epithelialized, with associated perivascular hyalinization and thickening of the intima. This leads to contraction and shrinkage of the stroma and contributes to the migration of the squamocolumnar junction up the endocervical canal. Eventually, the hyalinized stroma is replaced by a more normal histologic makeup, and this explains how some patients may regain a normal location of the squamocolumnar junction.

The cytologic changes that occur during this process reflect the histologic changes in the tissue. Karyorrhexis, perinuclear halo formation, and vacuolization are commonly seen, and these changes may persist for up to 1 year after treatment.[18] Also, in the first few months, it is not uncommon to see parabasal cells with hyperchromatic and irregular nuclei that may be confused with changes noted in cervical dysplasias.[12] Pap smears performed during this time may be mistaken for squamous atypia or even mild dysplasia. This misinterpretation can be avoided by noting that the nuclear changes associated with significant dysplasia are lacking. It has also been shown that many mild atypias and mild dysplasias noted on Pap smears within the first 6 months after cryosurgery spontaneously regress.[19] Whether this is because of misinterpretation of the smears secondary to the intense inflammatory changes or whether these represent true atypical Pap smears that regress spontaneously is not known.

Cryosurgery can also be used on the vulva, with little scarring. Histologic studies show that many of the same changes noted in cryonecrosis of the cervix are found in normal skin and epidermis after therapy. There is cellular disruption and death, with desquamation of the epidermis and hyalinization of the dermis; dead fat is replaced by collagen but the treated area eventually reepithelializes and heals with little visible scarring.[15]

Cryosurgery effectively destroys localized lesions through the effects of cryonecrosis. There is a high degree of safety with this procedure and little operative blood loss or discomfort. One should remain familiar, however, with the histologic and cytologic changes that occur after cryosurgery because they may lead to the diagnosis of recurrent or persistent disease.

TECHNIQUE FOR CRYOTHERAPY

Cervical Cryotherapy

As in other forms of surgery, technique is important in the implementation of cryosurgery. The most important aspect of this involves preoperative evaluation and selection of appropriate candidates. Many cases of treatment failure or progression to invasive disease can be traced back to improper or incomplete evaluation. Also, proper use of the equipment and an understanding of the biology of the cryosurgical lesions are necessary to properly and fully treat those patients who are candidates. If these methods are employed, cryosurgery carries a high success rate.

In the late 1970s, cryosurgery was being widely employed to treat benign and preinvasive lesions of the cervix. Several reports began to surface, however, regarding invasive cervical cancer after cryotherapy.[23,24] Townsend and coworkers set up a registry to attempt to determine the magnitude of the problem and allow analysis of the evaluation errors.[22] There was evidence of inappropriate preoperative evaluation of most of the patients who were diagnosed with cancer after cryotherapy. Some patients were treated based on symptoms and gross visualization of the cervix; others were treated based on Pap smear results alone or an incomplete colposcopic evaluation and some patients were treated despite having a positive endocervical curettage (ECC). From these registry findings, several recommendations were made regarding patient evaluation and selection: (1) all patients with cervical bleeding should be fully evaluated with colposcopy, cervical biopsy, and ECC before treatment; (2) all patients who have abnormal cytology should likewise undergo a colposcopic evaluation with cervical biopsy and ECC; if the ECC shows abnormal epithelium, a cervical conization should be performed; (3) those patients with benign cervicitis noted visually should have at least two negative Pap smears or one negative Pap smear and a negative colposcopic examination before treatment (Table 24-1). If these recommendations are followed closely, there should be few cases of inappropriate selection of candidates, alleviating a large source of failures.

Once those patients who are candidates are properly evaluated and selected, they are treated

Table 24–1
Preoperative Evaluation for Cryosurgery of the Cervix

Patients with cervicitis and no bleeding
Two normal Pap smears or one normal Pap smear and a negative colposcopic evaluation.
Patients with cervical bleeding or abnormal Pap smear
Satisfactory colposcopic evaluation identifying the entire lesion.
Biopsies of any abnormal appearing epithelium.
Endocervical curettage.

(Adapted from Townsend DE, Richart RM, Mark E, Nielsen J: Invasive cancer following outpatient evaluation and therapy for cervical disease. Obstet Gynecol 57:145, 1981)

using the proper technique. In performing the procedure, generally no analgesia or anesthesia is necessary. Most patients experience mild cramping pain but generally this is well tolerated. A nonsteroidal anti-inflammatory agent may be prescribed, however, and taken by the patient at home 3 to 4 hours before the procedure.

First, the lesion in its entirety must be identified to be sure that it can be entirely encompassed by the probe tip. There are several techniques one may employ. The procedure can be performed under direct colposcopic visualization after the application of 3% acetic acid, or Lugol's solution may be applied to the cervix and the procedure conducted under gross visualization. If the second method is used, the physician must ensure that the lesion identified with the Lugol's solution corresponds to the lesion identified colposcopically.

Once the lesion has been identified, a probe tip is selected that will completely cover the lesion (Fig. 24-3). As a general rule, a large nipple-tip probe is most effective in treating all lesions.[25] This allows greater coverage of the ecto- and endocervix. Also, coating the tip with a water-soluble lubricant allows a more uniform freeze.[25,26] This is particularly important in the parous cervix, in which there tends to be scarring and irregularities of the topography.

The double-freeze technique should always be employed when performing cryosurgery.[27,28] A 3- to 5-minute freeze, ensuring that the ice-ball formation extends 4 to 5 mm beyond the edge of the lesion, is followed by a 5-minute thaw and a second 3- to 5-minute freeze. This technique is superior to

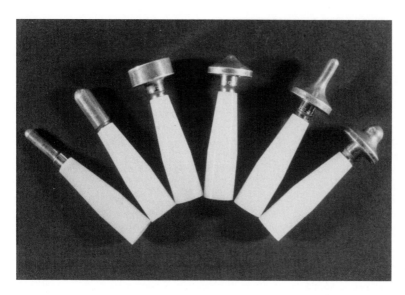

Figure 24–3.   Selection of tips for a cryoprobe.

the single-freeze method in eradicating the lesion in cases of preinvasive cervical disease.[27] Histochemically, water redistributes throughout the tissue mass once the cellular membranes have been disrupted. This leads to a more uniform distribution of ice crystals in the intra- and extracellular space with the second freeze, allowing further and more complete destruction of cellular membranes and organelles.[13] Electron microscopy has shown that membrane, mitochondrial, and nuclear changes are greater and more complete after using the double-freeze technique than after using the single-freeze technique.[29] During the freeze, ensure that the cryoprobe tip is less than −20°C and remains so throughout both freeze cycles. The temperature is 0°C at the edge of the ice ball; therefore, the ice ball must extend several millimeters beyond the edge of the lesion to ensure a temperature of −20°C to the abnormal epithelium. After the procedure, the patient should be counseled regarding the heavy vaginal discharge, which may last up to 4 to 6 weeks. Patients should also be instructed to avoid placing anything into the vagina during this time.

Vulvar Cryosurgery

Patient selection is again important when using cryosurgery on vulvar lesions. Diffuse or multifocal lesions are more likely to recur after cryosurgery than are a few well-demarcated lesions.[30] This is particularly true with vulvar intraepithelial neoplasia and vulvar condyloma, which tend to be multifocal. Colposcopic assessment after the application

of 3% acetic acid should be performed and appropriate biopsy samples taken to rule out invasion. Once identified, the base of the lesion should be infiltrated with 1% lidocaine. The probe tip should be wetted with a saline or water-soluble lubricant and applied to the lesion, with freezing continued until the ice ball extends 1 to 2 mm beyond the lesion.[31] The double-freeze technique should be employed to ensure adequate treatment. Because the probe tip does not adhere to the tissue without first wetting it, this step is important to ensure an adequate freeze. The patient should be instructed to use liberal sitz baths and application of 2% lidocaine jelly as needed for postoperative discomfort.

Urethral Cryotherapy

Patients with a urethral syndrome that does not respond to conservative therapy and patients with urethral condyloma are candidates for urethral cryotherapy.[32,33] Again, appropriate diagnostic procedures and biopsy should be part of the preoperative evaluation.

A specially designed 26 French cryoprobe is inserted into the urethra (Fig. 24-4). Treatment consists of a 90-second freeze, followed by a 180-second thaw, followed by a 60- to 90-second refreeze. The length of the second freeze is determined by the cryoprobe temperature. If it is less than −26°C, the second freeze should be shortened by 30 seconds to avoid excessive cryonecrosis. With this technique, the depth of cryonecrosis should not be greater than 2 mm. Two percent lidocaine jelly

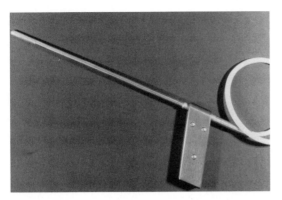

Figure 24–4.   Cryoprobe for urethral cryotherapy.

is inserted into the urethra and 50 mL of 4% lidocaine into the bladder preoperatively as anesthetic agents. A bladder pillar block should be considered if the urethra is particularly sensitive. Patients tolerate this procedure fairly well, with minimal discomfort.

After the procedure, an 8 French Foley catheter is placed because the resulting edema may lead to obstruction, and in-and-out catheterization may traumatize the fragile postfreeze urethral mucosa. On postoperative day 1, patients are instructed to push the catheter about 3 cm upward into the bladder and attempt to void around it. Once they are able to do this with postvoid residual urine being less than 100 mL, the catheter is removed. This usually takes 2 to 4 days. Patients are placed on suppressant antibiotics while the catheter remains in place. The patient should be counseled regarding the placement of this catheter preoperatively. Generally, postprocedure catheterization is well tolerated by the patients if they receive preoperative counseling regarding its use.

INDICATIONS

Cryosurgery enjoys widespread use for multiple indications in gynecologic practice. It has been extensively studied and applied in the treatment of cervical disease and has also been used to treat a wide variety of vulvar and urethral disease. Despite the abundant literature, however, there are still several questions remaining regarding its application. This section presents a relevant discussion on a wide variety of applications and allows the reader to decide how best to employ cryosurgery in his or her practice.

CERVICAL DISEASE

Cervicitis

Although some of the earliest literature on the use of cryosurgery involved cervical cancer therapy, these were largely case reports.[1,2] The first real application of cryosurgery was in the treatment of cervicitis.[3] Previously, patients with cervicitis and cervical erosions were treated with electrocautery but the results were less than satisfactory, with many patients requiring multiple treatments for complete healing.[34–36] Cryosurgery proved an effective alternative, with most patients requiring only a single treatment for resolution of their symptoms. In a study comparing the two, cryosurgery was also noted to have better patient tolerance and decreased postoperative bleeding.[37]

Complete healing of the cervix occurs in about 90% of patients by 6 weeks after a single treatment.[13,17,29] The results with single- or double-freeze techniques are comparable, and cervicitis is the one situation in which a single freeze may be employed. Cryosurgery has largely replaced electrocautery and is an accepted form of therapy in treating patients with cervicitis. Before treatment, however, the diagnosis of cervicitis should be confirmed by cytology or biopsy to rule out other disease processes.

Cervical Intraepithelial Neoplasia

In the early 1970s, cryosurgery was introduced as a method to treat preinvasive disease of the cervix. Since that time, there have been many reports with divergent opinions regarding its effectiveness in treating patients with advanced grades of dysplasia.[7,21,27,38,40–58]

There is general agreement that in treating patients with cervical intraepithelial neoplasia (CIN) grades I and II, cryosurgery offers an excellent low-cost form of therapy, with cure rates reported as greater than 90%.[21,38–43] There are reports in the literature of less-than-optimal cure rates; however, careful examination of these studies often reveals incomplete evaluation or treatment (ie, no ECC performed preoperatively or a single-freeze technique used).[28,44,45]

The controversy concerning the use of cryosurgery in preinvasive disease of the cervix surrounds its use in CIN III and CIS. In these cases, the literature is not in agreement and cure rates range from 61% to 96% (Table 24-2.) The reasons for this

Table 24–2
Results of Treatment of Advanced Grades of Dysplasia With Cryotherapy

Author	Type of Dysplasia	Failure Rate (%)
Townsend (1971)[7]	SD/CIS	11.8/10*
Tredway (1972)[46]	CIN3	30.6
Creasman (1973)[27]	CIN3	31.2
DiSaia (1974)[47]	SD/CIS	9.3/12*
Popkin (1978)[48]	SD/CIS	4/9
Kaufman (1978)[43]	SD/CIS	17.3/21.4*
Walton (1980)[49]	CIN3	31.6
Ostergard (1980)[38]	SD/CIS	7.1/38.8*
Hatch (1981)[58]	CIN3	7
Hammingsson (1981)[51]	CIS	18
Wright (1981)[40]	CIN3	25
Benedet (1981)[52]	SD/CIS	9/8*
Peckham (1982)[53]	SD/CIS	6.5/20*
Savage (1982)[50]	SD/CIS	9.5/33.3*
Stuart (1982)[54]	SD/CIS	18/0*
Townsend (1983)[21]	CIN3	10
Creasman (1984)[55]	CIN3	17.7
Arof (1984)[57]	CIN3	27.1
Bryson (1985)[56]	CIN3	7.1
Kwikkel (1985)[44]	CIN3	8
Ferenczy (1985)[41]	CIN3	29
Anderson (1988)[42]	CIN3	23

SD, severe dysplasia; CIS, carcinoma in situ; CIN3, cervical intraepithelial neoplasia.
*Where two failure rates are given this represents separate rates for SD and CIS in those studies where the distinction was made. SD failure rate/CIS failure rate.

disparity are many and usually involve (1) problems with proper evaluation and selection of candidates, (2) improper technique in treatment, (3) lack of uniform follow-up, (4) variable size of the lesion, (5) and the extent of endocervical gland involvement. Proper preoperative evaluation should include colposcopy with appropriate biopsies, visualization of the entire lesion, ECC, and general agreement between diagnoses by cytology and histology of biopsies. If the ECC is positive, the biopsies suggest invasion, or there is significant disparity between the cytology and the histology, then the patient should undergo a cervical conization (Table 24-3). In reviewing those studies with high failure rates, the above-mentioned criteria were not strictly followed. Several studies did not employ ECC as a routine preoperative evaluation or patients were treated with cryotherapy despite a positive ECC. In the studies that employed cryosurgery despite en-

docervical disease, significantly higher failure rates were noted when the lesion extended into the endocervical canal.[42,43,50,57] Therefore, the results of studies in which patients who either had existing endocervical disease or who were treated without endocervical sampling should be suspect.

Another problem noted in some studies involves the cryosurgical technique employed. Most of the studies employed the single-freeze technique in part or all of their treated population. The double-freeze technique has been shown to be superior and should always be employed.[27,28,56] In the study by Creasman and colleagues, the single-freeze technique only provided a 69% cure, whereas the double-freeze technique provided a greater than 80% cure.[27] Studies that employ only the single-freeze technique should be expected to have lower cure rates.

Also important in evaluating a study is the defi-

Table 24–3

Selection Criteria for Cryosurgery in Patients With Cervical Intraepithelial Neoplasia

Appropriate preoperative evaluation

General agreement between cytology and histology*

No endocervical involvement

No evidence of invasive cancer

No abnormal epithelium in inaccessible topographic abnormalities of the ectocervix†

Lesion size may play a role in the selection criteria but only in that larger lesions tend to have more endocervical involvement, or may be cumbersome to treat with overlapping cryoprobe applications.

*Pap smear and cervical biopsies should not be off by more than one grade of dysplasia.

†Such as the deep clefts commonly seen at 3 and 9 o'clock in the parous cervix.

---

nition of cure and the length and method of follow-up that are employed. Follow-up should be for at least 1 year because most failures occur within this time.[43,52,56,58] Some studies define cure as negative follow-up cytology without atypia or CIN for 6 months; this may include only one or two follow-up Pap smears. In this country, the incidence of false-negative Pap smears may be as high as 40%; consequently, if the cure rate is based on only one or two follow-up cytologic evaluations, the cure rates could be falsely elevated.[59] The definition of cure also needs to be stated. Some studies define cure as negative follow-up Pap smears, whereas others insist on negative follow-up colposcopic exams in addition to normal Pap smears. There are also a few studies that define failure as the presence of CIN II or higher grade dysplasia on follow-up cytology and consider the presence of CIN I or lesser pathology as being a cure.[7,56] Finally, there is the question of persistent atypia that most studies do not address.

As previously mentioned, cytology after cryosurgery may be misinterpreted because of the intense inflammation that occurs during healing. Accurate assessment of treatment should include colposcopic examination, cervical biopsy, and ECC if the Pap smear shows dysplasia or significant persistent atypia. The routine use of follow-up colposcopy with each exam is not warranted. It has been suggested that ECC should be performed as part of the post-treatment evaluation because the squamocolumnar junction frequently migrates up the en-

docervical canal and the addition of ECC to cytologic evaluation may detect up to 12% of failures that may be missed with cytology alone.[38,43] Figge and Creasman, in a review article, suggest that appropriate follow-up should include negative cytology and ECC for a minimum of 2 years and that this will reduce the incidence of undetected residual disease after treatment.[60] These reports predate the widespread use of endocervical brushes; because it is generally agreed that this is an excellent form of endocervical sampling, endocervical brush sampling may be all that is necessary for follow-up (Table 24-4).

With the above in mind, there are several large studies that include all or most of the criteria for appropriate selection, treatment, and follow-up. Even among these studies, however, the cure rates for cryosurgery in patients with CIN III and CIS range from 61% to 90%.[21,38,42,51,55,58] Therefore, it is difficult to determine with absolute assurance the effectiveness of cryosurgery in eradicating advanced grades of dysplasia.

Most studies in the literature demonstrate a decrease in cure rates with increasing grades of dysplasia. There may be several reasons for this but probably the most important is the natural history of the lesions. There is a regression to normal in many patients with untreated lower-grade lesions.[61] Also, lesions with higher-grade dysplasia tend to be larger and have deeper cervical glandular crypt extension.[28,49,55–57] This brings up another controversial point regarding lesion size and treatment failures. Several studies show that larger lesions are more prone to failure.[21,39,41,44] They used different methods, however, to describe the size of a lesion (ie,

Table 24–4

Recommended Follow-Up for Patients With Cervical Intraepithelial Neoplasia Treated With Cryosurgery

---

Pap smears every 3 months for the first year, then every 6 months for the second year, then yearly

Colposcopic evaluation for any significant atypia or dysplasia

Endocervical sampling at each visit*

---

*The endocervical sampling may be by either endocervical curettage or by endocervical brush.

Adapted from Figge DC, Creasman WT: Cryotherapy in the treatment of cervical intraepithelial neoplasia. Obstet Gynecol 62:353, 1983

number of involved quadrants versus a subjective small, medium, and large classification) and did not mention whether the larger lesions had endocervical extension or if the ice-ball formation covered the entire lesion with at least a 2-mm extension beyond the abnormal epithelium. Consequently, it is difficult to compare and evaluate these reports. Adding to the confusion are several studies that do not demonstrate any effect of lesion size on cure rates.[38,52,55–57] The size of the lesion may play a role but only that larger lesions are more likely to have endocervical extension or are incompletely frozen.

This should all be considered when selecting those patients who are candidates for treatment. If patients with CIN III and CIS are considered for treatment with cryosurgery they should undergo (1) appropriate preoperative evaluation, including ECC; (2) treatment with a double-freeze technique (3-minute freeze, 5-minute thaw, 3-minute freeze); and (3) frequent long-term follow-up with Pap smears and ECC (or endocervical brush sampling) at each visit, with colposcopy when indicated. Follow-up visits should be every 3 months for 1 year and then every 6 months for 1 year.

Despite the controversy regarding the role of cryosurgery in advanced grades of cervical dysplasia, compared with other conservative forms of therapy, it appears to have similar cure rates. Cervical conization carries a cure rate of 84% to 96% and is judged to be as effective as hysterectomy in treating patients with CIN III and CIS.[63–65] Cervical conization carries a higher morbidity rate, requires hospitalization with anesthesia, and even when the margins are free of dysplasia, there is residual disease in up to 16% of the hysterectomy specimens.[64] Also, the same arguments against cryotherapy in terms of migration of the squamocolumnar junction into the endocervical canal and difficulty detecting persistent disease by cytology apply to conization.[60]

Laser ablation of the transformation zone is a popular means of treating patients with CIN III and CIS and has been compared with cryotherapy in several studies (Table 24-5). From the data, it appears that cryosurgery compares favorably with laser therapy. Laser therapy is thought to be superior because the depth of destruction can be accurately gauged and destruction of all glandular crypts can be ensured. Most of the glandular crypts are less than 5 mm in depth and dysplastic epithelium is generally not found beyond a depth of 2.5 mm.[61,62] This is the rationale for the destruction to a depth of 5 to 7 mm with laser therapy. When cryosurgery is appropriately applied, destruction of tissue to a depth of 4 to 5 mm is obtained and is deemed adequate.[25] Therefore, it is not surprising that in comparing the two, the cure rates are similar. Laser therapy has the advantage of efficiently destroying larger lesions that would require overlapping of applications with the cyroprobe, which can be cumbersome. Also, if the lesions are located deep in the clefts (normally found at 3 and 9 o'clock) in the parous cervix, cryosurgery is inadequate in obtaining an appropriate depth of destruction to efficiently obliterate the dysplastic epithelium.[25] In properly selected cases, however, cryotherapy is as effective as other forms of therapy in treating advanced grades of dysplasia.

The loop excision of the transformation zone is a new mode of therapy for cervical dysplasia and is being extensively studied. There are no large studies that compare it with cryotherapy, however, and time and experience will determine its role in CIN.

Genital Human Papillomavirus Infection

Genital tract human papillomavirus (HPV) infection is a major problem and concern in the field of gynecology and is thought by many to play a role in dysplasia and cancer of the lower female genital

Table 24–5
Comparative Studies on Cryosurgery versus Laser Therapy in the Treatment of Cervical Intraepithelial Neoplasia III

Author	Laser Therapy Failure Rate (%)	Cryotherapy Failure Rate (%)
Wright (1981)[40]	8	25
Townsend (1983)[21]	13	10
Ferenczy (1985)[41]	6	29
Kwikkel (1989)[44]	19	8

tract. Cryosurgery has been used to treat condyloma of the cervix, vagina, and vulva, with mixed results, and its use in vaginal disease has for the most part been abandoned. The flacidity of the vaginal wall, the multifocal nature of HPV infections, and the concern regarding vesicovaginal and rectovaginal fistulas have precluded its use in vaginal disease.[66] Cryosurgery remains a popular form of therapy, however, for cervical, vulvar, and urethral condyloma and in the latter two, appears to be effective if properly applied.

Cervical Human Papillomavirus

In treating cervical condyloma, cryotherapy carries a success rate between 50% and 90% but recurrences are common.[45,67–69] The reason for the high recurrence rate is that the HPV reservoir is not adequately treated. In most studies, routine evaluation of the urethra and anus was not employed and these are known reservoirs of HPV. If these reservoirs are not adequately evaluated and treated at the time the cervical disease is treated, recurrences should be expected. Despite the high recurrence in cervical infections, cryotherapy effectively treats the CIN commonly associated with HPV lesions, resulting in adequate treatment of the dysplasia even though the HPV infection persists.[45] Therefore, the premalignant potential of the HPV lesions is eradicated. No long-term follow-up has been conducted, however, to determine the incidence of recurrent dysplasia in these patients. An interesting report in the literature by Myers and coworkers suggests an increased immune response against specific tumors after cryosurgical destruction of a portion of that tumor.[70] Thus, individuals may be more resistant to the carcinogenic effects of HPV after cryosurgery—an interesting hypothesis that needs to be confirmed. Cryosurgery may alter the natural course of an HPV infection of the cervix but it does not appear to be effective in eradicating the disease and has a limited role in treating cervical condyloma.

Vulvar Human Papillomavirus Infections

Although there are only a few reports in the literature regarding the use of cryosurgery in the treatment of vulvar condyloma, it appears to be effective in eradicating isolated lesions.[31,71] This may not eradicate reservoir infections and if recurrence is noted, a thorough evaluation should be performed that includes urethroscopy, anoscopy, and colposcopy. With large or multifocal disease, cryosurgery has not proved its efficacy and laser therapy has a distinct advantage. Applying the cryoprobe to large areas of multifocal disease is cumbersome compared with laser therapy, wherein large areas can be ablated quickly and easily. For isolated lesions, however, cryotherapy appears to be effective and produces little or no scarring.

Urethral Human Papillomavirus Infections

If urethral condyloma are detected on urethroscopic examination, cryotherapy offers an excellent mode of therapy. In a report by Sand and associates, eight patients with proximal urethral condyloma were treated with cryotherapy, with no recurrences at 6 months.[33] Although somewhat limited information is available in the literature, it appears that this is an excellent form of therapy.

Other Vulvar Disorders

There are several studies of cryotherapy for treatment of a variety of vulvar diseases. There is a case report of a 3-year-old Haitian female who had pediatric bowenoid papillosis of the vulva successfully treated by cryotherapy.[72] Another small study reported four patients with vulvar intraepithelial neoplasia grade II and III who were successfully treated with cryotherapy, with no recurrences after 5 years.[30] Cryotherapy has also been used in the treatment of patients with vulvar vestibulitis syndrome but it has not been shown to be significantly better than observation alone.[73]

Cryosurgery appears to be an effective treatment option for specific vulvar lesions. Other forms of therapy (eg, laser) are equally effective and better suited to treat a large field.

Other Urethral Disorders

One area in which cryosurgery has been found to be effective is the treatment of urethral disorders. In patients with urethral syndrome that is unresponsive to urethral dilation and massage, cryosurgery offers an alternative method of treatment, with excellent cure rates. After one treatment, 60% to 70% of patients reported improvement in their symptoms, increasing to more than 90% in patients who required a second treatment.[32,74] There have been no urethrovaginal fistulas or urethral stenosis reported with this form of treatment.

The use of cryosurgery to successfully treat urethral prolapse and caruncles has also been described.[75–77] It has also been used as adjunctive therapy in urethral cancer.[77] Cryotherapy has a role in treating patients with urethral disorders and is a safe and effective means of therapy, with excellent cure rates.

Cryosurgery is an effective form of therapy for a wide range of gynecologic diseases and in some situations (ie, urethral syndrome and urethral condylomata), it appears to be the optimal method. There remains some controversy regarding its use with high-grade cervical dysplasia but if used judiciously, it should remain an effective treatment option.

COMPLICATIONS

One of the major advantages of cryosurgery is the low incidence of complications associated with the procedure. However, the clinician should be aware of potential postoperative problems, however. Its use in vulvar and urethral disease is relatively uncommon and there is little literature regarding complications in these settings. In the few studies that employed urethral cryosurgery for treating the urethral syndrome and urethral condylomata, there were no reported instances of postoperative stenosis or urethrovaginal fistulas. The potential problems that may arise after cryotherapy for cervical disease have been extensively studied and can be divided into short-term sequelae and long-term changes in structure and function.

The most common complaint after cryosurgery of the cervix is the profuse watery discharge during healing that occurs in virtually all patients and may last for 2 to 13 weeks. This discharge is high in potassium salts and some suggest that it may lead to weakness from hypokalemia. One author recommends that patients eat foods high in potassium during this time.[29] It has been shown, however, that serum potassium remains stable during the postoperative course; therefore, this discharge does not appear to cause a significant electrolyte imbalance.[20]

Postoperative bleeding may be a frequent complication but is rarely of sufficient amount to warrant further therapy. Whereas up to 40% of patients may have some spotting, only a few (0% to 3%) have bleeding that requires hemostatic measures.[17,20,29,41] Throughout the healing process, the cervix is covered by granulation tissue and is susceptible to manipulation or trauma. Postcoital bleeding has been noted in up to 25% of patients after cryosurgery.[20] Therefore, patients should be counseled to avoid placing anything into the vagina (ie, tampons, douches, or intercourse) until the discharge has abated. Most instances of significant postoperative bleeding can be traced to patients not following the physician's counsel regarding pelvic rest.

Lack of significant hemorrhage with cryosurgery is a distinct advantage over other forms of therapy. In studies comparing it with laser therapy, (1) significant blood loss occurred only during laser treatment, (2) postoperative bleeding occurred in 20% to 31% of patients after laser surgery; (3) postoperative bleeding severe enough to require vaginal packing only occurred after laser therapy.[21,44] Some authors have described using cryotherapy to control bleeding from other cervical procedures and in cases of advanced malignancy with uncontrolled hemorrhage.[12] As described previously, cryosurgery brings about small-vessel sludging and thrombosis, and this makes it an ideal modality for achieving hemostasis. With appropriate counseling to avoid cervical manipulation, postoperative bleeding should remain an infrequent complication and cryosurgery can be employed in cases of significant hemorrhage after other forms of cervical therapy.

Cervical stenosis after cryosurgery of the cervix is another common concern. The diameter of the cervical canal is decreased by 10% to 20% in about half of the patients treated but not enough to produce symptoms.[17,20,29] There are a few cases of cervical stenosis reported in the literature, in which patients developed mucometra and hematometra but this is so rare as to warrant case reports.[78,79]

There are also concerns regarding fertility, pregnancy loss, and dysfunctional labor that may occur as a result of changes in the cervical canal after cryotherapy. Several reports demonstrate normal fertility and normal spontaneous pregnancy loss after cervical cryotherapy compared with the general population.[29,39,80,81] The course and outcome of labor have been evaluated; a study of 30 term pregnancies reported that 23 delivered vaginally, four required forceps, and three required cesarean section—only one of which was for failure to progress. The duration of labor in these patients was not increased over expected times.[39] Consequently, the literature suggests that there do not appear to be long-term sequelae from cervical cryotherapy on fertility or pregnancy management. There are a few reports of cryosurgery on the cervix in patients during pregnancy.[12,27] However, there is not enough experience to make recommendations, except that patients should be followed-up until after delivery before treatment.

One other area of concern involves the affect of cryosurgery on upper genital tract infection. Several studies show a flare-up in pelvic inflammatory disease (PID) after treatment but only in patients with a previous history of genital tract infections. In no instance was cryosurgery thought to be responsible for inciting an upper genital tract infection.[22,29,81] Patients with active PID, however, should have therapy delayed until the infection has been properly treated. Creasman and coworkers and Curry and associates reported on the use of cryotherapy in patients with an intrauterine device (IUD) in place.[27,82] They noted two cases of pyometra that developed after cryosurgery in patients with an IUD in place and a history of PID. They concluded that this was an uncommon occurrence and do not recommend removing an IUD before surgery. They do, however, recommend anaerobic and aerobic cultures in these patients before therapy.

Overall, cryosurgery has the advantage of a low complication rate. Except for the serous discharge that occurs in almost all patients and the spotting that may occur in many patients, there are few short-term or long-term sequelae that adversely affect the cervix. Most of the data on complications involve cervical cryotherapy but even with urethral and vulvar treatment, no serious postoperative complications are reported. Therefore, cryosurgery should be viewed as a safe form of therapy to which the only absolute contraindications would be active upper genital tract infection and suspected invasive cancer.

SUMMARY

Cryosurgery as a form of therapy in the practice of gynecology has a long history. It has a role in the treatment of cervical, urethral, and vulvar diseases and its advantages include low cost, high effectiveness when properly applied, and minimal postoperative complications. Although its use in the treatment of advanced grades of cervical dysplasia remains controversial, cryosurgery may be an option when used judiciously and patients are appropriately evaluated and selected. By fully understanding its effects on tissue, its proper applications, and its possible complications, the practicing

gynecologist can best decide how to employ cryosurgery in his or her practice.

REFERENCES

1. Openchowski PH: Sur l'actron localisee du froid, appliquee a la surface de le region corticale du cerveau. Compt rend Soc de Biol 5:38, 1883
2. Fay T, Henry GC: Correlation of body segmental temperature and its relation to location of carcinomatous metastasis. Clinical observation and responses to methods of refrigeration. Surg Gynecol Obstet 66:512, 1938
3. Weitzer K: The treatment of endocervicitis with carbon dioxide snow (dry ice). Am J Surg 48:620, 1940
4. Hall FE: The use of quick freezing methods in gynecologic practice. Am J Obstet Gynecol 43:105, 1942
5. Crisp WE, Asadourin L, Romberg W: Application of cryosurgery to gynecologic malignancy. Obstet Gynecol 3:668, 1967
6. Crisp WE, Smith MS, Asadourin LA, Warrenburg LB: Cryosurgical treatment of premalignant disease of the uterine cervix. Am J Obstet Gynecol 107:737, 1970
7. Townsend DE, Ostergard DR: Cryocauterization for preinvasive cervical neoplasia. J Reprod Med 6:55, 1971
8. Cahan WG: Cryosurgery of the uterus: description of technique and potential application. Am J Obstet Gynecol 88:410, 1964
9. Droegemueller W, Greer BE, Makowski EL: Preliminary observations of cryocoagulation of the endometrium. Am J Obstet Gynecol 107:958, 1970
10. Droegemueller W, Greer BE, Makowski EL: Cryosurgery in patients with dysfunctional uterine bleeding. Obstet Gynecol 38:256, 1971
11. Droegemueller W, Greer BE, Davis JR, et al: Cryocoagulation of the endometrium at the uterine cornua. Am J Obstet Gynecol 131:1, 1978
12. Sonek MG, Acosta AA, Collins RJ, et al: Cryosurgery in the treatment of abnormal cervical lesions; an invitational symposium. J Reprod Med 7:147, 1971
13. Collins RJ, Golab A, Pappas HJ, Palovceck FP. Cryosurgery of the human cervix. Obstet Gynecol 30:660, 1967
14. Cahan WG, Brockunier A: Cryosurgery of the uterine cavity. Am J Obstet Gynecol 99:138, 1967
15. Myers B, Donovan W: Cryohemorrhoidectomy: an experimental study and clinical appraisal. Am Surg 41:799, 1975
16. Cooper IS: Cold as a surgical instrument. N Engl J Med 268:743, 1963
17. Ostergard DR, Townsend DE: The use of freon for the cryosurgical treatment of chronic cervicitis. J Cryosurg 1:67, 1968
18. Gondos B, Smith LR, Townsend DE: Cytologic changes in cervical epithelium following cryosurgery. Acta Cytol 14:386, 1970
19. Gondos B, Ostergard DR: Cytologic Evaluation following cryosurgical treatment for severe dyspla-

sia and carcinoma-in-situ. J Reprod Med 11:68, 1973

20. Ostergard DR, Townsend DE, Hirose FM: Treatment of chronic cervicitis by cryotherapy. Am J Obstet Gynecol 102:426, 1968

21. Townsend DE, Richart RM: Cryotherapy and carbon dioxide laser management of cervical intraepithelial neoplasia: a controlled comparison. Obstet Gynecol 61:75, 1983

22. Townsend DE, Richart RM, Mark E, Nielsen J: Invasive cancer following outpatient evaluation and therapy for cervical disease. Obstet Gynecol 57: 145, 1981

23. Sevin B, Ford JH, Girtanner RD, et al: Invasive cancer of the cervix after cryosurgery. Obstet Gynecol 53:465, 1979

24. Tredway DR, Townsend DE, Hovland DN, et al: Colposcopy and cryosurgery in cervical intraepithelial neoplasia. Am J Obstet Gynecol 114:1020, 1972

25. Boonstra H, Koudstaal J, Oosterhuis JW, et al: Analysis of cryolesions in the uterine cervix: application techniques, extension, and failures. Obstet Gynecol 75:232, 1990

26. DiSaia PJ, Creasman WT: Clinical gynecologic oncology, 3rd ed, p 27. St. Louis, CV Mosby, 1989

27. Creasman WT, Weed JL, Curry SC, Johnson WW, Parker RT: Efficacy of cryosurgical treatment of severe cervical intraepithelial neoplasia. Obstet Gynecol 41:501, 1973

28. Charles EH, Savage EW: Cryosurgical treatment of cervical intraepithelial neoplasia: analysis of failures. Gynecol Oncol 9:361, 1980

29. Collins RJ, Pappas HJ: Cryosurgery for benign cervicitis with follow-up of six and a half years. Am J Obstet Gynecol 113:744, 1972

30. Basta A: Diagnostic and therapeutic procedures in the vulvar intraepithelial neoplasia (VIN) and early invasive cancer of the vulva. Eur J Gynaec Oncol 10:55, 1989

31. Ostergard DR, Townsend DE: The treatment of vulvar condyloma acuminata by cryosurgery. Cryobiology 5:340, 1969

32. Sand PK, Bowen LW, Ostergard DR, Bent A, Panganiban R: Cryosurgery versus dilatation and massage for the treatment of recurrent urethral syndrome. J Reprod Med 34:499, 1989

33. Sand PK, Shen W, Bowen LW, Ostergard DR: Cryotherapy for the treatment of proximal urethral condyloma acuminatum. J Urol 137:874, 1986

34. Beard RW: Diathermy coning and cautery in the treatment of the eroded cervix. J Obstet Gynecol Br Com 71:287, 1964

35. Mathews HB: Electric cautery versus Sturmdorf operation in the treatment of chronic endocervicitis. JAMA 87:1802, 1926

36. Payne FL: The treatment of leucorrhea. Am J Obstet Gynecol 17:841, 1929

37. Miller JF, Elstein M: A comparison of electrocautery and cryocautery for the treatment of cervical erosions and chronic cervicitis. J Obstet Gynecol Br Com 80:653, 1973

38. Ostergard DR: Cryosurgical treatment of cervical intraepithelial neoplasia. Obstet Gynecol 56:231, 1980

39. Monaghan JM, Kirkup W, Davis JA, Edington PT: Treatment of cervical intraepithelial neoplasia by colposcopically directed cryosurgery and subsequent pregnancy experience. Br J Obstet Gynaecol 89:387, 1982

40. Wright VC, Davies EM: The conservative management of cervical intraepithelial neoplasia: the use of cryosurgery and the carbon dioxide laser. Br J Obstet Gynaecol 88:663, 1981

41. Ferenczy A: Comparison of cryo- and carbon dioxide laser therapy for cervical intraepithelial neoplasia. Obstet Gynecol 66:793, 1985

42. Anderson EJ, Thorup K, Larson G: The results of cryosurgery for cervical intraepithelial neoplasia. Gynecol Oncol 30:21, 1988

43. Kaufman RH, Irwin JF: The cryosurgical therapy of cervical intraepithelial neoplasia. Am J Obstet Gynecol 131:381, 1978

44. Kwikkel HJ, Helmerhorst TJM, Bezemer PD, Quakk MJ, Stolk JG: Laser or cryotherapy for cervical intraepithelial neoplasia: a randomized study to compare efficacy and side effects. Gynecol Oncol 22:23, 1985

45. Yliskoski M, Saarikoski S, Syrjanen K, Syrjanen S, Castern O: Cryotherapy and CO_2-laser vaporization in the treatment of cervical and vaginal human papillomavirus (HPV) infections. Acta Obstet Gynecol Scand 68:619, 1989

46. Tredway DR, Townsend DE, Hovland DW, Upton RT: Colposcopy and cryosurgery in cervical intraepithelial neoplasia. Am J Obstet Gynecol 114:1020, 1972

47. DiSaia PJ, Townsend DE, Morrow CP: The rationale for less than radical treatment for gynecological malignancy in early reproductive years. Obstet Gynecol Surv 29:581, 1974

48. Popkin DR, Scali V, Ahmed MN: Cryosurgery for the treatment of cervical intraepithelial neoplasia. Am J Obstet Gynecol 130:551, 1978

49. Walton LA, Edelman DA, Fowler WC, Photopulos GJ: Cryosurgery for the treatment of cervical intraepithelial neoplasia during the reproductive years. Obstet Gynecol 55:353, 1980

50. Savage EW, Matlock DL, Salem FA, Charles EH: The effects of endocervical gland involvement on the cure rates of patients with cervical intraepithelial neoplasia undergoing cryosurgery. Gynecol Oncol 14:194, 1982

51. Hammingsson E, Stendahl U, Stenson S: Cryosurgical treatment of cervical intraepithelial neoplasia with follow-up of five to eight years. Am J Obstet Gynecol 139:144, 1981

52. Benedet JL, Nickerson KG, Anderson GH: Cryotherapy in the treatment of cervical intraepithelial neoplasia. Obstet Gynecol 58:725, 1981

53. Peckham BM, Sonek MG, Carr WF: Outpatient therapy: success and failure with dysplasia and carcinona-in-situ. Am J Obstet Gynecol 142:323, 1982

54. Stuart GCE, Anderson RJ, Corlett BMA, Maruncic MA: Assessment of failures of cryosurgical treatment in cervical intraepithelial neoplasia. Am J Obstet Gynecol 142:658, 1982

55. Creasman WT, Hinshaw MS, Clarke-Pearson DL: Cryosurgery in the managment of cervical intraepithelial neoplasia. Obstet Gynecol 63:145, 1984

56. Bryson PSC, Lenehan P, Lickris MB: The treatment of grade 3 cervical intraepithelial neoplasia

with cryotherapy: an 11-year experience. Am J Obstet Gynecol 151:201, 1985

57. Arof HM, Gerbie MV, Smeltzer J: Cryosurgical treatment of cervical intraepithelial neoplasia: four-year experience. Am J Obstet Gynecol 150:865, 1984

58. Hatch KD, Shingleton HM, Austin M, Soong SJ, Bradley DH: Cryosurgery of cervical intraepithelial neoplasia. Obstet Gynecol 57:692, 1981

59. DiSaia PJ, Creasman WT: Clinical gynecologic oncology, 3rd ed, p 4. St. Louis, CV Mosby, 1989

60. Figge DC, Creasman WT: Cryotherapy in the treatment of cervical intraepithelial neoplasia. Obstet Gynecol 62:353, 1983

61. Anderson MC, Hartley RB: Cervical crypt involvement by intraepithelial neoplasia. Obstet Gynecol 55:546, 1980

62. Boonstra H, Aalders JG, Koudstaal J, Oosterhuis W, Janssens J: Minimum extension and appropriate topographic position of tissue destruction for treatment of cervical intraepithelial neoplasia. Obstet Gynecol 75:227, 1990

63. Bjerre B, Eliasson G, Linell F, Soderberg H, Sjoberg NO: Conization as only treatment of carcinoma in situ of the uterine cervix. Am J Obstet Gynecol 77:769, 1970

64. Kolstad P, Klem V: Long term follow-up of 1121 cases of carcinoma in situ. Obstet Gynecol 48:125, 1976

65. Ostergard DR: Prediction of clearance of cervical intraepithelial neoplasia by conization. Obstet Gynecol 56:77, 1980

66. DiSaia PJ, Creasman WT: Clinical gynecological oncology, 3rd ed, p 35. St. Louis, CV Mosby, 1989

67. Patsner B, Day TG, Powers W: The use of cryosurgery in the treatment of human papillomavirus infections of the cervix. Colp Gynecol Laser Surg 2:163, 1986

68. Ghosh AK: Cryosurgery of genital warts in cases in which podophyllin treatment failed or was contraindicated. Br J Vener Dis 53:49, 1977

69. Benrubi G, Nuss RC, Holmes K, Lammert N: Efficacy of cryotherapy in the treatment of human papillomavirus infection of the uterine cervix. J Fla Med Assoc 73:188, 1986

70. Myers RS, Hammond WG, Ketchum AS: Tumor-specific transplantation immunity after cryosurgery. J Surg Oncol 1:241, 1969

71. Huffman JW: Vulvar disorders in premenarchal children. Clin Obstet Gynecol 3:154, 1960

72. Weitzner JM, Feilds KW, Robinson MJ: Pediatric bowenoid papulosis: risks and managment. Pediatr Dermatol 6:303, 1989

73. Peckham BM, Maki DG, Patterson JJ, Hafez GR: Focal vulvitis: a characteristic syndrome and cause of dyspareunia. Am J Obstet Gynecol 154:855, 1986

74. Borehham P: Cryosurgery for the urethral syndrome. J R Soc Med 77:111, 1984

75. Friedrich EG: Cryosurgery for urethral prolapse. Obstet Gynecol 50:359, 1977

76. Droegemueller W, Herbst AL, Mishell DR, Stenchever MA: Comprehensive gynecology, p 443. St. Louis, CV Mosby, 1987

77. Ostergard DR, Townsend DE: Malignant melanoma of the female urethra treated by cryosurgery with radical vulvectomy and anterior exenteration. Obstet Gynecol 31:75, 1968

78. Guijon FB: Mucometra: a rare complication of cryosurgery. Am J Obstet Gynecol 159:26, 1988

79. Galt CE: Iatrogenic hematometra: cryogenic corking of the cervix: case report. Rocky Mt Med J 72:72, 1975

80. Ostergard DR, Townsend DE, Hirose FM: The long-term effects of cryosurgery on the uterine cervix. J Cryosurg 2:17, 1969

81. Weed JC, Curry SL, Duncan ID, Parker RT, Creasman WT: Fertility after cryosurgery of the cervix. Obstet Gynecol 52:245, 1978

82. Curry SL, Weed JL, Creasman WT: Pyometra: a complication of cervical cryosurgery. Obstet Gynecol 40:499, 1972

Ambulatory Gynecology, Second Edition,
edited by David H. Nichols and Patrick J. Sweeney.
J. B. Lippincott Company, Philadelphia, © 1995.

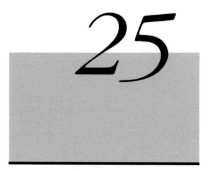

Laser Surgery of the Lower Genital Tract

Stephen M. Cohen

The laser is an extremely precise tool for removing lesions of the skin and mucous membranes. The application of this energy to female genital tract lesions has become a frequent treatment modality during the last decade. Lesions such as cervical, vaginal, and vulvar intraepithelial neoplasms and condylomata acuminata can accurately and safely be removed in an office or ambulatory setting, with significant reduction in tissue destruction and scarring.

"Laser" is an acronym for Light Amplification by Stimulated Emission of Radiation. In a laser, the electrons of a specific atom or molecule are excited to high, unstable energy levels. As the electrons fall back to their resting states, photons of a unique wavelength for that atom or molecule are released. These photons collide with other excited atoms/molecules in a mirrored chamber causing a cascade of photons to be released. When the laser is fired at its target, photons pass through a partially transmissive mirror at one end of the laser tube. These photons then travel down either a fiber, hollow wave guide, or mirrored tube to the impact site.

Laser light travels in waves. The wavelength depends on the atomic or molecular source of the photons. The wavelengths of light generated by medical lasers are found in the infrared-to-ultraviolet range of the light spectrum. Laser energy is nonionizing light, which may or may not be visible to the human eye. The general properties of laser light are similar for all lasers but specific basic properties vary by wavelength characteristics. Modern lasers can modify some of these basic properties by using advanced sophisticated delivery systems.

GENERAL PROPERTIES OF LASERS

There are three general properties of laser light that hold true for all medical lasers: all laser light is monochromatic, collimated, and coherent.

Monochromatic light is light all of one wavelength. Unlike common incandescent light or sunlight, which contains many wavelengths, the laser emits only one wavelength, which is specific for the type of laser used. These different wavelengths are the reason each specific laser device has unique interactions with matter, including fluids and tissue. Medical lasers have wavelengths that vary from 0.458 to 10.6 μm.

The coherent property of laser light means that the waves are in phase, both spatially and temporally. This means that the peaks and valleys of these waves all occur at the same time while the wave travels to the target.

Collimated light is light with rays all traveling parallel to each other. Parallel rays can be focused into a small space, which can then be captured by a lens system and further compressed. These properties of laser light give lasers the power and properties they possess.

SPECIFIC PROPERTIES OF LASERS

Although all lasers have the general properties just discussed, the specific properties of each laser are vastly different. The unique wavelength of each laser creates a wide variance in the photon–tissue interaction.

The ability to penetrate fluids depends on wavelength. Carbon dioxide laser energy is 90% absorbed by as little as 0.01 mm of water, whereas yttrium–aluminum–garnet (YAG), argon, and KTP laser wavelengths pass through water. Yttrium–aluminum–garnet, argon, and KTP laser wavelengths readily pass through substances that permit ordinary light to pass, such as glass and the cornea, whereas CO_2 laser light is absorbed by these substances, creating an immediate superficial effect. Certain laser wavelengths, such as that emitted by the argon laser, are preferentially absorbed by red-pigmented tissue.

EQUIPMENT

Laser ablation of lower genital tract lesions can be performed in the office or ambulatory surgery center. The CO_2 laser is most commonly used for destruction of these lesions.

Modern CO_2 lasers are self-contained, small, quiet machines that are powered by common electrical current and do not require water cooling. The CO_2 laser is composed of a high-voltage generator, a CO_2-gas laser chamber with mirrored ends, a hollow arm with mirrors at each knuckle, and an adaptor to connect to the handpiece, micromanipulator, and endoscope. Laser-beam firing is controlled by a foot pedal. A helium–neon finder beam marks the point of invisible CO_2 laser impact. The laser has settings that allow the operator to use single-pulse, repeat-pulse, or continuous laser power. Single-pulse power delivers one burst of energy when the foot pedal is depressed and does not fire again until the pedal is released and depressed again. The repeat-pulse setting fires intermittently, with a burst of energy—followed by a pause, followed by another burst—repeating as long as the operator keeps the pedal depressed. The continuous power setting allows photons to pass without interruption until the foot pedal is released.

The surgeon is able to control the length of time the laser is fired for both single and repeat pulses. Under the pulsed settings, laser-beam firing may be limited to 0.01 seconds. This allows extremely precise tissue removal by vaporization of only a few cells at a time. Limitation of tissue penetration is thus controlled by electronic circuitry rather than the by surgeon's reaction time.

The surgeon can also control the power of the laser by adjusting the wattage from low to high level. Carbon dioxide lasers can deliver power of up to 100 W for cutting through dense tissue or for ablating large areas of abnormal tissue. Laser power is measured as power density (W/cm²). The formula for calculating power density is:

$$PD = \frac{watts \times 100}{spot\ size^2\ (in\ min)} = \frac{watts}{cm^2}$$

Superpulse–ultrapulse settings cause ablation and vaporization of tissue, using high bursts of power many hundreds of times during 1 second. There is minimal tissue damage and reduced carbonization when these settings are used for ablation and tissue-removal procedures.

A colposcope is used to evaluate all lesions of the lower genital tract. A micromanipulator can be attached to the colposcope and used to control the laser beam, directing it to the tissue. The light leaves the rigid arm and hits the mirror in the micromanipulator. The mirror is controlled by a joystick. By moving the mirror, the beam is moved and aimed at the abnormal tissue. Micromanipulators can be fitted to all of the common colposcopes.

A plume evacuator is necessary to clear all

smoke from the impact site. The plume contains harmful carbon, cells, and viral DNA. Evacuating tubing may be attached to the speculum for intravaginal surgery or surgery on the cervix. Large-bore tubing is used to evacuate plume during vulvar disease removal.

For intravaginal or cervical lesions, a speculum that is ebonized is used to prevent inadvertent reflection and damage to unintended targets. It is important for all people in the room, including the patient, to wear protective glasses to prevent laser-light damage to the eyes from either direct impact or the reflected laser beam.

HUMAN PAPILLOMAVIRUS INFECTION OF LOWER GENITAL TRACT

Human papillomavirus (HPV) is a double-stranded DNA virus that infects humans and other animals. More than 60 strains of HPV virus have been identified. Human papillomavirus infections occur in various areas of the body; many of these viruses infect the lower genital tract. These viruses have been implicated as causative in most benign and malignant changes of squamous cells in the lower genital tract, including cervical intraepithelial neoplasia (CIN), vaginal intraepithelial neoplasia (VAIN), vulvar intraepithelial neoplasia (VIN), and condylomata.[1]

Host cells become infected by viral invasion through the cell wall. Under certain circumstances, the viral DNA may be inserted into the host cell chromosome. When this occurs, the viral DNA is replicated each time the cell divides and the viral DNA becomes immortalized. This infectious process appears to lead to more advanced benign and malignant conditions. It appears that other cofactors (eg, smoking, host health) may increase susceptibility to cell changes.

CERVICAL INTRAEPITHELIAL NEOPLASIA

The diagnosis of a cervical cell abnormality is almost always made by finding abnormal cells on the Pap smear. The Pap smear reporting system has been changed to divide cell abnormalities into three categories. Under the new Bethesda reporting system, Pap smear abnormalities are separated into

benign low-grade, benign high-grade, and malignant squamous intraepithelial lesions.

Once a lesion is discovered on Pap smear, a colposcopic examination must be performed. Basic rules of colposcopy must be satisfied if a lesion is to be removed by ablative techniques:

1. The squamocolumnar junction must be seen in its entirety.
2. The full extent of the lesion must be seen.
3. The endocervical curettage must be negative.
4. The Pap smear and biopsy must be in concordance.

Although most agree that CIN II and III should be treated, the best course of action for HPV–CIN I lesions has not been determined.[2] Some physicians observe and follow low-grade lesions, whereas others recommend removal.

Laser Treatment of Cervical Intraepithelial Neoplasia

Laser treatment of CIN is performed using the colposcope for visualization and the micromanipulator for control of the laser spot. The patient is placed in the dorsolithotomy position; her legs are placed in Allen stirrups. The colposcopic examination is performed and the transformation zone identified (Fig. 25-1). A suction catheter is attached to the speculum. The ablation procedure may be performed without anesthesia but local anesthesia eliminates the cramping sensation that is experienced by the patient during laser treatment. A 27-gauge Potocky needle is used to inject the cervix with lidocaine 1% plain, or lidocaine 1% with 1:200,000 epinephrine. The injection is placed directly intracervically. Usually, 3 mL of solution is enough to anesthetize the cervix.

Using the helium–neon aiming beam, the CO_2 laser beam is guided to the tissue. The transformation zone is completely outlined, using single pulses of about 25 W and a spot size of 1.5 mm (power density = 1100 W/cm²; Fig. 25-2). Once the spots are placed, they are connected using the continuous mode.

The power setting is usually between 25 to 35 W and spot sizes selected vary between 1.5 to 2.0 mm (power density = 1000 to 1500 W/cm²). With a random rapid sweeping motion, the operator begins to vaporize the cervical tissue, beginning at the 6 o'clock position and moving upward toward the

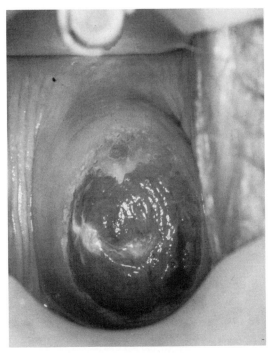

Figure 25–1. Before laser ablation of cervical intra-epithelial neoplasia, the transformation zone is identified, using the colposcope, with the patient in the dorsolithotomy position.

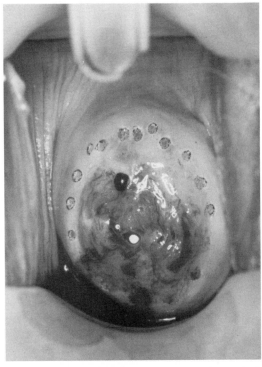

Figure 25–2. After the cervix is anesthetized, the transformation zone is outlined with spots, using single pulses, which are then connected.

os.[3] The lower half of the cervix should be vaporized to a final depth of 6 mm before beginning vaporization of the upper half (Fig. 25-3). The crater walls should be kept straight and parallel (Fig. 25-4). The base of the crater should be flattened. The depth of vaporization to 6 mm has been determined based on the classic article by Anderson and Hartley, showing that the maximum depth of cervical crypts involved in CIN changes are less than 6 mm (Fig. 25-5).[4] The endocervical canal should be vaporized to the same depth as the rest of the crater. No moat should be placed around the canal, nor should it be vaporized more deeply than the rest of the cervix.

Occasionally, troublesome bleeding may be encountered during the ablation procedure. At the first sign of bleeding, the beam should be directed to the bleeding site and rapidly passed over the surface, pausing only to see whether bleeding has stopped. It is important not to delay because once significant bleeding occurs, it is difficult to penetrate the pooled blood with the CO_2 beam. If one is unable to control the bleeding directly, the beam

may be used to form a moat in an inverted "U" surrounding the bleeding vessel. By approaching the vessel from above and from the sides, it is coagulated by the heat generated in the tissue. Other methods, such as direct injection of a vasoconstrictor and thermal or electrocautery, may be applied if the previous two methods fail. One should never "chase" a vessel deep into the stroma with the CO_2 beam because complications may occur if major vessels or other organs are penetrated inadvertently. If bleeding is not easily stopped within a minute or two, the patient should be grounded and the bleeding controlled with electrosurgical coagulation.

It is usually not necessary to place any substance in the bed of the defect to control bleeding. If minor bleeding is encountered, Avitene or Monsel's solution may be placed into the crater. As seen in Table 25-1, an overall cure rate of 90% to 95% can be expected in the treatment of CIN with the CO_2 laser. For the best results, the entire transformation zone must be destroyed. Patients should be followed-up postoperatively with Pap smears per-

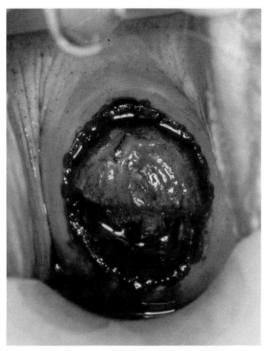

Figure 25-3. The cervical tissue is vaporized to a depth of 6 mm, starting with the lower half and moving to the upper.

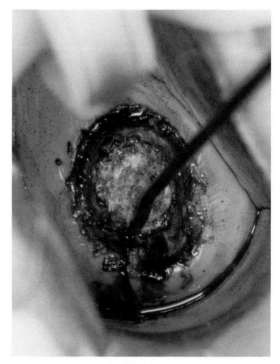

Figure 25-5. The maximum depth of vaporization should be 6 mm.

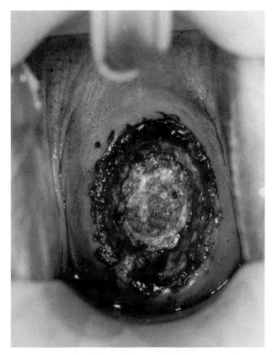

Figure 25-4. A crater is formed that has straight and parallel sides.

formed at 3-month intervals. After three negative Pap smears, patients may return to yearly smears.

Laser Cone Biopsy of Cervix

A cone biopsy of the cervix for removal of CIN disease may be necessary if the lesion is in the canal, the endocervical curettage is positive, the squamocolumnar junction is not seen, or the Pap smear shows significantly more advanced disease than the colposcopic biopsy. The CO_2 laser is an ideal tool for this procedure. The operative setup is the same as that for cervical ablation. The laser is attached to the micromanipulator, which is connected to the colposcope. A 300-mm lens is optimum for this procedure. This provides room to manipulate instruments but at the same time allows the colposcopist to reach the cervix.

The operator first determines the ectocervical boundary of the cone. If the squamocolumnar junction can be seen, the laser incision is placed about 3 to 4 mm outside this junction. If the squamocolumnar junction cannot be seen, the cone should begin 6 mm from the external os.

Table 25–1
Success of One Laser Treatment for Cervical Intraepithelial Neoplasia Using the Carbon Dioxide Laser

Diagnosis	Wright[3] Number (%)	Baggish[5] Number (%)	Townsend[6] Number (%)	Burke[1] Number (%)	Popkin[8] Number (%)	Benedet[9] Number (%)
CIN I	92 (97.8)	64 (92)	10 (90)	49 (85.7)	26 (89)	301 (96.5)
CIN II	137 (94.9)	106 (91)	37 (89)	42 (90.5)	82 (91.5)	428 (90.7)
CIN III	200 (94.5)	127 (87)	53 (87)	40 (85)	30 (90)	702 (90.8)
Total	429 (95.3)	297 (90)	100 (89)	131 (87)	138 (91.6)	1431 (91.9)

*Six patients treated twice.

Lidocaine with 1:200,000 epinephrine or a similar vasoconstrictor is injected into the stroma of the cervix, 360° around the os to the depth of the cone.[10] The border for the cone is placed using the single-pulse 20-W setting and 1-mm spot size. Once the laser-spots craters are placed, they are connected, using continuous mode. The cone biopsy is performed, using a spot size of 0.6 mm. Some find it is easiest to bring the incision down equally, 360° around. Others prefer to incise one quadrant completely to the final depth of the cone before moving to another. A small hook is used to manipulate and place traction on the specimen as the procedure continues.

Although called a "cone" the specimen is actually a cylinder because the walls of the incision are parallel and do not converge, as in a traditional cone. Once the planned depth of the cone is reached, the base of the specimen may be separated from the cervix by laser incision, knife, or tonsil loop. An endocervical curettage or cytobrush sampling may then be performed, if that is the practice of the operator. Minor bleeding can be controlled with Avitene or Monsel's solution.

Postoperative Instructions

Patients are told to report fever, severe or increasing pain, or excessive bleeding to their physician. Nothing should be placed into the vagina, and intercourse should be restricted for 4 weeks postoperatively. Antiprostaglandins are used for pain relief. Patients are seen for a postoperative visit 4 weeks after surgery. Pap smears are performed at 3-month intervals for the next year. Although some physicians perform a postoperative colposcopy, others rely on the Pap smear for detecting recurrence or persistence.

CONDYLOMATA ACUMINATA

Condylomata acuminata are an atypical benign cell proliferation occurring on the nonkeratinized tissues (vagina and labia minora) of the lower genital tract. The same process occurring on keratinized skin (labia majora) is called a wart. Condylomata and warts are other manifestations of HPV. Condylomata may be found at all ages—infants to postmenopausal women—but reach peak occurrence in 20- to 30-year-olds. Condylomata may be few and small or large and extensive. Some warts disappear without therapy; others persist and grow, requiring treatment to remove them.

Many local treatments are available to remove condylomata and warts. No treatment is uniformly successful. Some therapies include podophyllin, podophylox, trichloroacetic acid, bichloroacetic acid, cryocautery, liquid nitrogen, electrocautery, electrosurgery, and Efudex cream, and interferon.

The laser is a useful therapeutic tool for treating patients with extensive condylomata of the vulva. Condylomata of vagina, urethra, and anus may also be treated by laser. Laser is also the treatment of choice in patients who have failed more conservative methods of therapy.

Laser Treatment of Condylomata Acuminata

The setup for laser treatment of condylomata acuminata is similar to that for the treatment CIN. The colposcope should be used because it allows the physician to find lesions that would be missed otherwise. Using the micromanipulator, the operator is able to control the area and depth of vaporization with greater precision than if the laser is used with the handpiece.

Extensive condylomata should be treated under

general or regional anesthesia. Limited numbers of warts may be treated with a local anesthetic injection.[11] For vulvar lesions, the laser is set at about 15 W, and a spot size of 1.5 to 2.0 mm is selected (power density = 400 W/cm^2). A similar superpulse power-density may be used if the operator prefers. Superpulse produces less carbonization at similar powers.

A sweeping motion is used to vaporize the lesions.[12] The operator should begin moving the micromanipulator before firing the laser because this prevents deep penetration as the beam is started. The depth of vaporization should not exceed 1 mm below the surrounding skin (Fig. 25-6). In sensitive areas such as the clitoris, perianal, and periurethral areas, a repeat-pulse mode may be used. An assistant should hold wide-bore plume-evacuation tubing above and within 1 cm of the impact site. After laser vaporization is finished, wash the carbon off the surface of the tissue.

When treating vaginal lesions, the laser is set at about 15 W and a spot size of 1.5 to 2.0 mm (power density = 250 W/cm^2) is selected. The laser beam may be aimed down the center of the speculum or from the sides through the blades. Again, a sweeping motion is to be used. Superficial vaporization is all that is necessary to remove these lesions. Washing the vagina with 3% acetic acid before vapori-

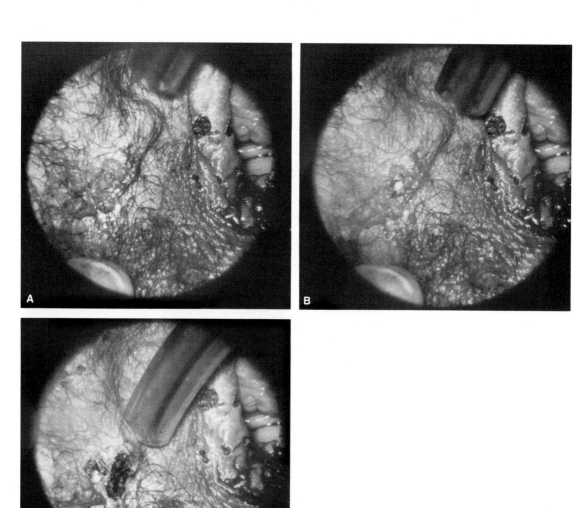

Figure 25–6. Laser treatment of condyloma acuminata (**A**) After local anesthesia, the wart is vaporized using continuous power. (**B**) Using the micromanipulator, the lesion is vaporized with a sweeping motion. (**C**) Depth of vaporization should not exceed 1 mm below surrounding skin.

zation helps to define lesions that may otherwise remain undetected.

VULVAR INTRAEPITHELIAL NEOPLASIA

Vulvar intraepithelial neoplasia is a more rare manifestation of HPV than condylomata or CIN. It may present in any age group. The lesion takes many forms and cannot be confidently diagnosed by gross appearance. If any questionable lesion on the vulva is seen, it should undergo biopsy for diagnosis. Large abnormal areas require multiple biopsies to confirm the diagnosis.

Vulva intraepithelial neoplasia is easily treated by laser vaporization if the lesion occurs on the nonhairy areas of the vulva. The nonkeratinized tissue is vaporized, using identical technique as that for vaporization of condylomata acuminata, with the depth of vaporization being about 1 mm. The epithelium must be removed in its entirety to treat VIN disease.[13]

If the hairy areas are involved with VIN changes, the procedure becomes more difficult, with tissue removal to a depth of 3 mm becoming necessary. In these areas, VIN changes follow the hair follicle into the dermis and if one does not vaporize to the base of the follicle, recurrence predictably occurs. Many operators have abandoned laser treatment of VIN disease in these areas, believing that it offers no advantages over traditional surgical techniques.

VAGINAL INTRAEPITHELIAL NEOPLASIA

Vaginal intraepithelial neoplasia is even more rare than other forms of HPV change. These lesions are diagnosed by colposcopic examination and biopsy. Laser treatment is conducted using the same techniques as those for vaginal condylomata. Cure rates for VAIN (Table 25-2) are slightly below those for CIN.[14] Follow-up visits for VIN and VAIN require frequent colposcopic examinations and liberal biopsy.

Postoperative Instructions for Vulva–Vaginal Laser

Immediately after laser treatment of the vulva, ice is applied to decrease immediate swelling and inflammation. After 24-hours, ice is discontinued and

Table 25–2

Results of Treatment of Vaginal Intraepithelial Neoplasia With the Carbon Dioxide Laser

Author	Patients Treated Successfully	Percentage Success
Stafl[15]	5/6	83
Petrilli[16]	9/10	90
Townsend[14]	33/36	92
Capen[17]	11/13	85
Totals	58/65	89

warm soaks are substituted two to three times a day. Many natural substances (eg, tea, epsom salts) and chemical products (eg, silvadene, antibiotic creams, local anesthetics) are recommended by various authors. Most importantly, this area should be kept clean, so that normal healing can occur. Intercourse and tampons are restricted until healing is complete. Analgesics are prescribed for pain relief. Patients are instructed to gently spread the labia twice a day to prevent coaptation of the labia. A postoperative check at 6 weeks is planned. Colposcopic examinations are performed at 6-month intervals in patients who have been treated for VIN or VAIN.

CONCLUSION

Laser treatment of lower genital tract disease has become a important treatment modality during the last decade. Precise, safe, rapid treatment of common benign cell changes can be performed in the office or ambulatory surgery center. The procedures are easily learned. High cure rates may be obtained. Regardless of other developing therapies, the laser will remain an important tool for treating HPV-related disease of the lower genital tract.

REFERENCES

1. Rotkin ID: A comparison review of key epidemiologic studies in cervical cancer related to current searches for transmissible agents. Cancer Res 33: 1353, 1973
2. Ferenczy A: Management of the patient with an abnormal Papanicolaou test, recent developments. Obstet Gynecol Clin North Am 20:189, 1993
3. Wright CV, Davies E, Riopelle MA: Laser surgery for cervical intraepithelial neoplasia: principles and results. Am J Obstet Gynecol 145:181, 1983

4. Anderson MC, Hartley RB: Cervical crypt involvement by intraepithelial neoplasia. Obstet Gynecol 41:501, 1973

5. Baggish MS: Management of cervical intraepithelial neoplasia by CO_2 laser. Obstet Gynecol 60:378, 1982

6. Townsend DE, Richart RM: Cryotherapy and the carbon dioxide laser management of cervical intraepithelial neoplasia: a control comparison. Obstet Gynecol 61:75, 1983

7. Burke L: The use of carbon dioxide laser in the therapy of cervical intraepithelial neoplasia. Am J Obstet Gynecol 144:337, 1982

8. Popkin DR, Scali V, Ahmed MN: Cryosurgery for treatment of cervical intraepithelial neoplasia. Am J Obstet Gynecol 130:551, 1978

9. Benedet JL, Miller DM, Nickerson KG: Results of conservative management of cervical intraepithelial neoplasia. Obstet Gynecol 79:105, 1992

10. Thomsen CF, Helkjaer PE, Skovdal J, et al: Acceptance of ambulatory laser conization under local anesthesia by danish women. Ugeskr Laeger 154:3590, 1992

11. Petersen CS: Local anesthesia in CO_2 laser treatment of disseminated therapy-resistant condylomata. Ugeskr Laeger 155:1861, 1993

12. Townsend EE, Smith LH, Kinney WK, et al: Condylomata acuminata. Roles of different techniques of laser vaporization. J Reprod Med 38:362, 1993

13. Baggist MS, Dorsey JH: CO_2 laser for the treatment of vulvar carcinoma in situ. Obstet Gynecol 57:371, 1981

14. Townsend DE, Levine RV, Crum CP, et al: Treatment of vaginal carcinoma in situ with the CO_2 laser. Am J Obstet Gynecol 143:565, 1982

15. Stafl A, Wilkinson EJ, Mattingly RF: Laser treatment of cervical and vaginal neoplasia. Am J Obstet Gynecol 128:128, 1977

16. Petrilli ES, Townsend DE, Morrow CP, et al: Vaginal intraepithelial neoplasia: biological aspects and treatment with topical 5-fluorouracil and the carbon dioxide laser. Am J Obstet Gynecol 138:321, 1980

17. Capen CV, Masterson BJ, Magrine JF, et al: Laser therapy of vaginal intraepithelial neoplasia. Am J Obstet Gynecol 142:973, 1982

Ambulatory Gynecology, Second Edition,
edited by David H. Nichols and Patrick J. Sweeney.
J. B. Lippincott Company, Philadelphia, © 1995.

26

Minor and Ambulatory Surgery

David H. Nichols and Karen L. McGoldrick

Most extraperitoneal diagnostic and many therapeutic procedures that involve the female genitalia can be accomplished in an ambulatory setting. Not only is this approach cost-effective but when preceded by a careful explanation of the procedure and accompanied by a compassionate and reasonably comfortable general physical examination, it is usually well-received by patients.

BIOPSY OF THE VULVA

If a vulvar lesion has failed to respond promptly to what was considered appropriate therapy and if the physician has even the slightest suspicion that the condition is malignant or premalignant, the patient should undergo biopsy to ensure an accurate diagnosis. Careful inspection with a hand lens or colposcope usually reveals the appropriate area for the biopsy. If there is any doubt about the proper site, however, the physician should paint the vulva with 1% toluidine blue, wait for it to dry, and rinse it off with 1% acetic acid. The tissues that retain the deep purple stain are the areas of the most intense nu-

clear activity and therefore the most appropriate sites for biopsy.

When the disease is obviously malignant, biopsies from the central portion and from the margin of the lesions may be sufficient. For widespread disease, such as suspected Paget's disease, the dyskeratoses, carcinoma in situ, or Bowen's disease, multiple biopsies from random sites are appropriate.

Using an epinephrine–lidocaine solution (lidocaine 0.5% in epinephrine 1:200,000), the physician carefully infiltrates the site from which the tissue is to be taken. After the anesthetic has taken effect, the physician brings a sterile Keyes biopsy punch to the surface of the site and, with gentle rotation of the punch in the manner of a drill, makes a circular incision through the skin (Fig. 26-1). When the punch reaches the desired depth through the complete thickness of the skin, the physician removes the punch, picks up the edge of the specimen disk with fine-pointed forceps, and gently cuts it away from the underlying subcutaneous connective tissue with either scissors or a scalpel. The specimen is promptly placed in a formalin solution. As

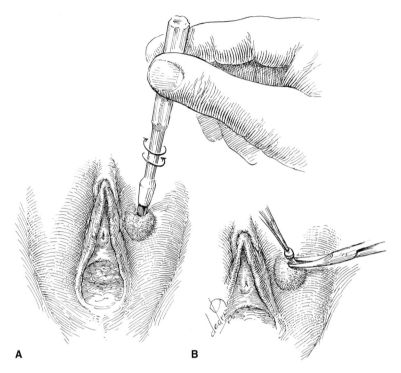

A   **B**

Figure 26–1. Biopsy of vulvar skin using a Keyes biopsy punch. The site has been infiltrated with a local anesthetic and the cutting end of the punch applied to the site selected for biopsy. Pressure is applied lightly and the punch rotated back and forth (*arrows*), drilling a hole through the full thickness of the skin. The specimen disk is elevated with fine pointed forceps and cut away from the subcutaneous tissue. The wound is cauterized for hemostasis.

many biopsies as are necessary may be performed on a single occasion but each specimen should be labeled separately and the area from which it was taken identified in the record.

Gentle pressure with a gauze compress often causes a clot to develop and thus relieves any bleeding. Cauterization with the tip of a silver nitrate applicator stick may halt any unacceptable oozing. The physician should instruct the patient to expect some soreness when the anesthetic has worn off but to resume normal physical activities. A small scab develops over the site of the biopsy but disappears within 2 to 3 weeks.

When a punch biopsy is inappropriate, the physician may excise a wedge of tissue with the scalpel and then approximate the tissue from side to side with one or more interrupted absorbable sutures.

VULVAR VESTIBULAR SYNDROME

The abrupt onset of severe dyspareunia, usually in a young Caucasian patient with no visible outlet obstruction or palpable endopelvic pathology, suggests vulvar vestibular syndrome (focal vulvitis). The patient may have one or more areas of exquisite tenderness in the vestibule, most commonly in the posterior portion between the hymen and the vulvar skin. Gently touching this area with the end of a cotton-tipped applicator produces instant discomfort and the site may be sharply demarcated. The condition has been identified from time to time for more than 100 years but it has received increased attention since 1981.

The gynecologist may suggest alternative or noncoital means of sexual gratification for the couple but 4% aqueous lidocaine (Xylocaine) saturating a cotton ball applied to the vestibular area some 15 minutes before coitus often provides sufficient temporary anesthesia for sexual relations.[1] For the non-acetowhite lesion not associated with coincident human papilloma-virus infection, a course of treatment may be initiated using 15-minute applications of these lidocaine-soaked cotton balls, four daily for a period of 6 months, if relief of symptoms is obtained. Xylocaine ointment may be applied to the area for temporary relief during the day. Because the use of oral contraceptives may exacerbate the condition for reasons unknown, the patient should stop taking them for at least 6 months. Remission occurs in about 50% of cases.

For acetowhite lesions, presumably associated with virus origin, local laser ablation may be curative.

Blazin and coworkers find no support for the idea that infection causes the vulvar vestibular syndrome and believe that hormonal factors such as early oral contraceptive use may be involved in the etiology.[2]

If the syndrome persists after 6 months of observation and treatment, vestibulectomy and perineoplasty provides relief in most cases. The gynecologic surgeon should reconfirm the diagnosis preoperatively by examining the vestibule with a magnifying glass or low-power colposcope. There is often a cluster of raised pinkish or yellowish papules in the area of pain, and this specific site of pain may be carefully delineated with a marking pen immediately before the administration of anesthesia to ensure that the affected area is totally excised (Fig. 26-2). The full epithelial thickness, including the adjacent hymen of this sensitive area within the vestibule, should be excised. The full thickness of the

posterior vaginal wall should be mobilized for 2 or 3 cm so that at the conclusion of the operation, it can be brought down to cover this raw area; it is attached to the skin of the perineum by two layers of interrupted sutures. Because postoperative oozing at this site is common, the patient may be kept in the hospital for a day or two postoperatively.

CHRONIC VULVAR PRURITUS

Kelly and coworkers find that subcutaneous injection of triamcinolone acetate (Kenalog) is useful if the patient without lichen sclerosus has responded (but *briefly*) to betamethasone cream or flurandrenolide cream applied topically for 1 to 2 weeks after biopsy has excluded vulvar malignancy.[3] Their

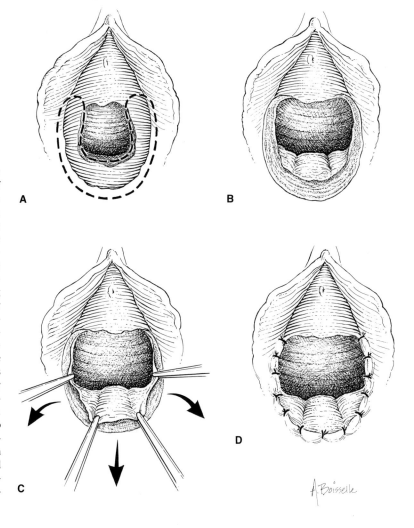

Figure 26–2. Vestibulectomy is illustrated. The painful area of vestibular skin is carefully demarcated preoperatively and an incision made lateral to this line of demarcation, as noted by the *dotted line* (**A**). The full thickness of the skin, including the adjacent hymen has been removed (**B**) and any bleeding vessels clamped and ligated or electrocoagulated. (**C**) The posterior vaginal wall has been mobilized and pulled down (*arrows*) to cover the raw area. The full thickness of the vagina is sewn to the skin of the vulva by two layers of interrupted synthetic absorbable sutures (**D**). Raw areas anterior or lateral to the urethra are left open to granulate and avoid stricture. (From Nichols DH, Randall CL: Vaginal surgery, 3rd ed. Baltimore, Williams & Wilkins, 1989; with permission.)

technique describes placing a small wheal of local anesthetic on the upper margin of the labium majora and, using a 25-gauge spinal needle, slowly injecting 15 to 20 mg of triamcinolone acetonide (10 mg/mL) as the needle is advanced toward the anal orifice (1.5 to 2 mL of the preparation on either side). The area is thoroughly massaged to diffuse the agent throughout the labia, and the patient is informed that it takes 24 to 48 hours for an effect.

MARSUPIALIZATION OF BARTHOLIN'S DUCT CYST

Obstruction of the duct of Bartholin's gland at the site of the vulvar orifice usually results in a cyst of the duct. When uninfected, such cysts are often asymptomatic. If they are causing no trouble, they need not be disturbed. If they are symptomatic or if it is possible to palpate areas of hardness within the lesions, however, treatment is in order.

An infected cyst is usually painful and leads to abscess formation. If not drained, the abscess may burst spontaneously.

Although such a rupture relieves the symptoms immediately, the rapid closure of the skin through which the rupture occurred and the continued obstruction of the duct orifice, which is likely, permit the reformation of the cyst or abscess. Because the lesion is a cyst of the duct and not of the gland, extirpation of the cyst without removal of the gland is often ineffective. After the skin heals, the gland continues to function without the duct and another cyst may gradually form. The gland may be difficult to find because the cyst has compressed and displaced it from its usual anatomic site but there is a 25% chance that the cyst will recur if the gland is not removed.

Therefore, when discomfort is present and surgical treatment is indicated, an effective treatment is for the operator to create a new orifice and duct for the gland on the affected side. The ideal site for the creation of a new stoma over the obstructed duct is at the former orifice of the duct. (This is not always visible but it can be identified by painting the area with iodine solution; the site of the former orifice does not take up the iodine stain.)

Either of two marsupialization procedures can be performed with the use of local anesthesia. The operator may excise the roof of the cyst, leaving a window-like opening 1 to 2 cm in diameter, and sew the margin of the cyst wall to the skin of the introitus. Alternatively, the operator may make a stab wound into the cyst cavity and immediately—before the cavity has emptied itself—insert the tip of a Word catheter through the wound. The bulb of the catheter is then inflated and allowed to remain in place for 4 to 6 weeks. The end of the catheter that projects from the stab wound may be tucked into the vagina so that it is out of the way (Fig. 26-3). When the bulb of the catheter is subsequently deflated and removed, it leaves behind a new epithelialized duct. If a Word catheter is not available, a pediatric-sized Foley catheter may be used. After the bulb of the Foley catheter has been inflated, the catheter is securely bent onto itself and tied about 2.5 inches from the bulb; the excess catheter is then cut off.

The "unroofing" technique of marsupialization is useful for other symptomatic vaginal cysts, especially for large inclusion cysts in the vaginal vault or wolffian-duct cysts, which may occur in the vault or along the lateral walls of the vagina. Generally, the technique of cutting a window and sewing the cyst wall to the vaginal wall is the more effective of the two procedures. It is also safer than surgical excision of the cyst because each a cyst is often adjacent to the ureter and may even have displaced the ureter from its usual position. Deep hemostatic sutures in this area, placed after the excision of a cyst, may unexpectedly occlude the ureter. If discovered more than 24 to 48 hours after surgery, ureteral occlusion requires not only deligation but also ureteroneocystostomy because of the likelihood of future ureteral necrosis as a result of the interference with its blood supply.

Occasionally (particularly when the initial cyst was acutely infected), scarring and fibrosis may close the orifice after several months and another cyst may form, requiring retreatment if it is symptomatic. To reduce the risk of this possibility, the physician should caution the patient against wearing tight undergarments made of synthetic fabrics, wearing undergarments to bed, and wearing tight slacks or shorts—all of which impede the evaporation of perspiration. Overheating of the local tissues results in congestion, and the trauma of friction against clothing increases susceptibility to infection.

HYMENOTOMY

When the hymenal ring is so rigid and inelastic that it prohibits coital entrance to the vagina or even progressive enlargement by graduated dilators, hymenotomy may be necessary. Superficial infiltration by lidocaine with epinephrine is permissible,

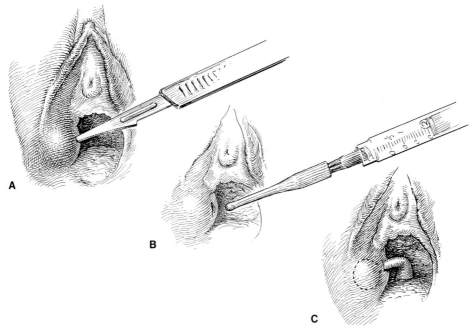

Figure 26–3. Marsupialization of Bartholin's cyst using a Word catheter. (**A**) A stab wound is made to the full thickness of the wall of the right Bartholin's cyst at the site chosen for the new duct. (**B**) A Word catheter has been attached to a syringe containing 2 mL of sterile saline, and the tip of the catheter is quickly introduced into the cyst cavity. (**C**) The catheter bulb is inflated, the syringe removed, and the free end of the catheter tucked back into the vagina. It should remain in place for several weeks until the new duct has become epithelialized. The bulk is then deflated and the catheter removed.

although a stoic patient may require only the superficial anesthesia induced by lidocaine jelly or Cetacaine spray. The operator makes two longitudinal incisions through the rigid hymenal membrane at the 4 and 8 o'clock positions. Suturing is rarely needed.

The physician should tell the patient that there may be a little bleeding for a few days and that she may bathe normally in the interim. When the initial soreness has gone, the patient herself may digitally increase the size of the hymenal opening by introducing first one, then two, and finally three fingertips through the hymenal ring until the opening has reached the desired size and healing has occurred. She can often perform this dilation most comfortably while tub bathing.

Treatment of an Obstructed Hemivagina

A hemivagina associated with a didelphic uterus or a bicornuate or septate vagina may be totally or partially obstructed. When the obstruction is complete, the patient has dysmenorrhea and the monthly blood accumulates as a palpable mass in the lateral wall of the vagina. (The patient may also have congenital abnormalities of the urinary tract.) The gynecologist can confirm the diagnosis by aspiration of old blood from the mass, and treatment is prompt marsupialization to create a large vaginal window that connects the two vaginal cavities.

PERINEOTOMY AND RELAXING INCISIONS

When the perineum is rigid and inflexible, perineotomy may be necessary. For this procedure, the patient should receive deep local or brief general anesthesia. The operator makes a mid-line perineal incision in the 6 o'clock position to a depth sufficient to permit the introduction of three fingers into the vagina. The application of gentle pressure posteriorly stretches the tissue. Any bleeding vessels must be clamped and ligated and using interrupted absorbable polyglycolic acid or catgut sutures, the apical edge of the vaginal incision should be sewn

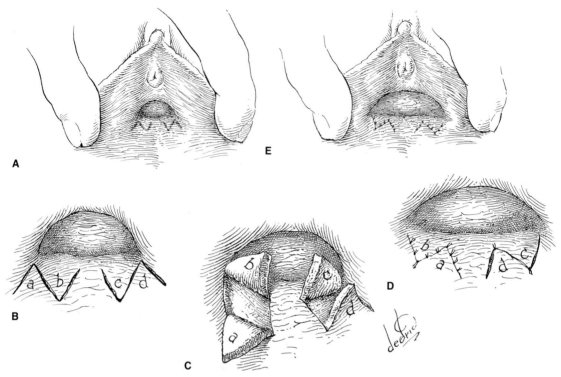

Figure 26–4. The Z-plasty. (**A**) Preoperative introital stenosis. The lines of incision are shown. (**B–D**) The full-thickness flaps are undermined and rotated. (**E**) At the conclusion of the procedure, introital enlargement is noted. (From Nichols DH, Randall CL: Vaginal surgery, 3rd ed. Baltimore, Williams & Wilkins, 1989; with permission.)

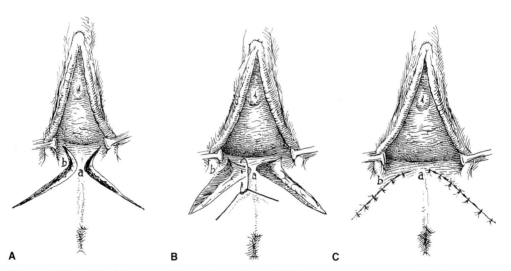

Figure 26–5. (**A**) A bilateral episiotomy is performed. (**B**) Repair begins at the medial edge in such a fashion that *b* is no longer adjacent to *a* but is moved laterally on each side enough for the introitus to be enlarged as much as necessary. (**C**) The end result shows the widened introitus. (From Nichols DH, Randall CL: Vaginal surgery, 3rd ed. Baltimore, Williams & Wilkins, 1989; with permission.)

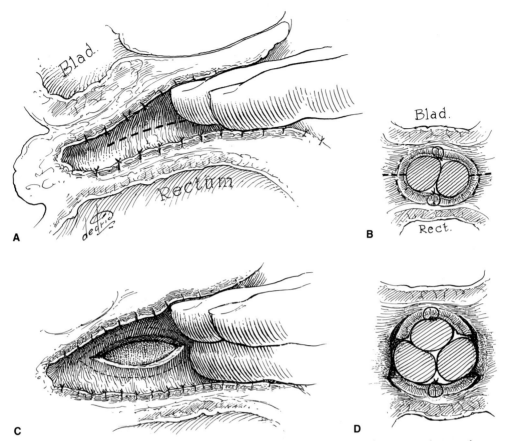

A

B

C

D

Figure 26–6. Lateral relaxing incisions in the vagina. (**A**) A mid-vaginal stenosis admits only two fingerbreadths. (**B**) The sites of lateral relaxing incisions are indicated by the *dotted lines.* (**C**) The incisions are made through the lateral vaginal walls to a length sufficient for the vagina to comfortably admit three fingerbreadths. (**D**) The vaginal wall is undercut 1 cm in each direction. A firm vaginal packing or obturator is inserted. (From Nichols DH, Randall CL: Vaginal surgery, 3rd ed. Baltimore, Williams & Wilkins, 1989; with permission.)

to the perineal skin in transverse fashion, perpendicular to the original incision. The physician should tell the patient that tenderness will persist for 2 or 3 weeks, that she may bathe, and that the knots fall off spontaneously when the underlying suture has been absorbed.

A carefully measured Z-plasty is useful for patients with a tight introitus (Fig. 26-4). If the vaginal introitus is not only rigid but also moderately small, as may occur in patients who are elderly or who have undergone lower pelvic radiation, the innovative resuturing of a bilateral mediolateral episiotomy may be beneficial (V-plasty; Fig. 26-5). Longitudinal lateral relaxing incisions through the full thickness of the vaginal wall relieve mid-vaginal strictures effectively (Fig. 26-6). During the healing process, the patient must wear at night an obturator

(eg, a 50-mL plastic syringe barrel with the tip cut off) lubricated with estrogen cream until re-epithelialization is well under way.

CONIZATION

Although colposcopically directed biopsy has largely replaced diagnostic conization, the latter continues to be of value in the investigation of patients with a malignant noninvasive lesion or an abnormal Papanicolaou smear when the squamocolumnar junction is so high that it is not clearly visible and thus does not permit a specimen to be taken by biopsy. The procedure is primarily diagnostic but it may be therapeutic under certain circumstances, such as when the entire noninvasive lesion of the cervix may be visualized and included within the surgical specimen. (Because intraepithelial neoplasia is commonly multicentric, the removal of this specimen does not preclude the future development of other areas of dysplasia or carcinoma in situ.)

Technique of Conization

A simple conization technique that provides acceptable hemostasis begins with the infiltration of the cervical stroma with not more than 50 mL of 0.5% lidocaine (Xylocaine) in 1:200,000 epinephrine (Adrenalin) solution. This produces a marked spasm of the cervical blood vessels, confirmed by a visible blanching of the cervix. Using a #11 pointed scalpel for the incision, the operator removes a cone of tissue up to but not including the internal cervical os. It is absolutely essential that the axis of the cone is parallel to the axis of the vagina and cervix; perforation of the uterus during a conization may damage the neighboring organs and tissues, including blood vessels, bladder, or rectum. Bleeding or oozing points should be coagulated with the electrosurgical unit. The operator may place a suture at the 12 o'clock position of the specimen for orientation in the pathology laboratory.

As an alternative procedure for preliminary hemostasis, the operator may use deep hemostatic sutures of absorbable material in the 3 and 9 o'clock positions. After obtaining the cone of the cervix and coagulating the numerous bleeding points, the operator packs the cervix with ½-inch iodoform gauze, which should remain in place for 24 to 48 hours. If significant oozing is immediate, which is rare, a more hemostatic "hot" electroconization may follow immediately. The difficulty with this procedure being used routinely is that, should the initial conization fail to remove the entire lesion, there is no more fresh adjacent tissue for study by immediate biopsy. Also, the additional tissue destruction increases postoperative cervical scarring.

If a patient who is having a conization is to undergo dilation and curettage (D&C) at the same time, the operator performs the D&C immediately after the conization—never before.

Complications of Conization

Hemorrhage may follow conization, either at surgery or within the first postoperative weeks. Visible bleeding points require electrocoagulation; general oozing requires suture ligation of the area. The use

of the tip of a silver nitrate stick or a cotton applicator soaked in ferric ammonium chloride or Monsel's solution may stop mild bleeding. If not, packing the affected area with microfibrillar collagen (Avitene) is generally effective. (Avitene exerts its hemostatic effect by attracting functioning blood platelets, which adhere to the microfibrils and trigger the formation of thrombi in the adjacent tissue. Although more expensive, it is more effective than Gelfoam or Surgicel.) A recurrence of bleeding may require transvaginal ligation of the uterine artery on both sides. Rarely, excessive recurrent postoperative bleeding mandates hysterectomy or iliac ligation, particularly if the conization has transected a major branch of the uterine artery that has subsequently retracted into the substance of the cervix or lower uterine segment.

Cervical stenosis is the principal long-range complication of conization. It follows inadvertent resection or trauma to the internal cervical os. Cervical conization heals by scar formation, and the associated contraction decreases the diameter of the canal. If stenosis or stricture results, long-term treatment by periodic endocervical dilation may be necessary until the surface of the cervix has been re-epithelialized and scar formation and healing have stabilized.

There is little place for hot electroconization in the treatment of chronic cervicitis. The procedure is not cost-effective in this case and carries additional risks, including scar-tissue formation and its troublesome sequelae. If endocervicitis causes a chronic leukorrhea that disturbs the patient enough to require treatment, strip cauterization or electrocoagulation of the affected area of the cervix may be the procedure of choice. Because infection often involves the depths of the endocervical glands, superficial cauterization of the cervix by local applications of a caustic agent or silver nitrate is not indicated. Electrodissection is useful and provides a specimen reliable for pathology study. Large-loop excision of the transformation zone has been reported by Hallam and coworkers to be an effective diagnostic and treatment alternative to conventional conization.[4] Diathermy loop excision of premalignant lesions of the vulva, vagina, and cervix is effective in an outpatient setting without sacrifice of uninvolved tissue.[5]

CULDOCENTESIS

If it is necessary to differentiate a hemoperitoneum caused by an ectopic pregnancy from one caused by a leaking dysfunctional ovarian cyst, culdocentesis can be useful. The fluid from a leaking or ruptured ectopic pregnancy is frank blood, whereas fluid from a leaking ovarian cyst is usually blood-tinged serum. If the fluid is purulent, pelvic abscess is likely and Gram staining and culture should be performed. Laparoscopy may be necessary to establish the diagnosis if the volume of intraperitoneal fluid is less than 250 mL, as estimated by ultrasound examination. Laparotomy may be necessary if the volume of fluid is more in the event of circulatory collapse.[6]

Culdocentesis, which rarely requires the administration of anesthesia, involves a minimum of preparation. It is most easily performed on a patient in whom the cul-de-sac is already distended by intraperitoneal fluid. A sterile, long, sharp 18- or 20-gauge needle is attached to a 10- or 20-mL syringe. With the patient in the lithotomy position, the physician performs a bimanual examination, including a rectovaginal examination. A speculum is gently inserted into the vagina and the posterior fornix painted with an antiseptic solution such as povidone–iodine (Betadine). The posterior lip of the cervix should then be grasped with a tenaculum, preferably in the anteroposterior direction, and slight traction applied to the cervix with the tenaculum in an upward and outward direction. The patient is asked to cough and the operator quickly advances the previously prepared needle by a sharp thrust through the vaginal mucosa of the posterior fornix and the peritoneum into the posterior cul-de-sac (Fig. 26-7). The safest area for the insertion of the needle is in the mid-line, between the uterosacral ligaments.

If the first attempted aspiration produces no fluid, the operator may reposition the tip of the needle or may withdraw and reinsert the needle. Repositioning the patient into a reverse Trendelenburg position may facilitate fluid collection. Some authorities advocate the introduction of several milliliters of air after the introduction of the needle, followed by an attempt to aspirate this air. The free flow of air into the cavity with inability to aspirate it indicates that the peritoneal cavity has been entered but is free of fluid.

When the physician is performing a culdocentesis under anesthesia in the operating room because of a suspected pelvic abscess and plans to follow the procedure with a colpotomy, it is helpful to localize where the abscess appears to be by bimanual and rectal examinations. The needle should be introduced into the abscess cavity at that point. If the expected pus is aspirated, a sample should be sent to the laboratory for Gram staining and culture and the needle should be left in place as a guide for prompt scalpel incision. After digitally breaking up any loculations, the operator places an appropriate drain and removes the needle.

REMOVAL OF A CERVICAL POLYP

Not only are cervical polyps a source of intermenstrual bleeding and leukorrhea but they occasionally contain cancer. Therefore, they should be removed. Anesthesia is not required. Polyps are sometimes multiple, in which case all should be removed.

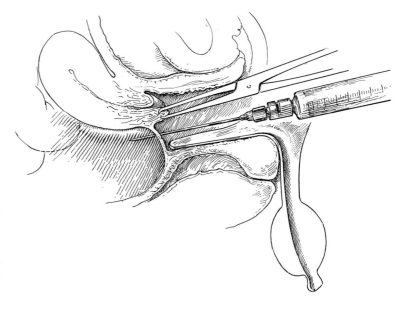

Figure 26–7. Culdocentesis. The cervix has been steadied with a tenaculum and a sharp 18-gauge needle attached to a syringe has been inserted directly into the bulging cul-de-sac. The fluid is then aspirated and examined.

A small polyp should be clamped across its base with a curved hemostat and the hemostat twisted until the polyp comes free. The polyp should be placed in fixative and sent for examination by a pathologist. Because there is a risk of recurrence if even a small portion of the base remains, the area should be sharply curetted or electrocoagulated at the next office visit—after the pathology report has been reviewed.

A larger polyp with a broader base is easily removed with a tonsil snare. The wire loop is opened wide and placed around the polyp. (The tip of a polyp tends to come to a point, whereas that of a pedunculated leiomyoma is round and smooth.) Steadying the tip of the polyp with a forceps, the operator advances the loop of the snare as high up the stalk as it will go (Fig. 26-8). When the loop can go no further, it has reached the point of attachment of the polyp base to the wall of the cervix or uterus. The operator then tightens the snare and slowly crushes the base to permit thrombosis of the transected blood vessels. If the base is estimated to be

1 cm or more in diameter, the tip of an active diathermy may be touched to the handle of the snare during this process. Occasionally, the tip of an endometrial polyp protrudes through the cervix; it should be similarly removed. The dependent tip of a polyp generally comes to a point, in contrast to that of a pedunculated leiomyoma which is globular. It too should be removed.

ENDOMETRIAL BIOPSY

A good endometrial biopsy is easier, faster, more convenient, more effective, and infinitely less costly than conventional curettage. Furthermore, the study of the tissue obtained by biopsy may establish in a timely fashion the diagnosis of an endocrinopathy (ie, by assessment of the phase of the endometrial cycle) and of malignant or premalignant disease of the genital tract. Thus, it may hasten the necessary treatment.

A popular curette for sampling of the endome-

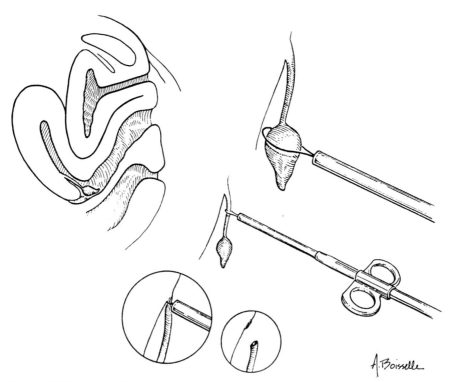

Figure 26–8. Removal of an endocervical or endometrial polyp. The polyp protruding through the cervix is seen in sagittal section through the pelvis. It is threaded through the eye of the wire of a tonsil snare, as shown, which is advanced along the stalk as far as it will go. The snare is tightened slowly (*insert*), first crushing and then transecting the stalk, and the polyp is removed for laboratory examination. (From Nichols DH, Randall CL: Vaginal surgery, 3rd ed. Baltimore, Williams & Wilkins, 1989; with permission.)

trium in the past has been the Randall-type metal suction biopsy curette. The serrated edge of the Novak curette is useful for obtaining samples of endocervical material when malignancy of this area is suspected but its use seems to cause too much pain for routine sampling of the endometrial cavity. Endometrial biopsy curettes are available in different diameters, from ³⁄₁₆- to ⁷⁄₁₆-inch, to accommodate varying degrees of endocervical size or cervical stenosis. Endometrial aspiration kits such as the Vabra or the Masterson are also convenient and effective but the softer and flexible plastic Pipelle (Unimar, Inc., Wilton, CT) suction curette (Fig. 26-9) is significantly less painful for the patient and is rapidly replacing the metal curettes.

A careful bimanual examination is essential to determine the size, shape, and position of the uterus, which indicates the likely direction and depth of the endocervical and endometrial canals. After passing a speculum into the vagina, the operator paints the cervix with povidone–iodine (Betadine) and places a tenaculum on the anterior lip of the cervix, usually in a transverse direction. The operator then uses a blunt Simpson sound to confirm the direction and depth of the endocervical and endometrial canals. The direction and depth to which the sound can be passed from the external cervical os must be carefully noted because this is the direction and maximum depth to which the endometrial biopsy curette can be passed. If the introduction of the sound reveals a stricture or stenosis, the operator may gently dilate the cervical canal with a small Hanks dilator at least as big as the diameter of the endometrial biopsy curette that will follow.

A paracervical or uterosacral block with a local

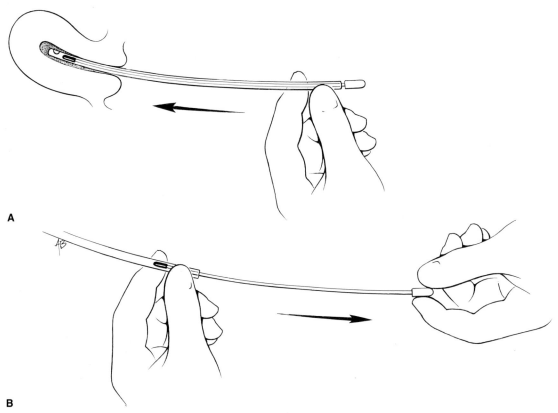

Figure 26–9. Endometrial biopsy, using the Pipelle suction curette. (**A**) The plastic curette (with sheath fully advanced) is inserted through the cervix into the full depth of the endometrial cavity. A tenaculum may be used to steady the cervix if necessary. (**B**) While holding the sheath, the piston is quickly and fully withdrawn until it is stopped and locked in position. The sheath is rotated as it is moved back and forth several times to sample the endometrium. It is then withdrawn and the tip is cut off and discarded. Contents of the hollow tube are expressed into a specimen jar by pushing the plunger to its original position. (From Nichols DH, Randall CL: *Vaginal surgery,* 3rd ed. Baltimore: Williams & Wilkins, 1989; with permission.)

anesthetic agent (eg, 0.5% lidocaine) relieves pain caused by the introduction of the sound. Alternatively, the biopsy curette can be attached to a sterile 10- or 20-mL syringe that contains 4 mL of 4% lidocaine and this agent may be quickly injected into the endometrial cavity. The anesthesia takes effect in 4 or 5 minutes. In addition to the paracervical block and the intrauterine instillation of lidocaine, two tablets of naproxen sodium (Anaprox) or other analgesic may be given 20 to 30 minutes before the procedure.

Once the anesthesia has taken effect, the operator withdraws the plunger on the syringe, creating negative pressure within the syringe, and makes several passes with the curette from the fundus of the uterus to the level of the internal os. To minimize patient discomfort, the operator should make these passes in rapid succession. Quickly withdrawing the curette with the syringe that contains the specimen, the operator then flushes the specimen into a bottle of formalin fixative. Generally, several "swipes" with the biopsy curette from different quadrants of the endometrium are advisable to obtain representative samples for study. The patient should be warned of momentary discomfort with each withdrawal.

The role of endometrial washings in providing diagnostic accuracy is being studied but a tissue diagnosis obtained from endometrial biopsy is preferable.

DILATION AND CURETTAGE

Conventional D&C of the uterus is indicated:

- To evaluate abnormal uterine bleeding when the cervical os is so tight that an endometrial biopsy is not possible
- To evaluate and diagnose the cause of postmenopausal uterine bleeding when endometrial biopsy has not clarified the diagnosis. Knowledge of the presence of an endometrial polyp or malignant tumor is essential to the patient's treatment
- To empty the uterus of its contents when the unwanted products of conception remain, as after an incomplete abortion
- To distinguish clearly between adenomyosis interna and uterine leiomyomata, particularly submucous leiomyomata, in the patient with intractable menorrhagia and an enlarged uterus
- To complete the work-up of an infertility patient who has leiomyomata when a hysterogram has not resolved the issues of location and types of leiomyomata (eg, submucous)

- To evaluate the condition of a patient who has an abnormal Papanicolaou smear when there is no gross or colposcopically visible lesion of the cervix
- To facilitate the staging of an endometrial malignancy
- To treat known or suspected intrauterine synechiae (Asherman's syndrome)

Adhesions may be freed and an intrauterine device inserted to keep the walls of the uterine cavity apart during the healing process.

Dilation and curettage of the uterus is ideally suited to an ambulatory setting. Although it is possible to perform a D&C while the patient is under analgesia only or under local anesthesia by paracervical block, brief general or regional anesthesia allows the physician to examine the internal genitalia carefully at a time when all painful stimuli have been removed.

There is both dogma and confusion in the operating room procedure manuals concerning the degree of surgical "prep" that a patient needs for a D&C. The site at which the procedure will take place often seems to determine the recommendations. In all instances, however, cleansing or bacteriostatic douches, pubic shaving, and enemas not only serve no useful purpose but add to the patient's discomfort.

Site of Dilation and Curettage

Ambulatory Surgical Center

For a D&C in an ambulatory setting, the vagina and cervix are painted with a solution of povidone–iodine (Betadine). Instruments are sterile, draping is minimal, and the surgeon, whose hands have been washed but not necessarily scrubbed, wears sterile gloves.

Hospital Operating Room

Dilation and curettage in the hospital operating room is generally performed under maximum aseptic techniques because there is a particular risk of uterine perforation and infection in some patients, such as those with a gravid uterus and those with an atrophic or cancerous uterus. After cleansing the area with a nonabrasive perineal and vaginal wash, the surgeon paints the operative area with povidone–iodine (Betadine). The patient is fully draped and the instruments are sterile. The surgeon is fully gowned, masked, capped, and gloved.

Technique of Dilation and Curettage

Suction curettage may be used to complete an abortion. If curettage is to be performed on a pregnant or recently pregnant uterus, an intramuscular or intravenous injection of an oxytocic should produce a firm contraction of the myometrium that increases its resistance to perforation. The administration of some analgesia or a paracervical block may precede outpatient curettage of the nonpregnant uterus with the Vabra suction apparatus. In most cases, the operator should perform diagnostic uterine curettage in a fractional manner with the sharp curette.

When the patient is under anesthesia, the first step is to perform a careful examination. This always provides vital information concerning diagnosis and future clinical management. For example, it may provide valuable details about the appropriate route and technique of a future hysterectomy. The physician should note the size, shape, and mobility of the uterus; the location and size of the cul-de-sac; and the strength and elasticity of the uterosacral ligaments, the cardinal ligaments, and the urogenital diaphragm.

After determining the axis and size of the uterus, the operator grasps the anterior cervical lip with a tenaculum for traction and carefully scrapes the endocervical canal with a small sharp curette (eg, the Duncan), up to but not beyond the internal cervical os. Most operators begin curettage at the 12 o'clock position and proceed in a careful clockwise or counterclockwise direction around the circumference of the cavity. The curettings are saved on a piece of Telfa or gauze, to be processed separately from the specimen obtained later from the endometrial cavity.

The malleable Simpson sound should then be bent to accommodate the anteflexion, anteversion, retroflexion, or retroversion of the uterus. It is best if the operator grasps the sound at its round shaft because grasping it at the flat part of the end may interfere with the sound's tendency to follow the path of least resistance, the axis of the uterus. The force exerted on both sound and curette during their insertion should be minimal, similar to that required to hold a pencil or a pen for writing, to decrease the risk of perforation.

After gently inserting the blunt-tipped malleable Simpson sound along the axis of the uterine cavity, the operator carefully measures the depth of the cavity from the external cervical os to the top of the fundus. Not only is this measurement important in establishing the size of the endometrial cavity but it also tells the operator the precise depth beyond which the curette should not be passed during the curettage. The passage of graduated dilators then expands the cervical canal and the internal cervical os to a size large enough to permit the introduction of the largest curette or polyp forceps that will be used during the procedure. Gradual dilation with the patient under anesthesia markedly reduces the risk of rupture or permanent damage to the musculature of the cervix.

After the gentle introduction of a sharp curette into the endometrial cavity to the top of the fundus, the operator grasps its handle firmly and by traction against the resisting uterus, scrapes the endometrial cavity down to but not through the presumed basal layer. In an orderly clockwise or counterclockwise direction, the operator scrapes all segments and quadrants of the endometrium. Scraping ceases when the passage of the sharp edge of the curette across the surface of the endometrium produces the delicate sensation of a "grating" resistance, which is characteristic of the basal layer.

When the endometrium has been curetted and any submucous irregularities, diverticula, or septa in the uterine cavity have been noted, the curettings are separately saved on a piece of Telfa or gauze and the specimen carefully examined and palpated. Benign tissue is soft and spongy; when squeezed, it is somewhat elastic and resists shattering. In contrast, malignant tissue tends to be hard and fragile; when squeezed even gently, it fragments and shatters.

The cavity of the uterus should then be explored with polyp or kidney stone forceps because the curette may miss an endometrial polyp of almost any size, particularly if it has a narrow base. After the introduction of the forceps, the operator opens and closes the jaws in various quadrants of the uterine cavity; after each closing, the operator tugs to see whether there is any resistance. If this procedure reveals the presence of a narrow-based polyp of a size that can negotiate the dilated cervical canal, the operator can safely remove it by twisting the forceps.

Hysteroscopy further clarifies the site and number of polyps, and the source of unusual bleeding (see Chapter 22).

After removing all instruments, the operator carefully inspects the uterus and cervix. If there is significant fresh bleeding from the endometrial cavity, the operator should sound the uterine cavity to ensure that neither perforation of the uterus nor laceration of the endocervix has occurred. Excessive bleeding from tenaculum marks on the cervix may be cauterized or a gentle, temporary packing may be placed against the face of the cervix.

The surgeon should dictate the operative report immediately while all the details of each procedure are fresh and should plan for the removal of any packing that was used. He or she should also convey to the patient or her family the operative findings and discharge instructions and make arrangements for postoperative office evaluation.

Complications of Dilation and Curettage

Although a minor surgical procedure, a D&C requires delicacy and precision if it is to be effective. Performed carelessly, forcefully, or thoughtlessly, the procedure may cause serious injury to the patient.

If a patient who is about to have a D&C has a severe endocervical stenosis that permits the insertion of only a small and narrow sound or probe and it is not possible to dilate the endocervical canal significantly, a small laminaria tent may be inserted along the path of the sound and the procedure rescheduled for 24 hours later. At that time, the laminaria tent may be removed. The cervix will be suf-

ficiently dilated to permit the insertion of a small curette.

Perforation of the wall of the uterus by either a sound or a curette is generally the result of a failure to identify the proper axis of the cavity of the uterus, which is often in anteflexion or retroflexion (Fig. 26-10). The operator forces the perforating instrument through the wall of the uterus, often on the presumption that it is negotiating a somewhat stenotic internal os. When the softness caused by pregnancy or invasion by a malignant tumor has compromised the myometrium, perforation occurs easily. It is recognized by the passage of the tip of the sound or curette beyond the known depth of the uterine cavity. It may be possible to introduce the instrument all the way to its handle without meeting any resistance.

If perforation occurs with the sound, the instrument should be promptly withdrawn. Usually, little of consequence follows. A careful bimanual examination should reveal the position of the uterus, after which the operator should bend the sound in a way that allows it to negotiate the uterine cavity safely. If gently reinserted along the axis of the uterine cavity, the sound generally stops when its tip has reached the fundus of the uterus. The operator may then complete the procedure. If it is impossible to determine the proper axis of the uterus

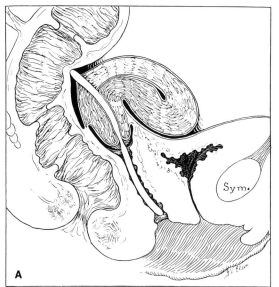 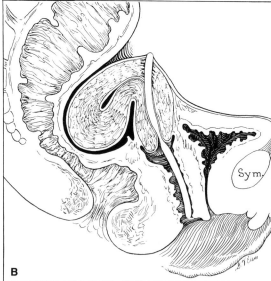

Figure 26–10. Perforation of the uterus at curettage. (**A**) Failure to recognize the axis of a markedly anteflexed uterus may lead to perforation by the curette of the posterior wall of the uterus. (**B**) Similarly, perforation of the anterior wall of the uterus may occur when retroflexion is present. (From Thompson JD, Rock JA [eds]: TeLinde's operative gynecology, 7th ed, p. 307. Philadelphia: JB Lippincott, 1992.)

after a perforation, it is best to discontinue the procedure and schedule it for a future date, after the myometrium has had an opportunity to heal.

If the tip of the sharp curette has perforated the uterus and the surgeon does not realize it, curettage may cause significant damage to the visceral contents of the pelvis. If the curette brings forth evidence of perforation, such as the recovery of tissue from the intestinal epithelium, bowel wall, or bowel contents, immediate laparotomy is essential to repair whatever damage has occurred. If the operator strongly suspects that there has been some damage but the character of the curettings fails to confirm this suspicion, preliminary diagnostic laparoscopy may be of value. If it appears that the bowel has not been damaged, the patient may be observed only.

The surgeon should tell the patient postoperatively about any perforation and should watch her carefully for tachycardia, hypotension, abdominal tenderness, fever, and other signs of intraperitoneal bleeding or uterine or pelvic infection. Any such sequelae make themselves known within 24 hours.

REFERENCES

1. McKay M, Frankman O, Horowitz BJ, et al: Vulvar vestibulitis and vestibular papillomatosis—report of the ISSVD Committee on Vulvodynia. J Reprod Med 36:413, 1991
2. Blazin S, Bouchard C, Brisson J, et al: Vulvar vestibulitis syndrome: an exploratory case-control study. Obstet Gynecol 83:47, 1994
3. Kelly RA, Foster DC, Woodruff JD: Subcutaneous injection of triamcinolone acetonide in the treatment of chronic vulvar pruritus. Am J Obstet Gynecol 169:568, 1993
4. Hallam NF, West J, Harper C, et al: Large loop excision of the transformation zone (LLETZ) as an alternative to both local ablative and cone biopsy treatment: a series of 1000 patients. J Gynecol Surg 9:77, 1993
5. Bloss JD: The use of electrosurgical techniques in the management of premalignant diseases of the vulva, vagina, and cervix: an excisional rather than an ablative approach. Am J Obstet Gynecol 169:1081, 1993
6. Raziel A, Ron-El R, Pansky M, et al: Current management of ruptured corpus luteum. Eur J Obstet Gynecol Reprod Biol 50:77, 1993

Suggested Reading

Brook I: Aerobic and anaerobic microbiology of Bartholin's abscess. Surg Gynecol Obstet 169:32, 1989

Cheetham DR: Bartholin's cyst: marsupialization or aspiration? Am J Obstet Gynecol 152:569, 1985

Friedrich EG: Vulvar vestibulitis syndrome. J Reprod Med 32:110, 1987

Goetsch MF: Vulvar vestibulitis: prevalence and historic features in a general gynecologic practice population. Am J Obstet Gynecol 164:1609, 1991

Grimes DA: Diagnostic dilation and curettage: a reapprisal. Am J Obstet Gynecol 142:1, 1982

Hale RW, Pion RJ: Laminaria: an underutilized clinical adjunct. Clin Obstet Gynecol 15:829, 1972

Haskins A: Questions and answers. JAMA 241:623, 1979

Heah J: Methods of treatment for cysts and abscesses of Bartholin's gland. Br J Obstet Gynaecol 195:321, 1988

Helmkamp BF, Denslow BL, Thomas AB, et al: Cervical conization: when is uterine dilatation and curettage also indicated? Am J Obstet Gynecol 146:893, 1983

Peckham BM, Maki DG, Patterson JJ, et al: Focal vulvitis: a characteristic syndrome and cause of dyspareunia. Am J Obstet Gynecol 154:855, 1986

Rock JA, Azziz R: Wolffian duct cyst at the vaginal vault. In Nichols DH (ed): Clinical problems, injuries and complications of gynecologic surgery, 2nd ed. Baltimore, Williams & Wilkins, 1988

Silver MM, Miles P, Rosa C: Comparison of Novak and Pipelle endometrial biopsy instruments. Obstet Gynecol 78:828, 1991

Smith JJ, Schulman H: Current dilation and curettage practice: a need for revision. Obstet Gynecol 65:516, 1985

Stovall TG, Ling FW, Morgan PL: A prospective, randomized comparison of the Pipelle endometrial sampling device with the Novak curette. Am J Obstet Gynecol 165:1287, 1991

Woodruff JD, Friedrich EG: The vestibule. Clin Obstet Gynecol 28:134, 1985

Woodruff JD, Genadry R, Poliakoff S: Treatment of dyspareunia and vaginal outlet distortions by perineoplasty. Obstet Gynecol 57:750, 1981

Woodruff JD, Parmley THG: Infection of the minor vestibular gland. Obstet Gynecol 62:609, 1983

Ambulatory Gynecology, Second Edition,
edited by David H. Nichols and Patrick J. Sweeney.
J. B. Lippincott Company, Philadelphia, © 1995.

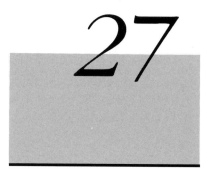

Laparoscopic Surgery

Harry Reich

Most gynecologic intraperitoneal procedures can be performed laparoscopically on an ambulatory basis. Surgical advantages of laparoscopy include (1) panoramic pelvic visualization and magnification, (2) techniques similar to microsurgery, (3) documentation of absolute hemostasis by underwater examination, and (4) steadily increasing surgical versatility because of progress in instrumentation that allows more sophisticated suturing and stapling techniques. The patient enjoys simultaneous diagnosis and treatment and all of the inherent benefits of minimally invasive surgery in terms of cosmetics and rapid recuperation. Laparoscopic surgery is distinctly advantageous because of the decreased risk of de novo adhesion formation.[1] The major limitation of the laparoscopic approach is the skill and experience of the surgeon.

Laparoscopic surgery enjoys a wide range of interventional potential. The most common problem encountered in ambulatory gynecologic health care is pelvic pain, usually with some degree of chronicity; it may be associated with a history of infertility. The second most common problem is infertility that may be associated with some degree of pelvic pain. Frequently at laparoscopy, pelvic adhesions or endometriosis are documented and excision of endometriosis and adhesiolysis is performed. Ovarian cysts are another common problem, discovered either during surgery or preoperatively by physical examination or ultrasound. Cystectomies may be undertaken for relief of pelvic pain, mass, or both. Chronic unilateral pain, however, in a woman who does not desire future fertility and who has demonstrated ovarian pathology (endometriosis, adhesions, persistent cyst) may require oophorectomy for permanent pain relief. This is particularly significant with left-sided involvement because this ovary has an increased susceptibility to healing by adhering to the rectosigmoid. Laparoscopic myomectomy may be requested by women who desire uterine preservation. This procedure carries an increased risk of adhesion formation and may be replaced by myolysis (myoma blood vessel coagulation) in the future.

Acute pelvic pain is best managed by early recourse to laparoscopy for definitive diagnosis and simultaneous treatment. Findings include hemorrhagic corpus luteum, ectopic pregnancy, appendicitis, adnexal torsion, and the spectrum of pelvic inflammatory disease (PID), from acute salpingitis to pelvic abscess.

Minimally invasive surgery will become the standard of operative care within the next decade. The drive to promote less-invasive surgical procedures has been fueled by media attention given to laparoscopic cholecystectomy and hysterectomy and is maintained by consumer interest.

This chapter discusses many techniques and applications of laparoscopic intervention. Laparoscopic hysterectomy is not an outpatient procedure in most centers but is also addressed. Laparoscopic hysterectomy is major surgery, albeit accomplished through minor incisions, and requires at least an overnight stay. The patient must be attended and observed for early postoperative problems.

EQUIPMENT AND TECHNIQUES

Discussion of standard equipment such as laparoscopes, light sources, and video systems is beyond the scope of this chapter. Equipment necessary for advanced procedures and energy sources are included.

High-Flow CO_2 Insufflators

High-flow CO_2 insufflation up to 10 L/minute is necessary to compensate for the rapid loss of CO_2 during suctioning. Models that filter smoke produced by electrosurgery or laser surgery from the CO_2 gas still work poorly. The ability to maintain a relatively constant intraabdominal pressure of between 10 and 15 mmHg during long laparoscopic procedures is essential. Higher pressure settings are used during initial insertion of the trocar (20 to 25 mmHg), with the setting lowered afterward to diminish subcutaneous emphysema. High-pressure settings may be used to control venous bleeding but only for short periods to avoid the possibility of CO_2 embolism and delayed bleeding.

30°-Tiltable Operating Room Table

For the past 16 years, I have used steep Trendelenburg's position (20° to 40°), with shoulder braces and the arms at the patient's sides. Operating room tables capable of a 30° Trendelenburg's position are necessary for advanced laparoscopic surgical procedures, especially when the deep pelvis is involved. The hand-controlled Champagne model 600 (Affiliated Table Company, Rochester, NY) is used; an electronically controlled table capable of this degree of body tilt is available (Skytron Model 6500, Grand Rapids, MI). My patients have experienced no adverse effects from steep Trendelenburg's position.

Uterine Manipulators

A Valtchev uterine mobilizer (Conkin Surgical Instruments, Toronto, Canada) is the best available single instrument to antevert the uterus and delineate the posterior vagina throughout complicated cases. The uterus can be anteverted to about 120° and moved in an arc about 45° to the left or right by turning the mobilizer around its longitudinal axis. With this device in the anteflexed position, the cervix sits on a wide acorn, which is readily visible between the uterosacral ligaments when the cul-de-sac is inspected laparoscopically. Interchangeable detachable uterine obturators and cannulas of various length and diameter are available.

Rectal and Vaginal Probes

If a Valtchev uterine mobilizer is not available, a sponge on a ring forceps is inserted into the posterior vaginal fornix and an 81 French rectal probe (Reznik Instruments, Skokie, IL) is placed in the rectum to define the rectum and posterior vagina, in cases of endometriosis and adhesions with some degree of cul-de-sac obliteration, and to open the posterior vagina (culdotomy). In addition, a 3 or 4 Sims curette or Hulka uterine elevator is placed in the endometrial cavity to antevert the uterus markedly and stretch out the cul-de-sac. The rectal probe and intraoperative rectovaginal examinations remain important techniques, even when the Valtchev is available. Whenever rectal location is in doubt, it is identified by placing a probe.

Trocar Sleeves

Trocar sleeves are available in many sizes and shapes. For most cases, 5.5-mm cannulas are adequate. Newer electrosurgical electrodes that eliminate capacitance and insulation failures (Electroshield, Electroscope, Boulder, CO) require ⅞-mm sleeves. Laparoscopic stapling is performed through $^{12}/_{13}$-mm ports.

Short, trapless 5-mm trocar sleeves with a retention screw grid around the external surface are used in most cases (Richard Wolf, Vernon Hills, IL; Apple Medical, Bolton, MA). These trocar sleeves facilitate efficient instrument exchanges and evacuation of tissue while allowing unlimited freedom during extracorporeal suture tying. With practice, a good laparoscopic surgical team makes instrument exchanges so quickly that little pneumoperitoneum is lost. Once placed, the portal of exit stays fixed at the level of the anterior abdominal wall parietal peritoneum, permitting more room for instrument manipulation.[2]

U.S. Surgical (Norwalk, CT) disposable trocar sleeves with adjustable locking retention collars (Reich screw-grid design) hold their position well for stapling but their trap makes extracorporeal suturing cumbersome. Their retention collars are used to prevent any company's 10-mm trocar sleeve from sliding out of the umbilicus and to stabilize their 12.5-mm sleeve during stapling.

Scissors

Blunt- or round-tipped 5-mm scissors with one stable blade and one movable blade are used to lyse thin and thick bowel adhesions sharply. Scissors that actually cut represent new laparoscopic instrumentation. Sharp dissection is the primary technique used in adhesiolysis to diminish the potential for adhesion formation; electrosurgery and laser surgery are usually reserved for hemostatic dissection of endometriosis or adhesions in which anatomic planes are not evident or vascular adherence is anticipated. Blunt-tipped sawtooth scissors (Richard Wolf), Manhes scissors (Karl Storz, Culver City, CA), and U.S. Surgical disposable scissors all cut. Hook scissors are used when the surgeon can get completely around the structure being divided but rarely maintain their sharpness.

Scissors are the best instrument to cut avascular or congenital adhesions and peritoneum. Blunt dissection can be performed with blunt tipped scissors. This includes ovary–pelvic sidewall and tubo-ovarian adhesions. Loose areolar tissue is separated by inserting a closed scissor and withdrawing it in the open position. Pushing tissue with the partially open or closed blunt tip is the technique used to develop natural planes.

Surgeons should select a scissor that feels comfortable in the hand. It should not be too long or

encumbered by an electrical cord to facilitate direction changes. I prefer to make rapid instrument exchanges between scissors and bipolar forceps through the same portal to control bleeding.

Aquadissection

Aquadissection is broadly defined as the use of hydraulic energy from pressurized fluid to aid in the performance of surgical procedures. The force vector with hydraulic energy is multidirectional within the volume of expansion of the noncompressible fluid. Installation of fluid under pressure displaces tissue, creating cleavage planes in the least resistant spaces. Aquadissection into closed spaces behind peritoneum or adhesions produces edematous, distended tissue on tension, with loss of elasticity, making further division easy and safe.

Aquadissectors (suction irrigators with the ability to dissect using pressurized fluid) should have a single channel to maximize suctioning and irrigating capacity. An aquadissector with a solid (not perforated) distal tip is necessary to perform atraumatic suction–traction–retraction, to irrigate directly, and to develop surgical planes (aquadissection). The shaft should be specially treated to provide a dull finish to prevent CO_2 laser-beam reflection, allowing it to be used as a backstop.

The Aqua-Purator (WISAP, Sauerlach, Germany, or Tomball, TX) was the first of the aquadissection devices. It delivers fluid at 200 mmHg pressure and a rate of 250 mL/10 seconds. One liter can be instilled in 35 seconds. The handle of the Aqua-Purator uses large staples to occlude separate suction and irrigation tubing, which funnel into a single-channel tube. The market is crowded with many aquadissection devices but few suction and irrigate with the speed of the original.[3]

Electrosurgery

Electrosurgical knowledge and skill are essential.[4,5] Monopolar cutting current is safe for laparoscopic use. At the same electrosurgical power setting, less arcing occurs at laparoscopy than at laparotomy because it takes 30% more power to spark or arc in CO_2 than in room air. Electrosurgical burns may occur, however, in areas outside the surgeon's laparoscopic view, from electrode insulation defects or capacitative coupling.

Cutting current is used to both cut or coagulate (desiccate), depending on the portion or configuration of the electrode in contact with the tissue. The tip cuts, whereas the wide body tamponades and coagulates. The voltage is too low with pure cutting current to arc or spark.

Coagulation current with conventional electrodes (80 to 120 W) may arc or spark about 1 mm and is used in close proximity to tissue (but not in contact) to fulgurate diffuse venous and arteriolar bleeding. It is not used in contact with tissue to coagulate because this waveform uses voltages more than 10 times those of cutting current. Coagulation current is modulated so that it is on only 6% of the time. The high voltage allows it to arc or spark for 1 to 2 mm, producing good hemostasis with venous and arteriolar bleeding while penetrating the tissue superficially. The argon beam coagulator (argon gas at 2 L/minute and high-voltage coagulation current) may be used to increase the spark or arc that is possible with conventional fulguration.

Bipolar desiccation for large-vessel hemostasis at laparoscopy was first reported in 1986.[6,7] A more uniform bipolar desiccation process is obtained by using cutting current. Coagulating current is not used because it may rapidly desiccate the outer layers of the tissue, producing superficial resistance that may prevent deeper penetration and cause sparking to surrounding tissue, cutting instead of coagulating. Large blood vessels are compressed and bipolar cutting current is passed until complete desiccation is achieved (ie, the current depletes tissue fluid and electrolytes until it ceases to flow between the forceps), as determined by an ammeter or current flow-meter (end point monitor, EPM-1, Electroscope, Boulder, CO).

Laser Surgery

Laser surgery in the 1990s means CO_2 laser devices. The newer CO_2 laser devices from Coherent (Palo Alto, CA); Sharplan (Tel Aviv, Israel); and Heraeus LaserSonics (Milpitas, CA) do fine work in an uncluttered field, with a collimated (parallel) beam traveling through the operating channel of the laparoscope. In the 1980s, poor CO_2 laser-beam alignment discouraged many surgeons, who switched to fiberoptic laser devices. The problem was not the CO_2 laser device arm; the laser laparoscope and its coupler did not connect with the laparoscope at precisely 90° (ie, 85° to 89°). New laser couplers correct this problem.

Major problems encountered when using CO_2 laser devices through the operating channel of an operating laparoscope are (1) jumping, (2) bloom-

ing, and (3) loss of the beam. If the laser laparoscope coupler does not connect with the laparoscope at precisely 90°, an asymmetric passage of the beam through the operating channel occurs. This beam energy heats the CO_2 purge gas unevenly, causing it to act as an asymmetric lens, refracting the CO_2 laser-beam energy to a different spot than where the aiming helium–neon beam was located.

The passage of CO_2 gas through the laparoscope lumen, a necessity to purge this channel of debris, results in a decrease in both power delivered to tissue and power density at tissue because the 10.6-μm wavelength of the laser beam is absorbed by the CO_2 purge gas, which has the same wavelength. Power to tissue is reduced by 30% to 50% with a 7.2-mm laparoscopic operating channel (12-mm scope) and by 60% with a 5-mm operating channel (10-mm scope).[8] Although it is desirable to operate at high-power density for a short time to minimize thermal damage to surrounding tissue, heating of CO_2 gas in the laparoscope lumen results in an increase in spot size and thus a reduction in power density (the concentration of laser energy on the tissue) at higher power settings. Setting the CO_2 laser device at high power (80 to 100 W) produces a large 3- to 4-mm spot that is extremely coagulative and provides hemostatic cutting. Considering these limitations of using the laser device through a 10-mm laparoscope with 5-mm operating channel, a setting of 20 to 35 W in the superpulse or ultrapulse mode is used for cutting (less than 1000 W/cm² at the tissue), and a setting between 80 and 100 W is used in the continuous mode to obtain a diffuse hemostatic effect for myomectomy and culdotomy.

Some terms need defining. Superpulse mode implies high power (500 W) released for brief surges (less than 50 mJ), theoretically allowing tissue to cool between spikes to reduce surrounding thermal effect. Higher energy pulses (more than 200 mJ) are generated with Ultrapulse (Coherent) or Pulsar (Sharplan), allowing longer cooling intervals between pulses, with resultant char-free vaporization.

The Coherent "L" laser device brings a new dimension to surgical precision, speed, and cutting ability through the operating laparoscope and will be welcomed by expert CO_2 laser surgeons. The Coherent 5000L ^{13}C isotope CO_2 laser device uses an 11.1-μm wavelength beam to circumvent absorption of laser energy by the CO_2 purge gas in the operating channel of the laparoscope. At all power settings, a 6-mm beam enters the coupler from the end of the laser device arm and emerges as a 1.5-

mm spot 350 to 400 mm away. The axis of the beam is the same as the axis of the laparoscope. At high-power settings, the power density at impact is 10 times more than at similar settings with a 10.6-μm wavelength beam that results in a 4-mm spot from heating of the CO_2 purge gas. With the isotope laser device, cutting without coagulation is obtained at 200 mJ per pulse. For some degree of coagulation with the cutting, 100 mJ or less should be used.

When using fiber laser devices, coagulation of tissue occurs before cutting is initiated. Fibers cannot be maneuvered with precision into places accessible with the collimated CO_2 laser beam, which is shot through the operating channel of an operating laparoscope across space perpendicular to the surgeon's field of vision. The argon, KTP-532, and Nd:YAG fiber laser devices have little advantage over electrosurgical electrodes for cutting, coagulation, or fulguration. They are more cumbersome, less versatile, and thus rarely justify their extreme expense. Less plume (smoke) occurs with these laser devices because the heat is dispersed into the tissue, causing greater tissue necrosis; studies are in progress to determine whether this effect may be used to shrink fibroids (myolysis).

Suturing

Suturing is facilitated by tying the knot outside the peritoneal cavity (extracorporeal) and passing it through a trocar sleeve without a trap.[2] An excellent technique for laparoscopic suturing was developed in 1972 by Clarke, using a knot-pusher (Marlow Surgical, Willoughby, OH) to tie in a manner similar to that used to hand-tie suture at open laparotomy.[9] This device performs like an extension of the surgeon's fingers.

To suture with a straight needle, the surgeon applies the suture to the tissue, pulls the needle outside, makes a simple half-hitch, and pushes the throw down to the tissue with the Clarke knot-pusher. A square knot is made by pushing another half-hitch down to the knot to secure it while exerting tension from above.

The Endoloop (Ethicon, Somerville, NJ) and SURGITIE (U.S. Surgical) are preformed knotted loops designed to fit over vascular pedicles and then be tightened. Over the last 15 years, I have used it for appendectomies and omentectomies but never for oophorectomy. Bipolar desiccation works better and eliminates any chance of slippage. Postoperative pelvic pain is less in desiccated pedicles; an endolooped pedicle leaves living cells distal to the loop to necrose and release lysozymes.

Suturing with large curved needles requires a technique to pull them into the peritoneal cavity through a 5-mm lower-quadrant incision.[10] The lower abdominal incisions are placed lateral to the rectus muscle, so that the trocar sleeve penetrates skin, external and internal oblique, transversalis, and peritoneum. A tract is obvious on removing the trocar sleeve and is easy to re-enter. To suture with a CT-1 needle, the trocar sleeve is taken out of the abdomen and loaded by grasping the end of the suture with a needle holder, pulling it through the trocar sleeve, reinserting the instrument into the sleeve, and grasping the suture about 2 to 3 cm from the needle. The needle driver is inserted into the peritoneal cavity through the original tract, as visualized on the monitor; the needle follows. Even large needles can be pulled into the peritoneal cavity in this manner. At this stage, the straight-needle holder is replaced with a Cook oblique curved-needle driver (Cook OB/GYN, Spencer, IN), and the needle applied to tissue. Afterward, the needle is stored in the anterior abdominal wall parietal peritoneum for later removal after the suture is tied. The suture is cut, the cut end of the suture pulled out of the peritoneal cavity, and the knot tied with the Clarke knot-pusher. To retrieve the needle, the trocar sleeve is unscrewed, after which the needle holder inside it pulls the needle through the soft tissue. The trocar sleeve is replaced easily, with or without another suture.

Underwater Examination

At the close of each operation, an underwater examination is performed to document complete intraperitoneal hemostasis in stages; this detects bleeding from vessels and viscera tamponaded during the procedure by the increased intraperitoneal pressure of the CO_2 pneumoperitoneum. The CO_2 pneumoperitoneum is discontinued and displaced with 2 to 5 L of Ringer's lactate solution, and the peritoneal cavity is vigorously irrigated and suctioned with this solution until the effluent is clear of blood products—usually after 10 to 20 L. Underwater inspection of the pelvis is performed to detect any further bleeding, which is controlled using the Vancaillie microbipolar forceps (Storz) to coagulate through the electrolyte solution.

To visualize the pelvis with the patient supine, the 10-mm straight laparoscope and the actively irrigating aquadissector tip are manipulated together into the deep cul-de-sac beneath floating bowel and omentum. During this copious irrigation procedure, clear fluid is deposited into the pelvis and circulates into the upper abdomen, displacing upper abdominal bloody fluid, which is suctioned after flowing back into the pelvis. An "underwater" examination is then performed to observe the separated tubes and ovaries and to confirm complete hemostasis.

A final copious lavage with Ringer's lactate solution is undertaken and all clot directly aspirated; at least 2 L of lactated Ringer's solution are left in the peritoneal cavity to displace CO_2 and to prevent fibrin adherence from occurring by separating raw operative surfaces during the initial stages of reperitonealization. Displacement of the CO_2 with Ringer's lactate diminishes the frequency and severity of shoulder pain from CO_2 insufflation. No other anti-adhesive agents are employed. Hyskon is not used because it pulls intravascular fluid into the peritoneal cavity. No drains, antibiotic solutions, or heparin are used.[11]

INCISIONS

Cutaneous

Only three laparoscopic puncture sites, including the umbilicus, are used for most laparoscopic procedures: 10- or 12-mm umbilical, 5-mm right, and 5-mm left lower quadrant. When a 12 mm laparoscopic stapler is used (rarely), it is inserted through the umbilical incision and the procedure is viewed through a 5-mm laparoscope in one of the 5-mm lower quadrant sites.

Placement of the lower quadrant trocar sleeves just above the pubic hairline and lateral to the deep epigastric vessels and the rectus abdominis muscle is preferred. These vessels, an artery flanked by two veins (venae comitantes), are located lateral to the umbilical ligaments (obliterated umbilical artery) by direct laparoscopic inspection of the anterior abdominal wall. The deep epigastric vessels arise near the junction of the external iliac vessels with the femoral vessels and make up the medial border of the internal inguinal ring. The round ligament curls around these vessels to enter the inguinal canal. If the anterior abdominal wall parietal peritoneum is thickened from previous surgery or obesity, the position of these vessels is judged by palpating and depressing the anterior abdominal wall with the back of the scalpel; the wall appears to be thicker where rectus muscle is enclosed and the incision site should be chosen lateral to this area, near the anterior superior iliac spine.

The umbilical incision is closed with 4-0 Vicryl (polyglactin 910). The lower quadrant incisions are loosely approximated with a Javid vascular clamp

(V. Mueller, McGaw Park, IL) and covered with Collodion (AMEND, Irvington, NJ) to allow drainage of excess Ringer's lactate solution.

Culdotomy

A posterior vaginal culdotomy is the preferred method for specimen removal. The CO_2 laser device at high power produces a large spot size (3 to 4 mm) for hemostatic cutting and is used to make a transverse culdotomy incision in the posterior vaginal apex, which is distended by a wet sponge on ring forceps inserted behind the cervix, without the bleeding that accompanies a vaginal colpotomy made with scissors. The incision is closed with interrupted or running 0-Vicryl applied laparoscopically or vaginally.

PROCEDURES

The procedures selected for discussion in this chapter are those most frequently encountered in ambulatory gynecology. Because many procedures can be performed laparoscopically, the list in Table 27-1 was developed to provide a frame of reference for relative difficulty.

Table 27–1

Gynecologic Laparoscopic Procedures or Conditions Treated According to Degree of Difficulty (Ascending)

1. Acute PID
2. Adnexal torsion
3. Ectopic pregnancy
4. Ureteral dissection
5. Pelvic abscess
6. Excision peritoneal endometriosis
7. Oophorectomy
8. Hysterectomy
9. Cyst excision, including dermoids without spill
10. Excision of ovarian endometrioma
11. Salpingostomy for hydrosalpinx
12. Tubal reversal
13. Salpingo-ovariolysis for thick "fused" tube–ovary complex
14. Large myomectomy
15. Lymphadenectomy
16. Cul-de-sac dissection, with excision of deep fibrotic endometriosis from anterior rectum and posterior vagina
17. Small bowel adhesions (partial bowel obstruction)

Peritoneal Cavity Adhesiolysis

Extensive peritoneal cavity adhesions are a frequent finding at laparoscopy for pain or infertility. Adhesions cause pain by entrapment of the organs they surround. Usually, the bowel and omentum are involved, the tube is stuck to the ovary, and the ovary is adhered to the pelvic sidewall and uterus. The extent, thickness, and vascularity of adhesions varies widely. In many cases, the rectosigmoid is involved. Adhesions may be the result of an episode of PID or endometriosis but most commonly are caused by previous surgery.

General Adhesiolysis, Including Enterolysis

Adhesions encountered initially that involve omentum and small bowel attachments to the anterior abdominal wall parietal peritoneum are released. If they extend above the umbilicus, another incision is made above the highest adhesion and the laparoscope inserted therein. Adhesions are easier to divide by working above them than below because of the panoramic view of the parietal peritoneum, omentum, and bowel. Gravity helps to delineate the plane for separation.

Special entry techniques may be necessary if extensive adhesions are suspected. If CO_2 insufflation is not obtainable through the umbilicus, Veress needle puncture is performed in the left ninth intercostal space, anterior axillary line. The trocar is then inserted at the left costal margin in the midclavicular line, giving a panoramic view of the entire peritoneal cavity. Thereafter, the adhesions can be freed down to and just beneath the umbilicus, making it possible to establish the umbilical portal for pelvic work.

Salpingo-Ovariolysis, Including Salpingostomy

The surgical procedures performed for tubal adhesions are salpingo-ovariolysis, fimbrioplasty, or salpingostomy. Small or large bowel enterolysis often accompanies these procedures. If both tubes are open and the fimbria of the tube are not involved in the adhesive process, the procedure is termed salpingo-ovariolysis. If the distal tube is completely blocked, the procedure is designated salpingostomy. If the fimbria are adhered to the ovary or the distal tube is partially occluded, the procedure is termed fimbrioplasty. Actually, there is overlap between these procedures. In performing salpingo-ovariolysis when the tube is completely blocked,

with its distal end stuck to the ovary, freeing this end from the ovary frequently results in a salpingostomy. (The salpingostomy was performed while doing the salpingo-ovariolysis.) This is an important point because if the surgeon makes a tubal incision before dissecting the distal tube off the ovary (ie, in the most dilated portion of what looks like the end of the tube), the opening seals just as a salpingotomy does after ectopic pregnancy surgery. In other words, linear incisions along the length of the tube seal; incisions at what was once the true tubal distal ostium stay open, if opened widely. Salpingo-ovariolysis for a retroperitoneal ovary or a fused tubo-ovarian complex is more difficult than a terminal salpingostomy with a free ovary, where the blockage was caused by tubes sealing at their distal end before extensive outpouring of purulent material occurs.

Laparoscopic tubal surgery must be as meticulous as that performed by laparotomy.[12] Tubo-ovarian adhesions are placed on traction and divided with scissors. Microbipolar forceps with irrigant are reserved for hemostasis after bleeding occurs. Laser surgery should be avoided during this dissection to prevent adhesions from thermal necrosis. The ability of laser incision to dissect with hemostasis makes it ideal for separating vascular fused tubo-ovarian complexes. In these cases, it is not possible to easily identify dissection planes with traction. Frequent tubal lavage distends the tube to aid in its identification. Aquadissection and CO_2 laser surgery are used to complete the dissection.

Chronic PID with hydrosalpinx may almost always be treated laparoscopically. Preoperative hysterosalpingogram to evaluate the proximal tube for salpingitis isthmica nodosa is helpful. This portion of the tube also requires careful intraoperative inspection.

Cystectomy

Ovarian cysts are discovered during pelvic examination or ultrasonography. If persistent, these cysts should be surgically evaluated because of the small risk of malignancy. Laparotomy with cyst excision is inappropriate because of the increased risk of ovarian adhesions.[13]

Laparoscopic inspection of a suspected ovarian cyst often reveals a parovarian cyst, hydrosalpinx, or inflammatory peritoneal pseudocyst. Parovarian cysts are excised if large enough to disrupt ovum pickup, and pseudocysts require excision of pelvic adhesions. The ovaries are evaluated for visual evic nce of malignancy. All cysts should be smooth-walled and without excrescence. Cysts with a translucent thin wall are usually functional. Most organic cysts have thick walls. All but the most benign-appearing cysts are removed intact through the cul-de-sac to avoid the potential risk of metastasis to the anterior abdominal wall.

All cysts opened during laparoscopic surgery, either intentionally or during mobilization of the ovary, require a careful examination of their inner walls. Cystectomy is preferable to puncture with biopsy to avoid recurrence of both functional and organic cysts.

Ovarian cystectomy for functional cysts (simple cysts, follicle cysts, or corpus luteum cysts) is not a common laparoscopic procedure, and laparoscopic excision should be considered only when persistence of the cyst or pain is documented. Even an actively bleeding hemorrhagic corpus luteum cyst can be excised with minimal bleeding. Hemostasis without excision of a bleeding corpus luteum may be obtained using electrosurgical fulguration (ie, noncontact high-voltage spray coagulation current [80 to 120 W]). Suture repair is sometimes indicated.

Simple cysts are aspirated with a needle attached to a syringe after cul-de-sac washings have been obtained. It must be emphasized that drainage with a needle does not prevent spill and is performed for only the most benign-appearing cysts. After documentation of clear or hemosiderin-filled fluid, the ovarian cortex is opened at its most dependent portion with a knife electrode at 70 W cutting current, and the cyst is excised.

Enlarged ovaries containing cysts are either free in the peritoneal cavity or attached to the pelvic sidewall, uterosacral ligament, or cul-de-sac. Frequently, the cyst proves to be an endometrioma when attached to the sidewall. During mobilization of the cyst from the pelvic sidewall, chocolate-like hemosiderin-filled fluid will spill from the ovary (Color Fig. 27-1*G*). If this occurs, the ovary is completely mobilized to its hilum, using aquadissection and careful blunt dissection to avoid unnecessary pelvic sidewall peritoneal damage. The endometrioma cyst wall is then excised; experience has proved that drainage is not enough. The cyst wall is most firmly attached to the ovarian cortex in the area of rupture during dissection or avulsion (ie, on the portion that was adhered to the pelvic sidewall or uterosacral ligament). A knife electrode at 70 to 100 W cutting current is used at the juncture of ovarian cortex and endometrioma cyst wall to develop a dissection plane in this firmly attached area.

If possible, this incision is extended through the visible 360° opening. The cutting current destroys endometriosis at the ovarian cortex–endometrioma junction while making a divot of separation between the two structures. Thereafter, biopsy forceps are placed on ovarian cortex and endometrioma cyst wall and traction exerted to peel the endometrioma cyst wall from the ovary.[14] Minimal bleeding occurs and usually stops spontaneously. Hemostasis is checked by underwater examination inside the ovary, and individual bleeders are identified by using irrigation through an irrigating channel and coagulated with microbipolar forceps. If removal results in a large asymmetric defect, the ovary is suture-repaired, usually with one purse-string suture applied close to the uretero-ovarian ligament in one direction and the infundibulopelvic ligament in the other.

If the ovary is free of the pelvic sidewall and other structures, a dermoid cyst or other benign neoplasm may be present and an attempt is made to excise the cyst without spill (Color Fig. 27-2). A superficial incision is made in the cortex with the CO_2 laser device set at 10 to 20 W. The incision is extended with scissors and undermined with scissors and aquadissection. If the cyst is neoplastic, it rarely ruptures; the thin wall of functional cysts (follicle or corpus luteum) rupture spontaneously. Forceps traction and aquadissection are used to separate the dermoid cyst from surrounding ovarian tissue. Laser incision and scissors are used to separate fibrous adherences and vessels near the hilum. After excision of the intact cyst from inside the ovary, electrosurgical fulguration is used, if necessary, inside the ovary to obtain complete hemostasis. Usually the edges reapproximate and suturing is not required; large ovarian defects are suture-repaired. The cyst is removed through the cul-de-sac, using the previously described culdotomy.

The intact cyst is pushed deep into the cul-de-sac, where it is aspirated vaginally, using a 14-gauge needle on a needle extender attached to a 50-mL syringe until it is small enough to pop out of the culdotomy incision. Thereafter, the laser culdotomy incision is closed with 2-0 Vicryl on a curved needle, vaginally or laparoscopically.

After laser culdotomy, an impermeable sack (LapSac: Cook OB/GYN) is inserted into the peritoneal cavity through the vagina. This 5″ × 8″ nylon bag has a polyurethane inner coating and a nylon drawstring. It is impermeable to water and dye. The free intact specimen is placed in the bag, which is closed by pulling the drawstring. The drawstring is delivered through the posterior vagina, the bag opened, and the intact specimen visually identified, decompressed, and removed.

If a dermoid cyst is encountered during syringe aspiration, cyst excision should be accomplished with as little spill as possible. Vigorous peritoneal cavity irrigation with at least 10 L of Ringer's lactate and underwater examination with direct suctioning of fatty and epidermal elements is recommended to prevent a chronic granulomatous reaction.[15]

Oophorectomy

Outpatient laparoscopic oophorectomy (Color Fig. 27-3) was first reported by Reich and McGlynn, using bipolar electrosurgical desiccation and culdotomy.[6,7] Semm and Mettler advocated using a loop ligature and a tissue punch morcellator, followed by inpatient observation.[16] The indications for laparoscopic oophorectomy (or salpingo-oophorectomy) include (1) pelvic pain secondary to ovarian adhesions from previous hysterectomy, (2) pain from ovarian adhesions unresponsive to laparoscopic lysis, (3) pelvic mass secondary to hydrosalpinx from PID or previous surgery, and (4) postmenopausal palpable ovary. In women who do not desire future fertility, oophorectomy should be considered for pain or mass arising from ovarian endometrioma, hemorrhagic corpus luteum cyst, or dermoid cyst if the contralateral ovary is normal—especially if the cyst is on the left because this ovary frequently heals adhered to the rectosigmoid. Postmenopausal cystic ovaries may be removed intact through a culdotomy. Women who have two or more first-degree relatives (mother or sister) with ovarian cancer may consider early prophylactic oophorectomy after age 35 years if childbearing has been completed.

Preoperatively, endovaginal ultrasound is performed to evaluate the ovaries in cases involving a pelvic mass, retrocervical nodules, or fibroids, and a CA-125 assay is obtained if persistent enlargement is documented. Intravenous pyelograms are rarely necessary preoperatively but are ordered postoperatively if abdominal pain persists after surgery on or near the ureter. There is no indication for computed tomography or magnetic resonance imaging scanning before laparoscopic ovarian surgery.

In all cases, careful inspection of the pelvis and abdomen is undertaken. The ovaries are evaluated for visual evidence of malignancy; washings are taken if indicated; endometriomas are drained. Be-

fore starting oophorectomy, it is imperative that the surgeon visualize the course of the ureter. It crosses the external iliac artery near the bifurcation of the common iliac artery at the pelvic brim and is usually lower on the left, where its entrance into the pelvis is covered by the inverted V-shaped root of the sigmoid mesocolon. The peritoneum above the ureter is opened with sharp scissors. Smooth grasping forceps are then opened parallel and perpendicular to the retroperitoneal structures until the ureter is identified. Scissors may be used to further dissect the ureter throughout its course along the pelvic sidewall.

Before removal, the ovary is released from all pelvic sidewall and bowel adhesions. The fallopian tube is grasped and pulled medially to stretch out the infundibulopelvic ligament containing the ovarian vessels. Kleppinger bipolar forceps are used to compress and desiccate the infundibulopelvic ligament, the broad ligament, the fallopian tube isthmus, and the utero-ovarian ligament with bipolar cutting current. In most cases, three contiguous areas are desiccated. Laparoscopic scissors are used to divide the pedicle. Alternatively, laparoscopic staples or suture may be applied. The free ovary is removed through the umbilicus or cul-de-sac.

If the ovary or ovarian remnant is fused to or within the pelvic sidewall peritoneum, a retroperitoneal approach for oophorectomy is considered. Scissors or CO_2 laser incision is used to incise the peritoneum lateral to the infundibulopelvic ligament, progressing parallel to the tube and ovary up to the uterine end of the round ligament. With traction on the tube, ovary, or peritoneum, the retroperitoneal space is entered and its loose areolar tissue dissected with scissors until the ureter is identified. At this time, the ovarian vessels may be desiccated just caudad to where they cross over the iliac vessels. After division of the infundibulopelvic ligament, it is placed on traction and the procedure continues caudad, with division of the peritoneum just below its ovarian attachments and lateral to its rectosigmoid attachments. Finally, the utero-ovarian ligament and proximal fallopian tube are desiccated and divided, freeing the specimen. The peritoneal sidewall defect is left alone.

Extensive Endometriosis

The surgical objective of laparoscopic treatment of endometriosis is the removal of all visible and palpable endometriosis by excising large superficial and deep lesions and vaporizing smaller deposits.

Cul-de-sac endometriosis causes partial or complete cul-de-sac obliteration from fibrotic deposits between the anterior rectum, the posterior vagina, and the cervix. The technique of freeing the anterior rectum from the posterior vagina to the loose areolar tissue of the rectovaginal septum before excising and vaporizing the deep fibrotic endometriosis is used.[17] This approach is possible, even when anterior rectal muscularis infiltration is present (see Color Fig. 27-1)

Complete cul-de-sac obliteration is diagnosed when the outline of a sponge on a ring forceps in the posterior vaginal fornix cannot be seen through the laparoscope. Partial cul-de-sac obliteration is determined when rectal tenting is visible but a protrusion of the sponge in the posterior vaginal fornix is identified between the rectum and the inverted "U" of the uterosacral ligaments.

Superficial fibrotic hemorrhagic peritoneal endometriosis implants and adjacent peritoneum are excised, using either a pulsed CO_2 laser beam at 20 to 35 W, an electrode at 80-W cutting current, or scissors. An elliptic incision is made in normal peritoneum surrounding the lesion, its edge lifted upward, and the lesion undermined using aquadissection. This pushes the rectum and other vital structures away and facilitates undercutting of the lesion. After peritoneal excision, the anterior rectal wall is checked and any superficial endometriosis excised or vaporized. Ovarian endometriomas are excised as discussed earlier.[14]

Endometriosis surgery is not made easier by perioperative medical therapy with gonadotropin-releasing–hormone agonists or danazol. Ovarian suppression is expensive, has a significant rate of side effects, and prohibits fertility during its administration. The hormonal responsiveness of deep endometriotic fibrotic lesions is unpredictable and inconsistent.[18,19] There is no conclusive evidence to suggest that hormonal suppression improves the long-term outcome in women with extensive disease.

Patients are informed preoperatively that they are at high risk for bowel injury during laparoscopic procedures if extensive cul-de-sac involvement with endometriosis or adhesions is suspected from the clinical presentation. A mechanical bowel preparation (Golytely or Colyte) is administered orally the afternoon before surgery to induce brisk, self-limiting diarrhea to cleanse the bowel without disrupting the electrolyte balance. Antibiotics are not given as preoperative prophylaxis for laparoscopic surgery but are administered during operative procedures that last more than 2 hours.

Endometriosis and deep fibrotic tissue that is assumed to contain endometriosis is excised or vaporized from the anterior rectum with the aid of multiple rectovaginal examinations. In most cases dissection to the loose areolar tissue of the rectovaginal septum reveals that the bulk of the fibrotic lesions are on the posterior vagina.

Laparoscopic Myomectomy

The major indications for myomectomy are secondary infertility, with a history of second trimester loss, and preservation of fertility in women with either hypermenorrhea leading to anemia or a large abdominal mass. The benefits of a myomectomy in an asymptomatic woman whose fibroid does not destroy the uterine or tubal portion of her reproductive system—even with a history of infertility—cannot be documented by existing literature.[20,21] Multiple myomectomy is usually more time-consuming than hysterectomy and is associated with postoperative adhesions and the risk of subsequent surgeries. In most cases, a 5-cm intramural fibroid may be removed from the uterus in less than 30 minutes but another hour may be necessary to obtain complete hemostasis and suture-repair the uterus. Ten-centimeter intramural myomectomies may take 4 hours. Women with a strong desire to avoid hysterectomy, although not desiring future fertility, require lengthy counseling about the risks and benefits of this procedure; laparoscopic hysterectomy is a better choice.

The preoperative use of gonadotropin-releasing–hormone analogs for at least 2 months before myomectomy should be encouraged because it may reduce the total uterine volume and shrink the leiomyoma.[22,23] More lengthy treatment may result in degeneration of the myoma, making it difficult to grasp adequately for traction during surgery. During treatment with depoleuprolide (Lupron Depot), at a dose of 3.75 mg intramuscularly once per month, anemia secondary to hypermenorrhea resolves, and autologous blood donation may be considered before the surgical procedure.

Myomectomy for hypermenorrhea can often be accomplished using a resectoscope to excise submucous myomas. Laparoscopic excision of submucous myomas, even when half of the myoma is submucous, often leaves an intact endometrium, with little risk of synechia.

Laparoscopic myomectomy requires a thorough knowledge of electrosurgical and laser surgery techniques for hemostasis because lower–uterine-segment tourniquets are not available to reduce intraoperative blood loss. Electrosurgical hemostasis is often supplemented by placing Surgicel inside the defect before suture repair. Bulldog clamps inserted through the 10-mm umbilical trocar sleeve may be applied to the infundibulopelvic ligaments for hemostasis in selected cases. Vasoconstrictive agents are not used because they may cause delayed bleeding in the myometrium. Solitary pedunculated myomas may be separated from the uterus after desiccating their pedicle with bipolar forceps. Adenomyosis may masquerade as an intramural myoma, with bulging of the serosa. When encountered, the bulk of the lesion should be removed with an electrosurgical wedge resection, hemostasis obtained with fulguration, and the defect closed as described below.

Myomectomy is ideal for video observation (Color Fig. 27-4). The serosa and surrounding myometrial shell are entered with a spoon electrode at 150-W cutting current. Arteriolar bleeding is controlled with cutting-current desiccation, and venous oozing is controlled with coagulation-current noncontact fulguration at 80 to 120 W. Persistent arterial bleeding from small or large vessels requires bipolar desiccation with cutting current. Thereafter, a 5-mm corkscrew (WISAP) is screwed into the myoma, which is pulled outward, so that the tip of the aquadissector can be inserted between the fibroid and surrounding myometrial pseudocapsule to aquadissect tissue planes. Fibrous adherences between the fibroid and its myometrial shell are divided with electrosurgery or laser surgery; large pedicles, usually at the base, are separately desiccated with bipolar forceps. If using CO_2 laser incision through the operating channel of an operating laparoscope, high-power settings between 50- and 100-W continuous mode produce large spot sizes, which control most arteriolar and venous bleeding. Throughout the procedure, the aquadissector with a solid distal tip is used to dissect the pseudocapsule cleavage planes, suction-retract both myometrium and myoma, and suction smoke.

After removal of the myoma, a myometrial defect of varying size results. Myometrial bleeding is controlled with unipolar fulguration through a spatula electrode, with resultant shrinkage of the defect. Kleppinger bipolar forceps or microbipolar forceps may also be necessary to obtain complete hemostasis. The defect is suture-repaired with curved needles to compress the full thickness of exposed myometrium. Surgicel is left inside the defect.

The myoma is removed from the peritoneal cavity through a culdotomy. The tenaculum or 11-mm corkscrew is inserted through the vagina to grasp the fibroid under direct laparoscopic vision by maneuvering it around the sponge. An 11-mm corkscrew device is screwed into the myoma vaginally through the culdotomy incision, the myoma put on traction at the incision, and further morcellated vaginally with scissors or scalpel if necessary, until removal is completed.

Laparoscopic Hysterectomy

Laparoscopic hysterectomy is a substitute for abdominal hysterectomy and not for vaginal hysterectomy. Most hysterectomies performed with an abdominal approach may be performed with laparoscopic dissection of part or all of the abdominal portion, followed by vaginal removal, including fibroids of more than 1000 g.

Because of the high degree of consumer interest, many more surgeons are attempting this procedure, sometimes without adequate information or support staff. Safety measures must be stressed and caution exercised. More experience than a 2-day course or video series is required. Support staff must also be trained, so that the operating room personnel work optimally as a team. If a surgeon becomes uncomfortable with laparoscopic technique, it is prudent to convert to abdominal or vaginal approach rather than place the patient at increased risk.

Ureteral isolation has always been advised. Although some criticize the time required for ureteral dissection, I find the time well spent if ureteral injury can be eliminated. As a further safeguard, a single "sentinel" stitch is placed on each side during uterine vessel ligation as a constant reminder of ureteral location.

Various procedures have been called "laparoscopic hysterectomy":

- Diagnostic laparoscopy with vaginal hysterectomy indicates that the laparoscope is used for diagnostic purposes when indications for a vaginal approach are equivocal to determine whether vaginal hysterectomy is possible.[24] It also assures that vaginal cuff and pedicle hemostasis is complete and allows clot evacuation.
- Laparoscopic vault suspension after vaginal hysterectomy is useful when vaginal hysterectomy alone cannot accomplish appropriate repair for prolapse. Ureteral dissection before vaginal hysterectomy aids in high uterosacral ligament identification.
- Laparoscope-assisted vaginal hysterectomy is a vaginal hysterectomy after laparoscopic adhesiolysis, endometriosis excision, or oophorectomy.

- Laparoscopic hysterectomy denotes laparoscopic ligation of the uterine arteries.[25] All maneuvers after uterine vessel ligation may be performed vaginally or laparoscopically, including anterior and posterior vaginal entry; cardinal and uterosacral ligament division; uterine removal, intact or by morcellation; and vaginal closure vertically or transversely.
- Laparoscope-assisted abdominal hysterectomy (Total laparoscopic hysterectomy) indicates that laparoscopic dissection continues until the uterus lies free of all attachments in the peritoneal cavity. The vagina is closed with laparoscopically placed sutures.
- Laparoscopic supracervical hysterectomy has regained advocates. The uterus is removed by morcellation from above or below.

The technique described in this chapter is for laparoscope-assisted abdominal hysterectomy (Color Fig. 27-5).

Ureteral Dissection

Immediately after exploration of the upper abdomen and pelvis, each ureter is isolated deep in the pelvis if possible. This is undertaken early in the operation, before the pelvic sidewall peritoneum becomes edematous or opaque from irritation by the CO_2, pneumoperitoneum, or aquadissection and before ureteral peristalsis is inhibited by surgical stress, pressure, or Trendelenburg's position. The ureter and its overlying peritoneum are grasped deep in the pelvis on the left to avoid division of the lateral rectosigmoid attachments required for high identification. An atraumatic grasping forceps is used from a right-sided cannula to grab the ureter and its overlying peritoneum on the left pelvic sidewall, below and caudad to the left ovary, lateral to the left uterosacral ligament. Scissors are used to divide the peritoneum overlying the ureter and are then inserted into the created defect and spread. Thereafter, one blade of the scissor is placed on top of the ureter, the buried scissor blade is visualized through the peritoneum, and the peritoneum is divided. This is continued into the deep pelvis, where the uterine vessels cross the ureter. Connective tissue between the ureter and the vessels is sharply divided with scissors. Bleeding is controlled with well-insulated bipolar forceps.

Bladder Mobilization

The left round ligament is divided at its mid-portion with a spoon electrode at 150-W cutting current. Persistent bleeding is controlled with unipolar ful-

guration at 80-W coagulation current or bipolar dissection at 30-W cutting current. Thereafter, scissors are used to divide the vesicouterine peritoneal fold, starting at the left side and continuing across the midline to the right round ligament. The right round ligament is divided in the same manner as was the left, with unipolar electrosurgery. The bladder is mobilized off the uterus and upper vagina using scissors.

Upper Uterine Blood Supply

If ovarian preservation is desired, the utero-ovarian ligament and fallopian tube are divided adjacent to the uterus after incising the broad ligament peritoneum and placing 2/0 vicryl suture ligatures around the vessels. If ovarian preservation is not desired, the infundibulopelvic ligaments and broad ligaments are sutured or coagulated until desiccated and then divided.

Uterine Vessel Ligation

The broad ligament on each side is skeletonized down to the uterine vessels. Each uterine vessel pedicle is suture-ligated with 0-Vicryl on a CT-1 needle or 0 POLYSORB on a GS-21 needle (27-inch). The needles are introduced into the peritoneal cavity by pulling them through a 5-mm incision. The curved needle is inserted on top of the unroofed ureter, where it turns medially toward the previously mobilized bladder. A short rotary movement of the Cook oblique curved-needle holder brings the needle around the uterine vessel pedicle. Sutures are tied extracorporeally, using a Clarke knot-pusher. A single suture placed in this manner on each side serves as a "sentinel stitch," identifying and watching over the ureter for the rest of the case.

Circumferential Culdotomy

Circumferential culdotomy is the division of cervicovaginal attachments. The cardinal ligaments on each side are divided using the CO_2 laser device, which is set at high power, or the spoon electrode at 150-W cutting current. Often, bleeding control is necessary, using bipolar forceps. The vagina is entered posteriorly over the Valtchev retractor, which identifies the junction of cervix with vagina. Continuing toward the left, the vaginal fornix is divided. Thereafter, it is possible to insert the Aqua-Purator into the anterior vagina above the cervix tenaculum on the anterior cervical lip. Following the Aqua-Purator tip and using it as a backstop, the anterior fornix is divided. The Aqua-Purator is inserted

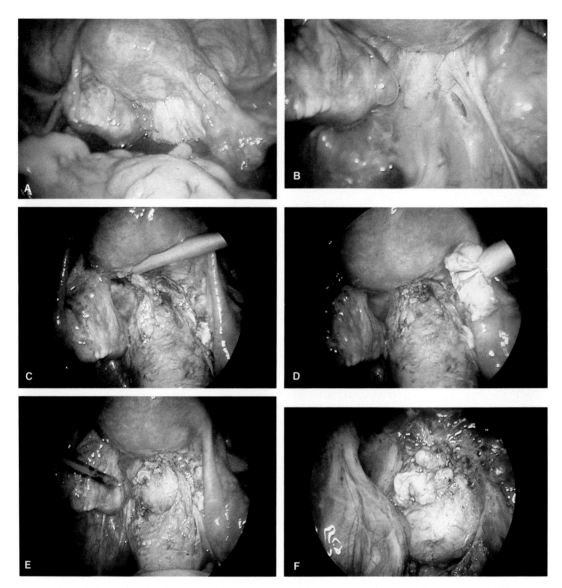

Color Figure 27–1. Cul-de-sac obliteration secondary to deep fibrotic endometriosis and bilateral endometriomas. (**A**) Cul-de-sac obliteration and bilateral ovarian endometriomas. (**B**) Close up of deep cul-de-sac, showing rectum stuck to back of cervix. (**C**) Dissection begins by freeing both ovaries. Rectum is then freed from posterior vagina down to rectovaginal septum (loose areolar tissue). Deep fibrotic endometriosis is excised from uterosacral ligaments, posterior vagina, and anterior rectum. (**D**) Rectovaginal septum, thick with deep fibrotic endometriosis, is excised. (**E**) Sponge in posterior vagina demonstrates its freedom from the anterior rectum and also additional endometriosis near junction of vagina with cervix. (**F**) Close-up of deep fibrotic endometriosis on posterior vagina near cervix before excision.

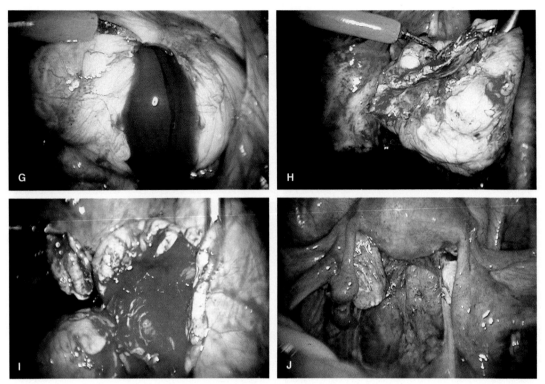

(**G**) After freeing of the ovary to its hilum, the most dependent portion of the ovary is incised with a knife electrode at 70-W cutting current. Chocolate-like fluid exudes from ovary. (**H**) The knife electrode is used to separate the closely adherent ovarian cortex from the endometrioma cyst wall. Once developed, this plane of dissection is used to separate the endometrioma cyst wall from ovarian cortex. (**I**) Using traction and countertraction, the endometrioma cyst wall is removed. (**J**) At the end of the procedure, all deep fibrotic endometriosis has been excised from the ovaries, posterior cervix, posterior vagina, and anterior rectum. Loose areolar tissue of rectovaginal septum is seen.

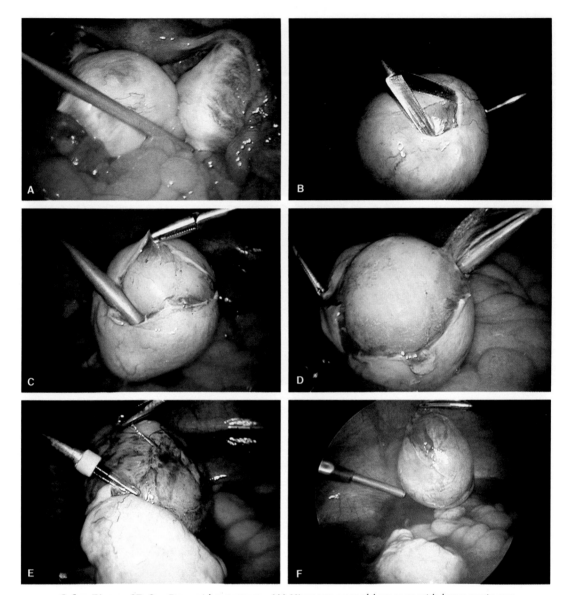

Color Figure 27–2. Dermoid cystectomy. (**A**) Nineteen-year-old woman with large cystic ovaries. Ultrasound suggested multiple dermoids in each ovary. (**B**) Microscissors or CO_2 laser is
used to open ovarian cortex without entering cyst. (**C**) A plane is established between the ovarian
cortex and the cysts. (**D**) Aquadissection is used during this portion of the procedure as the cyst
becomes mobilized down to its blood supply. (**E**) Bipolar forceps desiccate the cyst vascular
pedicle. (**F**) After excision of the first cyst, it is stored in the cul-de-sac while the others are
excised.

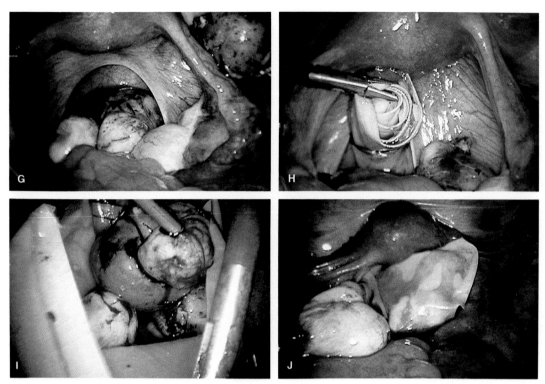

(**G**) Five dermoid cysts were excised in this case. (**H**) After laparoscopic opening of the cul-de-sac (culdotomy), an impermeable sack is pulled into the peritoneal cavity. (**I**) All of the cysts are placed in the sack. (**J**) The sack is delivered through the vagina. If cysts are too large to pull out, an 18-gauge needle on a needle extender is used for aspiration before their removal.

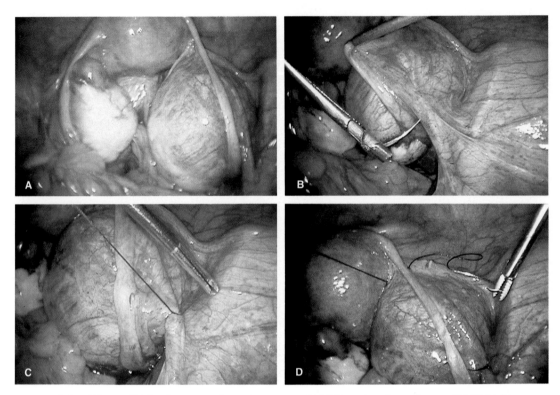

Color Figure 27–3. Laparoscopic oophorectomy. (**A**) Bilateral endometriomas. (**B**) Right fallopian tube is pulled medially. 0-Vicryl on a CT-1 needle (Ethicon) is applied to the right infundibulopelvic ligament, using the Cook oblique curved-needle holder. (**C**) Suture is secured, using the Clarke knot-pusher. (**D**) A second suture is placed around the right utero-ovarian ligament and fallopian tube pedicle.

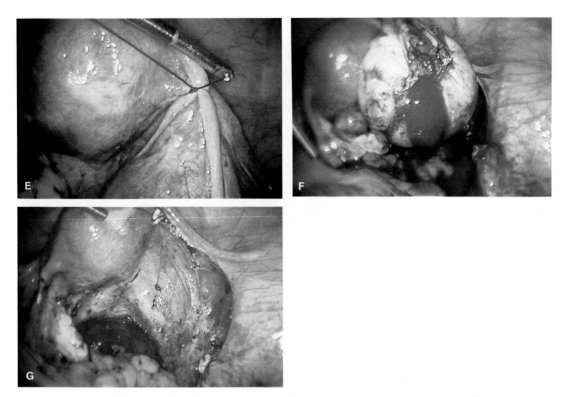

(**E**) This pedicle is also ligated, using the Clarke knot-pusher. (**F**) Some leakage occurs from the ovarian endometrioma after complete mobilization of the ovary from the pelvic sidewall. (**G**) Right oophorectomy is complete after culdotomy extraction. Left ovarian endometrioma has been excised, leaving a functional left ovary.

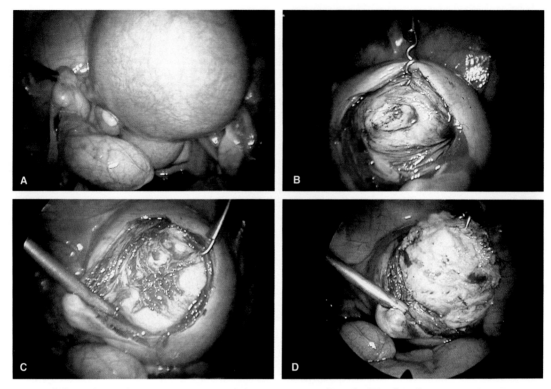

Color Figure 27–4. Myomectomy. (**A**) Large myoma (8 cm). (**B**) After the myometrium is opened with a spoon electrode, laparoscopic cork screw is inserted for traction. (**C**) Aquadissection, cutting current electrosurgery, and CO_2 laser used for dissection. (**D**) Operation proceeds slowly until half of the myoma is out.

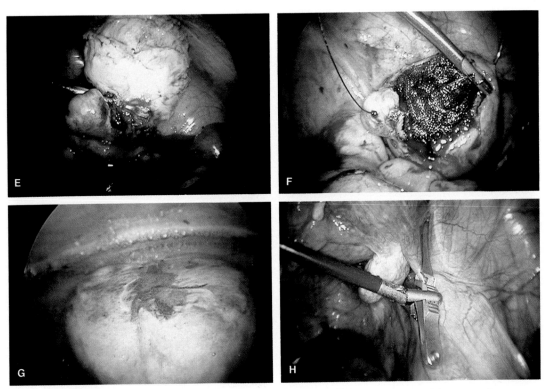

(**E**) Thereafter, the large pedicles at the base are desiccated with bipolar forceps. (**F**) Myometrium is suture-repaired with 0-Vicryl on a CTX needle (Ethicon) after operative surface area is covered with Surgicel. (**G**) Underwater examination confirms complete hemostasis of repair site. (**H**) Bull-dog clamp may be applied to infundibulopelvic ligaments to reduce blood loss (and fluid over-load during hysteroscopic and laparoscopic myomectomy procedures).

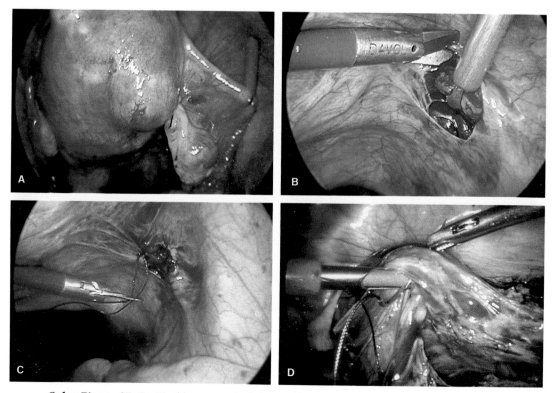

Color Figure 27–5. Total laparoscopic abdominal hysterectomy. (**A**) Laparoscopic photograph of large myomatous uterus. (**B**) Right ureter is isolated and unroofed. (**C**) Uterine vessels lying above ureter have been suture ligated. (**D**) Left uterine vessels are also ligated with 0-Vicryl on a CT-1 needle (Ethicon).

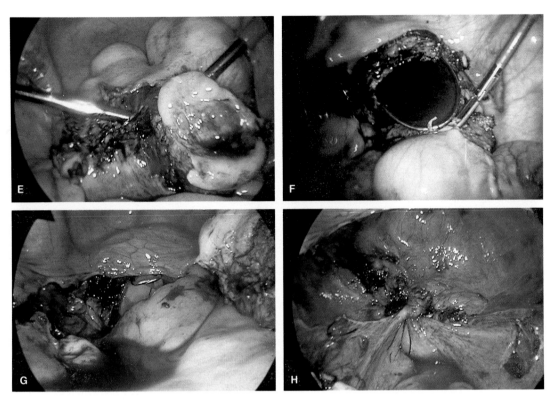

(**E**) The large fibrotic uterus lies free in the peritoneal cavity before vaginal morcellation. (**F**) View of vaginal cuff and cervix. Operating sigmoidoscope in the vagina occludes it, preventing loss of pneumoperitoneum. (**G**) Tenaculum introduced through the vagina is used to grasp the cervix and pull the uterus partially down into vagina, so that morcellation can proceed. (**H**) At the end of the procedure, both uterosacral ligaments have been brought together, with the vaginal apex to aid in support. Laterally, sutures are seen on the uterine vessels, with the ureter just medial and below the tie.

from posterior to anterior to delineate the right vaginal fornix, which is divided. The uterus may then be pulled out of the vagina.

Laparoscopic Vaginal Vault Closure and Suspension With McCall Culdoplasty

Vaginal repair is accomplished after packing the vagina. The left uterosacral ligament and posterolateral vagina are first elevated. A suture is placed through this uterosacral ligament and into the vagina; exits the vagina, including posterior vaginal tissue near the midline on the left; and re-enters just adjacent to this spot on the right. Finally, an opposite-sided oblique Cook needle holder is used to fixate the right posterolateral vagina to the right uterosacral ligament. This suture is tied extracorporeally and gives excellent support to the vaginal cuff apex, elevating it superiorly and backward toward the hollow of the sacrum. The rest of the vagina and overlying pubocervical fascia is closed vertically with a figure-eight suture.

Persistent Trophoblastic Tissue

Ambulatory treatment of tubal pregnancy is described in another chapter. Complications of tubal pregnancy management may also be treated on an ambulatory basis, including postoperative hemorrhage and persistent trophoblastic tissue. Declining quantitative levels of β-subunit human chorionic gonadotropin (β-hCG) are necessary to document successful conservative treatment of tubal pregnancy. Persistent titers imply further growth of the trophoblastic tissue, either within the tube or implanted on the peritoneum.

Persistent ectopic pregnancy implies the presence of viable trophoblastic tissue within the fallopian tube after salpingotomy or fimbrial expression. It should be suspected if serum levels of β-hCG are detectable 2 weeks postoperatively. Titers should be followed-up and a tentative diagnosis made if titers plateau or rise. A second laparoscopy should be performed to confirm diagnosis and institute treatment. At laparoscopy, a second salpingotomy procedure is usually effective. Alternatively, a salpingectomy may be performed using bipolar desiccation.

Persistent titers of hCG do not always imply that a conservative procedure for tubal pregnancy has failed. Trophoblastic implants capable of actively secreting hCG may occur outside the fallopian tube

or uterus, with no evidence of "persistent tubal pregnancy." Ectopic trophoblastic tissue implants on the pelvic side wall and cul-de-sac peritoneum are treated by excision with laparoscopic biopsy forceps and CO_2 laser vaporization of their bases. Laparoscopy has the advantage of documenting the location of the persistent trophoblastic tissue, treating it, confirming patency of the salpingotomized tube, and lysing early adhesions.[26]

Pelvic Abscess

The goals of managing acute tuboovarian abscess are prevention of infertility and the chronic sequelae of infection, including pelvic adhesions, hydrosalpinx, and pain—each of which may lead to further surgical intervention. The combination of laparoscopic treatment and effective intravenous antibiotics is a reasonable approach to the treatment of the total spectrum of PID, from acute salpingitis to ruptured tubo-ovarian abscess. Laparoscopic treatment is effective and economical. It offers the gynecologist 100% accuracy of diagnosis, including the extent of tuboovarian involvement, while simultaneously accomplishing definitive treatment with a low complication rate. This approach allows tubo-ovarian conservation, with subsequent fertility potential.[27,28]

A woman presenting with lower abdominal pain and a palpable or possible pelvic mass should undergo laparoscopy to determine the true diagnosis. The diagnosis of tubo-ovarian abscess should be suspected in a woman with a recent or prior history of PID who has persistent pain and pelvic tenderness on examination. Fever and leukocytosis may not be present. Ultrasound examination frequently documents a tubo-ovarian complex or abscess. The importance of laparoscopy cannot be overstated: even "obvious abscesses" may prove to be endometriomas, hemorrhagic corpus luteum cysts, or the result of a ruptured appendix. After presumptive diagnosis, hospitalization should be arranged, either on the day of diagnosis or the following morning, with laparoscopy soon thereafter.

Intravenous antibiotics are initiated on admission, usually a few hours before laparoscopy, to gain adequate blood levels to combat transperitoneal absorption during the procedure. Cefoxitin, 2 g intravenously every 4 hours, is frequently used from admission until discharge. Oral doxycycline 100 mg bid is started on the first postoperative day and continued for 10 days after hospital discharge on postoperative day 1 or 2. A single 1-g oral dose of azithromycin is given postoperatively, resulting in significant levels that are active against chlamydia infection persisting for a week or more in most tissues, including the endometrium and fallopian tubes.

The laparoscopic procedure uses either a blunt probe or an aquadissector to mobilize omentum, small bowel, rectosigmoid, and tubo-ovarian adhesions until the abscess cavity is entered. Purulent fluid is aspirated and inflammatory exudate excised with biopsy forceps. Afterward, aquadissection is performed by placing the tip of the aquadissector against the adhesive interface between bowel–adnexa, tube–ovary, or adnexa–pelvic sidewall to develop a dissection plane that can be extended either bluntly or with more fluid pressure. When the dissection is completed, the abscess cavity (necrotic inflammatory exudate) is excised in pieces, using a 5-mm biopsy forceps.

The importance of peritoneal lavage cannot be overemphasized. The peritoneal cavity is extensively irrigated with Ringer's lactate solution until the effluent is clear per underwater examination. The total volume of irrigant often exceeds 20 L. At the close of each procedure, at least 2 L of Ringer's lactate is left in the peritoneal cavity.

Acute Adnexal Torsion

Adnexal torsion is a rare cause of acute pelvic pain. Although torsion occurs most frequently if there is an adnexal lesion, healthy organs may twist.[29] The event may occur in the gravid or nongravid woman. Classically, management has been by laparotomy, with excision of the afflicted organ without untwisting the pedicle. The rationale for this approach is to avoid the risk of embolization from the occluded ovarian venous plexus.[30]

It has been suggested that ovarian preservation can be achieved if early diagnosis is made, before irreparable adnexal ischemia, and the pedicle is simply untwisted.[31,32] The torsed adnexa are untwisted, using a blunt probe or aquadissector and grasping forceps. After complete unraveling of the tube and ovary, often involving multiple turns, the affected adnexa is observed to assure viability of the involved structures, usually while additional surgical procedures are performed. No special precautions are taken in pregnant patients other than avoiding the placement of an intrauterine manipulator. Early recourse to laparoscopy permits accurate diagnosis and effective, safe ovarian conservation, while limiting hospital stay and hence cost.

FUTURE POSSIBILITIES

One of the most recent innovations in ambulatory surgery is in-office mini-laparoscopy. Mini-laparoscopy is defined as laparoscopy using instrumentation of 3 mm or less.

Medical Dynamics (Englewood, CO) has developed a small-diameter fiberscope imaging system (1.9 mm diameter) that can be introduced into the abdominal cavity through a special insufflation trocar (Adair/Veress Cannula). This cannula is a modification of the Veress needle; its metal trocar and "retractable" tip of the Veress needle can be removed, leaving a flexible plastic sheath capable of delivering CO_2 and introducing the imaging system.

This device is used for safe entry into the abdomen before the insertion of standard operative trocars in laparoscopic surgery. Not only can it be introduced in the same manner as the Veress needle but it can be manipulated through the abdominal wall under direct visual control. With the imaging system in place and after partial penetration of the abdominal wall, the device delivers small volumes of gas while being carefully advanced through the abdominal wall. When the peritoneal lining is reached, the determination is made whether there are opaque adherent structures inside the peritoneal cavity. The final penetration is made under visual control through translucent peritoneum. Insufflation is performed in the usual manner and the peritoneal cavity inspected (Edwin Adair, MD; personal communication).

Childers and coworkers used this optical catheter system for office laparoscopy and biopsy under local anesthesia to diagnose intraperitoneal breast, ovarian, and colon cancer as well as non-Hodgkin's lymphoma. In addition to its obvious economic advantages, this procedure allows the surgeon to obtain enough tissue for histologic evaluation and for special immunochemical studies. They have encountered no complications thus far and all patients have tolerated the procedure well.[33]

Dorsey and Tabb performed "mini-laparoscopy" on 15 patients under general anesthesia using 3-mm ancillary ports. They performed biopsies, lysis of adhesions, and used fiberoptic laser devices. There were no complications in their pilot series.[34]

Other applications for this procedure include emergency room use in conjunction with peritoneal lavage. With fluid in the abdomen, it is possible to perform routine inspection of the abdomen and to "run the bowel" with it floating on saline for a detailed inspection of the intestinal tract, which may include visualization of the inside of the lesser sac to view the pancreas and the spleen. Interventional radiologists have used this device to place trocars and guide wires into the common duct by a transhepatic insertion. The gallbladder has been entered under direct visual control for removal of gallstones in patients who were considered to be at high risk for conventional laparoscopic cholecystectomy. The device has also found use in the insertion of gastrostomy tubes in place of the more hazardous percutaneous endoscopic gastrostomy procedure (Adair, personal communication).

These experiences indicate that this is yet another horizon with widespread application for minimally invasive surgery. This optical catheter offers a simple, safe, effective, and economical means of evaluating and diagnosing intraperitoneal pathology. In addition, minor operative laparoscopic procedures can be performed under local anesthesia. Laparoscopists will soon incorporate this technique into gynecologic practice.

REFERENCES

1. Diamond MP, Daniell JF, Johns DA, et al: Postoperative adhesion development after operative laparoscopy: evaluation at early second-look procedures. Fertil Steril 55:700, 1991
2. Reich H, McGlynn F: Short self-retaining trocar sleeves. Am J Obstet Gynecol 162:453, 1990
3. Reich H: Aquadissection. In Baggish M (ed): Laser endoscopy, the clinical practice of gynecology series, vol 2, p 159. New York, Elsevier, 1990
4. Odell R: Principles of electrosurgery. In Sivak M (ed): Gastroenterologic endoscopy, p 128. New York, WB Saunders 1987
5. Reich H, Vancaillie TG, Soderstrom RM: In Martin DC, Holtz GL, Levinson CJ, Soderstrom RM (eds): Electrical techniques. Operative laparoscopy. Manual of endoscopy, p 105. Santa Fe Springs, American Association of Gynecologic Laparoscopists, 1990
6. Reich H, McGlynn F: Laparoscopic oophorectomy and salpingo-oophorectomy in the treatment of benign tuboovarian disease. J Reprod Med 31:609, 1986
7. Reich H: Laparoscopic oophorectomy and salpingo-oophorectomy in the treatment of benign tubo-ovarian disease. Int J Fertil 32:233, 1987
8. Reich H, MacGregor TS, Vancaillie TG: CO_2 laser used through the operating channel of laser laparoscopes: in vitro study of power and power density losses. Obstet Gynecol 77:40, 1991
9. Clarke HC: Laparoscopy—new instruments for suturing and ligation. Fertil Steril 23:274, 1972
10. Reich H, Clarke HC, Sekel L: A simple method for ligating in operative laparoscopy with straight and curved needles. Obstet Gynecol 79:143, 1992
11. Reich H: New techniques in advanced laparoscopic surgery. In Sutton C (ed): Bailliere's clinical

12. Reich H: Laparoscopic treatment of extensive pelvic adhesions including hydrosalpinx. J Reprod Med 32:736, 1987
13. Eddy CA, Asch RH, Balmaceda JP: Pelvic adhesions following microsurgical and macrosurgical wedge resection of the ovaries. Fertil Steril 56:1176, 1991
14. Reich H, McGlynn F: Treatment of ovarian endometriomas using laparoscopic surgical techniques. J Reprod Med 31:577, 1986
15. Reich H, McGlynn F, Sekel L, Taylor P; Laparoscopic management of ovarian dermoid cysts. J Reprod Med 37:640, 1992
16. Semm K, Mettler L: Technical progress in pelvic surgery via operative laparoscopy. Am J Obstet Gynecol 138:121, 1980
17. Reich H, McGlynn F, Salvat J: Laparoscopic treatment of cul-de-sac obliteration secondary to retrocervical deep fibrotic endometriosis. J Reprod Med 36:516, 1991
18. Metzgar DA, Olive DL, Haney AF: Limited hormonal responsiveness of ectopic endometrium: histologic correlation with intrauterine endometrium. Hum Pathol 19:1417, 1988
19. Cornillie FJ, Oosterlynck D, Lauweryns JM, et al: Deeply infiltrating pelvic endometriosis: histology and clinical significance. Fertil Steril 53:978, 1990
20. Berkeley AS, DeCherney AH, Polan ML: Abdominal myomectomy and subsequent fertility. Surg Gynecol Obstet 156:319, 1983
21. Collins JA, Wrixon W, Janes LB, Wilson EH: Treatment-independent pregnancy among infertile couples. N Engl J Med 309:1201, 1982
22. Schlaff WD, Zerhouni EA, Huth JA, Chen J, Damewood MD, Rock JA: A placebo-controlled trial of a depot gonadotropin-releasing hormone analogue (leuprolide) in the treatment of uterine leiomyomata. Obstet Gynecol 74:856, 1989
23. Freidman AJ, Hoffman DI, Comite F, Browneller RW, Miller JD: Treatment of leiomyomata uteri with leuprolide acetate depot: a double-blind, placebo-controlled, multicenter study. Obstet Gynecol 77:5, 1991
24. Kovac SR, Cruikshank SH, Retto HF: Laparoscopy-assisted vaginal hysterectomy. J Gynecol Surg 6:185, 1990
25. Reich H, DeCaprio J, McGlynn F: Laparoscopic hysterectomy. J Gynecol Surg 5:213, 1989
26. Reich H, DeCaprio J, McGlynn F, Wilkie W, Longo S: Peritoneal trophoblastic tissue implants after laparoscopic treatment of tubal ectopic pregnancy. Fertil Steril 52:337, 1989
27. Reich H, McGlynn F: Laparoscopic treatment of tuboovarian and pelvic abscess. J Reprod Med 32:747, 1987
28. Henry-Suchet J, Soler A, Loffredo V: Laparoscopic treatment of tuboovarian abscesses. J Reprod Med 29:579, 1984
29. Hibbard LT: Adnexal torsion. Am J Obstet Gynecol 152:456, 1985
30. Jeffcoate TNA: Torsion of the pelvic organs. In Principles of Gynecology. London, Butterworths, 1975
31. Mage G, Canis M, Mahnes H, et al: Laparoscopic

obstetrics and gynecology, vol 3, p 655. London, Harcourt Brace Janovich, 1989

management of adnexal torsion. J Reprod Med 34:52, 1982

32. Reich H, DeCaprio J, McGlynn F, Taylor PJ: Laparoscopic diagnosis and management of acute adnexal torsion. Gynaecological Endoscopy 2:37, 1992

33. Childers JM, Hatch KD, Surwitt EA: Office laparoscopy and biopsy for evaluation of patients with intraperitoneal carcinomatosis using a new optical catheter. Gynecol Oncol (in press).

34. Dorsey JH, Tabb CR: Mini-laparoscopy and fiberoptic lasers. Obstet Gynecol Clin North Am 18:613, 1991

Ambulatory Gynecology, Second Edition,
edited by David H. Nichols and Patrick J. Sweeney.
J. B. Lippincott Company, Philadelphia, © 1995.

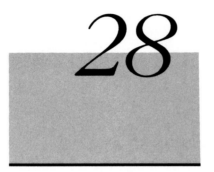

Ambulatory Hysterectomy

Thomas G. Stovall

In an era of health care reform, much has been written and said about cost containment in medicine and surgery. For most procedures performed in gynecologic practice, few cost-effectiveness data exist. During this same era, there has been an explosion in both hospital-based ambulatory surgery units and freestanding surgical centers across the nation. Another influence on gynecologic surgery has been the ever-increasing emphasis on minimally invasive surgery and an increased patient demand for outpatient surgery. The Association of American Hospitals estimates that the number of hospital-based outpatient surgical procedures has risen from 2.1 million in 1980 to 11.1 million in 1990, whereas the number of inpatient surgical procedures has fallen from 15.7 million to 10.9 million over the same period. This is also reflected in the percentage of hospital revenue that is generated from outpatient fees, compared with total hospital revenue. This number has increased from 13% to 22.6% during the 10-year period ending 1990. There is no question that costs associated with most medical procedures can be dramatically reduced by decreasing the need for hospitalization. In my esti-

mation, safety must precede cost considerations; thus, patient safety must be the prime concern when developing a program to perform hysterectomy on an outpatient basis.

A similar revolution has taken place in general surgery with cholecystectomy and in obstetrics with vaginal delivery. Furthermore, other surgical subspecialties (eg, orthopedics and plastic surgery) have increased their use of the outpatient surgical department. In the past, it was not uncommon to be hospitalized for 6 to 7 days after cholecystectomy. Studies demonstrate the feasibility of reducing the postoperative stay to 2 days with simple cholecystectomy and to only 1 day by using combined nasogastric drainage and enteral alimentation.[1-4] More recently, Saltzstein and coworkers report a series of 64 patients undergoing cholecystectomy, 44 (68.8%) of whom were discharged the day of the procedure.[5] In their experience, only one of 44 (2.3%) patients required readmission.

Over the last 2 decades, the length of hospital stay after vaginal hysterectomy has likewise been reduced. Moolgaoker and coworkers report that the average hospital stay after vaginal hysterectomy in their institution was 12.7 days before 1972.[6] During a period of 2 years, ending in 1974, the average postoperative stay was progressively reduced to 7.2 days.[6] During a similar period in the United States, the average stay after vaginal hysterectomy was 10.3 days.[7] Interestingly, the hospital stay after abdominal hysterectomy also averaged 10.3 days. Dicker and coworkers report a 2-year multicenter prospective observational study, which compared surgical morbidity in reproductive-aged women undergoing vaginal versus abdominal hysterectomy.[8] In this study, the overall rate of complications for abdominal hysterectomy was nearly twice as high as for vaginal hysterectomy (47% versus 25%). This report of a large multicenter experience is similar to that reported by other authors in smaller series from single institutions. The mean postoperative stay in this study was 5 days for vaginal hysterectomy and 7 days for abdominal hysterectomy. In review of data from our practice, the average postoperative stay after vaginal hysterectomy was 3 days, with about 30% of patients requesting discharge on the first postoperative day.[9] Although these studies are important to the individual patient, they also have implications in the public health arena. If more physicians would perform vaginal hysterectomy rather than abdominal hysterectomy, the reduction in morbidity and in length of hospital stay would result in substantial cost savings to the health care system as a whole. One must keep in mind that the patient populations in each of these studies are not necessarily comparable. Given this limitation, however, these studies clearly demonstrate that the average length of hospitalization after vaginal hysterectomy has decreased dramatically over the last 20 years.

During the planning phase before the initiation of the outpatient vaginal hysterectomy study, the available literature was reviewed. Moore reported a protocol used at the Ambulatory Surgery Center at Stringer Clinic, Tulsa, Oklahoma.[10] This freestanding surgical unit developed a protocol in which patients were discharged and accompanied by a private duty nurse, who stayed with the patient in her home for about 30 hours postoperatively. Patients in this center were instructed to remain at home for 2 weeks, to not drive for at least 3 weeks, and to not return to full-time work for 6 weeks after surgery. Reiner, in 1988, reported 66 patients from his private practice who were scheduled for vaginal hysterectomy, 58 of whom were considered eligible for early discharge.[11] Of these 50 enrolled patients, 41 (82%) were actually enrolled. Patients were transferred from the recovery room to the day-sur-

gery unit. Patients were offered the option of either discharge or transfer to the hospital's observation unit when the day-surgery area closed in the late afternoon. In this study, all 41 patients (100%) remained in the hospital, with all but one being discharged the next morning, or within 24 hours of hospital admission. Reiner routinely used postoperative Foley catheter drainage for several hours after surgery in addition to vaginal packing. In about 25% of patients, an anterior or posterior colporrhaphy (or both) was performed in conjunction with the hysterectomy. No postoperative complications were attributed to early discharge and no patient required blood transfusion or rehospitalization because of pain, bleeding, or infection.

Fayez and Dempsey report a series of 220 patients who had a laparotomy incision with either tubal reanastomosis, neosalpingoneostomy, or myomectomy and were subsequently discharged within 24 hours after the procedure.[12] No complications occurred in any of the patients and fewer than 1% of patients undergoing tuboplasty or reanastomosis complained of abdominal discomfort before discharge, whereas 4% had similar complaints in the myomectomy group. This study also supports the feasibility of decreasing hospital stay without compromising safety, even when an abdominal incision is required.

Lahti reported the hospital stay of 611 patients undergoing a variety of general surgical procedures.[13] He lists the following as being advantages of outpatient surgery: (1) customary foods and familiar surroundings for the patient, such as her own bed; (2) less exposure to foreign pathogenic bacteria; (3) fewer postoperative complications, such as gas pains, pneumonia, and thrombophlebitis; (4) shorter convalescence—patients return to normal activities sooner; (5) more efficient use of available hospital beds; (6) reduced cost per patient hospitalization; and (7) less strain on the surgeon—"rounds" take less time.

PATIENT ELIGIBILITY

Stovall and coworkers began a clinical trial in January 1991, in which selected patients requiring vaginal hysterectomy were offered the option of early discharge.[14] The protocol has been modified somewhat during the last 2 years to be less restrictive. The initial study group consisted of 35 patients who were considered to be candidates for outpatient vaginal hysterectomy. Patients who meet the inclusion criteria outlined in Table 28-1 are offered out-

Table 28–1

Table 28–1

Inclusion and Exclusion Criteria for Selecting Patients for Outpatient Vaginal Hysterectomy

- No medical condition requiring special postoperative care; examples include uncontrolled diabetes mellitus, class III or IV heart disease
- Have a condition that limits ambulation (eg, severe arthritis)
- Working telephone in the home
- Support person with patient for the first postoperative night
- Do not require anterior or posterior colporrhaphy

patient surgery. These inclusion and exclusion criteria have been modified over the last several months to allow patients who have had a previous conization to be included, and to allow for any additional postoperative intravenous antibiotics to be administered in the home. In addition to the preoperative inclusion and exclusion criteria, patients must also meet several postoperative criteria (Table 28-2).

PREOPERATIVE EDUCATION

Counseling during the preoperative visit is one of the most important means of ensuring patient acceptance and compliance during the immediate postoperative period. At the time of the preoperative visit and when scheduling the hysterectomy, we discuss the early discharge procedure. While emphasizing the benefits of early discharge, we also include an explanation of our experience and of the potential surgical complications. We explain to pa-

Table 28–2

Postoperative Criteria for Selecting Patients for Outpatient Vaginal Hysterectomy

- Does not sustain an intraoperative complication requiring hospital admission (gastrointestinal or urinary tract injury)
- Less than 3 vol% change in two hematocrits separated by at least 3–4 hours, with the first being at least 1 hour postoperation
- Understands the postoperative instructions
- Tolerates clear liquids
- Ambulates with assistance
- Temperature ≤100.4°F

tients that they will experience discomfort after surgery and that they initially may not believe that they are ready for discharge. Based on our past experience, however, we have found that once patients arrive home and are in familiar surroundings, they are glad that they chose early discharge. Patients are conditioned to being discharged as an outpatient. They are provided with positive statements, both preoperatively and postoperatively, such as "You will be discharged as soon after surgery as possible and although you might not feel 100% at that time, you will feel better when you get home in familiar surroundings." Patients are also reassured that they will not be discharged unless their vital signs and hematocrits are stable postoperatively and that we feel they will continue to do well at home. The procedure for an in-home nursing visit is also explained; the results of questionnaires provided to patients show that they find this both reassuring and comforting.

The nurse also explains that surgery and anesthesia will leave the patient feeling tired and not hungry. They are taught that anesthesia may leave them feeling as though they are not thinking clearly. Thus, patients are cautioned not to make any critical decisions for 48 hours after surgery. Postoperative instructions are also explained to the patient's support person during this preoperative visit, so that the postoperative instruction period is kept to a minimum.

SURGICAL PROCEDURE

Vaginal hysterectomy procedures are scheduled as early in the workday as possible. Although it is not always possible to have the patient scheduled as the first case of the morning, if possible, it is best to do this, so that the recovery time before discharge can be maximized. All patients are given a single dose of preoperative antibiotics, either 2 g of cefazolin (Ancef, Kefzol), intravenously, or 200 mg of intravenous doxycycline (Vibramycin) if the patient is allergic to penicillins or cephalosporins. The choice of either regional or general anesthesia is left to the discretion of the anesthesiologist after discussion with the patient; however, most patients choose general anesthesia. The vaginal hysterectomy is completed, using a standard Haney technique. When appropriate, uterine morcellation and oophorectomy are performed and do not affect the patient's ability to be discharged. The bladder is drained with an in-and-out straight catheter and the surgical procedure is performed. Synthetic absorbable sutures are used for all pedicles and for vaginal cuff closure. No vaginal packing or postoperative bladder drainage is used because this increases patient discomfort and is unnecessary.[12]

POSTOPERATIVE CARE

On completion of the hysterectomy, the patient is transferred to the recovery room, where she receives traditional postoperative care. About 25% of patients require a single dose of intramuscular narcotics during their 1.5 to 2 hour stay in the recovery room. A standardized set of postoperative orders are used (Table 28-3) to ensure that all patients receive similar management. Intravenous access is continued post-operatively at a rate of 50 mL/hour until the patient is discharged. This rate is used to ensure that there is minimal hemodilutional effect of the intravenous fluids on the patient's hematocrit.

Table 28–3

Postoperative Orders for Outpatient
Vaginal Hysterectomy

---

1. Admission to recovery room; transfer to outpatient recovery when approved by anesthesia staff
2. Diagnosis: S/P vaginal hysterectomy
3. Allergies: _____ (List) _____
4. IV D5LR at KVO
5. Clear liquid diet when fully awake
6. Ambulate when fully awake
7. Stat HCT on discharge from recovery room; call MD if HCT <30.0 vol%
8. Stat CBC with differential 3 hours after first HCT. Call MD as soon as results are available
9. Call MD if patient unable to void and/or for vaginal bleeding
10. Roxicet (Percocet), one or two tablets every 3–4 hours as needed for pain
11. Promethazine (Phenergan) suppository, 25 mg, one per rectum every 4 hours PRN nausea
12. Vital signs: pulse and BP every 1 hour times three, then every two hours until discharge; call MD for pulse >100/min and/or BP: systolic <90, diastolic <60
13. Temperature every 2 hours until discharge; call MD for oral temperature ≥101°F
14. Discharge instruction sheet and postoperative care kit to patient at discharge
15. Do not discharge until final evaluation is completed by Dr. _____ .

After this initial recovery period, patients are transferred from the recovery room to the ambulatory surgery unit. It appears that there are fewer barriers to discharge if the patients are cared for in an ambulatory surgery area. The environment in this area encourages patients to be mobile, and the nursing personnel are familiar with the care of this patient population. Patients are encouraged to begin a clear liquid diet and ambulate with assistance to the toilet. Only rarely are intramuscular narcotics or antiemetics required once the patient leaves the recovery room.

Hematocrits are obtained 4 hours apart, with the first hematocrit drawn about 11 AM, or 1.5 to 2 hours after the hysterectomy is completed. The second hematocrit is drawn about 3 PM, with a minimum of 2 hours between these two hematocrits. This timeframe enables the patient to be discharged by about 5 PM. The second hematocrit must be no less than 3 vol% below the first postoperative hematocrit to allow the patient to be discharged. This restriction was instituted as the protocol was designed and has served as an excellent measure of postoperative blood loss. That is, no patient has been readmitted because of a decreasing hematocrit on the first postoperative day. There are no restrictions, however, to the degree of blood loss or change between the preoperative and postoperative hematocrits.

Discharge Instructions

Patients are discharged only after postoperative hematocrits have been obtained and are stable and the patient has ambulated and is able to tolerate clear liquids. Discharge medications include (1) promethazine (Phenergan) suppository, 25 mg every 4 hours as needed for nausea (eight); (2) oxycodone–acetaminophen (Percocet) tablet, one or two every 4 hours as needed for pain; (3) docusate sodium (Colace), 100-mg tablet twice daily for 2 weeks, and (4) iron sulfate, 325 mg, one tablet twice daily for 1 month if the discharge hematocrit is lower than 35%. If the patient has undergone oophorectomy, estrogen replacement begins on the first postoperative day.

In evaluating early discharge, patients are asked to complete a questionnaire that seeks to evaluate their experience with outpatient hysterectomy. One of the most positive aspects from the patient's perspective is that the operating surgeon contacts the patient on the evening of surgery and early on the first postoperative day. This call serves two purposes: (1) to make certain the patient is clinically stable and has no major problems managing pain or nausea, and (2) to reassure the patient the physician is available and easily accessible if needed.

Before discharge, a commercially licensed home health care–agency visit is arranged for the morning of the first postoperative day. The nurse is asked to clinically evaluate the patient and to obtain a complete blood count to ensure that the patient's hematocrit is stable. These results are usually available by noon.

All patients and their support personnel are given a printed instruction sheet (Table 28-4). Although these instructions have been previously explained to the patient, the instruction sheet reinforces the postoperative instructions. The support personnel are instructed to record the patient's temperature and any problems experienced during the first 24 hours. In addition, patients are provided with a discharge kit, which contains supplies and items to ensure an easier transition from hospital to home (Table 28-5).

In a referral medical center, patients often travel more than an hour to obtain care. Although some

---

Table 28–4
Patient Discharge Instructions After Outpatient Hysterectomy

- Record your temperature every 4 hours for 2 days.
- If your temperature is greater than 100°F, notify your surgeon
- Drink at least six glasses of liquid during the first 24 hours after surgery
- Begin a regular diet after 24 hours
- Have a support person to assist and stay with you for the first 24 hours after surgery
- Refrain from heavy lifting or strenuous exercise for 1 week
- Do not drive for at least 48 hours and until you can turn quickly
- No douching or vaginal intercourse for 4 weeks
- Notify your surgeon if you develop vaginal bleeding heavier than a menstrual period, persistent nausea, vomiting, or pain not relieved by your pain medication
- You may contact your surgeon at: (Insert phone number).
- A nurse will visit you at your home in the morning about 9 AM
- You may return to work as soon as you are capable, usually 1 to 2 weeks.
- An appointment for an office visit is scheduled for you on (insert date) at (insert time).

Table 28–5
Contents of Discharge Kit

Card with emergency phone numbers
Discharge medications
  Colace
  Phenergan suppositories
  Percocet tablets
  Iron sulfate, if indicated
Discharge instruction sheet
Disposable bed sheet protectors
Emesis basin
Facial tissues
Oral thermometer
Pen
Perineal wash bottle
Sanitary napkins × 12
Support person's observation record
Washcloth

---

patients elect to return home after surgery, several patients have elected to stay in a nearby hotel overnight. Although this may seem strange at first, it still results in lower cost and allows patients to be in a home-like environment. If patients stay in a hotel, either the nursing visit is made there or the patient may be seen in the physician's office. An office visit is arranged for either 1 or 2 weeks after surgery. Patients are encouraged to return to normal activities as soon as practical and at the same time, they are encouraged to return to work. There are no data to support the previously held tradition that patients should wait 6 weeks before returning to work.

COST

The cost savings of this program depends on several variables, including the physician's traditional average stay after vaginal hysterectomy, the hospital room charges, the home nursing–care cost, and the charge structure of the hospital. Some hospitals actually charge more if the procedure is completed on an outpatient basis than if the same procedure is performed and the patient is hospitalized for more than 24 hours. In most institutions, however, there is a considerable cost savings when early discharge programs are used.

BARRIERS TO IMPLEMENTATION

Having been involved in instituting a program of outpatient vaginal hysterectomy in two medical centers, it is clear that change does not come easily. At both institutions, there was resistance to change among house staff, nursing, anesthesia, and administration personnel. Physicians and nurses did not automatically embrace the idea of outpatient hysterectomy and were concerned (as I was) about the possibility of postoperative hemorrhage, pain control, and medical–legal issues. As experience grew, so did confidence levels, with a concurrent decline in skepticism. This was especially true when those that were resistant to the idea began to realize that it was not too long ago that patients remained hospitalized for prolonged periods after vaginal delivery and hysterectomy. Resistance was also broken down when these persons began to realize that we actually do little for patients while they are hospitalized after vaginal hysterectomy. It is imperative that those responsible for instituting an early discharge program provide as much education as possible to all ancillary personnel so that their cooperation and help is obtained.

CLINICAL RESULTS

The initial experience with outpatient vaginal hysterectomy was reported in 1992. In this prospective study, 35 patients were enrolled and underwent vaginal hysterectomy. The study group was composed of both private insurance and public sector patients, with a mean age of 42.7 ± 7.6 years. The major indication for surgery was leiomyomata. The average anesthesia time was 109.8 ± 32.6 minutes, with 84% of patients having general anesthesia. The mean surgical time was 68.1 ± 32.7 minutes, with patients spending an average of 95.2 ± 34.7 minutes in the recovery room. Patients in this study spent an average of 9.4 ± 0.81 (7.8 to 10.6) total hours in the hospital time. The addition of oophorectomy or uterine morcellation did not exclude patients from participating in this pilot study or from being discharged on an outpatient basis.

No patients were readmitted to the hospital because of pain or nausea and the mean number of oral pain medication taken was about 20 tablets, whereas the mean number of antiemetic suppositories used was only five. Two patients required readmission: the first for a spinal headache and the second for a postoperative infection.

A questionnaire was given to all patients at their 1-week postoperative visit. This questionnaire sought to gain information regarding the patient's satisfaction with all aspects of her surgical experience, from her initial preoperative visit until her 1-week postoperative visit. Most patients completing this study found outpatient vaginal hysterectomy an acceptable method of having surgery. Patients gave favorable responses to the physician's call on the evening of surgery and subsequent follow-up calls as well as the home nursing visits. Only two patients—those who were readmitted—were dissatisfied regarding their discharge on the day of surgery.

Given these generally favorable results, the clinical trial was expanded to 133 patients and included patients undergoing vaginal and laparoscope-assisted vaginal hysterectomy.[15] In this trial, 12 of 133 (9%) were not discharged from the hospital on the day of surgery and five (3.8%) were readmitted. All but one of these patients was readmitted secondary to a postoperative infection. Surgical indications, the type of hysterectomy, and the requirement for postoperative pain medication were not associated with those patients who were or were not discharged as outpatients. Intraoperative transfusion and postoperative antiemetic requirements were statistically associated with the need for postoperative hospitalization. In addition, anemia and elevated temperature on the first and second postoperative day were factors associated with hospital readmission.

From this experience, it appears that outpatient–ambulatory vaginal or laparoscope-assisted vaginal hysterectomy can be safely accomplished on an outpatient basis, with appropriate safeguards. It also appears to be associated with acceptably low (30% to 40%) hospital readmission and decreased postoperative infection rates. More importantly, outpatient hysterectomy is well accepted by most patients.

SUMMARY

Although not applicable in all clinical situations, early discharge after vaginal hysterectomy or laparoscope-assisted vaginal hysterectomy is safe and well accepted by patients. When compared with an inpatient procedure, there appears to be decreased febrile morbidity, less postoperative pain and nausea, and decreased postoperative infection rate. This decrease in postoperative morbidity in addition to a shorter hospital stay results in substantial cost savings.

REFERENCES

1. Hall RC: Short surgical stay: two hospital days for cholecystectomy. Am J Surg 154:510, 1987
2. Merrill JR: Minimal trauma cholecystectomy (a "no-touch" procedure in a "well"). Am J Surg 54:256, 1988
3. Moss G: "Mini-trauma" cholecystectomy. J Abdom Surg 25:66, 1983
4. Saltzstein EC, Mercer LC, Peacock JB, Dougherty SH: Twenty-four hour hospitalization after cholecystectomy. Surg Gynecol Obstet 174:173, 1992
5. Saltzstein EC, Mercer LC, Peacock JB, Dougherty SH: Outpatient open cholecystectomy. Surg Gynecol Obstet 174:173, 1992
6. Moolgaoker AS, Rizvi JH, Payne PR: Reducing the hospital stay following vaginal hysterectomy. Obstet Gynecol 49:570, 1977
7. Ledger WJ, Child MA: The hospital care of patients undergoing hysterectomy: an analysis of 12,026 patients from the Professional Activity Study. Am J Obstet Gynecol 117:423, 1973
8. Dicker RC, Greenspan JR, Strauss LT, et al: Complications of abdominal and vaginal hysterectomy among women of reproductive age in the United States: the Collaborative Review of Sterilization. Am J Obstet Gynecol 144:841, 1982
9. Stovall TG, Ling FW, Henry LC, Woodruff MR: A randomized trial evaluating leuprolide acetate prior to hysterectomy as treatment for leiomyomas. Am J Obstet Gynecol 164:1420, 1991
10. Moore J: Vaginal hysterectomy: its success as an outpatient procedure. AORN J 48:1114, 1988
11. Reiner IJ: Early discharge after vaginal hysterectomy. Obstet Gynecol 71:416, 1988
12. Fayez JA, Dempsey RA: Short hospital stay for gynecologic reconstructive surgery via laparotomy. Obstet Gynecol 81:598, 1993
13. Lahti P: Early postoperative discharge of patients from the hospital. J Surg 63:410, 1968
14. Stovall TG, Summitt RL, Bran DF, Ling FW: Outpatient vaginal hysterectomy: a pilot study. Obstet Gynecol 80:145, 1992
15. Summitt RL Jr, Stovall TG, Lipscomb GH, Washburn SA, Ling FW: Outpatient hysterectomy: determinants of discharge and hospitalization in 133 patients. Am J Obstet Gynecol (In Press)

Ambulatory Gynecology, Second Edition,
edited by David H. Nichols and Patrick J. Sweeney.
J. B. Lippincott Company, Philadelphia, © 1995.

Breast Disease

George W. Mitchell, Jr.

Gynecologists routinely examine their patients' breasts at the time of the patients' first visit and at periodic intervals thereafter. The physician has the responsibility of advising patients about breast symptoms and any asymptomatic abnormalities that are discovered during an examination. Advice should include recommendations for or against diagnostic aids, medical treatment, and surgery, especially for a breast cyst or a solid tumor aspiration and breast biopsy. The failure of gynecologists to accept this responsibility has resulted in a substantial number of malpractice suits.

EXAMINATION

The examination of the breast is done with the patient both seated and supine, her arms up and down in each of these positions. The clinician should carefully inspect the skin, noting such common minor pathologies as striae, intertrigo, nevi, angiomata, furuncles, keratoses and warts; these are important, because the patient may equate them with malignancy. More serious signs, such as nipple or skin retraction, localized vascularity, melanoma, and Paget's disease of the nipple, should be charted on an appropriate diagram.

Breast inspection is important also for assessment of physical characteristics that may be of cosmetic concern to the patient. Breast size depends on the presence of steroid receptors and hormonal stimulation, as well as on age and amount of adipose tissue. Estrogen administered either topically or orally has a limited and temporary growth effect. Mechanical stimulation of the breast and muscular and postural exercises are not of great value. Augmentation mammoplasty, the insertion of prostheses containing silicone gel, is now proscribed for general use by the Food and Drug Administration (FDA) because of a paucity of data concerning possible serious complications from rupture of the capsule or long-term use. Prostheses containing saline have not been restricted but are now under critical scrutiny, making their use inadvisable except for the purpose of reconstruction after mastectomy, and then only under controlled conditions.

The ban on these devices is unfortunate for women with little or no breast tissue or with marked asymmetry. Various plastic procedures utilizing the transplantation of muscle, and even fatty tissue, are available for breast reconstruction, but major surgical intervention of this type for simple augmentation should be considered only in extreme cases. Complications of these plastic procedures include hemorrhage, infection and accumulation of excessive scar tissue.

Women of all ages with grossly hyperplastic breasts may benefit from reduction operations. Such breasts are often pendulous as well as heavy, and any attempt to correct the sagging with a supporting garment may place a severe strain on the neck, shoulders, and upper back, producing chronic discomfort. In cases of marked asymmetry in breast size, reduction of the larger breast may be necessary to make the two reasonably equal.

Reduction mammoplasty can now be accomplished by placing incisions around the areola, or in a submammary position, so that the future scar will be visible only on close inspection. The excision of redundant skin and breast tissue may necessitate the relocation of the nipple and areola, excision of the nipple or areola and replacement by a graft from the other nipple, or a tatoo. The result is usually satisfactory in terms of contour, and the patient is psychologically uplifted and physically relieved of strain. There is, however, a common side effect of sensation loss as well as loss of function.

Palpation of each breast proceeds either clockwise or counterclockwise around the breast perimeter. One technique is to press the breast tissue gently against the chest wall with the flats of the first and second fingers, making gradually smaller circles until the area beneath the areola is reached. Other techniques include using the tips of the fingers, gently stripping the breast tissue in parallel lines with the flats of all the fingers from the axilla to the sternum until the entire breast is encompassed. In order to rule out the possibility of disease close to the chest wall, the examiner horizontally compresses the superior and inferior skin attachments of the breast to the chest together, pulling the breast tissue outward and moving from the axilla to the sternum. It is important to examine with particular care any area to which the patient calls attention.

There is some debate among experts regarding the advisability of "milking" the nipple to ascertain the presence of a discharge. Milking is recommended only when there is a history of discharge; the examiner may thus confirm its presence, note its general characteristics, and obtain a specimen on a frosted or albumin-coated slide for cytologic evaluation. Such cytologic specimens, however, only rarely offer valuable information. Occasionally it is possible to determine the quadrant from which a sanguineous discharge exudes; this may be helpful later if it is necessary to explore the ductal system surgically.

All palpable lumps or masses should be diagrammed, with a description of their estimated size, consistency, mobility, and attachments to the skin, nipple, or chest wall. Dense, "lumpy" breasts should be characterized and the time between the date of examination and the date of the patient's last menstrual period noted because of expected premenstrual engorgement. Women whose periods are overdue often have the discomfort of excessive breast swelling as a result of either pregnancy or prolonged hyperestrinism, as do women receiving continuous estrogen replacement therapy.

The lobular thickening and ductal proliferation that occurs cyclically in the breasts of women of reproductive age, and sometimes in older women, is nearly universal but varies in degree among individuals. In general, it tends to be concentrated in the upper outer quadrant and axillary "tail" of the breast. The firm nodularity, coalescence, and ill-defined borders of these areas may be confusing to the examiner and to the patient who examines herself. Comparison with previous records, reexamination at a different time in the cycle, and experience are helpful in arriving at a conclusion concerning management, but mistakes are made nevertheless. Whenever there is reasonable doubt, a specimen must be obtained either by needle aspiration or biopsy. Of great importance is the presence of a so-called dominant mass, or well-circumscribed projection, in such an area, especially if it is a new finding in a regular patient. All such masses should be biopsied, regardless of size.

The lobular thickening and ductal proliferation described above has been referred to in the literature by many different names, such as chronic cystic mastitis and fibrocystic disease. The microscopic form of this "disease" is present in nearly all women in varying degrees of cellular activity, upon which depends the possibility of the future development of cancer. These cellular characteristics and their estimated risk factors are listed in Table 29-1. Since the different forms of this process are so common and the majority do not predispose to cancer, it seems desirable to refer to it as fibrocystic change, thus freeing the term from undesirable connotations to the patient. The grossly cystic form of this change (the development of a mass greater than 5 mm in diameter) occurs in approximately 20% of

Table 29–1

Histologic Indicators and Degree of Breast Cancer Risk

No Increased Risk

Adenosis
Apocrine metaplasia
Cysts, macro or micro
Hyperplasia, mild
Duct ectasia
Mastitis
Squamous metaplasia

Slightly Increased Risk (1.5 to 2 times)

Hyperplasia, moderate or florid
Sclerosing adenosis, florid
Fibroadenoma

Moderately Increased Risk (4 to 5 times)

Hyperplasia, atypical, ductal or lobular

(Adapted from Page DL, Dupont WD: Histologic indicators of breast cancer risk. Am Col of Sur 76:16, 1991)

women. Such a mass is usually dominant and must be further investigated by aspiration.

While the patient is seated, the lymphatic tissue in the anterior cervical and supra- and infraclavicular areas is palpated, and prominent nodes are charted. The left axilla is best palpated with the examiner's right hand and vice versa, with the patient's arm drawn in each instance across the front of the chest to relax the pectoralis major muscle. This procedure can be done with the patient either seated or supine. The examiner's fingers explore the pocket under the pectoralis major insertion, the high midaxilla, and the border of the latissimus dorsi. The size, number, and position of palpable lymph nodes are charted.

Throughout the examination, the patient should be reassured as much as possible by the attitude, voice, and expression of the examiner. In order to avoid creating unnecessary anxiety, the clinician should mention any findings realistically and calmly without waiting until the postexamination interview.

It is customary to teach previously uninformed patients how to perform breast self-examination. Although there is still some debate about the value of this procedure, the consensus is that it is helpful in detecting lumps before they reach a large size. In many offices the patient is taught by paramedical personnel with the aid of audiovisual equipment.

The entire examination should take not less than three minutes. It sometimes takes longer, depending on the size of the breasts and the presence of specific pathology. Patients frequently compare the examination they receive with what they have seen or read in film clips and magazines, and are likely to remember errors of omission.

NIPPLE DISCHARGE

The causes of nipple discharge are listed in Table 29-2. It is difficult to estimate from the character of the discharge the nature of the basic underlying pathology. Like blemishes, lumps and malformations, nipple discharge causes anxiety and most women seek an explanation. Lactation may persist for many months after nursing has stopped, especially if the breasts have been stimulated by jogging or sucking. However, galactorrhea which simulates lactation may also occur as the result of pituitary adenoma or the over-production of prolactin as well as by operations, including those around the chest area. When a milky discharge is seemingly unrelated to a recent pregnancy, blood should be drawn and assayed for serum prolactin. If elevated levels are found, the sella turcica should be investigated radiologically. Cytologic evaluation of galactorrhea is seldom productive.

A bloody or brownish discharge may be due to a variety of causes, the most common of which is intraductal papilloma, which may contain atypical or even frankly malignant cells. Some cancers pen-

Table 29–2

Causes of Nipple Discharge

Galactorrhea	Local Pathology
Pregnancy and childbirth	Cancer
Neonatal ("witchs'" milk)	Intraductal papilloma
Breast manipulation	Ductal extasia
Surgery	Gross cystic change
Stress	Infection
Sellar tumors	
Hypothyroidism	
Chronic renal disease	
Drugs*	

*Oral contraceptives, phenothiazines, tricyclic antidepressants, Rauwolfia alkaloids, methyldopa

etrating the ductal system give rise to a unilateral bloody discharge. When a discharge of this type is present, a mammography should be done and, regardless of whether the results are negative, the ductal system should be explored surgically. The preliminaries and incision are similar to those of an ordinary biopsy (see below), but the dissection is carried beneath the nipple until the main duct is identified, and this duct is traced downward until the offending lesion is reached, usually not more than 3 to 4 cm from the nipple. A block resection of the soft, friable papilloma is then done and the defect closed.

A yellowish, sticky discharge is often associated with either ductal ectasia or galactocele, both benign conditions requiring no treatment. Such a discharge, which occurs in elderly women, may be sporadic and temporary. Cytologic evaluation of the fluid is unlikely to provide useful information. Aspiration may be indicated, especially if the process is unilateral. Reassurance of the patient is important.

Any type of injury to the body, particularly to the chest, may produce a discharge, presumably from reflex stimulation of the phrenic nerve. The chafing of a poorly fitting bra or frequent bobbing of the breast as a result of athletic activity may produce the same phenomenon. In the same category are discharges produced by a variety of drugs that affect the central nervous system. The patient should always be asked about any medication she is taking.

DIAGNOSTIC AIDS

The gynecologist is responsible not only for performing an adequate breast examination but also for prescribing the necessary diagnostic aids. There is disagreement among various government agencies and professional societies, and the rules seem to change from one year to the next, making it difficult to decide what plan a conservative physician should adopt. The recommendations listed in Table 29-3 closely follow the American Cancer Society guidelines. Reports have recently appeared in the media to the effect that excessive mammographies may induce breast cancer. These reports are based on questionable clinical data. High-quality mammographies are done in hospitals and centers that use only equipment dedicated to this single purpose and are interpreted by subspecialists trained in mammography. The modern film-screen mammogram delivers only 0.5 cGy (rads) for the usual two

Table 29–3
Guidelines for Mammography

1. Baseline mammograms for all women at age 35 to 40 years.
2. Mammography at one to two year intervals from age 40 to 49.
3. Annual mammograms for women 50 years of age or older.

views. There are no human or animal data to indicate that breast cancer is induced by radiation at less than 5 cGy per year. The theoretical risk of breast cancer due to mammography has been estimated by the National Institutes of Health to be 3.5 excess cancers per million women per year per cGy. It is true, of course, that larger doses may be more dangerous, and such doses may be inflicted by technologists and equipment that have not been regularly tested and certified. The risk that exposure to x-rays will induce breast cancer has been calculated to be far less than the risk that minimal breast cancer will go undetected by physical examination.

Statistics indicate that a combination of mammography and physical examination is superior to either one alone but that mammography can detect lesions less than 1 cm in size that are not palpable. A positive mammogram is often based on the number and configuration of tiny calcifications in a cluster. This may be a sign of a very early cancer and must always be investigated by biopsy, regardless of whether a mass is palpable. Similarly, a palpable lesion is always an indication for histologic evaluation regardless of whether the mammogram is positive or not. Mammography has been refined to the point at which the incidence of false-negatives should be no higher than 10% in the hands of a specialist. Larger cancers may be missed by mammography, especially in breasts that are very dense as a result of fibrocystic change. The diagnosis is much easier in the fatty breasts of older women.

The interpretation of mammograms has been broadened to include not only minimal breast cancer but also so-called precancerous or dysplastic breast markings as well. The term dysplasia has been largely discarded since it has a different connotation to gynecologists, who relate the term to histology.

The interpretation of shadows on the mammographic film that vary in density and configuration from the normal, but do not conform to the standard criteria for malignancy, continues to be a subject for discussion and clinical research. The mammographic report may or may not emphasize the ominous aspect of these changes, and it is important for the clinician to develop a rapport with the mammographer so that a mutual understanding can be reached regarding the best future management of the patient.

The mammographic report should be straight forward, containing a description of the findings, a diagnosis with regard to those findings, and, usually, a disclaimer. The diagnosis must be in one of three categories: normal; dense normal (equivocal); and definitely abnormal (must biopsy). The disclaimer, if present, states in general terms the statistical accuracy of the method and tells the referring physician to use his or her own judgment in its clinical application. A follow-up date for a repeat examination may also be given, and this may occasionally be for time intervals of less than one year, based upon the mammographers' degree of concern. Recommended intervals of less than six months should be questioned, since architectural changes in the film within a brief period of time are unlikely. Unsatisfactory films must, of course, be repeated.

Techniques for the diagnosis of breast disease other than the standard two-view film-screen mammogram have been tested and applied, but to date none is as uniformly accurate at a reasonable cost. A form of mammography called xeroradiography was popular until ten years ago, but has now been discarded because of its relatively inferior imaging and the larger amount of radiation delivered. Computed tomography (CT) and magnetic resonance imaging (MRI) have been tested, and trials of the latter continue, but both would be prohibitively expensive as screening techniques, and there are few indications for their use in diagnosis.

Thermography involves the use of heat sensors to detect increased temperatures within the breast, which might indicate the presence of pathology, and it has been advertised as a desirable substitute for mammography because no radiation is involved. Variations of this method, all based on the same principle, have proliferated in so-called "breast health clinics" and in private offices. The diagnosis of non-palpable "minimal" breast cancer by these techniques has not been reliable, and the incidence of false-positive diagnoses has been too high. A positive thermogram should not lead to a surgical procedure until a mammogram has been done.

An unproved method of breast screening known as diaphanography updates the traditional transillumination of breast masses, using a fiberoptic light source and synchronized mapping of the breast to delineate areas through which the light does not pass. The potential of this tool is being studied prospectively, but the results to date have not been encouraging. It seems probable that most significant lesions will be palpable by the time they become evident through diaphanography.

Ultrasonography has become a useful adjunct to film-screen mammography, especially in the differentiation of cystic from solid masses, and it is not invasive. Its ability to detect "minimal" lesions is questionable, however, and it should not be used alone as a screening technique. Routine use would be unnecessarily expensive, and it should be confined to special indications in diagnosis.

Retrograde injection of contrast material into the ductal system has been used for many years to diagnose intraductal lesions, most of which are within 3 cm or 4 cm of the nipple and, therefore, in one of the larger branches. This technique is often uncomfortable for the patient; access to the ductal system is not always easy to obtain, and x-rays are difficult to interpret. Although duct injection still has its adherents and continues to be used in other countries, it has largely been replaced by mammography in the United States.

MEDICAL MANAGEMENT

Ductal and lobular proliferation, including epithelial hyperplasia, occur in response to stimulation by estrogen and progesterone. Since regular cyclic variations in the levels of these hormones occur in the normal menstrual cycle, it is not surprising that breast swelling and discomfort may occur near the end of the cycle in response to these changes. The symptoms may be minimal, or, in a minority of the female population, severe enough to require medical intervention. Higher serum levels of estrogen and progesterone have not been detected in those severely affected, but elevated levels of prolactin have been noted in some studies. In another small group of women, severe breast pain may be unremitting, casting some doubt on the cyclic hormonal etiology. Often the pain is associated with lumpiness, causing anxiety about the possibility of malignancy. Such symptoms are almost unknown in the postmenopausal age group.

For patients complaining of severe breast pain, the importance of a thorough examination can not be overemphasized, since in a significant number the pain is related to the chest wall rather than to the breast, especially in the costochondral junctions along either margin of the sternum. Injury to these areas as a result of a fall or a tight embrace is common, and tenderness to manual pressure over these areas confirms the diagnosis (Tietze's syndrome). Other causes of pain, such as inflammation and cancer must, of course, be ruled out. The absence of serious pathology necessitates strong and continuing reassurance of the patient.

The majority of women control their discomfort with analgesics, appropriate changes in supporting garments, and a grin-and-bear-it attitude. The minority are subjected to different hormonal regimens, which may have undesirable secondary effects even if effective. Those most commonly used are oral contraceptives and progestational agents in the second half or throughout the cycle. The benefits are variable but they may be worth a try. Drugs designed to lower estrogen, progesterone and prolactin production (Table 29-4) have been shown to improve symptoms for the duration of their use, but relapse is likely after discontinuance, and the undesirable side effects of the drugs are well known. Evening Primrose Oil has been shown to be helpful in some English studies, but has not been given a trial in this country. Mastectomy has been considered for non-cyclic pain in older women, but should not be implemented under any circumstances. The strong psychic component for pain of all kinds must be borne in mind.

Two other methods widely known to the public for the relief of fibrocystic changes are the administration of vitamin E and the withdrawal of methylxanthines from the diet. The ingestion of vitamin E in reasonable doses does no harm, but data indicating that it is beneficial are extremely sketchy. No well-controlled clinical study on vitamin E has been done; the assumption is that vitamin E alters the metabolic pathway from pregnenolone to pregnanediol, producing instead increased quantities of a 17-kerosteroid, which is androgenic. Megadoses of vitamin E are thought to increase the risk of thromboembolic phenomena, but patients who feel they have experienced improvement from smaller doses need not be discouraged. The same can be said about other vitamin supplements.

Abstinence from the methylxanthines (coffee, tea, cocoa, and cola) is a positive step in dietary regulation, but whether it is helpful in the management of fibrocystic changes or pain is moot. The scientific explanation is that the methylxanthines interfere with the action of phosphodiesterase, an enzyme that assists in the metabolism of cyclic adenosine monophosphate (AMP) and guanosine monophosphate (GMP), thus causing a buildup of these substances in breast tissue. The clinical studies that have been done to prove this hypothesis are not convincing, but satisfied patients do not need to know this.

The persistence of nipple discharge in the absence of demonstrated pituitary pathology may necessitate treatment. Bromocriptine reduces prolactin levels to normal and stops lactation in less than a week in 90% of cases. The drug must be continued, however, or milk production is likely to recur.

As in the case of surgical management, patients under treatment with drugs must be kept under close observation, be re-examined regularly, and receive frequent support and reassurance.

Table 29–4
Medical Therapy

Hormonal
Birth control pills
Medroxyprogesterone acetate
Danazol
Tamoxifen
GNRH analogues
Bromocryptine

Non-hormonal
Reassurance
Hypnosis
Nonsteroidal analgesics
Surgery

OFFICE PROCEDURES

When a dominant mass in the breast is demonstrated on mammography or palpated, the gynecologist may choose to refer the patient elsewhere for management, but the gynecologist also has other options. Only about one fifth of breast masses are malignant, and although 15% of cancers occur in women under 40, the majority are found in women with a median age of about 50. However, the incidence of malignant breast masses increases with age. Furthermore, an accurate diagnosis can often be made clinically through the following characteristics: malignant tumors tend not to be painful or tender, and they are likely to have well-defined margins and to be hard, irregular, and fixed to the skin or muscle. Benign tumors tend to be painful premenstrually, tender to the touch, rounded and mobile. They are likely to occur in areas of fibrocystic change and to be multiple in both breasts.

If clinical judgment supports the diagnosis of a benign cyst or fibroadenoma, and the mass is 1 cm in diameter or larger, aspiration should be attempted. After the patient has been counseled about the probabilities and the nature of the procedure, she is placed in a supine position, the skin over the mass is cleansed, and a 4-mm intradermal wheal is raised with 1% lidocaine administered through a #25-gauge needle. The same needle is then passed down through the wheal toward the mass, and 2 or 3 mL of local anesthetic is injected along its track. While the mass is stabilized with the thumb and forefinger of the clinician's left hand, a #20 needle attached to a 20-mL syringe is passed down the same track, tangential to the chest wall, until the tip penetrates the lesion. Aspiration of the contents of a typical cyst yields a cloudy, brownish fluid. The physician never points the needle directly at the chest wall to obviate the risk of penetration of the pleura and the development of pneumothorax.

Because of the relatively acellular nature of cystic fluid and the difficulty in cytologic evaluation, some experts believe that this fluid should be discarded. Very infrequently, however, cysts are associated with malignancy, and it is, therefore, best to forward all fluid to the laboratory. Should no fluid be obtained from a firm, well-circumscribed mass, it is likely to be a fibroadenoma, which most pathologists consider a variant of the same disorder.

Solid tumors may be aspirated by a similar technique. This involves the use of a somewhat longer #22 needle with a syringe attached to a syringe holder, which, when drawn upward by two fingers, keeps a constant vacuum in the syringe. Again by a tangential approach, the needle is passed to and fro 8 to 10 times through the tumor in various planes while constant suction is maintained [Fig 29-1]. The material thus aspirated is squirted on at least six separate slides, fixed, and sent immediately to the laboratory. The yield from benign tumors is frequently scanty, and what there is of it may be washed away by fixatives and sprays. "Skinny needle" aspiration is also applicable to malignant tumors and is highly accurate in establishing a diagnosis. No tumor spread has been shown to result from the aspiration of malignancies. The accuracy of the fine needle aspiration tech-

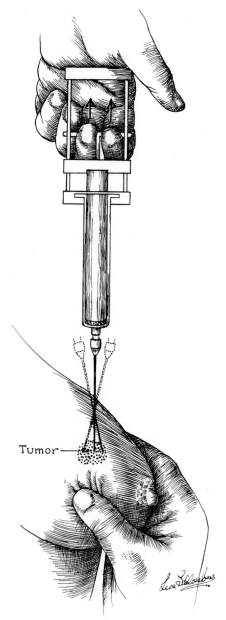

Tumor

Figure 29–1. Percutaneous needle aspiration of solid tumors. Using local anesthesia, a skinny needle (#22) is passed repeatedly through the lesion in different planes and directions while constant suction is maintained by means of the attached syringe holder. The aspirate is ejected on a slide and sent for cytologic analysis. A high degree of accuracy in diagnosis is possible, but the result is not definitive. (From Thompson JD, Rock JA: Te Linde's Operative Gynecology, 8th ed. Philadelphia, JB Lippincott 1992. Used by permission.)

nique is dependent to a large extent upon the skill of the operator, and this skill can be acquired only through long experience. The cytology laboratory and the cytologist must be specifically trained to interpret these specimens, some of which may be contaminated with gross blood. A definite positive diagnosis can be followed by definitive treatment; an equivocal diagnosis requires either another aspiration or histologic evaluation by open biopsy. A negative diagnosis may allow the physician to discontinue investigation if the report conforms to his clinical judgment, but if malignancy is strongly suspected, another attempt at aspiration or an open biopsy must be performed. In good hands the sensitivity of aspiration techniques approaches 90% and the specificity less than 5%. Material obtained by aspiration can also be used for receptor studies, DNA flow cytometry and electron microscopy. Good laboratories can send their diagnosis within the hour.

A variety of cutting needles capable of extracting a small but satisfactory core of tissue from a tumor are available for office or hospital practice. The use of such needles requires some skill; often two or three attempts must be made before a satisfactory specimen is obtained. The needle is inserted percutaneously, as described above, with the blunt end of the obturator to the fore inside of the needle sheath. Inside the tumor, the obturator is twisted to bring into play the scooped cutting side and is then withdrawn, bringing the fragment of tissue with it [Fig. 29-2.]

Open breast biopsy is a safe and effective ambulatory procedure. The delay between biopsy and definitive surgery, should the lesion prove to be malignant, has not been shown to affect the prognosis adversely, and patients are pleased to be able to discuss the problem with the doctor and to consider treatment alternatives. All that is required is a minor operating room, the necessary instruments and a nurse or qualified attendant.

The patient is counseled as to what she may expect and placed on the operating table in the supine position, with the arm on the affected side extended perpendicular to the chest. Patients who request analgesia may be given 5 mg of diazepam (Valium) and 25 mg meperidine (Demerol) intravenously. The majority of patients require no analgesia if the procedure has been properly explained to them. Although an assistant is handy, the operator can easily carry out the procedure alone while the attendant circulates and comforts the patient.

After appropriate cleansing and draping, a 5-cm intradermal wheal is raised along the path of the proposed incision. From this area, 5 to 10 mL of anesthetic is injected into the breast tissue surrounding the lesion. The anesthetic is renewed later as necessary. An incision 2 or 3 cm long is made with a #15 Bard-Parker blade. If the lesion is within 3 cm of the areolar margin or beneath the nipple, the incision should be circum-areolar at the perimeter of the pigmented area; by means of some tunneling, this usually gives adequate exposure. A properly placed scar in this area will subsequently be barely visible. When the lesion is further out in the breast, a curved invision is made over it parallel to the areolar margin. Radial incisions give poor cosmetic results; this is an important consideration for both young and old patients. The skin incision should be carried down through the dermis and into the subcutaneous fat. Once this soft tissue has been reached and a finger inserted, the tumor can usually be palpated, and subsequent sharp dissection with scissors can be directed down to and around it while traction is maintained.

The exposed mass can often be accurately diagnosed by its feel. If it is benign, it should be completely enucleated, with minimal loss of surrounding breast tissue so that there will be no pronounced defect after closure. Malignant or suspicious masses 4 cm or less in diameter should be excised with at least a 5-mm margin of surrounding fat and lobular tissue. In this day of lumpectomy for cure, it is important to remember that the biopsy may be the only surgical therapy, and the lesion must be completely extirpated. Representative wedge-shaped biopsies are taken from the surface of larger tumors, or such tumors can be further explored with the cutting biopsy needle if the frozen-section diagnosis of a surface biopsy is equivocal. Bleeding may be controlled with the Bovie unit or with ligatures, preferably with absorbable suture material beneath the skin. An attempt may be made to close a subsurface defect with sutures to obliterate dead space, but this is inadvisable if the sutures exert traction on the skin or subcutaneous tissues or in any way cause distortion of the breast. The skin is closed without drainage with 4-0 interrupted nylon, and a dry dressing, usually a Band-Aid or two, is applied. If bleeding has been excessive or a large amount of tissue has been removed, a pressure dressing over the entire breast is indicated.

The tissue removed is sent as rapidly as possible to the nearest laboratory for assay of estrogen and progesterone receptors and for frozen-section and histologic interpretation. The patient should have this information and, in the case of a diagnosis of

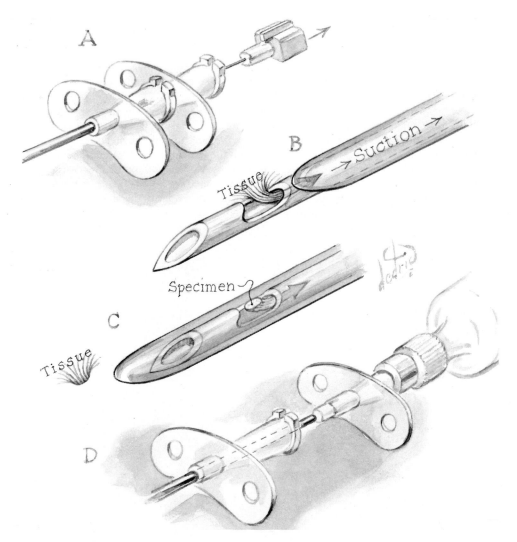

Figure 29–2. Tissue biopsy using the Lee biopsy needle. The assembled needle is advanced through the skin and into the breast until the point has entered the tissue from which the biopsy is to be taken. The stylet is then removed (**A**). The open, slotted inner needle protrudes beyond the tip of the outer cannula. A syringe partially filled with saline is attached to the inner needle and suction is applied (**B**), drawing the tissue to be biopsied into the main shaft of the needle. While the hub of the outer cannula is held, the entire syringe and attached inner needle are pulled outward 2 to 3 cm in a sharp, snapping motion, which neatly severs the tissue and deposits it in the inner-needle notch. Continued suction draws the tissue into the clear inner-needle hub or the fluid-filled syringe, where it can be visually identified (**C, D**). The process can be repeated as many times as required for additional biopsies. At no time should the assembly be advanced into a new track without the center stylet in place. At the conclusion of the biopsy, the entire assembly is removed and firm manual pressure is applied over the biopsy site.

malignancy, the benefit of preliminary consultation with the doctor before she leaves the office. The patient should always be accompanied from the office to her home.

Complications from this operation are relatively few, and the patient experiences little discomfort. She is allowed freedom of action and needs to return only to have the sutures removed in 5 or 6 days. Infrequently, there is a moderate amount of bleeding, always within the first 24 hours; in this case, the incision must be reopened and bleeding controlled. A small drain may be left in the operative site for 24 hours under these circumstances. Often there is ecchymosis of the skin surrounding the incision; the patient may be reassured that this will disappear in a few days. Accumulation of blood in a dead space may require repeated aspiration until it subsides. Infection is uncommon, as are large hematomas, but in both instances drainage or evacuation may be necessary.

As previously emphasized, every palpable dominant mass should be biopsied. When there is no palpable mass and mammography suggests the presence of a suspicious lesion, cytologic or histo-logic evaluation is indicated. The indiscriminate removal of a large quantity of breast tissue is avoided and excision of the suspicious lesion is ensured by localization of the area with preliminary x-ray imaging and the insertion of a guidewire in the desired area [Fig. 29-3]. Close cooperation with the radiologist in scheduling is necessary, and his instructions are important in enabling the surgeon to find the questionable spot in the breast.

With the patient under local anesthesia, the radiologist uses an image intensifier to insert a special needle through the skin and down to the lesion. A small wire with a hook on the end is passed through the needle; when it protrudes from the needle, it is

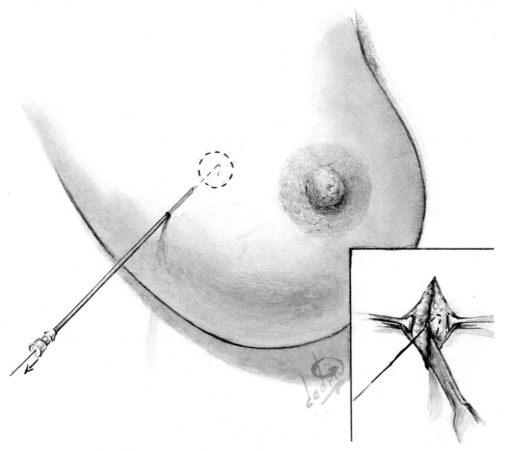

Figure 29–3. Insertion of a hooked needle for marking the biopsy site. The biopsy site has been identified on a mammographic film and a needle inserted at that location. A small wire with a hook on the end is passed through the needle so that the hook is fixed in the breast tissue. The needle is then withdrawn, and the wire is bent and fixed to the skin. The patient is sent to surgery after a confirmatory mammography has identified the portion of the hook in relation to the position of the lesion. In the operating room (*inset,* lower right), a circumferential incision follows the wire to the site of the hook, and a biopsy of the tissue containing the hook and the lesion is obtainead. The specimen containing the hook is sent to the radiology department for a confirmatory film that the suspected lesion has been excised, and the specimen is marked appropriately for identification of the lesion for sectioning.

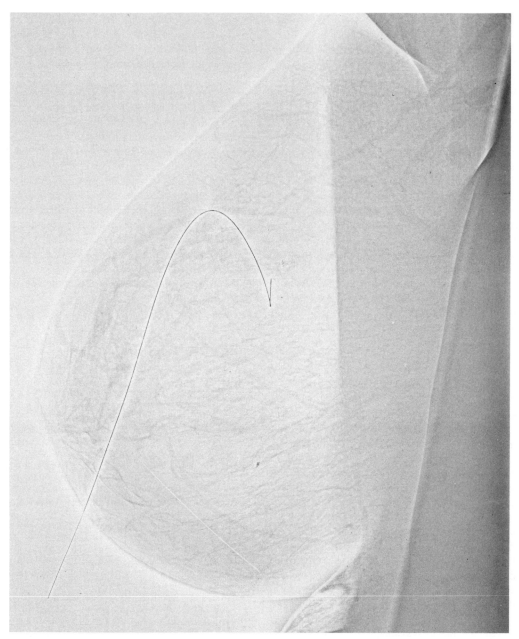

Figure 29–4. A mammogram showing excised microcalcifications and the hooked needle in place.

twisted and engaged at the proper spot. The needle is then withdrawn, the upper portion of the wire is bent and fixed to the skin to avoid undue motion, and the patient is sent to surgery (Fig. 29-4; see Fig. 29-3).

This procedure is done under the conditions previously described for biopsy. A block of tissue approximately 3 cm in diameter around the needle hook is removed and sent to the radiologist for x-ray confirmation that this is the area he saw originally. If it is not, another biopsy must be done. If it is, the tissue is sent on to the laboratory for further evaluation. Many very early cancers are found in this way, giving the patient the best possible prognosis.

Deep breast abscesses, though uncommon, are

usually seen postpartum or occasionally following trauma. Abscesses require incision and drainage, the latter being accomplished with a small wick or tube. The wall of a breast abscess should be biopsied since a carcinoma is occasionally associated with it. The drain should be removed in 24 hours. Lactation may continue after drainage.

Subcutaneous mastectomy has been advocated for women with advanced, generalized fibrocystic change, the so-called "dense breast," and a family history of breast cancer. The argument in favor of this procedure is that such breasts are difficult to read mammographically (which is true), that symptoms are relieved by the procedure, and that future cancer is prevented. Since prostheses for augmentation mammoplasty now are not readily available, patients undergoing subcutaneous mastectomy would have to be satisfied with a very poor cosmetic result. In addition, breast cancers have been known to occur in women who have had this operation. The final decision in such a situation would have to be based on the level of risk and consultation with the plastic surgeon.

BREAST CANCER IN PREGNANCY

It is important for the obstetrician to remember that breast cancer does occur during pregnancy and puerperium with an incidence from 10 to 30 cases per 100,000 deliveries, and with a mean age of 32 years. The incidence is likely to increase as women tend to delay pregnancy into the fourth decade. Accurate examination of the breast during pregnancy is difficult for both patient and physician, but both should be alerted to the possibility of cancer, especially in patients at high risk, and clinical examination and diagnostic aids should be employed when there is any suspicion of disease. Some experts have advised examination at each prenatal visit, but this seems excessive, particularly in the last trimester. Although breast cancer in pregnancy tends to be further advanced than in the nonpregnant state, probably because of delay in diagnosis, the prognosis is not adversely affected in stage-to-stage comparison.

ESTROGEN REPLACEMENT THERAPY IN WOMEN PREVIOUSLY TREATED FOR BREAST CANCER

The epidemiological evidence suggesting a role for estrogen in the etiology of breast cancer is convincing, and there is laboratory evidence of its enhance-ment of cellular activity, but many clinical studies and meta-analyses have failed to prove beyond reasonable doubt that exogenous estrogen use increases the incidence of breast cancer or promotes the recurrence of previously treated disease. Pregnancy after previously treated breast cancer, with the associated elevated hormone levels, has not been shown to lower the prognosis in terms of either early recurrence or longevity.

The problem thus posed is to balance the well-known advantages of estrogen replacement therapy after menopause against the possible risk of stimulating recurrent disease. Because new data incriminating estrogen in this circumstance may become available at any time, with unfortunate consequences to those who have provided it, and because fear of cancer probably overrides fear of osteoporosis and heart disease, a very conservative approach to this problem seems indicated for the time being.

Selected Readings

Angel M: Breast implants—protection or paternalism? N Engl J Med 326:1695, 1992

Barnes AB: Diagnosis and treatment of abnormal breast secretions. N Engl J Med 275: 1184, 1966

Barrett AH, Myers PC, Sadowsky NL: Microwave thermography in the detection of breast cancer. Am J Roentgenol 134:365, 1990

Berkel H, Birdsell DC, Jenkins H: Breast augmentation: a risk factor for breast cancer?. N Engl J Med 326:1649, 1992

Drukker BH: Nonsurgical treatment of breast disease. Obstet Gynecol Forum IV: 3, 1990

DuPont WD, Page DL, Parl FF, et al: Long-term risk of breast cancer in women with fibroadenoma. N Engl J Med 331:10, 1994

Estrogen replacement therapy in women with previously treated breast cancer. ACOG Comm Opin 135, 1994

Fentiman IS, Caleffi M, Hanred H, Chaudary MA: Dosage and duration of tamoxifen treatment for mastalgia: a controlled trial. Br J Surg 75:845, 1988

Fisher J: The silicone controversy—when will science prevail?. N Engl J Med 326:1696, 1992

Freundlich IM: Mammographic screening for breast cancer. Cancer Bull 44:17, 1992

Gabriel SE, O'Fallon WM, Kurland LT, Beard CM, Woods JE, Melton LJ: Risk of connective-tissue diseases and other disorders after breast implantation. N Engl J Med 330:1698, 1994

Gateley CA, Mansel RE: Management of the painful and nodular breast. Brit Med Bull 47:284, 1991

Geslien G, Fisher JR, DeLaney C: Transillumination in breast cancer detection: screening failures and potential. Am J Roentgenol 144:619, 1985

Goldberg IM, Schick PM, Pilch Y, Shabot MM: Contact plate thermography: A new technique for diagnosis of breast masses. Arch Surg 116:271, 1981

Hamed H, Caleffi M, Chaudary MA, Fentiman IS: LHRH analogue for treatment of recurrent and refractory mastalgia. Ann R Coll Sur Engl 72:221, 1990

Harris JR, Lippman ME, Veronest U, Willett W: Breast cancer. N Engl J Med 327:319, 1992

Hindle WH: The diagnosis of breast disease. Obstet Gynecol Forum IV:2, 1990

Homer MJ: Mammographic interpretation. New York, McGraw-Hill Inc, 1991

Homer MJ: Nonpalpable breast lesion localization using a curved-end retractable wire. Radiology 157:259, 1985

Longon RS, Solomon DM, London ED, et al: Clinical response and urinary excretion of 11-deoxy-17-ketosteroids and pregnanediol following α-tocopherol therapy. Breast Dis Breast 4:19, 1976

Mansel RE, Dogliotti L: European multicentre trial of bromocoriptine in cyclican mastalgia. Lancet 335:190, 1990

Minton JP, Foecking MK, Webster DJT, et al: Caffeine, cyclic nucleotides, and breast disease. Surgery 86:105, 1979

Mitchell GW: Benign breast disease and cancer. Clin Obstet and Gynecol 29: 705, 1986

Mitchell GW Jr, Homer JL: Outpatient breast biopsies on a gynecologic service. Am J Obstet Gynecol 144:127, 1982

Mitchell GW Jr, Bassett LW: The female breast and its disorders. Los Angeles, Williams & Wilkins, 1990

Moskowitz M: Mammographic screening: significance of minimal breast cancers. Am J Roentgenol 136:272, 1981

Moskowitz M, Feig SA, Cole-Beuglet C, et al: Evaluation of new imaging procedures for breast cancer: proper process. Am J Roentgenol 140:591, 1983

Nachtigall MJ, Smilen SW, Nachtigall RD, Nachtigall RH, Nachtigall LE: Incidence of breast cancer in a 22-year study of women receiving estrogen-progestin replacement therapy. Obstet Gynecol 80:827, 1992

Page DL, Dupont WD: Histologic indicators of breast cancer risk. Am Col of Sur 76:16, 1991

Peters R: Multicentre study of gestrinone in cyclical breast pain. Lancet 339:205, 1992

Rosner D, Blaird D: What ultrasonography can tell in breast masses that mammography and physical examination cannot. J Surg Oncol 28:308, 1985

Sickles EA: Mammographic features of "early" breast cancer. Am J Roentgenol 143:461, 1984

Stombler RE: Breast implants and the FDA. Am Coll Surg Bull 78:11, 1993

The role of the obstetrician-gynecologist in the diagnosis and treatment of breast disease. ACOG Comm Opin 140, 1994

The University of Texas MD Anderson Cancer Center: Cancer Bull 45:471–560, 1993

Vogel VG, Newell GR: Trends for screening mammography. Cancer Bull 41:5, 1990

Whitehead J, Carilie T, Koepecky K, et al: Wofle mammographic parenchymal patterns. Cancer 56:1280, 1985

Wolfe JN: Breast patterns as an index of risk for developing breast cancer. Am J Roentgenol 126:1130, 1976

Ambulatory Gynecology, Second Edition,
edited by David H. Nichols and Patrick J. Sweeney.
J. B. Lippincott Company, Philadelphia, © 1995.

30

The Use of Non-Physician Providers in the Ambulatory Gynecology Setting

Anne A. Stulik and Patrick J. Sweeney

Non-physician providers (NPPs) are an established part of the healthcare team. With the emphasis on healthcare reform, primary care, and cost consciousness, the demand for and use of these practitioners likely will increase. These health professions—nurse practitioners (NPs), physician assistants (PAs), and certified nurse midwives (CNMs)—were initially established in response to a national shortage and maldistribution of physicians and the need to provide primary health care to those in underserved areas. Since then, the number of NPPs has steadily grown. Most of them practice in public or privately funded clinics and hospitals serving low-income populations in medically underserved rural and urban areas in the United States.[1]

Non-physician providers perform many of the tasks that traditionally have been considered to be the work of physicians. These include health assessment, management of acute and chronic illness, minor surgical procedures, prescription writing, and collaboration with other licensed healthcare professionals. Non-physician providers often develop protocols in conjunction with physicians or healthcare organizations to allow independent practice and establish guidelines for referrals.

Most NPPs practice under the supervision of or in collaboration with a physician. Physician assistants work under the supervision of a licensed physician, with varying state and local regulations defining requirements for the physician's presence at the practice site. Nurse practitioners and CNMs work more in a "collaborative" role with the physician, ranging from direct supervision to working by protocol to independent practice. Although states vary widely in the legal and regulatory status of NPPs, national standards and credentialing for graduates of accredited programs are clearly defined.[1]

Many studies of NPPs in ambulatory healthcare

settings are reported in the literature. Competency in delivering healthcare and patient satisfaction and acceptance have all been repeatedly demonstrated. In addition, use studies and cost-effectiveness studies show positive economic results of NPP practice.[2-4]

In the ambulatory gynecology setting, NPPs provide gynecologic and family planning services. These include health history and screening examinations; complete physical examinations, including breast and pelvic examinations and Pap smears; screening and treatment of sexually transmitted diseases (STDs); and the prescription of contraceptives, including intrauterine devices and Norplant insertions. Nurse practitioners have sought education and training in procedures such as endometrial biopsy and colposcopy. In addition to providing direct healthcare services, NPPs in many settings play an important role in the education of future healthcare professionals, including medical students, NPP students, and residents.

This chapter is divided into two parts. The purpose of the first section is to outline some of the regulations governing the licensing and certification of three non-physician professions whose members frequently provide ambulatory gynecologic care—NPs, PAs, and CNMs. Appendix 30-1 contains more detailed, state-by-state information on NPs, who represent the largest of the three groups. Although regulations vary considerably among the states, and some may have changed since the preparation of this manuscript, information on prescriptive privileges and reimbursement guidelines are presented. For information on the status of these regulations in a specific locale, the reader should contact the respective licensing authority in his or her state. The second section, although not intended to be all-inclusive, discusses some of the traditional and contemporary roles NPPs can play in an ambulatory gynecologic practice.

LICENSING, CERTIFICATION, AND REIMBURSEMENT

Nurse Practitioners

Nurse practitioners—also known as advanced practice nurses or APNs—are registered professional nurses who have completed additional education in accredited institutions. This advanced education and expanded role training enables them to provide a broad range of primary healthcare services to patients, generally in collaboration with a physician.

The first program for training NPs began in 1965 in Denver, Colorado, under the direction of Dr. Henry K. Silver and Loretta C. Ford. Registered nurses were educated to perform additional functions in the field of pediatrics, enabling them to practice in expanded roles as NPs. Since then, colleges and universities have been training NPs to function in a variety of healthcare settings and medical specialties. There are 114 master's level programs and 26 certificate programs in the United States. Two thirds of NPs have received advanced education and training in 9- to 12-month certificate programs and a third in 2-year master's degree programs.[5]

Specialty area NPs are trained to practice in the following settings: adult, pediatric, and family health; gerontology; obstetrics and gynecology; and school health. Other areas in which NPs have developed special competencies include infant and school-age well-child care, adolescent health care, community health care for Southeast Asian refugees, care to disabled persons living in the community, personal fitness, and specialized inpatient settings (emergency rooms; medical, surgical, obstetrics and gynecology, and critical care units; rehabilitation and chronic care).[1]

This diversity of function illustrates the NP's potential for role expansion, often into areas where physicians are not involved. Most NPs are employed in ambulatory settings in the specialty areas of general practice, geriatrics, obstetrics and gynecology, family planning, adult health, school health, pediatrics, and psychiatry. Some NPs also practice in nurse-managed centers or are self-employed.[6]

Certification

Nurse practitioners are certified to practice by examination, according to specialty. The numbers of certified NPs is estimated to be 25,000 to 30,000 but certification is voluntary and not a prerequisite for practice in many states. Thirteen states require national certification to practice—Connecticut, Delaware, Maryland, Michigan, Montana, Nevada, New Hampshire, North Dakota, Oklahoma, Rhode Island, Tennessee, Virginia, and West Virginia.[7]

The American Nurses Association offers certification examinations in the following specialties: gerontologic NP, pediatric NP, adult NP, family NP, and school NP. The credential RNC (registered nurse, certified) is awarded to those who successfully pass the examination, including RNs who are not practicing as NPs.

The National Certification Corporation examination certifies obstetric, gynecologic, and neonatal NPs, and the RNC credential is awarded on successful completion of the examination. Pediatric NPs are examined and certified by the National Certification Board of Pediatric Nurse Practitioners and Nurses. The credential *Certified Pediatric Nurse Practitioner* is awarded on successful completion of the examination.

Legal Authority

Legal authority to practice as an NP is not nationally standardized. Recognition of NP advanced practice may be controlled by the states' Boards of Nursing, Boards of Medicine, or both. In some states, other state legislative bodies control NP practice, all granting differing degrees of autonomy. In Pearson's 1994 annual review article of legislative issues affecting advanced nursing practice, she reports that in 40 states NPs are regulated by their state boards of nursing through specified rules and regulations. In seven states, NPs function under a broad nurse-practice-act scope of practice, with no specific title protection; in four states, NPs are regulated by both the state board of nursing and the board of medicine. Nurse practitioners are authorized to practice under the Education Act in New York.[7]

Prescriptive Privileges

Prescriptive authority for NPs is authorized by state legislation, with varying degrees of prescriptive authority. Nurse practitioners are allowed to prescribe in 45 states (including the District of Columbia) and four more expect prescriptive authority in 1994. In the few remaining states without legislative prescriptive authority, NPs still prescribe by using pre-signed or co-signed prescription pads, calling in prescriptions under a physician's name and by using jointly written protocols.

On April 24, 1992, the Drug Enforcement Administration (DEA) withdrew regulations prohibiting nurse clinicians and physicians assistants from obtaining a DEA number. New regulations for NPPs are expected this year and reportedly will provide individual DEA numbers to all practitioners, including a code identifying the type of practitioner. By establishing a separate category of registration for NPPs, NPs will be allowed to dispense controlled substances, schedules II through V, as allowed by state law, which includes authorization through joint-practice protocols, guidelines, and agreements. Twenty-seven states grant federal DEA registration numbers and eight states grant dispensing authority.[7]

Third-Party Reimbursement

Reimbursement for NP services is authorized by state and federal legislation. State law identifies specific provider qualifications for reimbursement and most require certification and licensure. State statutes mandate that NP services be provided within the scope of practice, as determined by law. Reimbursement is provided through either direct or indirect payment. Indirect payment involves billing by or through a physician or institution, whereas direct payment allows NPs to bill directly for their services. In states that restrict direct reimbursement to NPs, physician supervision and physician participation in the billing process are required for reimbursement.[8]

Nurse practitioners have gained authority for reimbursement of their services under four federal health programs: Medicare, Medicaid, Civilian Health and Medical Program of Uniformed Services (CHAMPUS), and the Federal Employee Health Benefit Plan. Medicare reimburses NPs in a variety of settings, based on the NP specialty, type of healthcare setting, and the level of payment. Services covered include those performed in nursing homes, rural areas, rural health clinics, health maintenance organizations (HMOs), federally qualified health centers (FQHCs), and ambulatory care settings when the service is incident to a physician's service. Only NP services provided in nursing homes and rural areas are eligible for direct reimbursement.[9] Nurse practitioners working in rural areas may submit claims directly, whereas those working in nursing homes receive payment through their employers. In both settings, the NP must work in collaboration with a physician to receive payment. Payment levels are 85% of the Medicare fee schedule for services provided in nursing homes. Rural area providers receive 85% of the fee schedule for outpatient services and 75% for inpatient services.

Under Medicaid, federal legislation mandates that family and pediatric NPs be reimbursed for services. The payment rate is determined by the states and there is no requirement for supervision or collaboration. Individual states carry the option to cover additional types of NPs. Forty-nine states cover NP services, and 22 of them elect to cover NPs generally, rather than identifying their specific subspecialties. In 39 of these states, reimbursement is received at 80% to 100% of a physician's rate of reimbursement.

The Civilian Health and Medical Program of the Uniformed Services allows NPs to be directly reimbursed for services provided to members of the uniformed services and their dependents. The Federal Employee Health Benefit Plan offers health plans to federal employees. Nurse practitioners are directly reimbursed for their services without a supervision requirement.

Advance practice nurses receive third-party reimbursement in 34 states (10 states reimburse on a limited basis). Ongoing negotiations continue across the country to increase the number of states providing third-party reimbursement (see Appendix 30-1 for a state-by-state summary of prescriptive authority, legal authority, and reimbursement guidelines pertaining to NPs).

Physician Assistants

The PA profession began in the 1960s at Duke University. Shortly afterward, similar training programs were developed at the University of Washington, University of Colorado, and Wake Forest University. These programs were developed to meet a perceived shortage of primary care physicians, to control healthcare costs, and to compensate for the maldistribution of physicians, both geographically and by specialty area. Designed to expand the services of general practitioners, the first students were mostly former medical corpsmen.[10]

The profession grew in the 1970s with the Health Manpower Act of 1972 and the formation of the Committee on Allied Health Education and Accreditation, which accredits PA training programs. During this time, the American Academy of Physician Assistants (AAPA) was recognized by the American Medical Association.[1]

Training

Fifty-eight approved educational programs for training PAs are accredited in the United States, and they graduate about 1700 PAs each year. These programs are sponsored by schools of medicine and allied health and consist of 2- and 4-year programs. Most offer a baccalaureate degree or degree option; nine offer certificates and 12 offer Master of Science degrees. Postgraduate programs offering advanced training in medicine, surgery, and obstetrics and gynecology have been developed by some schools.[1]

The Accreditation Review Committee on Education for the Physician Assistant designates competency standards that educational programs must follow. The undergraduate PA program emphasizes teaching patient care in the primary care setting.

Curricula include courses in the basic sciences, pharmacology, physical diagnosis, and clinical laboratory procedures, followed by 9 to 15 months of clinical training.

Physician assistants are trained to:

1. Perform history taking and physical examinations
2. Perform uncomplicated diagnostic procedures
3. Gather data and formulate a diagnosis
4. Initiate basic treatment
5. Manage common acute and stable chronic conditions
6. Prescribe and dispense medication
7. Provide patient and family counseling and supportive functions[11]

The role of the PA is that of a dependent professional, functioning as a team member with the physician, not as a physician substitute. The supervising physician bears the legal responsibility for PA-provided services.[12]

Employment Settings

There are about 27,000 practicing PAs in the country. About 70% practice in outpatient settings (medical offices, HMOs, public and private clinics) and 30% in public and private hospitals. Other practice settings include correctional facilities, nursing homes, rural clinics, and the military. Most PAs (57%) practice in primary care. Of these, 33% work in family–general practice, 6% in internal medicine, 3% in obstetrics and gynecology, 2% in pediatrics, and 1% in geriatrics. The remainder practice in the primary specialties of industrial–occupational medicine, emergency medicine, general surgery and its subspecialties, and orthopedics.[13]

Like NPs, other specialty areas in which PAs have developed competencies include ophthalmic aides in state mental hospitals, junior house-staff in teaching hospitals, caring for disabled people living in the community, caring for federal prisoners, neonatal care, medical research, cardiothoracic surgery, pediatric bone marrow transplant units, military clinics, and health administration.[1]

Certification

The National Commission on Certification of Physicians Assistants offers qualifying examinations to graduates of accredited programs. Those who successfully complete the examination are allowed to use the title *Physician Assistant-Certified*. The certification is valid for 6 years. Every 2 years, a PA must reregister by documenting a required 100 hours of continuing medical education. Every 6 years, the recertification examination must be retaken and successfully completed to maintain certification. Special competency examinations in primary care and surgery are also provided by the commission. It is reported that more than 90% of PAs are certified.[1]

Legal Authority

Legal authority to practice as a PA is defined in varying state regulations, which may be generally or specifically defined. To qualify for practice as a PA, most states require graduation from an accredited training program and successful completion of the national certifying examination. Beyond these requirements, states vary widely regarding the scope of PA practice, performance tasks, and the definition of what constitutes adequate physician supervision. The term supervising physician may mean a physician must be present for the PA's performance of a task or must be in reasonable proximity by radio, telephone, or telecommunication (North Carolina); in some areas, the presence of a physician is not required.

Other provisions common to almost all state PA rules or statutes include the number of PAs that a physician may supervise, grounds for disciplinary action if the law is broken, penalties for violations, and requirements for identification.[14] Because laws and regulations are frequently amended, information is available from the AAPA or the PA regulatory authority in each state.

Prescriptive Authority

State regulations governing prescribing and dispensing rules for PAs vary widely. Legal authority to issue prescriptions has existed in some states since the 1970s but in the last few years, the number of states authorizing PA prescribing has rapidly increased. Physician assistants have prescriptive authority in 37 states and the District of Columbia. Included are Florida, Missouri, Pennsylvania, South Carolina, and Virginia, which are pending the publication of regulations to implement prescribing authority.[15] Although prescriptive authority is legally granted to PAs, in 20 of these states, prescriptions must be written either "with" or "under" a physician and three states require they be written on "behalf" of a physician. Still others provide specific stipulations for prescriptive writing. In Maine, prescriptive authority is limited; in North Dakota, authority is granted with specific rules; in South Dakota, prescriptions are allowed to be written only for symptomatic patients and temporary pain relief; and in Texas, only for underserved areas and the medically indigent.[15]

Twenty-one states authorize the prescribing of controlled substances, although varying schedule restrictions apply. In 24 states, PAs have also been authorized to dispense medications, although 13 states include various restrictions on dispensing. Attempts are being made to expand prescriptive authority to other states.

Third-Party Reimbursement

Reimbursement for physician services provided by PAs is authorized by the Rural Health Clinic Services Act of 1977 and varies with setting and geographic location. Under private insurance, PA services are covered when included as part of the physician bill or as a part of the fee for surgery. Reimbursement is made directly to the employing physician. Under Medicare, Part A (hospital services), PAs are reimbursed as employees of the institution. Billing is allowed directly in rural areas and indirectly in long-term care facilities.

In accordance with Medicare, Part B, physician services provided by PAs are reimbursed in special cases only. These include PA services provided in HMOs, certified rural health clinics, rural health manpower shortage areas, hospitals, skilled nursing facilities, intermediate care facilities, and those services provided to homebound patients in areas lacking home health agencies. Reimbursement rates vary from 65% to 85% of the physician's charge, depending on the setting. Efforts are underway to extend Part B coverage to all PA practice settings.

Under Medicaid, individual states mandate coverage of PA services. Forty-one states cover PA-provided services, with at least five states excluding coverage for assisting at surgery. Payment is made to the employing practice rather than directly to the PA, and the reimbursement rate varies from 65% to 100% of the rate paid to a physician.

The Civilian Health and Medical Program of Uniformed Services covers all medically necessary PA-provided services. The PA must be supervised in accordance with state law and the supervising physician must be an authorized CHAMPUS provider. The employer bills for the PA-provided services, and payment is 65% to 85% of the allowable physician charges, depending on the service provided. Payment is allowed in all states with PA licensure except Florida, Louisiana, Missouri, Oklahoma, and the District of Columbia.[16]

Certified Nurse Midwives

Certified nurse midwives are RNs who have completed a nurse-midwifery educational program at an accredited institution and have been certified through national examination to practice. The role was introduced in 1925 at the Frontier Nursing Service in Kentucky by Mary Breckenridge, a British nurse-midwife. It is one of the earliest models of the expanded role for nursing in providing primary health care for childbearing women. Initially, nurse-midwives conducted home births in rural and inner-city areas. In the late 1950s, Kings County Hospital in Brooklyn began hiring CNMs, and CNM-assisted hospital deliveries became the norm in the 1960s and 1970s. Recently some certified nurse midwives have returned to practice in birth centers (some associated with hospitals) and, to a lesser degree, in homes.

Nurse-midwifery practice, as defined by the American College of Nurse-Midwives (ACNM), includes the independent management of care of essentially healthy pregnant women and newborns and nonpregnant women seeking gynecologic care. These services occur within a healthcare system that provides medical consultation, collaboration, and referral. Certified nurse-midwives practice with jointly agreed on written protocols and guidelines developed in coordination with ACNM standards.[17] Many CNMs are considered to be independent from an administrative viewpoint but function clinically on an interdependent basis with physicians. Certified nurse-midwives have demonstrated the ability to reduce mortality rates, to be cost-effective, and to improve the birth experience of their clients.[18–20]

Training

The ACNM is the national organization for CNMs; its Division of Accreditation accredits all nurse-midwifery education programs. Programs grant either a degree (master's or doctorate) or a certificate to RNs who are studying midwifery. Courses cover clinical midwifery and advanced education in normal obstetrics and gynecology and newborn care.

There are 39 accredited educational programs at colleges and universities throughout the United States. Ten of these offer a certificate program (with five including the option of a master's degree through the affiliated institution) and 28 offer master's degrees. One other precertification program exists to prepare RNs trained in midwifery either in the United States or out of the country who need a refresher program to be eligible to practice in the United States.[21]

Employment Settings

There are more than 4500 CNMs in the United States and they practice in all 50 states. California has the largest concentration of CNMs (over 400), followed by New York, Florida, Massachusetts, Pennsylvania, Illinois, Georgia, and Texas. Most births attended by CNMs are in hospitals; in 1990, 3.6% of all births in the United States were delivered by CNMs.[22]

The scope of nurse-midwifery practice has expanded and includes services to normal healthy women and their infants in the areas of prenatal care, labor and delivery management, postpartum care, well-woman gynecology, and normal newborn care. Practice settings include home, hospital, and birthing centers for CNMs who provide childbearing care. Many CNMs choose to practice well-woman gynecologic care, including family planning, as an extension of their practice. These practice settings include ambulatory gynecology clinics, private gynecology offices, HMOs, public health departments, university healthcare services, and family planning clinics.[23]

Certification

Certification is by examination and is valid in every state. An affiliate of the ACNM offers the examination to individuals who have completed an accredited nurse-midwifery training program. After successful completion of the certifying examination, the initials "CNM" are awarded. Standards for the Practice of Nurse-Midwifery have been developed by the ACNM and unlike other nursing organizations, failure to comply with these standards can result in the revoking of certification.[24]

Legal Authority

Certified nurse midwives are licensed in every state, with varying privileges accorded to them. Individual states have their own licensing examinations and requirements for nurse-midwifery practice in addition to certification by the ACNM. Board regulation of nurse-midwifery practice also varies by state. Although most CNMs are regulated by Boards of Nursing, others are regulated by the Boards of Medicine or by joint regulation of both Boards of Nursing and Medicine. Still others are regulated by the Department of Health.

Prescriptive Authority

The laws governing the prescriptive practice of nurse midwives are complex and varied. Statutory definitions of which drugs, devices, and drug treatments that CNMs may prescribe also vary. Authorizing statutes may include the Medical Practice Act, Nurse Practice or Advanced Practice Act, State Pharmacy Act, and Controlled Substance Act in addition to the rules and regulations of these acts. Prescribing statutes include the category method, protocol method, exclusion formulary method, inclusion formulary method, or a list of scheduled substances. Often, a combination of prescribing methods is used.[24]

Generally, a CNM is granted prescriptive privileges after completing the educational requirements for state licensure as a nurse-midwife. In addition, in some states, a CNM must also apply to a designated state authority to obtain prescription privileges. In still other states, additional continuing education and academic preparation at the master's level is required for prescribing privileges. As of January 1994, 32 states (including the District of Columbia) have developed statutes or regulations governing prescription practice.[25] Several of these states also grant DEA numbers to CNMs, with varying schedules of controlled substances (II through V).

Third-Party Reimbursement

Nurse-midwifery services are covered by most private medical insurance carriers. In addition, nurse-midwifery services are also covered under Medicare, Medicaid, and CHAMPUS. Medicare covers the services of CNMs in rural health clinics and FQHCs. Since 1987, CNMs have been covered for services related to the maternity cycle as direct providers. The ACNM is lobbying congress to include reproductive health services also. To be reimbursed, CNMs must work in collaboration with a physician. They receive direct payment at 65% of the fee schedule. Under Medicaid, all state programs reimburse CNMs for services related to the maternity cycle. No supervision by a healthcare provider is required. The Civilian Health and Medical Program of Uniformed Services authorizes CNMs to provide services and directly reimburses for them.[9]

USE OF NON-PHYSICIAN PERSONNEL

Advanced practice nurses and their anticipated expanded roles have been proposed as an important component of healthcare reform. Unfortunately, most advanced practice nurses—like physicians—do not function as generalists; most are hospital-based and employed as clinical nurse specialists, nurse anesthetists, or nurse-midwives.[26] Consequently, the belief that increasing the numbers of APNs is a quick and simple solution to the shortage of primary-care providers is seriously flawed.

Nevertheless, the demand for NPPs will likely continue to increase secondary to needs generated by healthcare reform proposals and regulations governing the number of hours residents can work. One study that coded the activities of internal medicine residents discovered that the residents performed 67 kinds of activities. Based on contemporary medical management practices, 50% of the residents' time is spent in activities that *must* be done by a physician. If patient management is restructured, allowing NPPs enhanced responsibilities, it is estimated that this could be reduced to 20%. The study authors note, however, that a major advantage to using physicians is their ability to perform a wide range of tasks and their ability to move quickly from one type of task to another.[27]

Most NPPs working in a gynecologic practice setting are APNs. Only 3% of physicians assistants are concentrating their activities in the field of obstetrics and gynecology.[28] This relatively small percentage is likely to increase as the number of postgraduate educational opportunities for physicians assistants increases. Originally, in response to regulations limiting resident work hours, a postgraduate internship in gynecology and obstetrics was established in New York. Started in August 1986, the 15-month program begins with 3 months of didactics, followed by a clinical year similar to that of a rotating physician intern. Graduates perform histories and physical examinations, intravenous and central line placements, minor surgical procedures, and assist at major surgical procedures. They attend daily teaching rounds and take night call. Originally designed as an internship in gynecology alone, a rotation on labor and delivery was added to provide the interns with experience in assisting at cesarean sections, surgical sterilizations, and minor obstetric procedures. Intrapartum management is not included; graduates are prepared to work as part of a labor and delivery team.[29]

Obstetrics and gynecology is an ideal professional environment for the NP or nurse-midwife. Some patients prefer women providers for their gynecologic care (and 97% of nurses are women). In addition, because many of the health needs of adult women are wellness- rather than illness-oriented, the nursing emphasis on counseling and prevention is ideally suited to the primary care needs of this population.[30] In examining "sex versus role" in women's preferences for gynecologic examiners, Alexander and McCullough reported that sex appeared to be a more important factor than professional level of the provider. This was particularly important to low-income women, certain ethnic groups, and women who were reluctant to participate in screening programs.[31] Despite the fact that for the past 2 years slightly more than half of the medical students entering obstetrics and gynecology residencies were female, only 26% of the members of the American College of Obstetricians and Gynecologists are female.[32] Studies show that many women prefer a male gynecologist; those who prefer female providers may find their options continue to be limited for the next several years until the 50/50 gender distribution in residency programs begins to be reflected in practice settings.

Although studies have been undertaken to investigate the cost-effectiveness of using NPPs, the results are often difficult to interpret because of the inability to control for the many confounding variables. It is generally agreed that NPs spend more time per patient visit and see fewer patients than do physicians; the tradeoff, however, is that the NP provides services usually rendered by both the physician and the nurse.[33] It is also postulated that some of the cost savings could be explained by the fact that NPs order fewer laboratory tests and pay lower malpractice fees; however, these differences may largely be a function of the different case mix seen by NPs and physicians. Although NPs working in collaborative practice settings (HMOs, university-based clinics, group practices) likely result in a more cost-effective team, there are no published randomized patient studies that show that NPs working independently provide more cost-effective care than physicians.[26] Many believe that the emphasis on the cost-saving aspect of NPPs is ill-advised and detrimental, often depicting NPPs as cheaper substitutes for general practitioners. Such single-mindedness tends to detract from the NPPs' real value as additional resources for the development of innovative concepts of healthcare management and delivery.[34]

Most medical centers, HMOs, clinics, and large group practices have been using NPPs for several years. In many of these settings, they play a major role in the management and education of routine (or low-risk) prenatal patients. In the case of nurse-midwives, the continuity of care is extended to include labor and delivery. Although most NPPs working in an obstetrics and gynecology setting probably provide both prenatal and gynecologic care, this text limits its discussion to the latter. In many practice settings, NPPs have expanded their scope of practice to include inserting Norplant contraceptive devices, obtaining endometrial biopsies, and performing colposcopic examinations. Non-physician providers affiliated with academic medical centers or other practice settings in which health-profession students are trained often play a significant role in the clinical education of medical students and residents.

Whatever healthcare reform plan is ultimately enacted, there likely will be an increased emphasis on wellness and prevention and concomitantly, on patient education and screening. For many women, the obstetrician-gynecologist is the only physician they see regularly during their reproductive years. According to a 1993 Gallup poll, women are more likely to have had a physical examination within the last 2 years from an obstetrician-gynecologist than from any other type of doctor (72% versus 57%) and most of these women consider their obstetrician-gynecologist to be their primary-care physician.[35] Many of the primary–preventive health services provided by obstetrician-gynecologists can be enhanced or expanded through collaboration with NPPs. Some of these include:

1. Periodic health screening, including annual general physical examination plus pelvic and breast examinations
2. Pap smears
3. General health and lifestyle risk assessment, with appropriate counseling
4. Immunization
5. Family planning
6. Counseling or treatment of:
   Human sexuality and sexual dysfunction
   STDs
   Menopause and osteoporosis
   Hypertension and cardiovascular surveillance
   Domestic violence
   Substance abuse
7. Breast self-examination
8. General health education and promotion

In addition to these general primary–preventive services, in some settings, NPPs treat a variety of specific acute and chronic conditions, including but not limited to those that follow.

For Treatment of Vaginitis

The symptoms of vaginitis are not only annoying but can cause considerable anxiety, particularly for patients experiencing their first episode. Consequently, prompt evaluation and treatment combined with reassurance and appropriate educational intervention can go a long way toward improving patient satisfaction. The most common causes of vaginitis can be easily diagnosed by taking a careful history, performing a vaginal examination, and microscopically examining a wet smear. It is both convenient and cost-effective for NPs to see these patients. One group, composed of six obstetrician-gynecologists and one NP, reported that 61% of the more than 3300 wet smears evaluated in their office were seen by the NP.[36]

Once the diagnosis is made, patients need to be informed of the advantages and disadvantages of alternative therapies—oral antibiotics, vaginal creams, suppositories. All things being equal, receiving a method of one's choice is more likely to result in compliance. Also, patients who have questions about the use of the vaginal applicator may feel more comfortable asking them of a female provider.

To Provide Estrogen-Replacement Therapy

Increasingly, women are requesting information about the advantages and disadvantages of estrogen-replacement therapy. Ideally, the provider should take this opportunity to discuss the physical and emotional changes one might expect in the perimenopausal and postmenopausal years. The benefits of good nutrition and exercise should be explained. The initial health assessment and physical examination can be performed by either a physician or an NPP. If the patient is a good candidate for estrogen-replacement therapy, an appropriate regimen of estrogen replacement, with or without progesterone, is prescribed. Follow-up visits with the NPP can be arranged to check on the patient's response, to maximize compliance, and to identify potential problems early.

For Treatment of Premenstrual Syndrome

Premenstrual syndrome, a complex of symptoms with somatic, behavioral, and emotional components, is often managed by NPs. In many group practices or HMOs, NPs do all the screening and counseling. Once the possibility of underlying disease is ruled out, total nurse management is not unusual.[37]

To Perform Colposcopy

Many group practices, HMOs, community health centers, and academic medical centers encourage interested NPs to learn colposcopy, including endocervical and cervical biopsy techniques. Although individual NPs may obtain the requisite knowledge and skill through various mechanisms, several formal programs based on established educational curricula are available throughout the United States. The National Association of Nurse Practitioners in Reproductive Health (NANPRH), founded in 1980, is a nonprofit membership organization representing NPs who provide primary care in gynecology, obstetrics, and family planning in addition to specialty care in reproductive endocrinology and infertility. In collaboration with the American Society for Colposcopy and Cervical Pathology, NANPRH has established standards for the training of NP colposcopists, which outline the curriculum content, preceptorship–mentorship requirements, and evaluation.[38]

To Perform Abortions

Despite the evidence suggesting that the number of physicians willing and able to perform abortions is decreasing, information on the use of non-physician personnel to provide abortion services is extremely limited. Physicians assistants have been performing abortions in Vermont since 1973; a state law authorizes PAs to practice under a supervising doctor who can delegate tasks that he or she is qualified to perform and that the PAs have been trained to do. Montana has also permitted this practice. A 1986 Vermont study comparing the outcomes of nearly 2500 first-trimester abortions reported no differences in complication rates between those women who had abortions performed by a PA and those who had the procedure performed by a physician.[39] In October 1990, a national symposium was convened to explore the shortage of physicians willing to provide abortion and make recommendations to end it. The symposium's recommendations were (1) encourage physicians and clinics to train and integrate mid-level clinicians into abortion service delivery, and (2) encourage and facilitate national professional societies of mid-level clinicians to provide avenues and incentives for training in abortion care. At the same time, further research was encouraged to determine the content of training required for competency of NPPs.[40]

As one might expect, the above recommendations are not without controversy. Those who support training non-physicians to perform the procedure cite limited access as a major barrier to women seeking pregnancy termination. In 1988, 83% of counties in the United States had no abortion provider, and the number of doctors willing to provide the service has steadily declined in the past decade.[41] Although a 1985 survey reported that 72% of United States residency programs in obstetrics and gynecology included first-trimester abortion techniques in their training, only a third of these programs considered it a "routine" part of the residency; the other two thirds offered it as "optional" training.[42] A 1993 report of a survey of obstetrics and gynecology residency program directors and chief residents revealed that 47% of graduating residents had never performed a first-trimester abortion.[43]

Those who oppose the recommendations are concerned that non-physicians would not be able to handle the rare but potentially life-threatening complications that can occur. In addition to the medical reasons, several social and economic issues have been raised; a newspaper article posed the question—are physicians "abdicating their responsibilities and succumbing to political pressure?"[44] Will doctors for whom abortion is a significant part of their practice consider this a threat to their income? Is there evidence to indicate that NPPs *want* to perform abortions? In all likelihood, NPPs will be subjected to the same harassment physicians have endured.

SUMMARY

Healthcare reform is likely to have—directly or indirectly—a significant impact on the education, distribution, and use of health manpower in the United States. Greater emphasis will be placed on primary and preventive services, and the demand for non-physician healthcare professionals will continue to rise, at least for the near future. For the past two decades, thousands of obstetrics and gynecology residents have worked side by side with NPs and certified nurse midwives. The mutual respect generated by these experiences has resulted in many of these physicians establishing collaborative practices with NPPs. A survey of nearly 4000 members of the American College of Obstetricians and Gynecologists found that slightly more than half indicated they were in a collaborative practice ar-

rangement.[45] The American College of Obstetricians and Gynecologists has established a new Division of Collaborative Practice to serve as a resource to members interested in creating a collaborative practice environment. Although various definitions of collaborative practice exist, Sebas nicely states that, "The collaboration includes both independent and cooperative decision making and is based on the preparation and ability of each practitioner...Joint practice promotes a climate of trust and respect between the two professions based on their explicitly and jointly defined, mutually complimentary roles in patient care."[46]

As primary-care physicians for women, obstetrician-gynecologists have always provided continuous and comprehensive services to their patients. In addition to general health assessments, obstetrician-gynecologists provide annual physical examinations, including pelvic and breast examinations; general and specific screening (STDs, Pap smears, cholesterol); preventive services (prenatal care, family planning, immunizations); counseling (STDs, contraception, genetics, domestic violence); and education (breast self-examination, diet, exercise, menopause, osteoporosis). Non-physician providers can and do provide many of these services. Some NPPs have expanded their roles to include colposcopy, artificial insemination, endometrial biopsies, and other procedures generally performed in an ambulatory gynecology setting. Successful collaborative practice arrangements can be rewarding for both the healthcare professionals and the patients whom they mutually serve.

REFERENCES

1. Rodos JJ, Peterson B: Proposed strategies for fulfilling primary care professional needs. Part II: Nurse practitioners, physician assistants, and certified nurse-midwives, policy paper. Rockville, MD, United States Public Health Service, 1991
2. Nurse practitioners, physicians' assistants, and certified nurse-midwives: policy analysis. Washington DC, United States Congress, Office of Technology Assessment, Health Technology Case Study No. 37, December, 1986
3. Prescott P, Driscoll L: Evaluating nurse practitioner performance. Nurse Pract 5:28,31, 1980
4. McGrath S: The cost effectiveness of nurse practitioners. Nurse Pract 15:40, 1990
5. Directory of primary care nurse practitioner/specialist programs and nurse-midwifery programs for registered nurses. Washington DC, United States Department of Health and Human Services, Division of Nursing, July 1993
6. Waters S, Asbecker J: Nurse practitioners: how are they now? RN 48:38, 1985

7. Pearson LJ: How each state stands on legislative issues affecting advanced nursing practice. Nurse Pract 19:11, 1994

8. Caraher M: The importance of third-party reimbursement for NPs. Health Care Issues 13(4):50, 1988

9. Mittelstadt PC: Federal reimbursement of advanced practice nurses' services empowers the profession. Nurse Pract 18(1):43, 1993

10. Perry HB, Breitner B: Physician assistants: their contribution to health care. New York, Human Services Press, 1982

11. Curry RH, Luckie WR: The role of the primary care physician assistant. Physician Assistant 8:31, 1984

12. Bottom W: Physician assistants: current status of the profession. J Fam Pract 24(6):639, 1987

13. Physician assistants, partners in medicine. Washington DC, American Academy of Physician Assistants, July 1993

14. Gara N: State laws for physician assistants. American Academy of Physician Assistants, February 1–13, 1994, Alexandria, VA

15. Physician assistants: prescribing and dispensing. American Academy of Physician Assistants, July 1–14, 1993, Alexandria, VA

16. Third party reimbursement for physician assistant services. American Academy of Physician Assistants, April 1992, Alexandria, VA

17. Thompson JE: Nurse-midwifery care: 1925 to 1984. Annu Rev Nurs Res 153, 1986

18. Lops V: Midwifery: past to present. J Prof Nurs 4(6):402, 1988

19. Institute of Medicine: Preventing low birthweight: summary, p 25. Washington DC, National Academy Press, 1985

20. Nurse practitioners, physician assistants, and certified nurse-midwives: a policy analysis, p 5. Washington DC, United States Congress, Office of Technology Assessment, 1986

21. FACTS. Basic facts about certified nurse-midwives. Washington DC, American College of Nurse-Midwives, M & PR 94 - 1/31

22. FACTS. Statistics on certified nurse-midwives. Washington DC, American College of Nurse-Midwives, PR 93-2/4

23. Lichtman R, Papera S (eds): Gynecology: well woman care. Norwalk, CT, Appleton & Lange, 1990

24. Fennell K: Prescription authority for nurse-midwives: a historical review. Nurs Clin North Am 26(2):511, 1991

25. FACTS. States in which CNMs have prescriptive authority. Washington DC, American College of Nurse-Midwives, PR 94 - 1/24

26. DeAngelis CD: Nurse practitioner redux. JAMA 271:868, 1994

27. Knickman JR, Lipkin M, Finkler SA, Thompson WG, Kiel J: The potential for using non-physicians to compensate for the reduced availability of residents. Acad Med 67:429, 1992

28. 1993 membership census. Alexandria, VA, American Academy of Physician Assistants, 1993

29. McGill F, Kleiner GJ, Vanderbilt C, Nieves J, Keith D, Greston WM: Postgraduate internship in gynecology and obstetrics for physicians assistants: s 4-year experience. Obstet Gynecol 76: 1135, 1990

30. Barkaukas VH, Chen SC, Chen EH, Ohlson VM: Health problems encountered by nurse-practitioners and physicians in obstetric-gynecologic ambulatory care clinics. Am J Obstet Gynecol 140:393, 1981

31. Alexander K, McCullough J: Women's preferences for gynecological examiners: sex versus role. Women Health 6:123, 1981

32. 1994 membership data. Washington DC, American College of Obstetricians and Gynecologists, 1994

33. Safriet BJ: Health care dollars and regulatory sense: the role of advanced practice nursing. Yale J Reg 9:417, 1992

34. Salisbury CJ, Tettersell MJ: Comparison of the work of a nurse practitioner with that of a general practitioner. J R Coll Gen Pract [Occas Pap] 38: 314, 1988

35. 1993 Gallup poll of women's health practices. Washington DC, American College of Obstetricians and Gynecologists, 1993

36. Gietl KA: Role of the nurse practitioner in the management of vaginitis. Am J Obstet Gynecol 158: 1009, 1988

37. Frank EP: What are nurses doing to help PMS patients? Am J Nurs 86:136, 1986

38. Colposcopy education and clinical training standards. Washington DC, National Association of Nurse Practitioners in Reproductive Health, 1993

39. Freedman MA, Jillson DA, Coffin RR, Novick LF: Comparison of complication rates in first trimester abortions performed by physician assistants and physicians. Am J Public Health 76:550, 1986

40. Who will provide abortions? Ensuring the availability of qualified practitioners. Recommendations from a national symposium. Washington DC, National Abortion Federation and American College of Obstetricians and Gynecologists, 1991

41. Henshaw SK, Vav Vort J (eds): Abortion factbook, 1992 edition: readings, trends, and state and local data to 1988, p 190, 204. New York, Alan Guttmacher Institute, 1992

42. Darney PD, Landy U, MacPherson S, Sweet RL: Abortion training in United States obstetrics and gynecology residency programs. Fam Plann Persp 19:158, 1987

43. Westhoff C, Marks F, Rosenfield A: Residency training in contraception, sterilization, and abortion. Obstet Gynecol 81:311, 1993

44. Boodman SG: Should non-physicians perform abortions? The Washington Post, February 15, 1994

45. Parker S: Advanced practice nurses: partners or rivals? Ob Gyn News, January 15, 1994

46. Sebas MB: Developing a collaborative practice agreement for the primary care setting. Nurse Pract 19:49, 1994

Appendix 30–1

Prescriptive Authority, Legal Authority, and Reimbursement Guidelines for Nurse Practitioners, by State, 1994.

State	Prescriptive Authority	Legal Authority	Reimbursement
Alabama	No	Yes—MD collaboration required	No private insurance coverage; Medicaid covers only ped. services of family, PNP, and neonatal NPs
Alaska	Yes—including controlled substances; sched. II–V; receive DEA registration; may dispense drugs	Yes—no MD relationship required	Yes—private insurance coverage; PNPs and FNPs receive Medicaid reimbursement
Arizona	Yes—including controlled substances with individual DEA numbers, schedule II (48-hour supply); schedule III–V, 1-mo supply + no refills.	Yes—MD collaboration required	Yes—private coverage; no Medicaid AHCCC (Arizona Health Care Cost Containment) reimburses NPs; Medicare reimburses NPs in rural counties
Arkansas	Yes—limited number of drugs for women's health NPs only who work for Dept. of Health; Preprinted R$_x$s are cosigned by MD	Yes—MD collaboration required	Yes—some private carriers; Medicaid only to certified FNPs and PNPs
California	Yes—MD name required on container label; standardized procedures required (i.e., drug formulary); "drugs/devices" must be incidental to FP services, perinatal services, or routine health care to essentially healthy persons	Yes—MD collaboration required	No private insurance coverage to NPs; yes—Medi. Cal. reimburses FNPs and PNPs for Medicaid-covered services
Colorado	Yes, but not independent authority; prescriptive privileges under delegated medical acts; R$_x$ written per protocol; controlled substances require a physician cosign	Broad act covers NPs; no title protection or specifications for advanced practice; bill pending in 1/94 legislative sessions.	Yes—third-party reimbursement to all RNs; Medicaid reimbursements to PNPs, FNPs
Connecticut	Yes—including controlled substances; limitations based on setting and specialty	Yes—national certification required	Private insurers reimburse to certified NPs; Medicaid regulations for PNPs, FNPs currently being drafted; no direct Medicare reimbursement
Delaware	No current legislative authority; bill to be introduced in 1994 legislative session	Yes—national certification required and 1-yr post-basic education	Yes—private insurance reimbursements; FNPs and PNPs receive Medicaid reimbursement
District of Columbia	Yes—including class II–V drugs	Yes—specialty license granted by BON; must work in collaboration with MDs or DOs	Yes—private payors; no Medicaid reimbursement
Florida	Yes—no controlled substances; protocols used; R$_x$ lists NPs + physician's name and license number	Yes—with MD supervision and protocols	Yes—Medicaid, Champus, and third-party reimbursement; Medicare reimbursement to NPs in rural and underserved areas

(continued)

Appendix 30–1
(Continued)

State	Prescriptive Authority	Legal Authority	Reimbursement
Georgia	No independent authority; controlled substances ordered through protocol	Yes—must work with jointly written protocols by NP and MD	Yes—some private insurance but not required by law; Medicaid reimbursement to PNPs and FNPs and OB/GYN NPs
Hawaii	No—bill submitted in 1994 legislative session calls for prescriptive authority for APNs	Advanced practice not specified; 1994 langauge changes expected in the NPA	YES—CHAMPUS and Medicaid reimburses PNPs and FNPs
Idaho	Yes—no controlled substances	Yes—with proof of a supervisory physician	Medicaid reimbursement paid to physician employers; Medicare reimbursement per federal guidelines
Illinois	No	Yes—per legislation intent and position of Dept. of Professional Regulations	Some reimbursement for third-party payors; no Medicaid or Medicare reimbursement; cited out of compliance with federal guidelines
Indiana	No—legislation pending by late Spring '94; collaboration with MD would be required; controlled substances would be allowed if APN obtains a DEA number and state-controlled–substances registration	Yes	May receive direct third-party reimbursement and Medicaid reimbursement; Medicare reimbursement per federal guidelines
Iowa	Yes—controlled substances R_x pending in 1994 legislative session	Yes—national certification required	Legislation permits third-party reimbursement to certified RNs but no insurance companies have reimbursed ANPs; if NP practices independently, direct Medicaid reimbursement is received; indirect reimbursement if employed by physician or facility
Kansas	Yes—under jointly adopted protocols between NP and MD; excludes controlled substances; proposed 1994 legislation would add controlled drugs to prescribing authority	Yes	Reimbursement to all NPs providing services in health plans; Medicaid covers all services
Kentucky	Yes—only according to established protocols; no DEA number issued	Yes—with annually updated protocols between NP and MD	Medical Assistance reimburse NPs
Louisiana	No—APNs in public health clinics only may insert medications, implants, or deliver meds to treat STDs or prevent pregnancy; under approved protocols	NPA prohibits medical diagnosing or treating; NPs called Primary Nurse Associates (PNAs) and must practice under physician supervision	Medicaid reimbursement for pediatric and family NPs

(continued)

Appendix 30–1
(Continued)

State	Prescriptive Authority	Legal Authority	Reimbursement
Maine	Yes—limited to formulary supervised by physician: 1994 legislation pending to expand Nurse Practice Act (NPA)	Yes—only when medical diagnosis or prescription is delegated by MD to RN; 1994 legislation hopes to define APNs and expand their scope	Only for Master's-prepared psychiatric nurse/specialists; Medicaid reimburses FNPs and PNPs on a fee-for-service basis; Medicare reimburses per federal mandates
Maryland	Yes—including controlled substances; state and federal DEA numbers can be obtained by NPs; scope of authority defined by written agreement between NP and collaborating MD; NPs in most settings also legally dispense medications (as of 1993)	Yes—national certification exam and written agreement with an MD are required	Yes—entitled to private third-party and Medicaid reimbursement if practiced within legal scope; Medicare reimbursement per federal guidelines
Massachusetts	Yes—for schedule II–VI drugs; may apply for state and federal DEA numbers; supervising MDs name on prescription pad	Yes—with approved additional education by BON	No to private reimbursement; PNPs and FNPs reimbursed by Medicaid only if nonsalaried, independent, and accepted as primary-care providers under Mass. Medicaid
Michigan	Yes—with MD delegation; excludes controlled substances	Yes for NPs with specialty certification; no physician collaboration or supervision required	Pilot project to reimburse certified NPs in certain urban and rural areas; Medicaid reimburses certified PNPs and FNPs; Medicare reimbursement per federal guidelines
Minnesota	Yes—when delegated under annual updated, written agreement with MD; DEA numbers have been issued	Yes—under broad nurse practice act; no APN category	Yes—private insurance reimbursement: Medicaid reimburses NPs
Mississippi	Yes—per Board of Nursing–approved protocol; no DEA numbers issued	Yes—national certification and documentation of collaborative/consultative practice with MD is required; protocols also required	Yes—third-party reimbursement with MD co-signature; Medicaid reimbursement available; NPs in rural health clinics receive Medicare reimbursement
Missouri	Yes—in collaboration with MD; no controlled substances	Yes—collaborative practice with MD and use of protocol or written agreement	Yes—BC/BS; Medicaid reimbursement available; Medicare reimbursement for nursing home or rural visits if practice agreement
Montana	Yes—independent prescribing authority, including controlled substances II–V; DEA numbers issued	Yes—specific curriculum requirements and national certification required	Yes—third-party reimbursement; Medicaid reimbursement since 1986; Medicare reimbursement per federal guidelines
Nebraska	Yes—per practice agreement and protocol; includes controlled substances III, IV, V	Yes—collaborative practice with MD; practice agreement and protocols required	No third-party reimbursement; Medicaid reimbursement available; Medicare reimburses per federal guidelines

(continued)

Appendix 30–1
(Continued)

State	Prescriptive Authority	Legal Authority	Reimbursement
Nevada	Yes—with documentation of 1000 hours worked with collaborating MD and annually updated protocol; no controlled substances; dispensing privileges also	Yes—national certification or BSN required in addition to signed agreement with collaborating MD	Yes—third-party reimbursement: Medicaid reimbursement; Medicare reimburses for nursing home and rural areas per federal guidelines
New Hampshire	Yes—may prescribe controlled and noncontrolled meds from Joint Health Council formulary; DEA numbers issued	Yes—certification required; no requirement for MD collaboration or supervision	Yes—for legally performed services; Medicare reimburses NPs
New Jersey	Yes—collaborative practice with MD and annually updated protocol required	Yes—national certification and pharmacology education required; no controlled substances	Yes—third-party reimbursement; Medicaid reimburses pending rules and regulations by BON
New Mexico	Yes—may independently prescribe and dispense controlled substances, schedule II–V; state-controlled substance license, DEA number, and formulary required	Yes—may practice independently without MD supervision or collaboration	Yes—third-party reimbursement; Medicaid reimburses FNPs and PNPs; Medicare reimbursement for long-term care and some rural areas
New York	Yes—collaboration with MD, practice agreement, and protocols required; includes controlled substances; DEA numbers issued	Yes—collaboration with MD, practice agreement, and protocols required; state certification also required	Medicaid reimburses all NP specialties; Medicare reimburses for services in rural areas
North Carolina	Yes—from approved formulary; no controlled substances	Yes—contract with supervising MD if in independent practice	Third-party reimbursement for services within scope of practice; Medicaid and CHAMPUS reimbursement; Medicare reimburses nursing home visits and rural areas
North Dakota	Yes—including controlled substances; MD collaboration and pharmacology education required; DEA numbers issued	Yes—national certification required	Third-party reimbursement for APNs in mental health; Medicaid reimburses FNPs and PNPs; Medicare reimburses per federal guidelines
Ohio	No	No per Nurse Practice Act; APNs only recognized in 3 pilot university programs under MD advisement; pilot registration ends in 1996	Some NPs receive reimbursement through direct negotiation with insurance companies; NPs in pilot programs not considered independent Medicaid providers; physician co-signature on charts required
Oklahoma	No current legislative authority; bill to be introduced in 2/94 legislative session	Yes—national certification required	No third-party reimbursement; Medicaid reimburses only to PNPs and FNPs

(continued)

Appendix 30–1
(Continued)

State	Prescriptive Authority	Legal Authority	Reimbursement
Oregon	Yes—formulary determined by BON; includes controlled substances III–IV; DEA numbers issued; NPs in college health centers may dispense pre-packaged medications	Yes—Master's degree required; NPs granted hospital privileges	Third-party reimbursement and Medicaid reimburses to NPs
Pennsylvania	Yes—prescriptions must be co-signed by collaborating MD	Yes—with MD supervision	Third-party reimbursement is available to state or nationally certified NPs; Medicaid reimburses all NPs
Rhode Island	Yes—with collaboration from MD and annually updated practice guidelines; no controlled substances	Yes—no MD collaboration or supervision requirements for practice	Third-party reimbursement to NPs working in licensed health center; Medicaid legislation approved but not implemented
South Carolina	Yes—may R$_x$ meds in NPs specialty field with MD authorization and approved protocols: NPs may prescribe schedule V	Yes—MD preceptor and co-written protocols required	Medicaid reimburses all NPs; treatment plans required
South Dakota	Yes—as designated medical act; MD supervision and approved practice agreement required; no schedule II controlled substances	Yes—with MD supervision and approved practice agreement	Third-party reimbursement and Medicaid reimburses NPs
Tennessee	Yes—Master's degree, national certification, pharmacology education and approved practice site required; no controlled substances; no DEA number issued	Yes—co-written medical protocols required	No third-party reimbursement; FNPs and PNPs are eligible for Medicaid reimbursement
Texas	Yes—per MD supervision and protocol at sites serving medically underserved populations	Yes	Third-party reimbursement varies by company and type of NP; Medicaid reimburses all NPs
Utah	Yes—with consulting MD; includes controlled substances III–V; DEA numbers issued	Yes—Master's degree required; no MD collaboration required unless prescribing	Third-party reimbursement by some companies; Medicaid reimbursement to PNPs and FNPs; Medicare reimbursement per federal guidelines
Vermont	Yes—collaborating MD and annually updated protocols required; includes controlled substances; DEA numbers issued	Yes	BC/BS only reimburses to psychiatric NPs; Medicaid reimburses FNPs and PNPs
Virginia	Yes—with practice agreement listing categories of drugs to be prescribed; no controlled substances	Yes—national certification required	No third-party reimbursement; Medicaid reimburses FNPs and PNPs; Medicare per federal guidelines; no independent billing

(continued)

Appendix 30–1
(Continued)

State	Prescriptive Authority	Legal Authority	Reimbursement
Washington	Yes—pharmacotherapeutic education required; schedule V and legend drugs; DEA numbers issued	Yes	Private insurers and healthcare service contractors reimburse NPs; Medicaid reimburses all NPs; Medicare reimburses per federal guidelines
West Virginia	Yes—collaboration with MD and written protocols required; includes controlled substances with exclusionary formulary; anticipated DEA number issuance	Yes—national certification required; MSN required as of 1/94; no collaboration required unless prescribing	No third-party reimbursement; Medicaid reimburses FNPs and PNPs
Wisconsin	Yes—as delegated medical act; includes controlled substances; BON-controlled NP prescribing authority is anticipated in early 1994	Yes—with written protocols or verbal orders and consultation with MD; general supervision required (MD not required to be on-site)	No third-party reimbursement; Medicaid reimburses all Master's-prepared certified ANPs, PNPs, and OB/GYN NPs; Medicare reimburses NP services in nursing homes or rural areas; CHAMPUS reimburses NPs
Wyoming	Yes—legend and controlled substances III–V included; pharmacology education, liability insurance, written collaboration practice agreement, and 400 hours of APN practice required; DEA numbers issued	Yes—advanced education or national certification required	Third-party reimbursement per state statute; Medicaid reimburses all NPs

*All states by federal mandate must cover the services of certified pediatric (PNP) and family (FNP) nurse practitioners per section 6405, OBRA '89.

†Medicare coverage—based on NP specialty and type of setting.

‡Data from Pearson LJ: How each state stands on legislative issues affecting advanced nursing practice. Nurse Prac 1994;19:11; American Nurses Association: Advanced practice nursing reimbursement tables, status of Medicaid federal mandate, use of UPINs and new Medicare practitioner fees. Washington, DC 1992.

ANP, adult nurse practitioner; *APN,* advanced practice nurse; *BC/BS,* Blue Cross/Blue Shield; *BON,* board of nursing; DEA, Drug Enforcement Administration; *FNP,* family nurse practitioner; *MSN,* master of science in nursing; *NP,* nurse practitioner; *NPA,* nurse practice act; *PNP,* pediatric nurse practitioner; *RN,* registered nurse; *STD,* sexually transmitted disease.

Ambulatory Gynecology, Second Edition,
edited by David H. Nichols and Patrick J. Sweeney.
J. B. Lippincott Company, Philadelphia, © 1995.

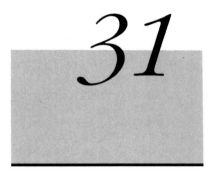

31

Quality Assurance in Ambulatory Gynecology

Beth E. Quill

Ambulatory care has experienced dramatic changes in the past 10 years. Driven primarily by the hospital-cost–containment movement, the variety and number of ambulatory care organizations have proliferated. Ambulatory care settings (where most patients receive care) include freestanding ambulatory care centers, outpatient care centers, health-maintenance organizations, physician practices, home healthcare agencies, hospital-based ambulatory care centers, urgent care centers, community health centers, managed-care organizations, and hospices. Freestanding ambulatory care centers, for example, are expected to treat 85 million patients in 5000 centers in 1991 (more than emergency rooms), compared with 50 million in 4000 centers in 1988.[1]

The American Hospital Association predicts that by the mid-1990s, 60% of all surgeries will be performed on an outpatient basis. Furthermore, expenditures on home care are increasing. By the year 2000, Americans will spend $60 billion dollars on home care—up 328% from 1986. Managed-care programs and physician–hospital joint ventures, such as preferred provider organizations, are also expected to experience growth.[1]

Primary care is predominantly delivered in multiple widely scattered independent facilities, with practitioner-owned offices being the most common site, followed by hospital outpatient departments, health-maintenance organizations, and other managed-care plans.[2] Although a small proportion of care is secondary and tertiary level care, technologic advances permit an increasing number of procedures to be performed in the outpatient setting at lower costs and in a setting that offers more convenience and comfort for the patient. The in vitro fertilization process, extraperitoneal laser surgery, urodynamic evaluation, and oncology treatments highlight the changing profile of diagnostic and therapeutic procedures that are available in ambulatory gynecology. The emerging technology of stereotactic aspiration cytology for the care of women with breast lesions, and the use of loop excision in the diagnosis and treatment of cervical disease both promise cost-effective, efficient ambulatory care alternatives. The future holds unlimited opportunities for technologic advances in ambulatory gynecologic care.

The rapid growth of alternative healthcare-delivery systems and the increasing shift from inpatient to outpatient settings emphasize the critical role of ambulatory care in the delivery of health services. Physicians have an opportunity to play a major role in defining ambulatory practice as they face pressures from employers, government, professional organizations, and consumers to demonstrate that they can provide cost-effective and efficient care without sacrificing quality. It is no surprise, therefore, that fundamental changes in quality assurance and quality improvement are taking place.

THE QUALITY ASSURANCE IMPERATIVE

Ambulatory care has traditionally been assigned a lower priority than hospital inpatient care, which has received the largest share of resources to acquire and implement complex technologies and interventions. As a result, quality assessment and quality assurance systems have been underdeveloped for ambulatory care settings and generally lag behind acute-care hospital programs.[2,3] Present quality assurance programs are ill-equipped to monitor the structural diversity, procedural risks, and high volume of ambulatory care settings. The inherent risks in ambulatory practice settings make it critical to establish relevant programs to respond to these special characteristics. William F. Jessee, MD, Vice President for Education, Joint Commission on Accreditation of Healthcare Organizations (JCAHO) notes the following risk characteristics of ambulatory settings:

Episodic nature of visits
Discontinuity of the patient–provider relation and the multiplicity of providers
Patients not known to staff in some settings
Long delays in obtaining an appointment and in being seen during appointment, inadequate examinations, and impersonal care because of high patient volume
Deceptive appearance of wellness in patients
Intraorganizational communication and coordination problems
Diagnostic difficulties with social deviations such as drug abuse and alcoholism[4,5]

Furthermore, tools for evaluating care, uniform data sets, and clinical standards have not kept pace with the dynamic growth of technology in ambulatory care settings.

The challenge to develop quality control programs is compelling. The stakes are high and the benefits are many because ambulatory care affects many people and has cost-savings implications. A program that strives to improve patient care by developing opportunities for identifying problems and taking appropriate actions affords physicians in gynecology numerous benefits. A quality assurance program minimizes the risk of malpractice, a major concern for practicing physicians. Moreover, the program documents the effectiveness of ambulatory care, enhances the competitive ability of the organization, attracts physicians who are dedicated to quality, and improves the organization's ability to plan and market services. Organizations benefit from improved internal communication and morale. Documentation of care identifies potential problems and satisfies external review and accreditation requirements. It also establishes problem-solving capabilities in the organization. In addition, areas of patient dissatisfaction are identified and may be corrected, subsequently improving public relations.[5] Physicians have the opportunity to influence the quality of care, develop a proactive system for preventive action, and reduce the risk of malpractice through participation in quality assurance and quality improvement efforts.[6]

Quality is a fundamental premise of medical practice. The definition of quality, however, has remained inherently subjective and the attributes of quality lack consensus. The JCAHO suggests seven characteristics of quality; these include, efficacy, appropriateness, accessibility, acceptability, effectiveness, efficiency, and continuity.[5]

The methods to assess the characteristics of quality of care, however, remain imprecise and traditionally focused on the narrow, clinical, technical aspects of the care process—exemplified by the emphasis on clinical outcomes and provider competence under the peer-review framework.[5,7,8] The American Medical Association, the American Hospital Association, and the American College of Obstetricians and Gynecologists have joined other professional associations in highlighting the importance of quality assurance activities for physicians.[9] The publication titled *Quality Assurance in Obstetrics and Gynecology* presents practical clinical indicators in gynecology that are particularly useful for inpatient care.[10] Physician leadership in the quality assurance program is essential to achieve corrective action and to improve the process of care.[11]

The evaluation of quality of care is further confounded by differing expectations of consumers, practitioners, and payors. Consumers place a high priority on responsiveness to their perceived need, level of communication, concern, courtesy, degree of symptom relief, and level of functional improvement. Practitioners measure quality by the degree to which care meets the technical state of the art and the degree of freedom that they have in acting in the patient's interest. The purchasers; primarily insurers, employers, of health care value the efficient use of funds available for health care, appropriateness of the use of health care resources, and the maximal contributions of health care to reduction in the cost of productivity.[5]

Intense interest has been generated regarding the patient's perception of and satisfaction with care. Including this previously ignored dimension of care in the quality of care plan will result in behavioral and system changes that are favorable for the patient.

Quality assurance is the continuum of actions, processes, and skills that contribute to the maximum health status given the available resources.[8] This contemporary view of an expanded concept of quality that includes an entire care process is illustrated by the evolution of Continuous Quality Improvement and Total Quality Management plans in the health care setting. These approaches underscore a framework that is multidisciplinary and incorporates a continuous process and system of care as well as the outcome of care. It promises to address the diversity of settings and the disparate perceptions of quality by different groups.[8,9]

UNDERSTANDING THE FRAMEWORK

The framework of structure, process, and outcome—noted by Donabedian and others—continues to be useful in developing individualized quality assurance plans. *Structure* refers to the system of providers, tools, and resources (human and fiscal) that are organized in a setting to deliver care. A solid, stable structure strongly contributes to protecting and promoting quality care.[12] Specific examples of structural components are personnel (training, qualifications, availability, humane qualities); facilities; equipment; hours worked; organization (leadership, policies, planning, goals, operations, consumer involvement); information flow

(medical records, educational resources, communication); and finances.[7] Structural components have significant influence on the delivery of quality care, yet often these elements are beyond the control of the providers. The medical record, for example, which is frequently used as the primary document for assessing the quality of care, rarely includes information on structural components of care and often omits process components.

The *process* component of this framework is the dynamic, active dimension of the assessment relation that links structure to care and the consequences to health and welfare. In the process, providers and staff give care and the patient receives care. Examples of process components include access; waiting time; diagnostic capabilities (epidemiology, history, physical, tests); management (manual skills, suitable prescriptions, patient education, follow- up, client–provider interaction); prevention, and cost control. Process components are often not included in measuring quality, particularly when clinical care is the only dimension that is considered.[7,12]

Outcome reflects the endpoint of the interaction between the patient, the provider, and the healthcare system. Outcome data reflect relief from disease or changes in comfort, actively level, or survival. Did the care change the status of the patient and was the patient pleased with the results?[7,12]

Developing assessment and monitoring mechanisms to ensure quality of care must include all three components to provide an objective, balanced profile of the care delivered. Unidimensional approaches have characterized medical assessments of the past, focusing on gynecologic clinical outcomes. These have been primarily designed to measure the effectiveness and appropriateness of surgical procedures but have neglected many aspects of gynecologic care in the ambulatory setting.

The application of the structure–process–outcome framework to ambulatory settings requires special consideration. First, the structural diversity of ambulatory settings is a challenge. Patients presenting to ambulatory settings have a variety of conditions, many of which are self-limited and may be ultimately related to lifestyle, such as sexually transmitted diseases. Patients may have chronic conditions (pelvic pain) wherein a good outcome may be the arrest of the natural disease process or restoration of a function. In either case, the outcome may partially depend on nursing intervention or social support. Many conditions in ambulatory settings require short-term counseling or reassurance—interventions that alter the patient's health and emotional status but are often undocumented. Acute infections, for example, may be appropriately treated medically with antibiotics but the follow-up condition of the patient is unknown.[7]

General guidelines in applying this framework include (1) selecting aspects of care that are common, occur frequently, or are high-risk aspects of care; (2) assessing aspects that are important to the practice setting; (3) considering aspects of care that are changeable and in which an improvement can be demonstrated; (4) using available resources and personnel to integrate the quality philosophy into the practice settings; and (5) a comprehensive approach that encompasses several methodologies and assessment tools.

ESTABLISHING STANDARDS

The cornerstone of quality of care is the triad of defining, implementing, and evaluating the standards that will assure adherence to the defined level of quality. Standards are statements that include societal, professional, institutional, and individual values that define accountability and the quality of patient care. Standards are dynamic and change with technology. They define an acceptable level of achievement at a specific time and are distinguished by predetermination, established by authority, and communicated and accepted by others. Notably, they are consistent with national norms, regulations, and legal practice. Furthermore, they must be both achievable and measurable. These standards may be voluntary or mandatory.[13]

The development of standards for a particular practice setting may emphasize one or all of the components of the quality assurance framework: structure, process, outcome. Structural standards identify characteristics of the healthcare system that are considered good and acceptable patient care—qualified staff, appropriate equipment and facilities. Process standards focus on the dynamics of the patient experience and specifically on the patient–provider interaction. The patient is given and receives care. Outcome standards measure the results in improved health status, increased survival, relief of discomfort, and patient satisfaction. Structural standards are most frequently omitted and dimensions of patient care experienced outside the provider interaction are rarely addressed. It is assumed, for example, that the medical record as the primary document of the patient experience contains sufficient information to measure the quality of care. Usually, the medical record identifies some

process and significant outcome parameters but it is woefully inadequate with respect to nonclinical data. Thus, if a broader circle of standards is not defined, essential aspects of quality will be ignored. The important contribution to quality of all the components of care cannot be overestimated and underscores the value of a comprehensive, continuous monitoring system.

Ambulatory care settings benefit from the development of standards that define the level of effective, acceptable practice. The American College of Obstetricians and Gynecologists has published a document that outlines the establishment of clinical indicators and criteria.[10] In addition, JCAHO has issued guidelines for quality assurance in ambulatory care settings.[5] These recommendations can be adapted to many practice models. Both documents emphasize the critical decision process in defining the standard (level of acceptable practice), selecting the indicator (events), and identifying a target level of acceptance practice or success (thresholds) criteria. This process is valuable in noting areas that need further investigation or in which variations in process or outcome reflect a change in quality. Table 31-1 presents several standards appropriate to the ambulatory gynecology setting.

IMPLEMENTING A PLAN

Irrespective of the type of setting, the demand for quality assurance documentation is escalating. Several key recommendations in developing and implementing a plan are advantageous. First, the plan should be an integral part of the delivery of health care. It should be a planned, systematic process that is comprehensive and continuous. Second, the plan should be based on the development of acceptable standards and thresholds. Third, the measurement of these results is critical. Identification and remediation of problems that compromise the quality of care to the gynecologic patient are the most fundamental benefit of a successful program.

Organizationally, the ambulatory care setting must determine a plan appropriate to the practice setting. The following steps should be be followed:

1. Establish a group or institution commitment to quality of care, with defined leadership
2. Define goals or care, with consensus on the priorities; high-volume services or high-risk procedures should be given priority
3. Develop standards, emphasizing the improvement of patient services

Table 31–1
Ambulatory Gynecology Standards

Standard	Indicator	Continuous Monitoring
Norplant Insertion Structural indicator Threshold, 100%	All physicians/nurse practitioners who insert Norplant are approved to perform the procedure by a physician certified in Norplant insertion	1. Existing employees will attend a training course 2. New employees will receive training 3. Documentation of the course attendance will be maintained by the employer 4. Medical records of patients who receive Norplant will receive periodic review, noting provider
Papanicolaou Smear Process indicator Threshold, 100%	All new gynecologic patients and gynecologic patients at their annual visit will receive a Papanicalaou smear	1. Medical record review of new, annual visits made by gynecologic patients 2. Laboratory log review every 6 months
Gonococcus Infection Process Indicator Threshold, 100%	All patients with a positive gonorrhea culture will be notified of the results and need for treatment within 48 hours of receipt of the test results	1. Medical record review of patients who were positive every year 2. Review of laboratory log every 3 months 3. Review of "Test Result Log" every 3 months
Patient Waiting Time Structural/process indicator Threshold, 90%	Routine gynecologic patients will be seen by the provider within 1/2 hour of their arrival time	1. Patient scheduling system: review every 6 months 2. Patient flow/routing sheet: review every 6 months
Chlamydia Treatment Outcome indicator Threshold, 90%	Chlamydia culture will be negative after completion of treatment per clinical standard at post-treatment visit	1. Medical record review: annually 2. Laboratory log: review every 6 months 3. Test result log: review every 6 months

(Modified from Joint Commission on Accreditation of Healthcare Organizations: Quality assurance in ambulatory care, 2nd ed, p 60. Oakbrook Terrace, IL, JCAHO, 1990)

4. Instruct all personnel on the standards and expectations for performance
5. Assign responsibility for data collection, observation, and reporting
6. Define the review and reporting process (eg, committee, peer review)
7. Establish the process to evaluate results, with plans of action and problem resolution, emphasizing continuous improvement of the process
8. Develop a mechanism for measuring and evaluating patient satisfaction
9. Communicate results to others

The intent of a quality assurance plan is to be proactive in establishing processes that assure quality of care. Many methods of assessment of care

have been suggested. Within the development of the plan, several methodologies may be selected to assess care. The "tracer" method reviews the outcomes of a few common, important conditions amenable to simple interventions; the "staging" method describes the clinical stages for many conditions (percentage of encounter), from no symptoms to death; the "microsampling" method reviews all records (medical, flow sheets, appointment sheets, encounter forms, phone logs) of a particular day, focusing on problems of care or organization of care; "criteria mapping" attempts to capture the logical flow of the minimal decision-making steps that are needed to provide care to each individual patient.[7]

Most methodologies such as these have weaknesses that limit their broad applicability. Existing methods have relied on the medical record and focused on the provider portion of care. Retrospective approaches have been predominant, with noted delays in remediation and little recognition of the multiple factors that contribute to the quality of care.[7] Furthermore, systems approaches that recognize client behavior, provider behavior, and system efficacy in the achievement of quality of care are lacking. Tools exist in most ambulatory care settings to begin the establishment of a plan that maximizes existing data sources. The following are all examples of existing valuable resources in defining and monitoring care:

- Peer-review committees
- Administrative committees
- Continuous medical-record monitoring
- Clinical review forms
- Safety–infection control committees
- Board meetings
- Community market surveys
- Patient satisfaction surveys
- Staffing plans
- Scheduling systems
- Occurrence screens and complaint inquiry
- Discharge summaries
- Use review
- Third-party audits
- Credentialing processes
- Employment records
- Telephone interviews
- Exit interviews
- Observations
- Patient quizzes to monitor education
- Staff surveys
- Logs, lab results, and computer analysis

Ambulatory care medical records are generally poor, compared with hospital medical records. Computerized quality assurance may be a mechanism for group practices to minimize the risks of providing ambulatory care to gynecology patients. Patient satisfaction requires increased attention to the development of data collection instruments. Emphasis of peer reviews on defining quality practice, not provider sanctioning, may be a productive monitor. Ambulatory visits are logical units of measurement but do not track individual experiences. Present standards are not well-defined systems that consider case mix; therefore, they may not reflect acceptability or expectations of all population groups.

A plan that provides comprehensive continuous monitoring of several key high-volume high-risk indicators, documents the patient experience, and notes structure process and outcome components satisfies external accreditation and external and internal review processes.

QUALITY OF CARE: THE FUTURE

Several external forces ensure the development of quality assurance for ambulatory care. Medicare regulations have moved toward inclusion of private practices in the review process. A fundamental tenet of managed care, particularly when government funds are used, is quality assurance. Third-party payors will continue to demand quality as a fundamental component of care, particularly as competition increases. Quality assurance (continuous quality improvement) programs signal a system that monitors costs as well as competency and reflects consumer (patient) satisfaction. The organization of medical practice is forecast to grow in both number and complexity, with attendant elevation of expectations. Malpractice concerns, which have played in increasingly significant role in the organization of medical services, will continue to loom over the delivery and quality of care.

The future holds many opportunities to develop more sophisticated systems of quality assessment in the ambulatory care setting. Practice guidelines must be modified to be applicable to ambulatory care. Tools to measure quality must be refined to suit the diversity and complexity of settings, and data systems to identify and track significant events of care must be developed that are practical and applicable to ambulatory situations.

In summary, three points are critical: (1) the physician must take a leadership role in determining and evaluating quality of care, (2) quality of care must include nonmedical aspects of care in the evaluation process, and (3) continuous quality monitoring must be integrated into the medical practice and practice environment to provide the maximum benefits for physicians, patients, and communities.

REFERENCES

1. Flory J (ed): Ambulatory care: a management briefing, p 35. Chicago, American Hospital Association, 1990
2. Palmer H: The challenges and prospects for quality

assessment and assurance in ambulatory care. Inquiry 25:119, 1988

3. Strain R, Palmer H, Maurer J, Lyons S, Thompson S: Implementing quality assurance studies in ambulatory care. Qual Rev Bull 10:168, 1984
4. Berman S: Quality assurance in ambulatory health care. Qual Rev Bull 14:18, 1988
5. Joint Commission on Accreditation of Healthcare Organizations: Quality assurance in ambulatory care, 2nd ed, p 11. Oak Brook Terrace, IL, Joint Commission on Accreditation of Healthcare Organizations, 1990
6. Eisenberg JM, Kabcenell A: Organized practice and the quality of medical care. Inquiry 25:78, 1988
7. Hirschorn N, Lamstein J, Klein SF, McCormack J, Warner TN: Quality by objectives: a model of quality of care assessment and assurance for ambulatory health centers. J Ambulatory Care Management 1:55, 1978
8. Warner P: Quality assurance: an evolving concept. Outreach 12:1, 1991
9. Joint Commission on Accreditation of Health Care Organizations: Transitions from Q.A. to C.Q.I., p 3. Oakbrook Terrace, IL, Joint Commission on Accreditation of Healthcare Organizations, 1991
10. The American College of Obstetricians and Gynecologists: Quality assurance in obstetrics and gynecology, p 1. Washington, DC, American College of Obstetricians and Gynecologists, 1989
11. Goodspeed RB, Goldfield N: Quality assurance in a preferred provider organization. J Ambulatory Care Management 10:2, 1987
12. Donabedian A: The definition of quality and approaches to its assessment, p 80. Ann Arbor, MI, Health Administration Press, 1980
13. Meisenheimer CG (ed): Quality assurance: a complete guide to effective programs, p 45. Rockville, MD, Aspen Publications, 1985

Index

Page numbers followed by *f* indicate figures; page numbers followed by *t* indicate tables. Page numbers in *italics,* preceded by the notation *color fig.,* indicate Color Figures, which are found at the end of their respective chapters.